a LANGE medical book

SECOND EDITION

The Patient History

An Evidence-Based Approach to Differential Diagnosis

Edited By

MARK C. HENDERSON, MD, FACP
Professor of Clinical Medicine and Vice Chair
Department of Internal Medicine
Associate Dean for Admissions
University of California, Davis School of Medicine
Sacramento, California

LAWRENCE M. TIERNEY, JR., MD
Professor of Medicine
University of California, San Francisco
Associate Chief of Medical Service
Veterans Affairs Medical Center
San Francisco, California

GERALD W. SMETANA, MD
Division of General Medicine and Primary Care
Beth Israel Deaconess Medical Center
Associate Professor of Medicine
Harvard Medical School
Boston, Massachusetts

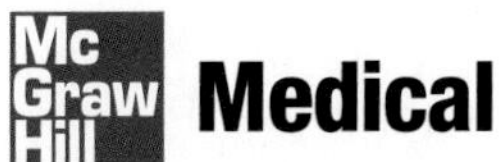

New York Chicago San Francisco Lisbon London Madrid Mexico City
Milan New Delhi San Juan Seoul Singapore Sydney Toronto

The Patient History: An Evidence-Based Approach to Differential Diagnosis, Second Edition

1 2 3 4 5 6 7 8 9 0 CTP/CTP 17 16 15 14 13 12

ISBN 978-0-07-162494-7
MHID 0-07-162494-5
ISSN 1552-1206

Notice

Medicine is an ever-changing science. As new research and clinical experience broaden our knowledge, changes in treatment and drug therapy are required. The authors and the publisher of this work have checked with sources believed to be reliable in their efforts to provide information that is complete and generally in accord with the standards accepted at the time of publication. However, in view of the possibility of human error or changes in medical sciences, neither the authors nor the publisher nor any other party who has been involved in the preparation or publication of this work warrants that the information contained herein is in every respect accurate or complete, and they disclaim all responsibility for any errors or omissions or for the results obtained from use of the information contained in this work. Readers are encouraged to confirm the information contained herein with other sources. For example and in particular, readers are advised to check the product information sheet included in the package of each drug they plan to administer to be certain that the information contained in this work is accurate and that changes have not been made in the recommended dose or in the contraindications for administration. This recommendation is of particular importance in connection with new or infrequently used drugs.

This book was set in Times LT Std. by Cenveo Publisher Services.
The editors were James F. Shanahan and Robert Pancotti.
The production supervisor was Catherine H. Saggese.
Project management was provided by Vastavikta Sharma, Cenveo Publisher Services.
The text designer was Elise Lansdon.
China Translation & Printing Services, Ltd. was printer and binder.

To John-John: skier, artist, explorer.

Contents

SECTION VI | CARDIOVASCULAR SYSTEM

SECTION VII | GASTROINTESTINAL SYSTEM

SECTION VIII | GENITOURINARY SYSTEM

SECTION IX | WOMEN'S HEALTH

SECTION X | MUSCULOSKELETAL SYSTEM

SECTION XI | NEUROLOGY

SECTION XII | PSYCHIATRY

SECTION XIII | COMMUNICATING THE HISTORY

Contributors

Naheed R. Abbasi, MD
Summit Medical Group
Berkeley Heights, New Jersey

Sandra G. Adams, MD, MS
Associate Professor of Medicine, Pulmonary/Critical Care Division, University of Texas Health Science Center at San Antonio;
Staff Physician, South Texas Veterans Health Care System
San Antonio, Texas

Miya E. Allen, MD
Fellow, Division of Endocrinology, Department of Internal Medicine, University of California, Davis
Sacramento, California

Antonio Anzueto, MD
Department of Pulmonary/Critical Care Medicine, University of Texas Health Science Center and the South Texas Veterans Health Care System
San Antonio, Texas

Kenneth A. Arndt, MD
Co-director, SkinCare Physicians
Chestnut Hill, Massachusetts;
Adjunct Professor of Dermatology, Brown Medical School;
Adjunct Professor of Medicine (Dermatology), Dartmouth Medical School
Hanover, New Hampshire;
Clinical Professor of Dermatology Emeritus, Harvard Medical School
Boston, Massachusetts

Paul B. Aronowitz, MD
Program Director, Internal Medicine Residency, California Pacific Medical Center
San Francisco, California

Matthew C. Baker, MD
Harvard Medical School, MS IV
Boston, Massachusetts

Jason J. S. Barton, MD, PhD, FRCPC
Professor and Canada Research Chair, Departments of Medicine (Neurology), Ophthalmology and Visual Sciences, and Psychology, University of British Columbia
Vancouver, British Columbia, Canada

Carol K. Bates, MD
Division of General Medicine and Primary Care, Beth Israel Deaconess Medical Center; Associate Professor of Medicine; Assistant Dean for Faculty Affairs, Harvard Medical School
Boston, Massachusetts

Thomas E. Baudendistel, MD
Program Director, Internal Medicine Residency, Kaiser Oakland
Oakland, California

John Wolfe Blotzer, MD
Clinical Associate Professor of Medicine, Department of Medicine, Pennsylvania State College of Medicine
Hershey, Pennsylvania;
Rheumatology, York Hospital
York, Pennsylvania

Alexander R. Carbo, MD
Assistant Professor of Medicine, Harvard Medical School;
Hospitalist, Division of General Medicine, Beth Israel Deaconess Medical Center
Boston, Massachusetts

Dayana Carcamo-Molina, MD
Resident Physician, Internal Medicine Department, Kaiser Permanente Medical Center
Oakland, California

Deborah Lynn Cardell, MD
Clinical Assistant Professor, Division of General Medicine, University of Texas Health Science Center at San Antonio
San Antonio, Texas

Gina R. Chacon, MD
Professor of Internal Medicine, Michigan State University
East Lansing, Michigan

Helen K. Chew, MD, FACP
Professor, Department of Internal Medicine, Division of Hematology and Oncology, University of California, Davis
Sacramento, California

Roger Chou, MD, FACP
Associate Professor, Department of Medicine and Department of Medical Informatics and Clinical Epidemiology, Oregon Health & Science University
Portland, Oregon

Virginia U. Collier, MD, MACP
Hugh R. Sharp, Jr. Chair of Medicine, Christina Care Health System
Newark, Delaware;
Professor of Medicine, Jefferson Medical College
Philadelphia, Pennsylvania

Michelle V. Conde, MD, FACP
Staff Physician, South Texas Veterans Health Care System, Audie L. Murphy Division;
Clinical Associate Professor, Division of General Medicine, University of Texas Health Science Center
San Antonio, Texas

Filippo Cremonini, MD, MSc, PhD
Assistant Professor of Medicine, Division of Gastroenterology, Beth Israel Deaconess Medical Center
Boston, Massachusetts

Richard A. Deyo, MD, MPH
Kaiser Permanente Professor of Evidence-Based Family Medicine, Department of Family Medicine and Department of Medicine, Oregon Health & Science University
Portland, Oregon

Francesca C. Dwamena, MD, MS
Professor of Medicine, Interim Chair, Department of Internal Medicine, Michigan State University
East Lansing, Michigan

Nephertiti Efeovbokhan, MD
Resident Physician, Department of Internal Medicine, Michigan State University
East Lansing, Michigan

Aaron E. Falk, MD
Chief Resident, Department of Internal Medicine, California Pacific Medical Center
San Francisco, California

Tonya L. Fancher, MD, MPH, FACP
Associate Professor and Associate Program Director, Department of Internal Medicine, University of California, Davis
Sacramento, California

Sara B. Fazio, MD, FACP
Associate Professor of Medicine, Harvard Medical School; Clerkship Director, Department of Internal Medicine, Beth Israel Deaconess Medical Center
Boston, Massachusetts

David S. Fefferman, MD
Clinical Instructor in Medicine, Harvard Medical School
Boston, Massachusetts;
Private Practice, Digestive Health Associates
Stoneham, Massachusetts

David Feinbloom, MD
Hospital Medicine Program, Beth Israel Deaconess Medical Center, Assistant Professor of Medicine, Harvard Medical School
Boston, Massachusetts

Robert D. Ficalora, MD
Senior Associate Program Director, Internal Medicine Residency Associate Professor of Medicine,
Mayo Clinic College of Medicine
Rochester, Minnesota

Faith T. Fitzgerald, MD
Professor of Medicine and Director of Humanities and Bioethics, University of California, Davis School of Medicine
Sacramento, California

Auguste H. Fortin VI, MD, MPH
Associate Professor of Medicine, Department of Internal Medicine, Yale University School of Medicine
New Haven, Connecticut

Steven Gelber, MD, MPH
Physician, Kaiser Permanente
Santa Rosa, California

Mona A. Gohara, MD
Assistant Clinical Professor of Medicine, Department of Dermatology, Yale School of Medicine
New Haven, Connecticut

John D. Goodson, MD
Associate Professor of Medicine, Harvard Medical School;
Physician, Massachusetts General Hospital
Boston, Massachusetts

Laurie M. Gordon, MD
Instructor, Department of Neurology, Harvard Medical School, Beth Israel Deaconess Medical Center
Boston, Massachusetts

Emmy M. Graber, MD
Assistant Professor of Dermatology, Boston University School of Medicine and Boston Medical Center;
Director, Cosmetic and Laser Center, Boston University;
Associate Director, Resident Training Program, Boston University School of Medicine
Boston, Massachusetts

Michelle M. Guidry, MD
Assistant Professor, Tulane University Health Science Center
New Orleans, Louisiana

David R. Gutknecht, MD
Associate Program Director, Internal Medicine Residency, Geisinger Health System
Danville, Pennsylvania

Mary E. Harris, MD
Internal Medicine Residency Director, Geisinger Health System
Danville, Pennsylvania

Mark C. Henderson, MD, FACP
Professor of Clinical Medicine and Vice Chair, Department of Internal Medicine, Associate Dean for Admissions, University of California, Davis School of Medicine
Sacramento, California

Calvin H. Hirsch, MD, FACP
Professor of Clinical Internal Medicine (Geriatrics) and Public Health Sciences, Division of General Medicine, University of California, Davis Medical Center
Sacramento, California

Zachary B. Holt, MD
Associate Physician, Department of Internal Medicine, University of California, Davis
Sacramento, California

David F. Jacobson, MD, FACP
Associate Program Director, Department of Medicine, California Pacific Medical Center
San Francisco, California

Craig R. Keenan, MD
Associate Professor, Department of Medicine, University of California, Davis Medical Center
Sacramento, California

Ciarán P. Kelly, MD
Professor of Medicine, Harvard Medical School, Gastroenterology Fellowship Program Director, Beth Israel Deaconess Medical Center
Boston, Massachusetts

Melanie M. Kingsley, MD
Assistant Professor, Director of Cosmetic Dermatology & Laser Surgery, Department of Dermatology, Indiana University School of Medicine
Indianapolis, Indiana

Veera Pavan Kotaru, MD, FACP
Assistant Professor of Medicine, Department of Medicine, Michigan State University
East Lansing, Michigan

Helaina Laks Kravitz, MD
Student Health and Counseling Services, University of California, Davis
Sacramento, California

Richard L. Kravitz, MD, MSPH, FACP
Division of General Medicine, University of California, Davis
Sacramento, California

Randall E. Lee, MD, FACP
Staff Gastroenterologist, Veterans Affairs Northern California Healthcare System, Associate Clinical Professor of Medicine, University of California, Davis School of Medicine
Sacramento, California

Anthony Lembo, MD
Associate Professor of Medicine, Harvard Medical School;
Director of Gastrointestinal Motility Center, Beth Israel Deaconess Medical Center
Boston, Massachusetts

Peter A. Lio, MD
Assistant Professor of Dermatology and Pediatrics, Department of Dermatology, Northwestern University, Feinberg School of Medicine
Chicago, Illinois

Timothy S. Loo, MD
Instructor, Harvard Medical School, Division of General Medicine and Primary Care, Beth Israel Deaconess Medical Center
Boston, Massachusetts

Catherine R. Lucey, MD, FACP
Vice Dean for Education, University of California, San Francisco School of Medicine
San Francisco, California

Iris Ma, MD
Department of Internal Medicine, Stanford University Medical Center
Stanford, California

Diego Maselli, MD
Department of Pulmonary/Critical Care Medicine, University of Texas Health Science Center and the South Texas Veterans Health Care System
San Antonio, Texas

Kenneth R. McQuaid, MD
Chief of Gastroenterology, San Francisco Veterans Affairs Medical Center, Professor of Clinical Medicine, University of California
San Francisco, California

Felipe J. Molina, MD
Instructor, Harvard Medical School, Division of General Medicine and Primary Care, Beth Israel Deaconess Medical Center
Boston, Massachusetts

Jason A. Nieuwsma, PhD
Assistant Professor, Duke University Medical Center;
Associate Director, Veterans Affairs Mental Health and Chaplaincy Program
Durham, North Carolina

Thuan Ong, MD, MPH
Acting Instructor, Department of Medicine, Division of Gerontology and Geriatric Medicine, University of Washington
Seattle, Washington

Jane E. O'Rorke, MD, FACP
Professor, Division of General Medicine, Department of Medicine, University of Texas Health Science Center
San Antonio, Texas

Jay I. Peters, MD
Professor of Medicine; Chief, Pulmonary and Critical Care Medicine, University of Texas Health Sciences Center at San Antonio
San Antonio, Texas

Sumanth D. Prabhu, MD
Mary Gertrude Waters Chair of Cardiovascular Medicine, Director, Division of Cardiovascular Disease;
Professor of Medicine, Physiology, and Biophysics, University of Alabama
Birmingham, Alabama

Daniel Press, MD
Staff Neurologist, Beth Israel Deaconess Medical Center;
Assistant Professor of Neurology, Harvard Medical School
Boston, Massachusetts

Erika E. Reid, MD
Dermatology Resident, University of Pennsylvania
Philadelphia, Pennsylvania

Michael Ronthal, MB, BCh, FRCP
Professor, Department of Neurology, Beth Israel Deaconess Medical Center, Harvard Medical School
Boston, Massachusetts

Stephany Sanchez, MD
Physician, Sacramento County Department of Health and Human Services and Department of Internal Medicine, University of California, Davis
Sacramento, California

Amarpreet S. Sandhu, DO
Department of Internal Medicine, Kaiser Permanente
Oakland, California

Mysti D. W. Schott, MD, FACP
Associate Professor, Department of Medicine, Division of General Medicine, University of Texas Health Science Center
San Antonio, Texas

Jessica Sheehan, MD
Dermatologist and Mohs Surgeon, North Shore Center for Medical Aesthetics,
Lake Forest Northwestern Hospital
Chicago, Illinois

Amandeep Shergill, MD
Assistant Clinical Professor of Medicine, Division of Gastroenterology, Department of Medicine, San Francisco Veterans Affairs Medical Center and University of California
San Francisco, California

Amy N. Ship, MD
Assistant Professor of Medicine, Harvard Medical School, Division of General Medicine and Primary Care, Beth Israel Deaconess Medical Center
Boston, Massachusetts

Richard J. Simons, MD
Professor of Medicine, Vice Dean for Educational Affairs, Pennsylvania State College of Medicine
Hershey, Pennsylvania

Gerald W. Smetana, MD
Division of General Medicine and Primary Care, Beth Israel Deaconess Medical Center;
Associate Professor of Medicine, Harvard Medical School
Boston, Massachusetts

M. E. Beth Smith, DO
Assistant Professor, Department of Medicine, Department of Medical Informatics and Clinical Epidemiology, Oregon Health & Science University
Portland, Oregon

Robert C. Smith, MD, MS
Professor of Medicine, Division of General Internal Medicine, College of Human Medicine, Michigan State University
East Lansing, Michigan

Malathi Srinivasan, MD
Associate Professor, Department of Medicine, School of Medicine, University of California, Davis
Sacramento, California

Daniel J. Sullivan, MD, MPH
Division of General Medicine and Primary Care, Beth Israel Deaconess Medical Center;
Assistant Professor of Medicine, Harvard Medical School
Boston, Massachusetts

Nicole A. Swallow, MD, FACP
Associate Director, Internal Medicine Residency Training Program;
Assistant Professor of Medicine, Pennsylvania State University, Hershey Medical Center
Hershey, Pennsylvania

Sara L. Swenson, MD
Associate Program Director, Department of Medicine, California Pacific Medical Center
San Francisco, California

Daniel Tarsy, MD
Professor, Department of Neurology, Harvard Medical School, Beth Israel Deaconess Medical Center
Boston, Massachusetts

Anjala Tess, MD
Assistant Professor, Harvard Medical School, Hospital Medicine, Beth Israel Deaconess Medical Center
Boston, Massachusetts

Lawrence M. Tierney, Jr., MD
Professor of Medicine, University of California, San Francisco;
Associate Chief of Medical Service, Veterans Affairs Medical Center
San Francisco, California

Emily S. Wang, MD
Staff Physician, South Texas Veterans Health Care System, Clinical Assistant Professor of Medicine, University of Texas Health Science Center at San Antonio
San Antonio, Texas

Jeff Wiese, MD, FACP
Professor of Medicine, Associate Dean, Graduate Medical Education, Tulane University Health Sciences Center
New Orleans, Louisiana

John W. Williams, Jr., MD, MHSc
Professor of Medicine, Psychiatry, and Behavioral Science, Duke University Medical Center and Durham Veterans Affairs Center for Health Services Research in Primary Care
Durham, North Carolina

Mark C. Wilson, MD, MPH
Professor of Medicine, and Associate Dean for Graduate Medical Education, University of Iowa Carver College of Medicine
Iowa City, Iowa

Christopher M. Wittich, MD, PharmD
Assistant Professor, Department of Medicine, Division of General Internal Medicine, Mayo Clinic College of Medicine
Rochester, Minnesota

Michael H. Zaroukian, MD, PhD, FACP, FHIMSS
Professor of Medicine, Michigan State University;
Vice President & Chief Medical Information Officer
Sparrow Health System
Lansing, Michigan

Preface

Give a man a fish and you feed him for a day.
Teach a man to fish and you feed him for a lifetime.

—Chinese Proverb

Welcome to the second edition of *The Patient History: An Evidence-Based Approach to Differential Diagnosis.* The purpose of this book is to introduce aspiring healthcare professionals to the timeless art of history taking, the gateway to establishing a diagnosis for a patient's symptoms. The patient's unique story lies at the heart of this endeavor and defies the categorization inherent to the printed page. There are, however, fundamental principles that can, and should, be articulated to start the novice on the correct path.

What makes this book different from other books on primary care? First and foremost, we use a patient-centered approach and have organized the book by *symptoms* rather than by diseases. Symptoms, after all, bring patients to the clinician. Second, we apply principles of evidence-based medicine to the clinical history; we highlight from the medical literature the most fruitful lines of questioning for making a diagnosis.

Despite the proliferation of modern diagnostic and imaging techniques, there is recent evidence that clinicians can still make a diagnosis for most patients using the history *alone* (Paley et al. *Arch Intern Med.* 2011;171:1394–1396). In this book, authors describe how historical data help to confirm or refute a particular diagnosis. Where aspects of the history have not been formally studied, the epidemiology, prevalence, and prognosis of the most common underlying conditions are reviewed. Such information, integrated with clinical experience, helps guide the interviewer toward the most important diagnostic considerations for a given symptom.

The book's introductory chapters cover general principles of history taking and the evidence-based method. The remaining symptom-based chapters tackle 59 common clinical symptoms, including the following elements: clinical case scenario, background and key terminology, differential diagnosis, interview framework and tips, alarm symptoms (features that alert the clinician to the most serious diagnoses), focused questions (with respective likelihood ratios), prognosis, caveats or clinical pearls, and references. Each chapter concludes with a Diagnostic Approach section that includes color algorithms and several multiple-choice questions to test your knowledge of the material. We conclude the book with a chapter on how to communicate the history to colleagues or consultants.

In each chapter, we include multiple actual questions for practical usage, ranging from basic queries to those that an experienced clinician might employ. We have not covered the physical examination or laboratory evaluation, lest we detract from the focus of the book—history taking.

Learning the clinical history requires communication, clinical experience with patients, and observation of master historians. Faith Fitzgerald and Larry Tierney, two such masters, open and close the book covering critical but often ignored aspects of this ancient art. We hope that this book gives you the fishing gear, or tools, for a successful journey to clinical excellence.

Mark C. Henderson, MD
Sacramento, California
Lawrence M. Tierney, Jr., MD
San Francisco, California
Gerald W. Smetana, MD
Boston, Massachusetts

Acknowledgments

I thank my wife, Helen, and my parents, Donna and Starr Henderson, without whose patience and love I would never have become a physician; and my children, Jessica, Paul, and John for their constant inspiration. I thank my tireless colleague, Dr. Jerry Smetana, and all authors for their thoughtful, practical, and scholarly contributions. I thank my teacher, colleague, and friend, Dr. Larry Tierney, who decades ago instilled in me the critical importance of a careful history. Finally, I salute my students and residents, who over the years have taught me as much as I have taught them.

Mark C. Henderson, MD
Sacramento, California

SECTION

I

INTRODUCTORY CONCEPTS

Chapter 1

History and Physical Examination: Art and Science

Faith T. Fitzgerald, MD

The medical history and physical examination are ***not*** separate entities, but necessarily continually enrich one another at every point. The patient's history leads the skilled doctor, even as he or she is eliciting it, to think of "things to look for" on physical examination, and physical findings—some of which are immediately obvious when one first meets the patient—stimulate further historical questions. This fluid oscillation, the ongoing back-and-forth between these two pillars of diagnosis, is, perhaps, the most difficult thing for students of medicine to grasp because it is learned only by evaluating real patients. Standardized patients do not have "true" physical findings that match the history or may have physical signs not "in the script." The techniques and some findings of physical examination can be described in books, seen on video, heard on audio, and demonstrated on simulacra or on well people, but the essential clues given by the physical findings in subsequent real patients, and their intertwining relationship with the history, cannot.

The medical history, say venerable clinicians righteously, is the core art of patient care. They continue to cite references that maintain that the patient's history provides the diagnosis in 85% of cases. That often-quoted figure of 85% is in doubt, however, because many of the histories now given by patients and taken by doctors are in actual content a compendium of data from the laboratories and radiology suites from previous visits to their doctors and admissions to hospital. So, for example, patients bring folders of laboratory studies with them to consultants' offices; house staff and students present patients with chief complaints of "fever, leukocytosis, and mitral vegetations on echo"; and a first concern given by a patient in clinic may be "high cholesterol." It is hard to escape the implicit conviction that laboratory and technologic data are more objective, and therefore more scientific, than the subjective information gathered by listening to a patient tell his or her story. Furthermore, the wondrous advances in technologic diagnosis appear to justify the reverence in which the results they generate are held.

DEVELOPING SKILL IN LISTENING AND LOOKING

Without a careful history, without knowing patients' stories of what happened to them and their unique circumstances and personality, the practice of medicine becomes neither art *nor* science. Consider what opinion we would have of a bench investigator who plated known microorganisms upon an unknown medium. Would we credit a geneticist who intercalated even the most intimately analyzed base pairs into an otherwise unknown genome? The study of the patient begins with the history, a history taken by a skilled listener too, for it is only the skilled listener who can hear the vocal inflections that suggest the importance of things to the patient. It is only she who can read the nonverbal clues that illuminate the meaning of the words. It is only he who can understand not only what is said but the often vitally important information gathered when things go unsaid by patients. It is only she who from the first moment can integrate the history and the physical examination so that they make sense, as in a patient who complains of anxiety but who has on first glance the bulging eyes and tremor of hyperthyroidism or the patient who moves slowly and stiffly, speaks monotonically and softly, and has minimal facial expression who tells you he has trouble swallowing, which are common symptoms of Parkinson's disease. In the first case, the examiner would make a mental note to ask for a history of weight loss and a family history of thyroid disease and, on the physical examination, would seek confirming signs, such as a rapid pulse and an enlarged thyroid gland. In the second case, the historian would ask about other parkinsonian risk factors and seek physical findings of resting tremor, cogwheel rigidity, or abnormal gait. The "complete physical" is not a list of things to do by rote; it is a search for things directed by the history. That is what makes it interesting for the doctor, as well as good for the patient.

The ability to take a good history cannot be acquired by lecture or syllabus, standardized patient exercises, CD-ROM, or even texts such as this one. It is an experientially acquired art, learned over time with each successive patient story and the careful observation of what follows from it. It is often frustrating for students and junior doctors who want to know what the so-called good history should include. They mistake structure for substance. The good history varies depending not on how one orders its component sections (such as present illness, review of systems, and the like) or on mastering the current jargon and multiple acronyms that more often obscure than facilitate understanding, but on the story that the patient needs to tell and the doctor needs to hear, so that they together may go further along the path of understanding what to do next. Like any art—and like science—the ability to do a patient assessment builds on the practitioner's past and requires *practice*. Knowing what to emphasize and what to discard, what question to ask next, and how to direct the discourse (subtly and without markedly influencing or altering its content) is difficult, and the lessons are never-ending. The only way to learn it is to do it, with real patients, again and again and again.

MORE THAN THE FACTS

Here we are, doctors in the 21st century, equipped with truly miraculous tools of diagnosis and therapy, and patients complain about us. Even the best educated, or especially the best educated, go to quacks. They do not trust us. Why? Perhaps it is because the greatest afflictions of our patients—fear, despair, fatigue, and pain—may have no "objective" findings. No laboratory result or image can portray them. Only through the history and the evidence of their bodies do patients tell us how they need our help and how best that help can be given.

Patients have also told us time and again in surveys that their greatest discontent with physicians of our era is that *they do not listen*. This has been markedly worsened, it appears, by the increasing demands of the electronic health record systems, which are wondrous and very useful but *cannot* be the main focus of any good doctor's attention during the patient visit. An increasingly heard lament of patients is that the doctor concentrates less on them than on putting "data" into computers and that all the patient sees is the doctor's back as he or she types the patient's story in formulaic language onto screens.

The history is more than the elucidation of the facts of the case, more than a construct of symptoms. It also tells the tale of the reaction a unique human being has to those symptoms and their impact on the patient's mind and life, their family, and their hopes. Listening to patients is more than an ingathering of indications for further studies or filling in the required spaces in the electronic health record. It is, in and of itself, a major therapeutic act, and the physician, himself or herself, is a potent therapeutic instrument. In conjunction with the laying on of hands that follows in the physical examination, the meeting of doctor and patient fulfills some primal need of vulnerable and often fearful people to be attended to, cared for, and cared about.

The history and physical examination also gives doctors much of the richness of their professional lives. Decades from now, a physician in retrospective reverie about his or her career in medicine will not remember the chemistry panels, the MRI results, or even the majority of the medical scientific facts of their past practice (just as well, since so many of these "facts" will have changed). What they will remember and tell to their potentially bored students are the stories of their patients, about who they were and how they acted, and what their physical examinations showed that surprised or confirmed history-generated hypotheses. If endurance in memory is any indication of the importance of events, it is the history and physical examination, that story of how the patient responded to duress both in spirit and in body, that is existentially most important to *both* doctor and patient.

The 20th century poet T.S. Eliot once wrote, "Where is the wisdom we have lost in knowledge? Where is the knowledge we have lost in information?" Laboratory studies and imaging are, without doubt, essential and informative; knowledge, however, comes only with their integration with the patient's story as told by history and physical examination; wisdom is what doctors acquire when they recognize this truth.

Chapter 2

Subtleties of Medical History Taking

Helaina Laks Kravitz, MD, and Richard L. Kravitz, MD, MSPH

When first seeing patients in clinics and on the wards, the learning curve is steep. During these early encounters, it is often a struggle to ask the right questions, follow up on the answers, and sort the information into the appropriate categories. On the other hand, when watching a seasoned clinician take a medical history, it all seems natural and effortless. The interview flows smoothly and the medical history falls seamlessly into place. Over time, clinicians develop a personal interview style, integrating the information in this book and experience with patients. The following guidelines are some "tricks of the trade" that may help the student—at whatever stage of training or practice—to dodge some of the usual obstacles to efficient, effective medical history taking.

FIRST IMPRESSIONS COUNT

The initial interview with your patient is a unique opportunity to lay a solid foundation in the patient–physician relationship. Spending extra time and paying special attention to patient concerns up front will save time in the long run and lead to better medical care.

MAKE THE MOST OF YOUR LIMITED TIME WITH THE PATIENT

In the course of everyday clinical care, there are occasions when you are pressed for time. There are several patients to see, laboratory results to check, and a presentation to rehearse for morning rounds. Patients are very perceptive and sense when you are in a hurry. When rushed, it is especially important to be completely present for the patient. Greet the patient by name. Sit down rather than stand. Maintain eye contact as much as possible, looking up at the patient frequently as you jot down notes or make an occasional entry into the electronic medical record (EMR). All of these things will help the patient feel heard, nurtured, and cared for, and will generally not require extra time.

TAKE A FEW MINUTES WITH THE CHART (PAPER OR ELECTRONIC) BEFORE YOU SEE THE PATIENT

There is a wealth of information in the chart, and it makes sense to use it. It takes much less time to extract dates of past surgeries from the medical record than to ask a typical patient to develop the list de novo. Making use of secondary sources does not release you from the obligation to confirm key points directly (eg, "I see from your record you were hospitalized in 1966 for kidney disease. Can you tell me more about that?"). Additionally, in patients with poor cognitive function or organizational skills, it is helpful to expand secondary sources and verify information with friends, family, and other physicians. Finally, beware of "chart lore" (eg, the patient who carries a diagnosis of "lupus" passed down from one discharge summary to the next but who has no corroborating physical or laboratory evidence of the disease). Recognizing these caveats, it is always appropriate and usually necessary to "interview the chart" as well as the patient.

THE COMPUTER IS NOT THE PATIENT

EMRs are increasingly available, and many clinics have installed computers in every examining room. The potential benefits of EMRs are numerous. However, if not used judiciously, computers can intrude upon and distort the physician–patient relationship. When accessing the EMR in the patient's presence, do not forget that the patient is also in the room with you. Some experienced clinicians do their electronic charting during breaks in the visit (eg, while the patient is changing). Others position the computer screen at an angle so it can be viewed by both patient and physician. And some maintain a dialogue with the patient while clicking away at the computer keys, looking up frequently to re-establish eye contact. If you choose this approach, refrain from commenting to the chart "hmm," "uh oh," or "that's good." Rather, let the patient know what you are finding out. "Your blood sugars seem to have been stable until a few months ago." "You have maintained your weight nicely since the last visit."

IT IS NOT NECESSARY TO GATHER INFORMATION IN THE SAME ORDER THAT IT WILL BE PRESENTED

Oral and written presentations should be delivered in a standard format, generally beginning with the reason for consultation or the chief complaint, then moving on through the history of present illness (HPI), past history (including medications and allergies), family history, personal and social history, review of systems, physical examination, and assessment and plan. Following a standard format for presentation helps organize your thoughts about the patient, reduces the likelihood of omitting critical data, and makes a presentation easier to follow. However, just because one *presents* information in a particular order does not mean one has to *gather* it that way.

Rigid adherence to a template means missing potential opportunities, such as noticing the stare of Graves disease (ordinarily part of the physical examination) as the patient describes the evolution of her abdominal complaints; asking about medications, drugs, and alcohol (usually reserved for the past medical history) right after the patient complains of insomnia; responding to a glint of sadness elicited during the HPI by inquiring about depressed mood and recent losses (points that might otherwise be relegated to the social history or review of systems). Waiting to follow up such observations until the "correct" time is artificial and may sacrifice diagnostic efficiency (or the interviewer may overlook them altogether).

ADMIT WHEN YOU ARE CONFUSED

Patients will not mind repetition. They want the doctor to get the story right. Do not be afraid to say, "I'm sorry, I didn't quite understand that." Occasionally, a meandering and inconsistent history is a clue to cognitive impairment. More often, misplaced details simply reflect the complexity of human experience; however, critical details must be clarified to effectively treat the patient. Was the onset of the pain or dyspnea instantaneous, acute (hours), subacute (days to weeks), or chronic (longer)? Did the nausea and anorexia precede the pain or vice versa? Is the patient who complains of frequent urination voiding relatively small volumes each time (frequency) or large volumes (polyuria)? If something does not make sense, persist until it becomes clear.

CHRONOLOGY IS KING: CREATE A TIME LINE WITH THE PATIENT

No dimension of the medical history is more important than the chronologic relation of one event to another. It can be useful to draw out a time line, indicating when symptoms started, how they have affected the patient, and what treatments have helped or been ineffective. The chronologic pattern of symptoms not only helps establish a diagnosis but also informs the urgency of response. Recurrent headaches unchanging in pattern over a period of years are unlikely to represent serious anatomic illness, whereas a new-onset headache of moderate severity may be a sign of increased intracranial pressure. Chronic stable angina can be managed as an outpatient; chest pain increasing in frequency or severity may warrant urgent intervention.

When the patient's story seems hopelessly confused, ask the patient about the last time he or she remembers feeling completely well. Then ask what the patient first noticed as he or she began to feel ill. Then ask what the patient noticed next, and the next, and so on. A solid chronology is the foundation of diagnostic accuracy.

BE ALERT FOR HIDDEN FEARS

Most clinicians recognize that a diagnosis of cancer is frightening and will appropriately prepare themselves to deal with the patient's emotional reaction. However, there are many situations that, while seemingly trivial, are in fact overwhelming to the patient. It is important to explore the patient's own ideas and feelings about the illness. For instance, an otherwise innocuous bout of upper abdominal pain might feel ominous to a 53-year-old male patient whose father died of a myocardial infarction. Failure to address the patient's worries may lead to further escalation of his or her complaints. One approach is to say, "Many patients have thoughts about what might be causing their symptoms. I was wondering if you were concerned about anything in particular?" If the response is vague, you could add, "What do *you* think is going on?"

TRUST, BUT VERIFY

Do not take every answer at face value. Many one-word answers demand follow-up, especially if they do not fit with other data. For instance, a 48-year-old woman with chronic cough who answers the question "Do you smoke cigarettes?" with a "no" may have "quit" yesterday after a 30-pack-year history. Sometimes definitions need to be quantified. The alcoholic might report "one or two" drinks a night, but only the persistent clinician will learn that he considers a "drink" to be 8 oz of hard liquor (or a 32-oz beer).

CLARIFY WHAT MEDICATION THE PATIENT IS ACTUALLY TAKING

It is important to review the chart and ask the patient to provide a list of prescribed medications, but this list does not always match what the patient actually takes. It is often helpful to ask the patient to bring all medications to a subsequent appointment. Sometimes a medication "is not working" simply because the patient skips doses of medications that need to be taken three or four times daily. Adding yet another medication or increasing the dose is not going to solve this problem, whereas good history taking will.

FOLLOW YOUR INSTINCTS

The doctor–patient interview is ultimately a conversation between two people. If something does not seem quite right, there usually is a reason. Note whether the affect of the patient matches the content of what is said. If the patient is describing pain in her chest, does she seem unduly worried or casually indifferent? Does the patient look away or wring her hands when she answers certain questions? She may be withholding something. Without being accusatory, making a simple observation or conjecture is often all that is needed: "You seem worried about something." "I was wondering if it feels uncomfortable to talk about this." Your instincts will often be right and may yield crucial information.

JUDICIOUSLY APPLIED, SILENCE IS GOLDEN

Eager not to miss anything, most beginning interviewers talk too much. Even seasoned clinicians interrupt a patient on average after 23 seconds.[1] Although it is important to clarify points of confusion, try not to interrupt the patient. As William Osler is frequently quoted as saying, "Listen to the patient. He is telling you the diagnosis." This crusty aphorism often rings true! It is easier to let the patient tell the story on his or her own terms if you remember that you will have a chance to rearrange the facts into a coherent presentation later.

ANYTHING ELSE?

Patients have an average of three concerns per office visit. Asking, "Anything else?" (or your version of the question) during the interview gives the patient a chance to fill in details or ask questions.[2] The sooner you can elicit the patient's agenda for the visit, the more likely you will have time to address the concerns.

GOOD HISTORY TAKING SERVES A TWOFOLD PURPOSE

Incorporating these guidelines into history taking will increase the likelihood of obtaining the correct information while forming a critical connection with the patient which is, in itself, therapeutic.

Test Your Knowledge

1. It is always important to verify the medications actually being taken because:
   A. the patient's chart may be inaccurate
   B. the patient may be receiving additional medications from another provider
   C. the patient may be taking a higher or lower dose than prescribed
   D. the patient may have stopped taking the medication due to side effects
   E. All of the above

2. When a patient gives an incomplete or one-word answer to a sensitive question, the interviewer should:
   A. pause until the patient provides a more detailed answer
   B. assume that the issue is not important to the patient and move on
   C. gently ask the question in a different way
   D. demand to know why the patient is withholding information

References

1. Marvel MK, Epstein RM, Flowers K, Beckman H. Soliciting the patient's agenda: have we improved? *JAMA*. 1999;281:283–287.
2. Beckman HB, Frankel RM. The effect of physician behavior on the collection of data. *Ann Intern Med*. 1984;101:692–696.

Chapter 3

Patient-Centered Interviewing

Francesca C. Dwamena, MD, MS, Auguste H. Fortin VI, MD, MPH, and Robert C. Smith, MD, MS

CASE SCENARIO

You are a primary care clinician seeing patients in your office. You glance at the intake form of your last patient of the day and notice that she is a 38-year-old woman with left-sided neck pain for 1 week. She is a colleague's patient whom you have never met before. You have 15 minutes for her visit.

- **How can you elicit the patient's full agenda for the visit in 1 minute or less?**
- **How can you elicit a patient-centered description of her neck pain?**
- **How can you obtain the personal and emotional context of her neck pain?**

INTRODUCTION

Effective medical interviewing is a skill that must be systematically learned and practiced. Traditionally, students were trained to use a primarily clinician-centered approach to elicit biomedical data.[1] The interviewer asked specific, often closed-ended, questions in order to help make a diagnosis. Unfortunately, this approach often resulted in an incomplete and/or inaccurate database and limited the ability of the interviewer to establish rapport with the patient. Patient-centered interviewing[2] focuses on the personal and emotional context and encourages the patient to spontaneously describe his or her symptoms. The interviewer efficiently establishes a relationship with the patient by focusing on the patient's emotions and concerns. When integrated with more traditional clinician-centered interviewing, patient-centered interviewing enables the interviewer to obtain a more complete biopsychosocial story.[1]

Unfortunately, many healthcare providers still use an exclusively clinician-centered style that discourages patients from expressing their concerns.[3] The data collected are skewed toward physical symptoms and often misinterpreted because of missing psychosocial context. In contrast, interactions that encourage patients to freely express their concerns yield more valid data and tend to improve patient satisfaction, compliance, knowledge, and recall.[4–6] They also decrease doctor-shopping and lawsuits.[7] Interactions that use a patient-centered style have also resulted in better blood pressure and diabetic control,[8] better perinatal outcomes,[9] shortened lengths of stay and improved mortality in critically ill patients,[10] and improved cancer outcomes.[11]

KEY TERMS

Biopsychosocial (BPS) model	The BPS model describes the patient as an integrated mix of his or her biologic, psychological, and social components. It differs from the biomedical model, which describes the patient only in terms of disease (physical or psychiatric).
Patient-centered interviewing	The interviewer encourages the patient to express what is most important to him or her and facilitates the narration of the patient's story.
Clinician-centered interviewing	The clinician takes charge of the interaction to acquire specific details not provided already by the patient, usually to diagnose disease or to develop the database (see Chapter 4).
Integrated patient-centered and clinician-centered interviewing	The interviewer uses both patient-centered and clinician-centered interviewing to elicit physical, personal (includes social), and emotional data from the patient and then synthesizes the data into the biopsychosocial story.

This chapter describes a step-by-step, behaviorally defined, patient-centered interviewing method that has been shown in a randomized controlled trial to be effective.[2]

FACILITATING SKILLS

In order to conduct an effective patient-centered interview, the interviewer must master a core set of questioning and relationship-building skills.

Open-Ended Questioning Skills

These skills generate the patient's agenda and elicit personal descriptions of symptoms and concerns. They encourage the patient to express what is on his or her mind (eg, questions, feelings, fears) rather than responding to what is on the interviewer's mind. In contrast, closed-ended questions focus on specific issues in the interviewer's mind (eg, diagnoses) and are used in the clinician-centered part of the interview (see Chapter 4).

Skill(s)	Description or Definition of Skill(s)
Nonfocusing questioning skills	Allow patient to talk freely without controlling the direction of the interview.
• *Silence*	Saying nothing while remaining attentive. Note: Prolonged silence may make a reticent patient uncomfortable.
• *Nonverbal encouragement*	Encouraging the patient to continue speaking by using gestures, sympathetic facial expressions, and/or other indications by body language.
• *Neutral utterances*	Brief, noncommittal statements like "oh," "uh-huh," "yes," or "hmm" that encourage a patient to keep talking.
Focusing questioning skills	Directs patient to a particular topic that the patient has already mentioned. They are critical to maintaining effectiveness and efficiency of the interview.
• *Echoing*	Encouraging a patient to elaborate by repeating a word or phrase.
• *Open-ended requests*	Direct invitations to provide more information on a particular subject.
• *Summarizing or paraphrasing*	Briefly restating the patient's expressed story in order to check accuracy or refocus the interview.

Relationship-Building Skills

These skills are used to encourage the patient to express his or her emotions and to nurture the patient. Once the patient shows or verbalizes an emotion, the interviewer can respond empathically using the following empathy skills: naming, understanding, respecting, and supporting (which can be recalled with the mnemonic "NURS").

Skill(s)	Description or Definition of Skill(s)
Emotion-seeking skills	Used to prompt the patient to express emotions.
Direct inquiry	Asking the patient directly how he or she feels.
Indirect inquiry	Used when direct inquiry is not immediately effective. It is usually followed with inquiring again about emotion.
• *Self-disclosure*	Sharing a related experience or emotion that may resonate with patient.
• *Impact of problem*	Asking how the problem has affected the patient or the patient's companion(s).
• *Patient's explanatory model*	Asking the patient what he or she thinks or is concerned might be causing the problem.
Empathy skills (NURS)	Verbal empathic responses to patient's expressed emotions.
Name	Repeating an expressed emotion to show you have heard the patient.
Understand	Verbally indicating comprehension of an expressed emotion after learning more about it.
Respect	Praising the patient or acknowledging the patient's plight.
Support	Offering partnership or concrete solutions to problems.

THE PROCESS OF PATIENT-CENTERED INTERVIEWING

Step 1: Setting the Stage for the Interview (30–60 seconds)

The interviewer begins the interaction by recognizing the patient, introducing himself or herself, and ensuring the patient's readiness to proceed with the interview. This step is usually done reflexively in less than a minute.

Step 1: Set the Stage	Explanation of Substeps
1. Welcome the patient.	With a greeting and handshake if appropriate.
2. Use the patient's name.	Address patient with the name by which he or she prefers to be called.
3. Introduce yourself and identify your specific role.	Students should explain that they are a part of the healthcare team, while being honest about their particular roles (eg, student doctor).
4. Ensure patient readiness and privacy.	This may include discretely excusing third parties and/or closing a door or curtain.
5. Remove barriers to communication.	Address any physical, emotional, or environmental circumstances that may preclude an effective interaction.
6. Ensure comfort and put the patient at ease.	This may include conducting light conversation (eg, asking about the weather or hospital food) to put the patient at ease.

Example of Step 1: "Good morning, Mrs. Green. I am Dr. Smith, and I will be your doctor today. (Shakes patient's hand; positions chair so that he is at the same eye level with the patient; closes the door to ensure privacy; and puts the patient at ease with some small talk.) "I hope you had no trouble getting here today."

Step 2: Obtaining the Agenda Including the Chief Complaint (30–60 seconds)

After orienting the patient to the expected duration and process, the interviewer briefly negotiates an agenda for the visit. With practice, the clinician can effectively negotiate an agenda in 1 minute.

Step 2: Obtain the Chief Complaint and Set the Agenda	Explanation of Substeps
7. Indicate time available.	This orients the patient to the duration of the interaction and helps both the patient and the interviewer to be efficient.
8. Indicate interviewer's needs.	Review the items the interviewer needs to have or to do in order to effectively address the patient's needs.
9. Obtain a list of all issues the patient wants to discuss.	This minimizes the chance of important issues arising at the end of the allotted time and may preclude patient complaints about not being given a chance to discuss important issues. It is accomplished by asking the patient to provide a list of the items for discussion and asking "Is there something else?" until a complete list has been obtained. The interviewer may need to respectfully discourage the patient from offering too many details about agenda items at this point.
10. Summarize and finalize the agenda.	Clarifies the chief complaint if it is not already apparent, prioritizes the list obtained, and empowers the patient to decide what will be addressed and what will be deferred to the next visit.

Example of Step 2: "We have 15 minutes together. I will need about 5 minutes to examine you and go over some of your vital signs. But before I do that, I'd like to get a list of what you want to talk about today.... Is there something else? So you'd like to talk about your headache and get some refills; anything else?"

Step 3: Opening the History of Present Illness (HPI) (30–60 seconds)

In Step 3, the interviewer asks an opening question and then listens attentively (using nonfocusing open-ended skills), while taking note of clues from the patient's environment and nonverbal behaviors.

Step 3: Open the History of Present Illness	Explanation of Substeps
11. State opening question.	Ask an open-ended question or invite the patient to tell his or her story.
12. Listen attentively for clues to the patient's personal circumstances.	Use nonfocusing questioning skills to encourage patient to talk freely.
13. Obtain additional data from nonverbal sources.	Make a mental note of the patient's physical characteristics, appearance, and environment for additional clues.

Example of Step 3: "Okay, tell me all about the headache." (Remains silent while the patient talks; nods head, leans forward, and intermittently says "uh huh" to encourage the patient to keep talking. Listens for at least 30 seconds, or longer if the patient is giving a coherent, nonrepetitive story.)

Step 4: Continuing the Patient-Centered HPI (3–5 minutes)

The biopsychosocial story consists of a symptom story (physical and/or psychological symptoms), an emotional story (how the patient feels about the symptoms and in general), and a personal story (details of the story that cannot be described as either symptoms or emotions). The goal in Step 4 is to help the patient to tell his or her unique symptom, personal, and emotional stories. With practice, the keen interviewer can use focusing open-ended and relationship-building skills to help the patient describe his or her most important concerns. In the process, the interviewer will also generate rich diagnostic data that likely will not be obtained by closed-ended questions. The challenge, therefore, is to resist asking clinician-centered questions at this time.

Step 4: Continue the Patient-Centered History of Present Illness	Explanation of Substeps
14. Obtain the patient's description of his or her symptom or problem.	If needed, use **focusing questioning skills** to encourage patient to describe the **physical problem.** Avoid asking clinician-centered questions about details of symptom description such as onset and duration at this point so that the patient may continue to lead the interaction. The goal is to obtain a good overview of the problem in the patient's own words.
15. Develop the personal context of the patient's story.	Use **focusing questioning skills** to direct the patient to talk more about **personal clues** from his or her opening statements or nonverbal sources.
16. Develop the emotional context of the patient's story.	Use **emotion-seeking skills** to encourage the patient to talk about his or her **emotions.**
17. Address the patient's expressed emotions.	Use **empathy skills (NURS)** to respond to the patient's emotions and express **empathy.**
18. Expand the patient's story.	Use the **questioning and relationship-building skills** in multiple cycles to learn about the **clues** offered by the patient's words and nonverbal sources and to deepen the **connection** with the patient.

Example of Step 4: Continuing from above, the interviewer focuses on a symptom mentioned by the patient: "You said the headache was really painful…." This invites the patient to expand on the symptom description. Then the interviewer picks up a **personal issue** mentioned by the patient: "work…say more about that…." The interviewer listens for the first opportunity to naturally ask for **emotion**, "How do you feel about that?" When the patient responds with an emotion (eg, scared), the interviewer NURSes emotion by (1) naming ("scared"), (2) understanding ("I can see how that would be scary."), (3) respecting ("It's been a hard time for you."), and (4) supporting ("Let's work together to get to the bottom of it."). The interviewer then expands on the patient's story by focusing on another symptom or personal issue previously mentioned by the patient: "You mentioned your son; tell me about him." The interviewer continues with cycles of focusing-emotion-seeking-NURS.

Step 5: Transition to the Clinician-Centered Process (30 seconds)

The interviewer closes the patient-centered portion of the interview and begins the clinician-centered process to obtain the details needed to complete the patient's biopsychosocial history.

Step 5: Transition to Clinician-Centered Process	**Explanation of Substeps**
19. Summarize patient-centered HPI.	Review the gist of the patient's symptom, personal, and emotional story in two or three sentences.
20. Check accuracy.	Ask the patient whether summary is accurate.
21. Indicate that both content and style of inquiry will change if the patient is ready.	Ask the patient whether it is okay to ask more specific questions.

Example of Step 5: "You are having headaches that get worse at work and you are worried about losing your job—is that right? Is it okay if I ask you some more specific questions about the headaches?"

5-Step, 21-Substep Patient-Centered Interviewing

Step 1: Set the Stage

1. Welcome the patient.
2. Use the patient's name.
3. Introduce yourself and identify your specific role.
4. Ensure patient readiness and privacy.
5. Remove barriers to communication.
6. Ensure comfort and put the patient at ease.

Step 2: Obtain the Chief Complaint and Set the Agenda

7. Indicate time available.
8. Indicate interviewer's needs.
9. Obtain a list of all issues the patient wants to discuss.
10. Summarize and finalize the agenda.

Step 3: Open the History of Present Illness

11. State opening question.
12. Listen attentively for clues to the patient's personal circumstances.
13. Obtain additional data from nonverbal sources.

Step 4: Continue the Patient-Centered History of Present Illness

14. Obtain the patient's description of his or her physical symptom or problem.
15. Develop the personal context of the patient's story.
16. Develop the emotional context of the patient's story.
17. Address the patient's expressed emotions.
18. Expand the patient's story.

Step 5: Transition to Clinician-Centered Process

19. Summarize patient-centered HPI.
20. Check accuracy.
21. Indicate that both content and style of inquiry will change if the patient is ready.

SUMMARY

The patient-centered interview consists of 5 steps and 21 substeps. The interviewer prepares the patient for the interaction with Steps 1 and 2. In Steps 3 and 4, the interviewer facilitates the sequential development of the patient's physical, personal, and emotional stories using nonfocusing skills followed by focusing, emotion-seeking, and empathy skills. The story is expanded and deepened by focusing the patient on revealed personal and emotional information and repeating the cycles in Step 4, while monitoring the patient's reaction to the interview. The interviewer uses Step 5 to transition to the clinician-centered process (described in Chapter 4), which elaborates the HPI and other routine historical data.

CASE SCENARIO | Resolution

You are a primary care clinician seeing patients in your office. You glance at the intake form of your last patient of the day and notice that she is a 38-year-old woman with left-sided neck pain for 1 week. She is a colleague's patient whom you have never met before. You have 15 minutes for her visit.

ADDITIONAL HISTORY

The pain started after a restless night 1 week ago. There is no history of trauma, fever, chills, neck stiffness, or any other red flags. With proper facilitation, she reports that she had a fight with her husband a week ago after discovering that he was having an affair. She tossed and turned the night of the fight and woke up with the neck pain, which is only getting worse. She feels betrayed and angry, and she is worried that her marriage may be ending. The last thing she needs is a neck pain that won't go away.

Question: What is the most efficient way to establish rapport and make this patient feel supported and cared for?

A. Use nonfocusing, open-ended skills.
B. Ask her how she feels emotionally and use NURS.
C. Set an agenda.
D. A and C
E. A, B, and C

Test Your Knowledge

1. A patient comes to your office with abdominal pain.
   Which of the following questions/statements is most likely to elicit a patient-centered description of the abdominal pain?
   A. How does that make you feel?
   B. On a scale of 1 (not painful) to 10 (worst pain you ever had), how severe is the pain?
   C. Is it a dull or sharp pain?
   D. Abdominal pain; tell me more about that.

2. A patient with a mild frontal headache and uncontrolled blood pressure admits to "forgetting" a dose of his blood pressure medication several times a week, including this morning, because he has "a lot on my mind." With proper facilitation by the interviewer, he admits to frequent arguments with his wife because of her drinking problem. He is worried about the marriage and feels helpless about the current escalation in their fighting.
   Which of the following is a "personal story"?
   A. Problems with wife
   B. Uncontrolled blood pressure
   C. Bad memory
   D. Feels worried and helpless

3. A 60-year old woman presents with abdominal pain and painful urination. During the interview, she mentions that she became really worried when she noticed blood in her urine.
   Which of the following statements is most likely to make her feel supported?
   A. How much blood was there in your urine?
   B. I'm glad you decided to come in today.
   C. Tell me more about the abdominal pain.
   D. You probably just have a urinary tract infection.

References

1. Engel GL. The need for a new medical model: a challenge for biomedicine. *Science.* 1977;196:129–136.
2. Smith RC, Lyles JS, Mettler J, et al. The effectiveness of intensive training for residents in interviewing. A randomized, controlled study. *Ann Intern Med.* 1998;128:118–126.
3. Beckman HB, Frankel RM. The effect of physician behavior on the collection of data. *Ann Intern Med.* 1984;101:692–696.
4. Ambady N, Laplante D, Nguyen T, et al. Surgeons' tone of voice: a clue to malpractice history. *Surgery.* 2002;132:5–9.
5. Hall JA, Roter DL, Katz NR. Meta-analysis of correlates of provider behavior in medical encounters. *Med Care.* 1988;26:657–675.
6. Kasteler J, Kane RL, Olsen DM, Thetford C. Issues underlying prevalence of "doctor-shopping" behavior. *J Health Soc Behav.* 1976;17:329–339.
7. Levinson W, Roter DL, Mullooly JP, et al. Physician-patient communication. The relationship with malpractice claims among primary care physicians and surgeons. *JAMA.* 1997;277:553–539.
8. Kaplan SH, Greenfield S, Ware JE Jr. Assessing the effects of physician-patient interactions on the outcomes of chronic disease. *Med Care.* 1989;27(Suppl):S110–S127.
9. Shear CL, Gipe BT, Mattheis JK, Levy MR. Provider continuity and quality of medical care. A retrospective analysis of prenatal and perinatal outcome. *Med Care.* 1983;21: 1204–1210.
10. Lilly CM, Sonna LA, Haley KJ, Massaro AF. Intensive communication: four-year follow-up from a clinical practice study. *Crit Care Med.* 2003;31(5 Suppl):S394–S399.
11. Spiegel D, Sephton SE, Terr AI, Stites DP. Effects of psychosocial treatment in prolonging cancer survival may be mediated by neuroimmune pathways. *Ann NY Acad Sci.* 1998;840: 674–683.

Suggested Reading

Fortin AH VI. Communication skills to improve patient satisfaction and quality of care. *Ethn Dis.* 2002;12:S3-58–61.

Fortin AH VI, Dwamena FC, Frankel RM, Smith RC. *Smith's Patient-Centered Interviewing: An Evidence-Based Method.* 3rd ed. New York: McGraw-Hill, 2012.

Smith RC. Videotape of Evidence-Based Interviewing: (1) Patient-Centered Interviewing and (2) Doctor-Centered Interviewing. Marketing Division, Instructional Media Center, Michigan State University. P.O. Box 710, East Lansing, MI 48824.

Chapter 4

Clinician-Centered Interviewing

Auguste H. Fortin VI, MD, MPH, Francesca C. Dwamena, MD, MS, and
Robert C. Smith, MD, MS

CASE SCENARIO

You have completed the patient-centered part of the interview of the patient from Chapter 3 (38-year-old woman with left-sided neck pain for 1 week after discovering that her husband was having an affair). Now you need to transition to the clinician-centered interview to learn more about the patient and her neck pain.

- **What further details about the neck pain do you need to know?**
- **Which aspects of the social history will be most important?**
- **How will you respond if the patient starts to cry when you inquire about her home life?**

INTRODUCTION

The patient-centered part of the interview yields the patient's personal description of his or her symptom and its impact on the patient's life, including any resulting emotional response. Consider this the patient's story of the history of present illness (HPI) (see Chapter 3).

Although the patient-centered interview provides important psychosocial information, it is rarely sufficient to make the diagnosis for a given symptom. More details (eg, symptom characteristics, the family history and social history) are needed to fill in the database, which is usually done in the clinician-centered interview.[1] Here clinicians inquire about symptom information not yet mentioned by the patient in order to complete the HPI. Other aspects of the patient's life and history are explored to consider diseases apart from the present illness, assess for disease risk, and get to know the patient better.

In the clinician-centered interview, the patient is led through a series of open-ended followed by closed-ended questions, moving from general information to specific details.

KEY TERMS	
Clinician-centered interviewing	The clinician takes charge of the interaction to acquire specific details not provided already by the patient, usually to diagnose disease or to fill in the routine database.
Closed-ended questions	Can be answered with "yes," "no," a number, or a short answer. For example, "When did your headache start?" "Where is it located?"
Open-ended questions/requests	Encourage the patients to tell a narrative or story. For example, "Tell me more about your headache." "Go on."

FILLING IN THE HPI

The clinician expands the symptom description and obtains any related symptoms, details, and other relevant data (eg, medications, hospitals, doctor's visits) not yet introduced by the patient (Table 4–1).

Expanding Description of Symptoms

Symptoms already mentioned by the patient usually need further explanation. To fully understand a symptom, clinicians need to know its 7 "cardinal features": **O**nset and chronology, **P**osition and radiation, **Q**uality, **Q**uantification, **R**elated

Table 4–1. Filling in the history of present illness.

1. Define the cardinal features of the patient's chief concern.
2. Define the cardinal features of other symptoms (those already mentioned by the patient and those not yet introduced) in the organ system of the patient's chief concern.
3. Inquire about relevant symptoms outside the involved system.
4. Inquire about relevant nonsymptom (secondary) data.

symptoms, **S**etting and **T**ransforming factors (the mnemonic **OPQQRST** may help)[1–3] (Table 4–2).

Even the most articulate patient is unlikely to have mentioned all important elements of his or her story. Therefore, the clinician must obtain additional details. Start with an open-ended request ("Tell me more about what your chest pain is like."), and then ask more specific closed-ended questions to elicit all the cardinal features ("You pointed to the left side of your chest; does the pain travel anywhere?"). For nonpain symptoms (eg, weakness, dizziness), all cardinal features may not apply (eg, location, radiation).

Table 4–2. The 7 cardinal features of symptoms.

1. **Onset and chronology**
   a. Time of onset of symptom and intervals between recurrences
   b. Duration of symptom
   c. Periodicity and frequency of symptom
   d. Course of symptom
      i. Short-term
      ii. Long-term
2. **Position and radiation**
   a. Precise location
   b. Deep or superficial
   c. Localized or diffuse
3. **Quality**
   a. Usual descriptors
   b. Unusual descriptors
4. **Quantification**
   a. Type of onset
   b. Intensity or severity
   c. Impairment or disability
   d. Numeric description
      i. Number of events
      ii. Size
      iii. Volume
5. **Related symptoms**
6. **Setting**
7. **Transforming factors**
   a. Precipitating and aggravating factors
   b. Palliating factors

Data from Fortin AH VI, Dwamena FC, Frankel RM, Smith RC. *Smith's Patient-Centered Interviewing: An Evidence-Based Method*. 3rd ed. New York: McGraw-Hill, 2012.

Precise position of symptoms should be determined. The location of a symptom and whether it radiates can be diagnostically important (eg, low back pain radiating to the buttock and down the posterolateral thigh and lateral calf suggests L5–S1 nerve root impingement from a herniated disk).

The quality of a symptom can assist with diagnosis. For example, burning substernal chest pain is more likely to be due to esophageal reflux, while squeezing or crushing chest pain is more likely to be angina or myocardial infarction. Patients sometimes describe their symptoms in unusual ways (eg, "It feels like someone is reaching inside me and tearing me apart."). Such language may suggest psychological problems but can indicate serious illness as well.

When quantifying a pain symptom, a numeric rating scale is used: "On a scale of 1 to 10, with 1 being no pain and 10 being the worst you can imagine, what number would you give the pain you're describing?"

Chronology provides the structure for the rest of the patient's disease story: the primary problem(s), when it began, its course to the present, and any previous treatment. All relevant details of this structure must be filled in to best understand the big picture—the interacting biologic, psychological (personal, emotional), and social dimensions of the patient. The student or clinician usually organizes the rest of the features to fit within the chronology.

Inquiring About Symptoms in Same Body System

After obtaining all relevant cardinal features of the symptom, ask about related symptoms within the same body system. In essence, one performs a "focused review of systems" for that system, ascertaining which other symptoms are present and which ones are absent. For example, the absence of dyspnea in a patient with chest pain weighs against a diagnosis of pulmonary embolism.

Asking About Other Relevant Symptoms

It is also important to ask about symptoms outside the involved body system if they are pertinent to a diagnosis you are considering. For example, when evaluating a patient with rheumatoid arthritis and fatigue, one asks about gastrointestinal bleeding symptoms ("Any black stools?") even though such symptoms are outside the musculoskeletal system, because bleeding may be caused by nonsteroidal anti-inflammatory agents. In patients with more than one problem, inquiry in multiple systems will be required.

Inquiring About Relevant Nonsymptom Data

Ask about the relevant secondary data not yet introduced by the patient including medications, diagnoses, treatments, doctors, and hospital stays. Clarify possible etiologic explanations for diagnoses being entertained to narrow the differential diagnosis. For example, if pulmonary embolism is a concern, asking about recent long car rides or air travel is warranted.

Scanning Without Interpretation Versus Hypothesis Testing

When interviewing is first being learned, students often do not know what might be causing a patient's symptom. By using the patient-centered and clinician-centered approaches, you will gather sufficient data to guide your search of texts and other resources to discover the most likely diagnosis. Novice interviewers must be exhaustive in their interviewing ("scanning" approach) because they are not interpreting the patient's responses in real time to guide further questioning.[4] It is often necessary to return to the patient with additional questions after reading about the problem and developing new hypotheses about what is causing the symptoms.

As medical knowledge and interviewing experience increase, students begin to develop "hunches" about what might be causing a patient's symptoms. Interviewers can then ask specific questions to test these hypotheses.[5] For example, a patient with sudden shortness of breath and chest pain following a long car ride might prompt consideration of pulmonary embolism. To test this hypothesis, ask about hemoptysis, leg pain, whether the chest pain is pleuritic in quality, and if there is a prior history of deep venous thrombosis. The symptom-based chapters in this book will help students develop hypotheses and test them. With time and practice, knowledge and skills develop to allow the hypothesis-driven approach to be blended with the scanning approach, improving efficiency.

Becoming Patient Centered When Necessary

Remember, clinician-centered interviewing is only a part of the interview. The interviewer must become patient-centered if the patient expresses emotion, using the NURS skills (**n**aming, **u**nderstanding, **r**especting, and **s**upporting; see Chapter 3) to communicate empathy. For example, if the patient suddenly becomes tearful when asked about her parents and then indicates that her father recently died, the interviewer must switch back to the patient-centered approach and use the NURS skills to learn more about this event, providing support and empathy: "That's very **sad;** I can **understand.** It's sure **been a hard time** for you. Is there anything **I can do to help?**"

Overview of the History After the HPI

At this point, all relevant details of the HPI have been obtained. Although you may have a reasonable idea about the diagnosis, ancillary data are still needed. Some of it will be related directly to the HPI (eg, prior history of myocardial infarction will be very germane in a patient with bloody stools if he requires major surgery). Much of the data will not relate directly to the HPI, but will nonetheless provide very important information about the patient (eg, personal exercise habits, education, family history of tuberculosis).

The approach to the remainder of the history is similar to the clinician-centered part of the HPI. Questioning should begin in an open-ended fashion in each major area and then be followed by closed-ended questions to obtain the relevant details, always returning to patient-centered skills and NURS when necessary.

PAST MEDICAL HISTORY

In the past medical history, inquire about medical issues and events not directly related to the HPI (Table 4–3). Start with

Table **4–3. Past medical history.**

- Inquire about general state of health and past illnesses.
  - — Childhood: measles, mumps, rubella, chicken pox, scarlet fever, and rheumatic fever
  - — Adult: hypertension, cerebrovascular accident, diabetes, heart disease, heart murmur, tuberculosis, sexually transmitted infections, cancer, blood transfusions
- Inquire about past injuries, accidents, psychotherapy, and unexplained problems.
- Elicit past hospitalizations (medical, surgical, obstetric, and psychiatric).
- Review the patient's immunization history.
  - — Childhood: measles, mumps, rubella, polio, hepatitis B, chicken pox, tetanus/pertussis/diphtheria, haemophilus B
  - — Adult: tetanus boosters, hepatitis B, hepatitis A, influenza, pneumococcal pneumonia
- Obtain the patient's obstetric history and menstrual history.
  - — Age of menarche, cycle length, length of menstrual flow, number of tampons/pads used per day
  - — Number of pregnancies, complications; number of live births, spontaneous vaginal deliveries/cesarean sections; number of spontaneous and therapeutic abortions
  - — Age of menopause
- List current medications, including dose and route.
  - — Ask specifically about over-the-counter medicines, alternative remedies, contraceptives, vitamins, laxatives
- Review allergies.
  - — Environmental, medications, foods
  - — Ensure that medication "allergies" are not actually expected side effects or nonallergic adverse reactions

open-ended questions (eg, "How was your health as a child?"), and then focus as needed with closed-ended questions to establish details (eg, "Did you have chicken pox? Measles?").

Medications

Determine the medications the patient takes, including both dosages and routes of administration. Be sure to ask about over-the-counter medications and herbal or alternative remedies. Ask specifically about birth control pills, hormones, laxatives, and vitamins, as these are sometimes not considered medications by patients. Assess for adherence with an open-ended, nonjudgmental question such as, "How is it going with your medication?" This gives the patient an opportunity to talk about whether or not he or she is taking the medication as prescribed and any difficulties such as side effects or excessive cost.

Allergies

Ask about environmental, food, and medication allergies. Determine exactly what reaction the patient had to a medication; many medication "allergies" are actually expected side effects (eg, itching with morphine) or nonallergic adverse reactions (eg, gastric bleeding from aspirin).

SOCIAL HISTORY

The social history describes behaviors and other personal factors that may impact disease risk, severity, and outcome; it also helps the interviewer to get to know the patient (Table 4–4).

As students gain experience, they learn the most important questions for a given patient encounter. Discussing the highlighted items will identify targets for risk factor modification and assist in building the clinician–patient relationship. Such issues, although rarely brought up by patients, should be discussed openly and in a nonjudgmental fashion to both garner trust and obtain accurate information. This type of information may need to be obtained over multiple patient encounters.

Ask about the nonbolded items in Table 4–4 if time allows and when directed by the patient's illness. For example, if the patient has an acute febrile illness, ask about travel and pets.

The psychosocial data collected in the social history complement the personal and emotional information obtained in the patient-centered portion of the interview. Hearing a patient's story and responding to his or her emotions is therapeutic and crucial to the clinician–patient relationship.

Some of the most important areas of the social history are detailed below.

Habits

Ask about tobacco use, including all forms of tobacco (eg, pipe, snuff, chewing tobacco) and number of pack-years of cigarette use (packs smoked per day multiplied by number of years of smoking).

Determine whether the patient consumes alcohol and whether it may be a health problem. Ask, "Do you drink beer, wine, or spirits? How much alcohol do you drink? Has alcohol ever been a problem in your life? When was your last drink?" A response to the last question indicating that the last drink was within 24 hours has a positive predictive value of 68% and a negative predictive value of 98% for alcohol abuse.[6] If the patient consumes alcohol, follow up with the "CAGE" questions.[7,8]

- "Have you thought about **C**utting down?"
- "Have you ever gotten **A**nnoyed when people talk to you about your drinking?"
- "Have you ever felt **G**uilty about your drinking?"
- "Do you ever have a drink first thing in the morning (**E**ye opener)?"

An affirmative answer to 2 or more CAGE questions has a sensitivity and specificity of > 90% for alcohol dependence.[6]

Determine whether the patient uses or abuses either "street" drugs or prescription drugs, and quantify the amount.

Personal Life

Occupation

A patient's occupation can affect health.[9] Ask, "Do you work outside the home?" "Tell me about your work." "What kind of work do you do?" "How long have you done this work?" "What other jobs have you had?" "Have you ever been exposed to fumes, dust, radiation, or loud noise at work?" "Do you think your work is affecting your symptoms now?" If so, ask, "Do your symptoms improve away from work?" "Are others at work having similar symptoms?" If the patient does not work outside the home, ask him or her to describe a typical day.

Home Life and Sexuality

A good way to inquire about home life is to ask, "Does anyone else live at home with you? Tell me about him or her." "Tell me about your support systems at home." This may provide a comfortable segue into asking about sexuality.[10] Suggested questions include:

- "Is there someone special in your life? Are you and this person having sex?"
- "Do you have sex with men, women, or both?"
- "Do you have sex with people who might be at risk for having sexually transmitted diseases or HIV (injection drug users, cocaine users, prostitutes, unknown partners, gay or bisexual men)?"
- "Are you using condoms to prevent disease? What percentage of the time?"

Table **4–4. Social history.**[a]

Habits	— Daily routine and schedule
• **Caffeine use**	— Health hazards
• **Tobacco use**	— Occupational exposures
— Forms	— Stress
— Pack-years	— Satisfaction
• **Alcohol use**	• **Hobbies, recreation**
— Type and amount consumed at 1 time/daily/weekly	• **Home life**
— "CAGE" questions	• **Personal relationships and support systems**
• **Drug use**	• **Sexuality**
— "Recreational" or "street" drugs	— Orientation
— Illicit use of prescription drugs	— Practices
Health promotion	— Any difficulty
• **Diet**	• **Intimate partner violence/abuse**
• **Physical activity/exercise history**	• **Stress**
• **Functional status**	— At home and work
• **Safety**	• **Health beliefs**
— Seatbelt use	• **Spirituality/religion**
— Safety helmet use	• **Exposures**
— Smoke detectors in home	— Pets
— Safe gun storage	— Travel
• **Screening**	— Illness at home, in the workplace
— Cervical cancer	— Sexually transmitted infections
— Breast cancer	• **Important life experiences**
— Prostate cancer	— Upbringing and family relationships
— Colon cancer	— Schooling
— Lipids	— Military service
— Hypertension	— Financial situation
— Diabetes	— Aging
— HIV	— Retirement
— Syphilis	— Life satisfaction
— Tuberculosis	— Cultural/ethnic background
— Glaucoma	• **Legal issues**
Personal life	— Living will or advance directives
• **Occupation**	— Power of attorney
— Workplace	— Emergency contact
— Level of responsibility	

[a]Items in bold should be asked about in most new patient encounters: They have high yield for risk factor modification, assist in building the clinician–patient relationship, and/or are important to patients but rarely brought up by them. Ask about other items as time allows and as indicated by the patient's symptom(s).

- "Do you have any other questions or concerns about sex?"
- "Are there any other sexual relationships that I should know about?"

To detect sexual problems, ask:

- "Have you noticed any recent changes or problems in your sexual functioning?"
- Men: "Do you have any problems having or maintaining an erection?" "Do you have any trouble having an orgasm?"
- Women: "Do you have pain during intercourse?" "Do you have any problems with lubrication or becoming aroused?" "Do you have difficulty having an orgasm?"
- "Has your illness affected your sexual functioning?"

Do not assume a patient's sexuality. Avoid questions such as, "Are you married or single?" or (to a woman), "Do you have a boyfriend?" Gender-neutral language (eg, "partner" and "spouse") communicates to gay, lesbian, bisexual, and transgender patients that it is safe for them to be honest and open with the interviewer.

As with the rest of the medical interview, questions must be tailored to the particular encounter. For example, it is not appropriate to take a detailed sexual history from a person experiencing acute heart failure in a crowded emergency department. Once the patient is stabilized and in a more private setting, return to these questions as indicated.

Intimate Partner Violence

An estimated 2 to 4 million US women are physically abused each year, with domestic violence occurring in as many as 1 of every 4 US families. Although it may feel uncomfortable, clinicians must learn to sensitively inquire about domestic partner violence, since patients are unlikely to broach this important issue. One suggested approach[11] is asking, "Have you ever been hit, slapped, kicked, or otherwise physically hurt by someone? Has anyone ever forced you to have sexual activities?"

Spirituality and Religious Beliefs

Spirituality and religious beliefs are important to many patients, especially in times of illness. One suggested mnemonic for asking about such issues is FICA[12]:

F: Faith and belief: "Do you consider yourself to be a spiritual or religious person?" "What is your faith or belief?" "What gives your life meaning?"

I: Importance and influence: "What importance does faith have in your life?" "Have your beliefs influenced the way you take care of yourself and your illness?" "What role do your beliefs play in regaining your health or coping with illness?"

C: Community: "Are you a part of a spiritual or religious community?" "Does the community support you? If so, how?" "Is there a group of people you really love or who are important to you?"

A: Address in care: "Would you like me to address these issues in your healthcare?"

FAMILY HISTORY

The family history, outlined in Table 4–5, is a critical source of information. Ask about the age and health of the patient's immediate family as well as the causes of death and ages of first-degree relatives. Patients with recent losses may exhibit emotion, which should be addressed with NURS.

Screen for genetic and environmental illnesses by asking about a family history of diseases such as cancer, heart disease, diabetes, tuberculosis, alcoholism, and asthma.

Table **4–5. Family history.**

1. Inquire about age and health (or cause or death) of grandparents, parents, siblings, and children.
2. Ask specifically about family history of:
   - Diabetes
   - Tuberculosis
   - Cancer
   - Hypertension
   - Stroke
   - Heart disease
   - Hyperlipidemia or high cholesterol
   - Bleeding problems
   - Anemias
   - Kidney disease
   - Asthma
   - Tobacco use
   - Alcoholism
   - Weight problems
   - Mental illness
     - — Depression
     - — Suicide
     - — Schizophrenia
     - — Multiple somatic concerns
   - Symptoms similar to those the patient is experiencing

REVIEW OF SYSTEMS

The review of systems (ROS) is a head-to-toe survey to uncover symptoms not elicited earlier in the interview. Part of the ROS was already performed (see Filling in the HPI). Now, the remaining body systems are surveyed to ensure that the database is complete (Table 4–6). At this point, the interviewer should already have a reasonable idea about the major diagnostic possibilities from data gathered in the HPI and past medical history. The ROS is not used to elucidate key features of the present illness.[1] Rather, it is used to screen for any additional symptoms *unrelated* to the HPI (eg, abnormal vaginal bleeding in a patient with suspected pneumonia). Do not extensively probe for every possible symptom in the ROS; try to identify only those symptoms that cause significant problems for the patient.

Table **4–6. Review of systems.**

General
Usual state of health
Fever
Chills
Night sweats
Appetite
Weight change
Weakness
Fatigue
Pain
Anhedonia
Skin
Rashes
Itching
Hives
Easy bruising
Change in moles
Loss of pigment
Change in hair pattern
Head
Dizziness
Headaches
Trauma
Fainting
Eyes
Use of glasses
Change in vision
Double vision (diplopia)
Pain
Redness
Discharge
History of glaucoma
Cataracts
Ears
Hearing loss
Use of hearing aid
Discharge
Pain
Ringing (tinnitus)
Nose
Nosebleeds (epistaxis)
Discharge
Loss of smell (anosmia)
Mouth and throat
Bleeding gums
Painful swallowing (odynophagia)
Difficulty swallowing (dysphagia)
Hoarseness
Tongue burning (glossodynia)
Tooth pain
Neck
Lumps
Goiter
Stiffness
Chest
Cough
Pain
Shortness of breath (dyspnea)
Sputum production
Coughing blood (hemoptysis)
Wheezing
Breasts
Lumps
Bloody discharge
Milky discharge (galactorrhea)
Pain
Self-examination
Cardiac
Chest pain
Palpitations
Shortness of breath (dyspnea)
• On exertion
• Lying flat (orthopnea)
• Awakening from sleep (paroxysmal nocturnal dyspnea)
• Swelling of feet or other regions (edema)
Vascular
Pain in legs, calves, thighs, hips, buttocks when walking (claudication)
Leg swelling (edema)
Blood clots (thrombophlebitis)
Ulcers
Gastrointestinal
Appetite
Nausea
Vomiting (emesis)
Vomiting blood (hematemesis)
Swallowing difficulty/pain
Heartburn (dyspepsia)
Abdominal pain
Constipation
Diarrhea
Change in stool color/caliber
Black, tarry stools (melena)
Rectal bleeding (hematochezia)
Hemorrhoids

—Continued next page

Table **4–6. Review of systems.** *(continued)*

Urinary	Numbness
Frequent urination (frequency)	Tingling
Urinating at night (nocturia)	Tremors
Abrupt urge to urinate (urgency)	Loss of memory
Difficulty starting stream	Mood changes
Incontinence	Sleep
Blood in urine (hematuria)	Nervousness
Painful urination (dysuria)	Speech disorders
Female genital	Poor balance (ataxia)
Lesions/discharge/itching	Hallucinations
Age at menarche	Seizures
Interval between menses	**Musculoskeletal**
Duration of menses	Weakness
Amount of flow	Pain
Last menses	Stiffness
Bleeding between periods	**Endocrine**
Pregnancies	***Diabetes mellitus***
Abortions/miscarriages	Excessive thirst
Libido	Frequent urination
Dyspareunia	Numbness or tingling of hands/feet
Orgasm function	Weight gain or loss
Age at menopause	Episodes of confusion, sweating, light-headedness (hypoglycemic reaction)
Menopausal symptoms	Blurred vision
Postmenopausal bleeding	Date of last eye examination
Male genital	***Thyroid***
Lesions/discharge	Swelling in neck
Erectile function	Weight gain or loss
Orgasm function	Palpitations or racing heart
Testis swelling/pain	Tremulousness
Libido	Hair loss (alopecia)
Hernia	Dry skin
Neuropsychiatric	Heat or cold intolerance
Fainting	Loss of skin pigment (vitiligo)
Paralysis	Constipation or diarrhea

SUMMARY

Clinician-centered interviewing helps uncover diagnostically important information and develops a routine database about the patient. Coupled with information from the patient-centered interview, the clinician develops the patient's biopsychosocial story, encompassing not only the patient's disease problems but also the personal and emotional context in which they occur.[12]

CLINICIAN-CENTERED PORTION OF THE INTERVIEW*

Fill-in the HPI	Family History
Past Medical History	Review of Systems
Social History	

*always be prepared to revert to patient-centered interviewing skills if needed

CASE SCENARIO | Resolution

You have completed the patient-centered part of the interview of the patient from Chapter 3 (38-year-old woman with left-sided neck pain for 1 week after discovering that her husband was having an affair). Now you need to transition to the clinician-centered interview to learn more about the patient and her neck pain.

ADDITIONAL HISTORY

In the patient-centered interview, the patient already related that her neck pain was present upon awakening 1 week ago and has worsened (onset and chronology) after having discovered that her husband was having an affair (setting). The pain is located in her right posterior neck and right shoulder at the base of the neck but does not radiate down the arm (position and radiation). The pain is tight and burning, and it feels "like it's in the muscles" (quality). She rates the pain as 7/10 in intensity (quantification). She has no fever, chills, headache, or weakness, tingling, or numbness of her arms or hands (related symptoms). The pain is worsened by turning her head or squeezing her neck and shoulder muscles, and it is relieved by ibuprofen and a heating pad (transforming factors). She denies feelings of depression or loss of interest (related symptoms outside of the involved body system). She has never had a pain like this before (secondary data). She is otherwise healthy and takes no medicines (past medical history).

In the social history, you learn that the patient has not turned to alcohol or drug use in response to her increased stress. She has many supports, including a sister who lives nearby and a pastor with whom she plans to talk. She has no history of domestic violence and feels safe in the relationship with her husband. She was shocked to discover her husband's affair, but in retrospect recognizes that he had grown distant over the past few months and that their sexual encounters had become less frequent. She becomes tearful when discussing the relationship.

Question: What is the best way to respond at this point?

A. I'm sure you'll be able to patch things up.
B. This is really a tough time that you are going through.
C. How frequently are you having sex?
D. I know just how you feel.

Test Your Knowledge

1. What is the best way to begin asking about the past medical history?
   A. Have you had measles, mumps, rubella, chicken pox, scarlet fever, or rheumatic fever?
   B. Did you get all your shots growing up?
   C. Were you hospitalized as a child?
   D. How was your health as a child?

2. A patient comes to the office concerned about loss of smell. Which of the 7 cardinal features would **not** apply to this symptom?
   A. Radiation
   B. Onset and chronology
   C. Related symptoms
   D. Transforming factors

3. A 22-year-old woman presents with a bruise around her cheekbone and eye. "I'm such a klutz—I fell down the stairs again," she says, avoiding your gaze. You wonder about the possibility of domestic violence, but she doesn't mention anything in response to your patient-centered questions. What should you do or say next?
   A. Keep it in the back of your mind and see if she brings it up at the next visit.
   B. Ask, "You're not being hit, are you?"
   C. Ask, "Have you ever been hit, slapped, kicked, or otherwise physically hurt by someone?"
   D. Refer her to a psychiatrist to help determine whether she is a domestic violence survivor.

References

1. Fortin AH VI, Dwamena FC, Frankel RM, Smith RC. *Patient-Centered Interviewing*. 3rd ed. New York, NY: McGraw-Hill, 2012.
2. Bickley LS, Hoekelman RA, Bates B. *Bates' Guide to Physical Examination and History Taking.* 7th ed. Philadelphia, PA: Lippincott, 1999.
3. Morgan WL, Engel GL. *The Clinical Approach to the Patient.* New York, NY: WB Saunders, 1969.
4. Barrows HS, Pickell GC. *Developing Clinical Problem-Solving Skills: A Guide to More Effective Diagnosis and Treatment.* New York, NY: W.W. Norton, 1991.
5. Elstein AS. Psychological research on diagnostic reasoning. In: Lipkin M, Putnam SM, Lazare A, eds. *The Medical Interview.* New York, NY: Springer-Verlag, 1995:504–510.
6. Fiellin DA, Reid MC, O'Connor PG. Screening for alcohol problems in primary care: a systematic review. *Arch Intern Med.* 2000;160:1977–1989.
7. Ewing JA. Detecting alcoholism. The CAGE questionnaire. *JAMA.* 1984;252:1905–1907.
8. Clark W. Effective interviewing and intervention for alcohol problems. In: Lipkin M, Putnam SM, Lazare A, eds. *The Medical Interview.* New York, NY: Springer-Verlag, 1995:284–293.
9. Landrigan PJ, Barker DB. The recognition and control of occupational disease. *JAMA.* 1991;266:676–680.
10. Williams S. The sexual history. In: Lipkin M, Putnam SM, Lazare A, eds. *The Medical Interview.* New York, NY: Springer-Verlag, 1995:235–250.
11. MacCauley JG, Kern DE, Kolodner K, et al. The "battering syndrome": prevalence and clinical characteristics of domestic violence in primary care internal medicine practices. *Ann Intern Med.* 1995;123:737–746.
12. Puchalski C, Romer AL. Taking a spiritual history allows clinicians to understand patients more fully. *J Palliat Med.* 2000;3:129–137.

Suggested Reading

Engel GL. The need for a new medical model: a challenge for biomedicine. *Science.* 1977;196:129–136.

Fortin AH VI, Dwamena FC, Frankel RM, *Smith RC. Smith's Patient-Centered Interviewing: An Evidence-Based Method.* 3rd ed. New York, NY: McGraw-Hill, 2012.

Smith RC. Videotape of Evidence-Based Interviewing: (1) Patient-Centered Interviewing and (2) Doctor-Centered Interviewing. Marketing Division, Instructional Media Center, Michigan State University. P.O. Box 710, East Lansing, MI 48824.

Chapter 5

Evidence-Based Clinical Decision Making

Mark C. Wilson, MD, MPH, Mark C. Henderson, MD, and Gerald W. Smetana, MD

MANAGING UNCERTAINTY IN DIFFERENTIAL DIAGNOSIS

Clinical decision making is laced with uncertainty, and efficiently sorting out an underlying diagnosis as the cause of a patient's ailment can be difficult. Novice clinicians may attempt a stepwise assessment of all possible explanations for a patient's concerns until finally arriving at the diagnosis. More seasoned clinicians make use of extensive clinical experience, pattern recognition, and a range of approaches to save patients from the potential delays, risks, and costs of inefficient diagnostic strategies. The wisest clinicians seek out best evidence from clinical research and use it to complement their clinical experiences.[1] In this chapter, we introduce the concepts of differential diagnosis, pretest probabilities, and test performance characteristics to bolster our abilities to make diagnoses.

Patients come to us for help with their concerns. As clinicians, we seek out additional information about the chief complaint and synthesize key findings into a clinical problem. To accomplish this efficiently, we must be well versed in the typical manifestations of various diseases, the frequency of the potential underlying causes, and the value of specific historical features in arriving at the most likely diagnosis.[2–5] The purpose of this book is to provide this kind of information.

If a patient's complaint is headache, it helps to know which diseases cause headache, their principal clinical manifestations, and the relative frequency of each possibility ordered from the most common to the rarest. We generate further questioning based on how powerful or predictive certain findings are to either increase or decrease our suspicion for a specific diagnosis.

This process is known as differential diagnosis, in which a clinician uses prior knowledge alongside unique clinical findings from the patient, to prioritize the list of possibilities into a leading suspicion or working diagnosis, a few potentially active alternatives, and other possibilities that do not merit further consideration because they are not sufficiently likely or serious.[4,6,7] Rather than memorizing an exhaustive list, differential diagnosis is a dynamic process in which clinicians use certain information or test results to modify their suspicion for a given disorder until the diagnosis can be identified with confidence.

Key clinical findings commonly include epidemiologic factors such as age and gender. For instance, your suspicion of migraine as the cause of a recent-onset headache in a 25-year-old woman is much higher than for a 65-year-old man with the same symptom.[8] Experienced clinicians use each piece of additional epidemiologic and clinical information to continually narrow the diagnostic possibilities. Think of this process as moving through a funnel. Initial considerations are broad, but as the history progresses, a smaller number of plausible diagnoses remains.

Consider the use of specific questions during focused history taking as analogous to performing diagnostic tests. Each question should either increase or decrease the likelihood of the suspected underlying disorder. Returning to our headache example, the presence of nausea, photophobia, and throbbing pain each increase the chance that migraine is the underlying diagnosis. In contrast, a headache occurring bilaterally makes migraine less likely.[9,10]

KEY TERMS

Sensitivity	Of everyone with disease, the proportion who possess a clinical finding (or positive test). Also known as the true positive rate.
Specificity	Of everyone without disease, the proportion who do not possess a clinical finding (ie, the proportion of healthy people who test negative). Also known as the true negative rate.

—Continued next page

Continued—

Prevalence	The proportion of people with the disease in question in a given population.
Pretest probability	Prior to further testing, an estimate of how suspicious (from 0%–100%) a clinician is that a certain disorder is responsible for a patient's clinical problem.
Posttest probability	Revision of the pretest probability by incorporating the impact of a new clinical finding or test result.
Positive predictive value	Of everyone with a positive test or clinical finding, the proportion who actually have the disease.
Negative predictive value	Of everyone with a negative test or clinical finding, the proportion who do not have the disease.
Likelihood ratio	The ratio of the likelihood of a given test result or clinical finding in patients with disease to the likelihood of the same test result in patients without disease.

DEALING WITH PROBABILITIES AND ACTION THRESHOLDS

One of the most important lessons in clinical decision making is juggling uncertainty. Because the clinical information we gather—and most diagnostic testing we order—cannot determine the presence or absence of a disease with absolute certainty, we must become comfortable thinking and speaking about the *probability* of disease.

Probability can be expressed mathematically as a spectrum from 0 to 1, where 1 represents absolute certainty that a given disease exists, and 0 represents certainty that the disease does not exist. Often clinicians live in the "gray zone" between these 2 extremes. The best clinicians judiciously use the most efficient, effective questioning (and diagnostic testing) to help move their suspicion of a given condition closer to either end of this spectrum.

0 -- 1

Probability of disease

This probabilistic approach is particularly important when considering disorders for which no diagnostic "gold standard" (eg, confirmatory laboratory, pathologic, or imaging test) exists. In these cases, our diagnostic confidence is based almost entirely on the history and physical examination. Migraine is such a condition. Migraine is a clinical diagnosis, in which diagnostic testing is completely normal.

Accurately interpreting how each new piece of clinical information affects the probability of disease is the basis of clinical decision making. By thinking probabilistically, we can identify where we are on this spectrum in relation to 2 key clinical action thresholds.[2] We use our clinical examination skills to further refine our estimate of the probability of the disorder to above a *testing* threshold or, if even more certainty exists, above a *treatment* threshold (Figure 5–1).

ORDERING PRETEST PROBABILITIES

There may be multiple plausible diagnoses to explain our patient's concern. For common clinical problems such as headache, it is helpful to use evidence from systematic research to estimate the probability of a given condition *before* performing the clinical examination. Arriving at this level of "suspicion" is known as setting the pretest probability.

We could estimate pretest probabilities for the leading possibilities based on our personal experience with similar patients in the past. However, our memories are imperfect, and previous clinical experiences usually represent an incomplete sample of patients. Estimating pretest probabilities in this fashion is biased further by recent or particularly vivid experiences (eg, patients with a poor outcome). Recalling such experiences can cause clinicians to overestimate the probability of certain disorders.

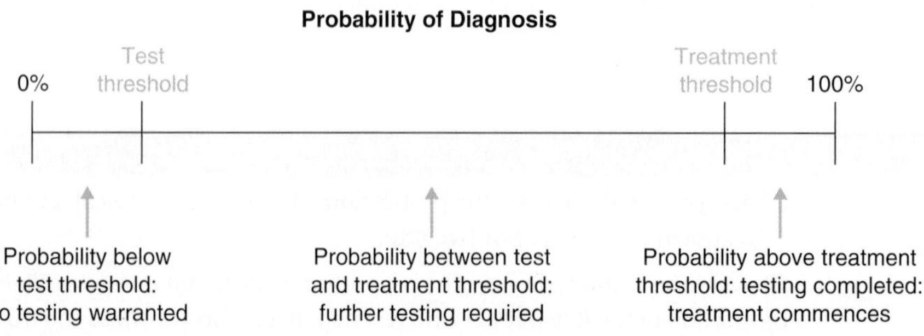

FIGURE 5–1 The two key action thresholds in probabilistic decision making. (Reproduced from: Guyatt G, Rennie D, Meade MO, Cook DJ. *Users' Guides to the Medical Literature: A Manual for Evidence-Based Clinical Practice*. 2nd ed. New York: McGraw-Hill; 2008. http:www.jamaevidence.com. Originally published in: JAMA. 1999;281(13):1214-1219. Copyright © 1999 American Medical Association. All rights reserved.)

Prevalence data from population-based studies can help us more rationally estimate a pretest probability of disease. More robust estimates come from clinical research that includes a well-defined patient population who all undergo standardized diagnostic evaluation to determine the eventual diagnosis.[4] Another source for pretest probabilities are clinical prediction rules, which quantify the contributions of historical and examination findings to predict an underlying diagnosis.

As clinicians, we must learn how to integrate these types of systematic research evidence into our clinical reasoning. Returning to our example, among 25-year-old women with headache, the prevalence or pretest probability of migraine is about 18%, whereas prevalence among 65-year-old men is 7%.[8] Thus the probability of migraine, based only on age and gender, is *already* 2.5 times greater in the young woman.

USING TEST PERFORMANCE CHARACTERISTICS[1,5]

The presence or absence of certain historical (or physical examination) findings may have been studied in patients with and without a disease. We can use test characteristics from these studies (sensitivity and specificity, predictive values, and likelihood ratios) to refine our initial probability estimates of disease.

The relationship between a clinical finding and the existence of a given disease process can be expressed in a simple 2 × 2 table.

	Disease present	Disease absent
Clinical finding present	True positives (TP)	False positives (FP)
Clinical finding absent	False negatives (FN)	True negatives (TN)

Using this format, there are 4 diagnostic possibilities or outcomes:

1. The clinical finding is present and the patient has the disease (true positive).
2. The clinical finding is present but the patient does not have the disease (false positive).
3. The clinical finding is absent but the patient has the disease (false negative).
4. The clinical finding is absent and the patient does not have the disease (true negative).

Sensitivity and Specificity

These terms are derived from the columns of the 2 × 2 table and express how the test performs in studies of patients with and without the disease of interest. **Sensitivity** refers to how frequently a clinical finding or test result is present in patients *known to have the disease*. Clinical findings with high sensitivity are useful for excluding diagnoses because as sensitivity increases, the number of false negatives (FN) decreases. With a very low number of FN, whenever a patient tests negative, they are much more likely to fall into the second column (ie, those without the disease). Going back to the 2 × 2 table:

Sensitivity = True Positives/(True Positives + False Negatives)

Specificity expresses the frequency of a negative finding or test result in patients *without the disease*. Clinical findings with a high specificity are useful for confirming diagnoses because as specificity increases, the number of false positives (FP) decreases. With a very low number of FP, a patient who tests positive is much more likely to have the diagnosis under consideration.

Specificity = True Negatives/(True Negatives + False Positives)

A large systematic review investigating historical features in patients with headaches found that the presence of nausea had a sensitivity of 81% and a specificity of 96% for detecting migraine.[9] The high specificity indicates that the presence of nausea should increase our suspicion that the underlying etiology of a patient's headache is migraine (ie, the finding of nausea is much more likely to represent a true positive [TP] than a FP).

Predictive Values

Unfortunately, clinicians do not have the luxury of already knowing who has disease and who does not (ie, the perspective of sensitivity and specificity). We must make inferences about the presence or absence of disease by knowing which tests have high specificity or sensitivity, respectively. We can also consider the 2 × 2 table from the perspective of a clinician who receives a positive or negative test result—that is, looking across the *rows*.

Positive predictive value (PPV) refers to how frequently a positive clinical finding or test result correctly identifies patients with disease (looking across the first row). Hence, PPV is the proportion of patients with disease (TP) out of all patients with a positive test (TP + FP).

Negative predictive value (NPV) refers to how frequently a negative clinical finding or test result correctly identifies patients without disease (looking across the second row). NPV is the proportion of patients without disease (true negative [TN]) out of all patients with a negative test (FN + TN).

Interpreting test results from the clinician's perspective is very appealing. However, it is reliable only if we have systematic evidence about PPV and NPV from patient populations similar to our own practice. Predictive values vary widely depending on the frequency or prevalence of disease in various populations.

PPV is inflated in populations with high disease prevalence; hence, a positive finding is more likely to be a TP (ie, occurring in patients *with* disease). Conversely, a positive test result in settings with lower disease prevalence is more likely to be a FP (than a TP) result; therefore, the resultant PPV plummets.

Likelihood Ratios

The **likelihood ratio (LR)** is a test performance characteristic that circumvents the vulnerabilities of predictive values. The LR also reflects the perspective of the clinician receiving a test result, but is *independent* of disease prevalence. LRs are "the doctor's friend" because they help us make sense out of test results we encounter in clinical practice.

The LR is merely a ratio of likelihoods ($LR = L_1/L_2$), comparing how likely a given test result is to occur in patients *with* disease relative to those *without* disease. Because we regard clinical findings as test results, we can calculate LRs using the following formula:

$$LR = \frac{\text{Likelihood of a clinical finding in patients } \textit{with} \text{ disease}}{\text{Likelihood of the same clinical finding in patients } \textit{without} \text{ disease}}$$

When LRs are greater than 1, the numerator is larger, meaning the test result occurs more frequently in patients with disease than in those without disease (thus *increasing* the probability of disease). When LRs are less than 1, the denominator is larger, meaning the test result occurs more frequently in patients without disease (thus *decreasing* the probability of disease). An LR near 1 has no diagnostic utility, because the test result is equally likely to occur in diseased and nondiseased individuals.

When considering dichotomous outcomes from a 2 × 2 table, we refer to a LR for a positive clinical finding or test result (LR+) and a LR for a negative test (LR–). LRs can easily be calculated from the classic test performance characteristics of sensitivity and specificity:

LR+ = Sensitivity/(1 – Specificity)
LR– = (1 – Sensitivity)/Specificity

Regarding our 2 patients with headache, the clinical finding of nausea had a sensitivity of 81% and a specificity of 96%. Therefore, the associated LRs are:

LR+ = Sensitivity/(1 – Specificity) = 0.81/(1 – 0.96) = 20.2
LR– = (1 – Sensitivity)/Specificity = (1 – 0.81)/0.96 = 0.20

So nausea (LR+) is 20 times more likely to occur in patients with migraine than in patients with other causes of headache. The absence of nausea (LR–) is 0.2 times as likely

Table 5–1. Impact of various likelihood ratios on the posttest probability of disease.

Likelihood Ratio	Effect on Posttest Probability of Disease
10	Large
5	Moderate
2	Slight
1	None
0.5	Slight
0.2	Moderate
0.1	Large

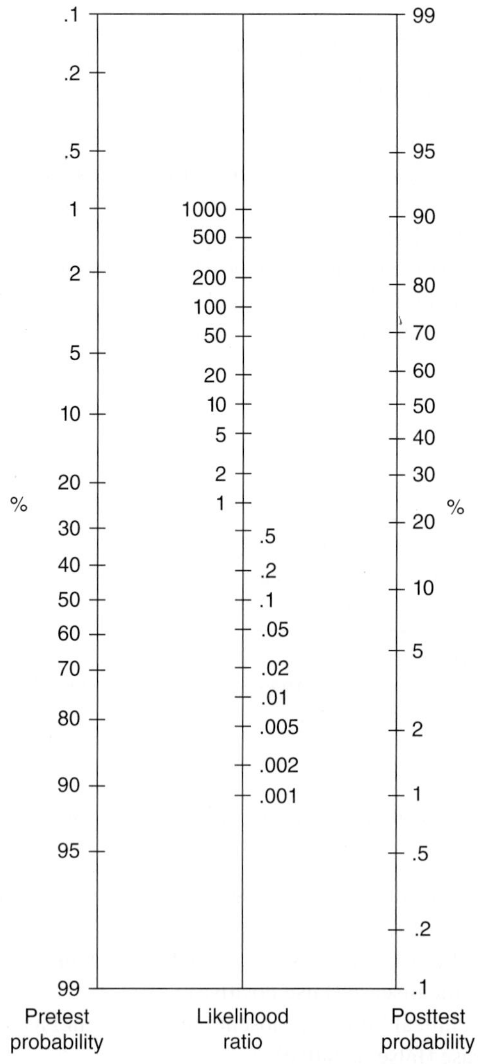

FIGURE 5.2 Nomogram for determining posttest probability from pretest probability and likelihood ratios. To figure the posttest probability, place a straightedge between the pretest probability and the likelihood ratio for the particular test. The posttest probability will be where the straightedge crosses the posttest probability line. (Reproduced from Fagan TJ. Nomogram for Bayes's theorem. *N Engl J Med.* 1975;293(5):257. Copyright Massachusetts Medical Society.)

to occur in patients with migraine as compared to other causes of headaches, or the absence of nausea is 1/0.2 or 5 times more likely to occur in patients with other causes of headache (not migraine).

CONSIDERING POSTTEST PROBABILITIES

LRs help us convert the pretest probability of disease into a posttest probability. As LRs get larger or smaller, they have greater impact on posttest probability (Table 5–1).

Beyond this qualitative understanding of LRs, the quickest way to use LRs to quantify a posttest probability is to use a nomogram (Figure 5–2).[11]

For a 25-year-old woman with headache, the prevalence or pretest probability of migraine is 18%. When we direct a straightedge from this anchoring pretest probability through the LR for a new clinical finding, we arrive at the posttest probability that she suffers from migraines. Because nausea is a powerful clinical finding (LR+ = 20), our posttest probability moves to 80%, which is high enough to make a presumptive diagnosis of migraine and to begin appropriate treatment. Similarly, nausea increases suspicion of migraine in our 65-year-old man from 7% (pretest) to almost 60% (posttest). While this clinical finding significantly increases the posttest probability of migraine, we still have significant uncertainty and will likely need to seek other clinical findings before arriving at a diagnosis.

This example illustrates explicitly how a clinician's diagnostic and therapeutic decision making is influenced by key clinical findings. Developing expertise in clinical reasoning skills, while challenging, underlies how savvy clinicians make wise diagnostic and management decisions for their patients.[12–14]

CAVEATS

- Differential diagnosis is a dynamic process in which clinicians actively adjust their consideration of plausible diagnoses by weighing the impact of new clinical findings and laboratory tests.
- When investigating a clinical problem, clinicians inform their pretest probabilities by using clinical experience *and* the best evidence about disease prevalence.
- Arriving at a working diagnosis necessitates that we understand—and can use—the test performance characteristics of key clinical findings and test results.
- LRs are "the doctor's friend"; they help clinicians interpret a test result by converting the pretest probability of disease into a new posttest probability.
- Clinicians should seek out clinical findings with the greatest ability to move the posttest probability toward the important clinical action thresholds of either testing further or initiating treatment.

Test Your Knowledge

1. The sensitivity of nausea in patients with migraine headaches is 81%.

   What is the best interpretation of this information?

   A. Nausea occurs 19% of the time in patients without migraine headaches.
   B. The false-negative rate for nausea as a "test" for migraine headaches is 19%.
   C. Nausea occurs in 81% of patients with headaches.
   D. Of all headache patients with nausea, 81% have migraines.
   E. The presence of nausea reliably diagnoses migraine.

2. You are investigating whether an elderly patient with anemia has iron deficiency. The serum ferritin level returns at 30, and the likelihood ratio for that result in iron deficiency is 3.0.

   What is the best interpretation of this result?

   A. Three percent of the general population has iron deficiency anemia.
   B. It is unlikely that your patient has iron deficiency anemia.
   C. A ferritin level of 30 is 3 times more likely to occur in patients with iron deficiency than is a ferritin result greater than 30.
   D. A ferritin level of 30 is 3 times more likely to occur in patients with iron deficiency than in patients with other causes of anemia.

3. Likelihood ratios (LRs) can be described as "the doctor's friend" because:

   A. LRs help clinicians interpret the meaning of test results.
   B. Doctors order lots of tests.
   C. LRs can reliably rule in or rule out disease.
   D. LRs are independent of sensitivity and specificity.

References

1. Straus SE, Richardson WS, Glasziou P, Haynes RB. *Evidence Based Medicine. How to Practice and Teach EBM.* 3rd ed. London: Churchill Livingstone, 2005.
2. Richardson WS, Wilson MC. Chapter 14. The process of diagnosis. In: Guyatt G, Rennie D, Meade MO, Cook DJ, eds. *Users' Guides to the Medical Literature: A Manual for Evidence-Based Clinical Practice.* 2nd ed, New York, NY: McGraw-Hill, 2008.
3. Richardson WS, Wilson MC, Moyer V, Guyatt GH, for the Evidence-Based Medicine Working Group. User's guides to the medical literature XXIV: how to use an article about clinical manifestations of disease. *JAMA.* 2000;284:869–875.
4. Richardson WS, Wilson MC, McGinn TG. Chapter 15. Differential diagnosis. In: Guyatt G, Rennie D, Meade MO, Cook DJ, eds. *Users' Guides to the Medical Literature: A Manual for Evidence-Based Clinical Practice.* 2nd ed. New York, NY: McGraw-Hill, 2008.
5. Furukawa TA, Strauss SE, Bucher HC, Guyatt GH. Chapter 16. Diagnostic tests. In: Guyatt G, Rennie D, Meade MO, Cook DJ, eds. *Users' Guides to the Medical Literature: A Manual for Evidence-Based Clinical Practice.* 2nd ed. New York, NY: McGraw-Hill, 2008.
6. Sox HC, Blatt MA, Higgins MC, Marton KI. *Medical Decision Making.* 2nd ed. Philadelphia, PA: American College of Physicians, 2007.
7. Sackett DL, Haynes RB, Guyatt GH, Tugwell P. *Clinical Epidemiology: A Basic Science for Clinical Medicine.* 2nd ed. Boston: Little, Brown, 1991.
8. Rasmussen BK, Jensen R, Schroll M, Olesen J. Epidemiology of headache in a general population—a prevalence study. *J Clin Epidemiol.* 1991;44:1147–1157.
9. Smetana GW. The diagnostic value of historical features in primary headache syndromes: a comprehensive review. *Arch Intern Med.* 2000;160:2729–2737.
10. Simel DL. Make the diagnosis: does this patient with headaches have a migraine or need neuroimaging? In: Simel DL, Rennie D, eds. *The Rational Clinical Examination: Evidence-Based Clinical Diagnosis.* New York, NY: McGraw-Hill, 2010.
11. Sackett DL. Original article: a primer on the precision and accuracy of the clinical examination. In: Simel DL, Rennie D, eds. *The Rational Clinical Examination: Evidence-Based Clinical Diagnosis.* New York, NY: McGraw-Hill, 2010.
12. Bowen JL. Educational strategies to promote clinical diagnostic reasoning. *N Engl J Med.* 2006;355:2217–2225.
13. Norman G. Building on experience: the development of clinical reasoning. *N Engl J Med.* 2006;355:2251–2252.
14. Kassirer JP. Teaching clinical reasoning: case-based and coached. *Acad Med.* 2010; 85:1118–1124.

SECTION

II

GENERAL SYMPTOMS

Chapter 6

Dizziness

Michelle V. Conde, MD, Emily Wang, MD, and Mark C. Henderson, MD

CASE SCENARIO

A 61-year-old woman comes to your office for intermittent dizziness for the past 2 weeks. At times, she misses work due to the dizziness. When she awakens in the morning, she states, "The entire room spins." Nausea accompanies the dizziness. The episodes last less than a minute.

- **What other components of the history are important to ask?**
- **How would you classify the patient's dizziness?**
- **What alarm symptoms should you ask about to determine the severity of the diagnosis?**

INTRODUCTION

Dizziness is classically categorized into 4 subtypes: vertigo, presyncope or syncope, dysequilibrium, and light-headedness (undifferentiated dizziness).[1] However, it may be difficult to identify a single category in every patient, particularly in the elderly, who often manifest more than 1 subtype. Medications may also cause more than 1 subtype of dizziness.

KEY TERMS

Dysequilibrium	Impaired walking due to difficulties with balance. It is sometimes described as dizziness "in the feet." Formally speaking, dysequilibrium does not occur in the nonambulatory patient.
Light-headedness	Dizziness that is not vertigo, syncope, or dysequilibrium; this form is also called **undifferentiated dizziness.**
Presyncope	The feeling that one is about to faint or lose consciousness, but actual loss of consciousness is averted. **Syncope** is defined as sudden, transient loss of consciousness (see Chapter 29).
Vertigo	An illusion or hallucination of movement, usually rotation, either of oneself or the environment.[2]
Benign paroxysmal positional vertigo (BPPV)	BPPV is a common peripheral vestibular disorder that is usually caused by migration of inner ear otoliths (calcific particles) to the posterior semicircular canal. The otoliths amplify any movement in the plane of the canal, resulting in brief episodes of vertigo following changes in head position.
Ménière's disease	A peripheral cause of vertigo characterized by the triad of fluctuating hearing loss, tinnitus, and episodic vertigo. Aural fullness or pressure is often present. Excess endolymph results in increased pressure within the semicircular canals.[2]
Vestibular neuronitis	A peripheral acute vestibular syndrome that typically lasts for a day or longer and is often accompanied by nausea, emesis, and unsteadiness.[2] Some episodes are associated with a preceding infectious illness. **Labyrinthitis** has a similar presentation but also includes hearing loss.[3]

—Continued next page

Continued—	
Vertebrobasilar insufficiency (VBI)	Reduced blood flow to the brainstem that can manifest as the following: vertigo, cranial nerve dysfunction (eg, diplopia, hoarseness, dysarthria, dysphagia), or cerebellar dysfunction (eg, ataxia). Sensory and motor impairment may also occur. VBI (from artery-to-artery embolization, low flow, or vertebral artery dissection) may result in transient ischemic attack (TIA) or stroke.

ETIOLOGY

The etiology of dizziness depends on the clinical setting. A systematic review including over 4500 patients from 12 clinical settings (primary care offices, n = 2; specialty clinics, n = 6; and emergency departments, n = 4) showed that dizziness was due to peripheral vestibular or psychiatric causes in roughly 60% of cases.[4] The cause was unknown in approximately 1 in 7 patients. In contrast, in a study of patients with acute dizziness in an emergency department setting, a significantly higher percentage of cases of dizziness were due to a cardiovascular or other medical cause.[5] In this emergency department study, general medical diagnoses comprised roughly 50% of dizziness etiologies. Otovestibular and psychiatric diagnoses were 32.9% and 7.2%, respectively.

Differential Diagnosis

Predominantly Outpatient Setting	**Frequency[a,4]**
Peripheral vestibulopathy	***44%***
BPPV	16%
Vestibular neuronitis/labyrinthitis	9%
Ménière's disease	5%
Other (including medication-related, recurrent vestibulopathy)	14%
Central vestibulopathy	10%
Cerebrovascular	***6%***
Tumor	< 1%
Other (including multiple sclerosis, migraine headache)	3%
Nonvestibular, nonpsychiatric	***24%***
Presyncope (including volume depletion, cardiac arrhythmia, or other cardiovascular etiology)	6%
Dysequilibrium	5%
Other (including anemia, metabolic causes, parkinsonism, medication-related)	13%
Psychiatric	***16%***
Psychiatric disorder	11%
Hyperventilation	5%
Unknown	***13%***

[a]Data from a review of 12 studies that included primary care offices (n = 2), specialty clinics (n = 6), and emergency departments (n = 4). Total percentage is greater than 100% because dizziness is attributed to more than 1 cause in some patients.

Emergency Department	Frequency[5]
Otologic/vestibular	32.9%
Cardiovascular	21.1%
Respiratory	11.5%
Neurologic	11.2% (4% cerebrovascular)
Metabolic	11%
Injury/poisoning	10.6%
Psychiatric	7.2%
Genitourinary	5.1%
Infectious	2.9%

GETTING STARTED WITH THE HISTORY

- Review medication list before seeing the patient and validate during the interview.
- Avoid leading questions. It may be necessary to follow up with a few closed-ended questions directed at the most likely disorder.

Open-Ended Questions	Tips for Effective Interviewing
Tell me about your symptoms. Describe the sensation you've been having without using the word dizzy.	Let patients use their own words.
Go over the last time you had this sensation, from start to finish.	Avoid interrupting.
Let's review all your medications, including over-the-counter medications, nutritional supplements, or herbal medicines.	Listen to the patient's description for diagnostic clues.

INTERVIEW FRAMEWORK

- Assess for alarm symptoms.
- Review medication list.
- Categorize into 1 or more dizziness subtypes: vertigo, presyncope/syncope, dysequilibrium, or light-headedness (undifferentiated dizziness).
- In determining the etiology of each subtype, consider temporal pattern and duration of symptoms, accompanying symptoms, precipitating factors, atherosclerotic risk factors, and comorbidities.
- Be aware that patients may not be able to reliably and reproducibly describe quality of dizziness, especially in the emergency department setting. Timing, duration, associated symptoms, and triggers are more reliably reported than quality.[6]

IDENTIFYING ALARM SYMPTOMS

Serious causes of dizziness are uncommon. However, most studies have oversampled persons with chronic dizziness and underrepresented persons with acute forms of dizziness who may be more likely to have life-threatening illnesses.[7] So these data may underestimate the prevalence of serious disorders in patients with acute dizziness.

Identification of these serious disorders requires detailed questioning aimed at eliciting cardinal symptoms of heart disease, neighborhood neurologic symptoms, and associated risk factors. **Any** focal neurologic symptoms should prompt immediate brain imaging to rule out serious central nervous system causes of vertigo, such as VBI. Other serious diagnoses, such as anemia, hypoglycemia, and carbon monoxide poisoning, are suggested by selected laboratory tests.

Selected Serious Diagnoses	Frequency[a,4]
Cerebrovascular disease (stroke, TIA)	6%
Cardiac arrhythmia	1.5%
Brain tumor	< 1%

[a]Derived from frequencies of specific causes of dizziness across 12 studies in a predominantly outpatient setting.

Alarm Symptoms	Serious Causes	Benign Causes
Chest discomfort or presyncope/ syncope	See Chapter 27 on chest pain and Chapter 29 on syncope.	
Acute-onset vertigo plus neurologic deficits (eg, diplopia, hemiparesis, dysarthria)	VBI Brainstem mass Meningoencephalitis Cranial polyneuritis Vasculitis (involving the eighth nerve) Multiple sclerosis or other demyelinating diseases Partial seizure	Basilar artery migraine
Acute-onset vertigo plus neck or occipital pain plus neurologic deficits	VBI (such as from vertebral artery dissection)	
Acute vertigo (lasting > 1 day), nausea, vomiting, severe imbalance	Cerebellar stroke/mass (patient usually unable to walk without falling)	Acute vestibular neuronitis/labyrinthitis (patient tilts to one side but is still able to walk)
Sudden-onset severe vertigo, facial paralysis, otalgia, external ear vesicular eruption, hearing loss	Ramsay Hunt syndrome (herpes zoster oticus)	
History of diabetes mellitus (insulin and/or oral hypoglycemic use)	Hypoglycemia	

Selected Clinical Situations in Patients Presenting With Dizziness	Positive Likelihood Ratio of Detecting Cause	Consider...
No vertigo, neurologic deficit present, or age > 69 years	1.5[8,9] (serious cause)	Serious causes, including seizures, stroke, cardiac arrhythmia, endocrine, medication adverse effects. If neurologic deficit is present, **always** consider serious cause.
Vertigo present, no neurologic deficit, and age ≤ 69 years	0.3[8,9] (serious cause)	Nonurgent causes, including peripheral vestibular disorder; less likely central causes
Matutinal vertigo (vertigo upon arising in the morning)	1.6[9,10] (peripheral cause)	Peripheral vestibular disorders, **but** presence does not confidently rule out central causes of vertigo

FOCUSED QUESTIONS

After having the patient tell his or her own story, follow up with a few closed-ended questions directed at the most likely subtype.

QUESTIONS	THINK ABOUT...
When you have these spells, do you see the world spin around you, as if you had just gotten off a merry-go-round?	Vertigo (if answer is "spin")[2]
Do you feel these spells in your head or in your legs? Do you have trouble with your balance?	Dysequilibrium (if answer is "in the legs")
Have you ever passed out?	Syncope, seizure
Have you ever felt you might pass out but did not (like the feeling you get when you stand up too quickly)?	Presyncope
Patient responses are vague; nonspecific descriptions that do not fit into above categories (eg, "I'm just dizzy")	Light-headedness or undifferentiated dizziness

APPROACH TO DIFFERENTIAL DIAGNOSIS FOR THE 4 TYPES OF DIZZINESS

Vertigo

Once vertigo is identified, knowing the temporal pattern and duration may help narrow the differential diagnosis. Further characterize the vertigo by assessing its quality, time course, associated symptoms, and modifying symptoms.

QUESTIONS	THINK ABOUT...
Quality	
Is the vertigo mild?	Central causes (vertigo less intense in central causes versus peripheral causes)
Is the vertigo intense? Does it confine you to bed or make you stop what you are doing?	Ménière's disease Vestibular neuronitis/labyrinthitis BPPV Recurrent vestibulopathy
Time course	
Was the onset abrupt?	VBI BPPV Ménière's disease Perilymphatic fistula (versus gradual onset, as in acoustic neuroma)
Did the symptoms begin over a few hours and then peak after 1 day?	Vestibular neuronitis
Do the symptoms recur?	BPPV (episodes last seconds) Ménière's disease Recurrent vestibulopathy VBI (assess for other neurologic symptoms)

—Continued next page

Continued—

Does the vertigo occur more commonly in the morning? (matutinal vertigo)	Peripheral causes (eg, vestibular neuronitis or labyrinthitis)
Associated symptoms	
Do you have nausea, vomiting, or sweating?	Usually peripheral disorders (eg, Ménière's disease vestibular neuronitis/labyrinthitis, or recurrent vestibulopathy); occasionally VBI
Do you have discharge from ear?	Suppurative otitis media
Do you have double vision, weakness, or numbness on 1 side of the body?	VBI Brainstem mass Basilar artery migraine Partial seizure
Do you have headache?	Basilar artery migraine Cerebellar mass
Is there ringing in your ear?	Ménière's disease Acoustic neuroma Drug toxicity (eg, aminoglycoside antibiotics, salicylates, and loop diuretics)
Ear fullness or stuffiness before the vertigo?	Ménière's disease Other ear disorders
Do you have hearing loss?	Ménière's disease (episodic vertigo) Other ear disorders (eg, otitis media, otosclerosis) Acoustic neuroma Drug toxicity Labyrinthitis (persistent vertigo) Labyrinthine concussion (basilar skull fracture traversing inner ear) Labyrinthine infarction (with associated neurologic signs) Perilymphatic fistula Stroke (complete ipsilateral deafness)
Have you had a preceding viral illness?	Vestibular neuronitis or labyrinthitis
Do you have severe imbalance?	Cerebellar stroke/mass
Is there bleeding from your ear canal?	Temporal bone fracture
Modifying symptoms	
Does rolling over in bed make your symptoms worse? Or bending over and straightening up or extending your neck to look up?	BPPV
Does coughing, sneezing, or straining worsen your symptoms?	Perilymphatic fistula (disruption of membranes separating the middle and inner ear with resultant perilymph leakage into middle ear, usually following barotrauma or ear surgery)

Presyncope/Syncope

In a dizzy patient who has lost consciousness, syncope must be distinguished from seizure. See Chapter 29 for the diagnostic approach to presyncope/syncope.

Dysequilibrium

Visual impairment, hearing loss, peripheral neuropathy, and musculoskeletal abnormalities all contribute to the **syndrome of multiple sensory deficits,** which is a common geriatric syndrome. Ask specific questions to further delineate any sensory and/or motor impairment.

QUESTIONS	THINK ABOUT...
Are you having any trouble seeing?	Visual impairment (eg, cataract)
Are you having any trouble hearing?	Conductive hearing loss (eg, impacted cerumen, otitis media, otosclerosis) and/or sensorineural hearing loss (eg, presbycusis, the degenerative hearing loss of aging)
Are you having any tingling or numbness in your legs or feet?	Disorders of nerve roots, plexi, or peripheral nerves
Do you feel weak in your legs or have incoordination in your legs?	Musculoskeletal abnormalities (eg, cervical spondylosis, osteoarthritis, cervicogenic dizziness accompanied by headache), cerebellar dysfunction, spinal stenosis, spinal cord disorders, movement disorders (eg, Parkinson's disease)

Common disorders that may cause dysequilibrium include the following:

- Diabetic peripheral neuropathy
- Parkinson's disease
- Alcoholic cerebellar degeneration
- Vitamin B_{12} deficiency
- Sequelae of vertebrobasilar stroke
- Bilateral vestibular hypofunction (alcohol, aminoglycoside toxicity; aminoglycoside toxicity may be accompanied by oscillopsia, which is the sensation that the eyes bounce up and down)

Light-headedness (Undifferentiated Dizziness)

Frequently, underlying psychological disorders are associated with this subtype of dizziness, which is difficult for patients to describe. In addition, prescription drug toxicity and substance abuse are associated with this subtype.

Four clinical cues (S4 model) predict a subgroup of ambulatory patients likely to have underlying depressive and anxiety disorders.[11] The presence of 2 or more of these clinical cues signals the need for a more detailed psychological evaluation.

S4 Model (Cues: Symptom Count, Stress, Severity, Self-Rated Health)[11]

Ask	Cue	Positive Likelihood Ratio
Tell me what symptoms you've been experiencing.	Symptom count (positive response if ≥ 6 symptoms)	
During the past week have you been under stress?	Stress	1.9 (2 cues present)
Describe how bad your symptom is, from 10 (unbearable) to 0 (none at all).	Severity (positive response if ≥ 6)	5.4 (3 cues present)

—*Continued next page*

Continued—

In general, would you say your health is excellent, very good, good, fair, or poor?	Self-rated health (positive response for "fair" or "poor" responses)	36.3 (ALL 4 cues present)

DIAGNOSTIC APPROACH (INCLUDING ALGORITHMS)

Keep in mind that the causes of dizziness may overlap the different subtypes. Some patients cannot describe their symptoms in a way that fits neatly into the 4 subtypes. Half of elderly patients describe 2 or more dizziness subtypes.[7] Psychiatric causes often coexist with other causes of dizziness.[12] Dysequilibrium may follow disorders that produce vertigo. Vestibular neuronitis or labyrinthitis initially presents with vertigo but may subsequently cause unsteadiness in the legs (dysequilibrium) lasting for several weeks or months. Likewise, vertebrobasilar stroke can present with vertigo followed by dysequilibrium because some patients (particularly the elderly) may also have reduced compensatory multisensory and circulatory systems.

See the algorithms (Figures 6–1 and 6–2) for evaluating patients with dizziness and assessing those with vertigo.

CAVEATS

- A single etiology may result in more than 1 subtype of dizziness.
- Positional vertigo may be confused with postural hypotension. Both can occur on arising; however, positional vertigo occurs with a change in position that does *not* result in global cerebral hypoperfusion. For example, positional vertigo (but not postural hypotension) may occur with rolling over in bed or bending forward to put on socks or tie shoes.
- Although uncommon, cerebellar stroke may present only with vertigo and ataxia and thus be mistaken for vestibular neuronitis.[13] The ataxia is severe, and most patients are unable to walk without support. Acute onset and atherosclerotic risk factors should heighten clinical suspicion.

PROGNOSIS

In a community-based study, 3% of patients with persistent dizziness were severely incapacitated by their symptoms.[14] History of fainting, vertigo, or avoidance of situations that provoke dizziness predicted chronic, handicapping dizziness.

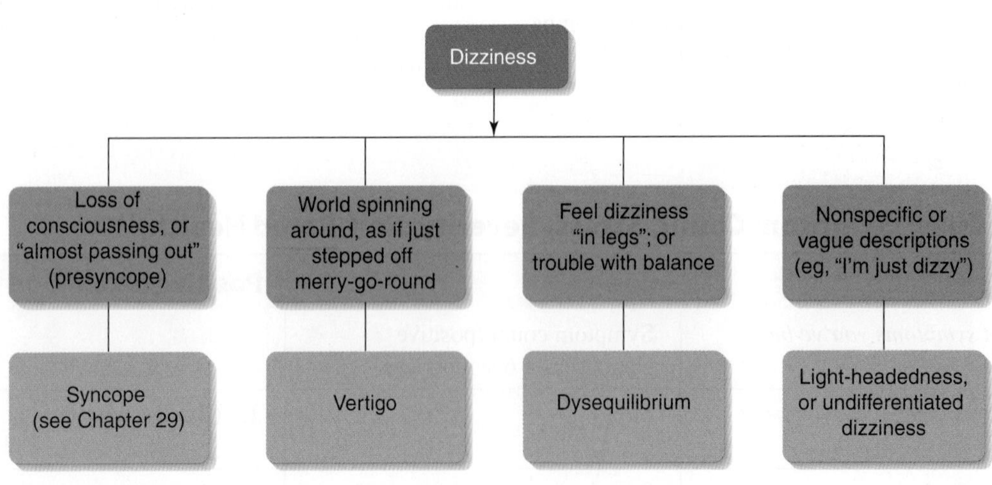

FIGURE 6–1 Diagnostic approach: Dizziness.

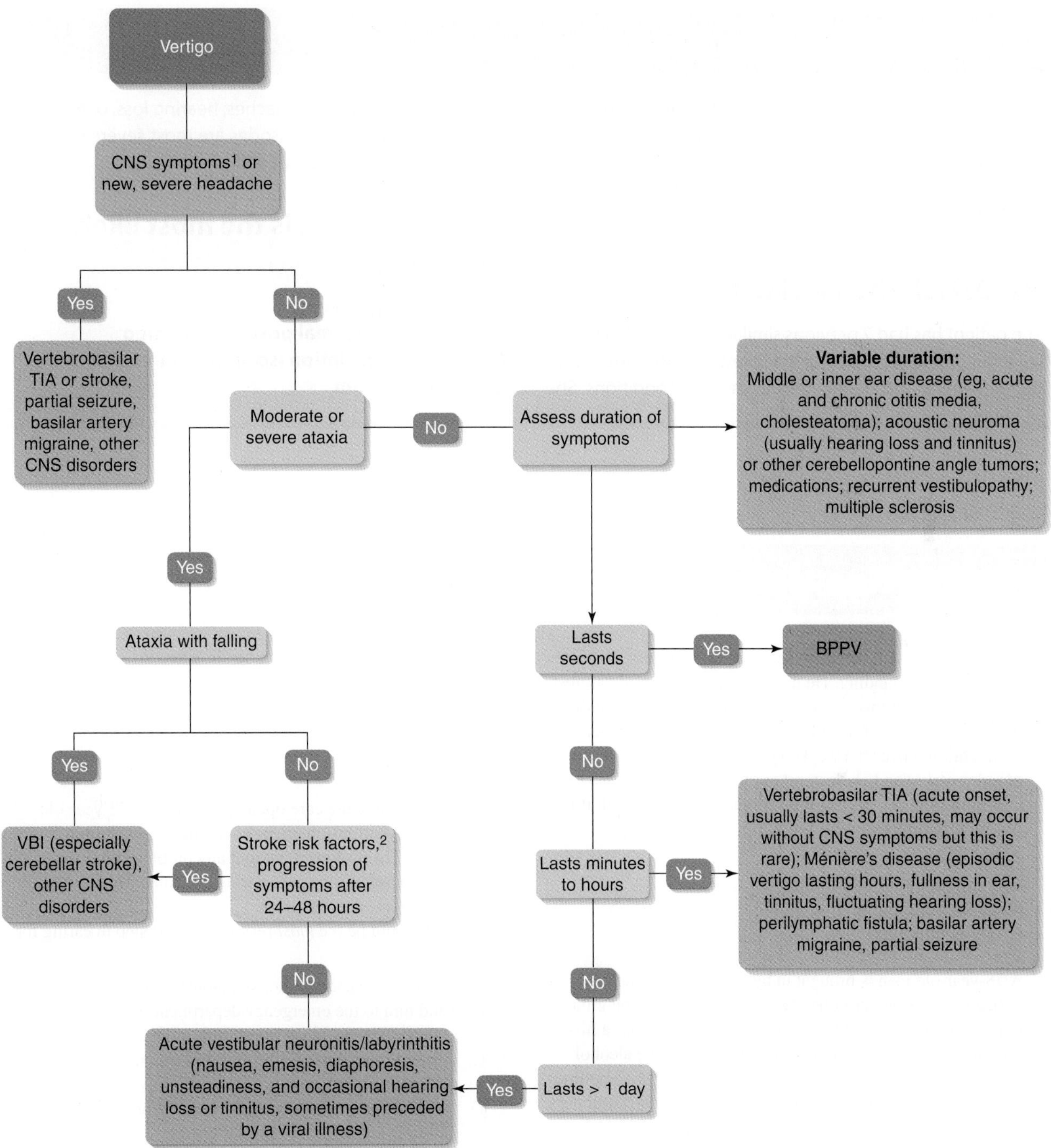

FIGURE 6–2 Diagnostic approach: Vertigo. BPPV, benign paroxysmal positional vertigo; CNS, central nervous system; TIA, transient ischemic attack; VBI, vertebrobasilar insufficiency. [1]CNS symptoms: Focal sensory or motor deficits; brainstem findings, eg, dysarthria, diplopia, dysphagia, hoarseness. [2]Stroke risk factors: Advanced age, smoking, dyslipidemia, family history, diabetes mellitus, hypertension, atrial fibrillation, coronary artery disease, congestive heart failure, peripheral vascular disease.

CASE SCENARIO | Resolution

A 61-year-old woman comes to your office for intermittent dizziness for the past 2 weeks. At times, she misses work due to the dizziness. When she awakens in the morning, she states, "The entire room spins." Nausea accompanies the dizziness. The episodes last less than a minute.

ADDITIONAL HISTORY

The patient has had 2 previous similar episodes of dizziness over the past year that resolved spontaneously. She is otherwise healthy and has no chronic medical conditions. She reports no associated headaches, hearing loss, or focal neurologic symptoms. The episodes are most severe when she rolls over in bed or gets out of bed.

Question: What is the most likely diagnosis?

A. Postural hypotension
B. Benign paroxysmal positional vertigo
C. Posterior circulation ischemic infarct
D. Dysequilibrium

Test Your Knowledge

1. A 65-year-old man comes to see you for dizziness. He states it occurs upon standing. He describes the feeling of "almost passing out," but this is averted by seating himself. He did have diarrhea for a few days after taking care of his sick grandchildren over the weekend. He continues to take his blood pressure and cholesterol medications.

   Which category of dizziness is most consistent with this patient's symptoms?

   A. Vertigo
   B. Presyncope
   C. Light-headedness
   D. Dysequilibrium

2. A 78-year-old man is brought in by his daughter who has noticed bruises on her father. He is falling and bumping into objects around him. He is well-known to you and has a history of long-standing diabetes mellitus and remote alcohol abuse. When queried, he states, "I get a little dizzy sometimes and slip." He has problems with his vision and also numbness and tingling in his feet. He is hard of hearing.

   This form of dizziness can be classified as:

   A. Vertigo
   B. Presyncope
   C. Light-headedness
   D. Dysequilibrium

3. In one of your acute care openings, you see a 72-year-old man with hypertension, diabetes mellitus, and chronic tobacco use. He awakened without any problems but developed the acute onset of dizziness during breakfast. He can barely walk. He notes double vision.

   What would be the *most* reasonable next step in caring for this patient?

   A. Return home and monitor symptoms of vestibular neuronitis
   B. Send him to the emergency department for urgent evaluation of acute vertebrobasilar infarct
   C. Perform maneuvers in the office to realign inner ear otoliths for BPPV
   D. Hold all blood pressure medications to prevent syncope

References

1. Drachman DA, Hart CW. An approach to the dizzy patient. *Neurology.* 1972;22:323–334.
2. Hanley K, O'Dowd T, Considine N. A systematic review of vertigo in primary care. *Br J Gen Pract.* 2001;51:666–671.
3. Kentala E, Rauch SD. A practical assessment algorithm for diagnosis of dizziness. *Otolaryngol Head Neck Surg.* 2003;128:54–59.
4. Kroenke K, Hoffman RM, Einstadter D. How common are various causes of dizziness? A critical review. *South Med J.* 2000;93:160–167.
5. Newman-Toker DE, Hsieh YH, Camargo CA, Pelletier AJ, Butchy GT, Edlow JA. Spectrum of dizziness visits to US emergency departments: cross-sectional analysis from a nationally representative sample. *Mayo Clinic Proc.* 2008;83:765–775.

6. Newman-Toker DE, Cannon LM, Stofferahn ME, et al. Imprecision in patient reports of dizziness symptom quality: a cross-sectional study conducted in an acute care setting. *Mayo Clin Proc.* 2007;82:1329–1340.
7. Sloane PD, Coeytaux RR, Beck RS, Dallara J. Dizziness: state of the science. *Ann Intern Med.* 2001;134:823–832.
8. Herr RD, Zun L, Mathews JJ. A directed approach to the dizzy patient. *Ann Emerg Med.* 1989;18:664–672.
9. Froehling DA, Silverstein MD, Mohr DN, Beatty CW. Original article: does this dizzy patient have a serious form of vertigo? In: Simel DL, Rennie D, eds. *The Rational Clinical Examination: Evidence-Based Clinical Diagnosis.* New York, NY: McGraw-Hill, 2009.
10. Berkowitz BW. Matutinal vertigo: clinical characteristics and possible management. *Arch Neurol.* 1985;42:874–877.
11. Kroenke K, Jackson JL, Chamberlin J. Depressive and anxiety disorders in patients presenting with physical complaints: clinical predictors and outcome. *Am J Med.* 1997;103:339–347.
12. Clark MR, Sullivan MD, Fischl M, et al. Symptoms as a clue to otologic and psychiatric diagnosis in patients with dizziness. *J Psychosom Res.* 1994;38:461–470.
13. Lee H, Sohn S-I, Cho Y-W, et al. Cerebellar infarction presenting with isolated vertigo. Frequency and vascular topographical patterns. *Neurology.* 2006;67:1178–1183.
14. Nazareth I, Yardley L, Owen N, Luxon L. Outcome of symptoms of dizziness in a general practice community sample. *Fam Pract.* 1999;16:616–618.

Suggested Reading

Baloh RW. Vestibular neuritis. *N Engl J Med.* 2003;348:1027–1032.

Froehling DA, Silverstein MD, Mohr DN, Beatty CW. Original article: does this dizzy patient have a serious form of vertigo? In: Simel DL, Rennie D, eds. *The Rational Clinical Examination: Evidence-Based Clinical Diagnosis*. New York, NY: McGraw-Hill, 2009.

Hanley K, O'Dowd T, Considine N. A systematic review of vertigo in primary care. *Br J Gen Pract.* 2001;51:666–671.

Hoffman RM, Einstadter D, Kroenke K. Evaluating dizziness. *Am J Med.* 1999;107:468–478.

Chapter 7

Fatigue

Richard J. Simons, MD, and Nicole A. Swallow, MD

CASE SCENARIO

A 45-year-old woman presents to your clinic after suffering from "months" of feeling bad. She feels tired all the time and is finding it difficult to keep up daily activities. Her tiredness is interfering with her ability to play an active role in the lives of her husband and 2 children. She has no significant past medical history and has not seen a physician in several years.

- **What additional information about her "tiredness" do you need?**
- **How would you classify her fatigue?**
- **What alarm symptoms would you look for in this patient?**
- **Would laboratory testing help you to make a diagnosis?**

INTRODUCTION

Fatigue is one of the most common symptoms encountered in primary care settings. Twenty-four percent to 32% of adult patients report significant fatigue during visits to their primary care physicians.[1,2] Fatigue is a sensation that everyone experiences from time to time; however, it is the *persistence* of fatigue that is considered abnormal. Common descriptors from patients with fatigue include a lack of energy to complete tasks, exhaustion, and tiredness. Fatigue often signifies underlying medical or psychiatric disease.

KEY TERMS

Chronic fatigue — Generally implies fatigue persisting for 6 months.

Chronic fatigue syndrome (CFS) — Unexplained, persistent, or relapsing fatigue that is of new or definite onset; is not the result of ongoing exertion; is not alleviated by rest; and results in substantial reduction in previous levels of occupational, educational, social, or personal activities ***and*** 4 or more of the following symptoms that persist or recur during 6 or more consecutive months of illness and that do not predate the fatigue:

1. Self-reported impairment in short-term memory or concentration
2. Sore throat
3. Tender cervical or axillary nodes
4. Muscle pain
5. Multiple joint pain without redness or swelling
6. Headaches of a new pattern or severity
7. Unrefreshing sleep
8. Postexertional malaise lasting 24 hours[4]

Idiopathic fatigue (IF) — Fatigue that has not been attributed to a psychiatric or medical illness.

Persistent fatigue — Fatigue that generally persists for more than 1 month.

The chronic fatigue syndrome (CFS) represents a very small subset of patients with chronic fatigue. CFS remains a controversial subject but probably has existed for centuries under various labels, including effort syndrome (soldier's heart described in 1870), neurasthenia (1890), and more recently, the Gulf War syndrome (1991). Recently, the Centers for Disease Control and Prevention (CDC) developed a tool to assist in the more definitive diagnosis of CFS, expanding upon previous work in this field.[3] Unfortunately, because fatigue may accompany almost any medical or psychological illness, evaluating and treating a patient with fatigue can be particularly challenging and sometimes frustrating for the clinician. A careful history with special attention to psychosocial issues, the physical examination, and a few selected laboratory tests should reveal the cause in most patients.

ETIOLOGY

Approximately 70% of patients with chronic fatigue are found to have a medical or psychological explanation.[2,5] Psychiatric disorders (depression or anxiety) are the predominant causes of fatigue. In approximately 25% patients, an acute or chronic medical condition is responsible. Although the CDC case definition has resulted in a prevalence as high as 2.5%,[6] CFS is responsible for fatigue in a small number of patients. More recent studies suggest that social or personal factors may be important causes of fatigue. For example, a survey of women attending a women's health symposium in Toronto, Canada attributed their fatigue to a combination of home and outside work, poor sleep, relationship problems, care of ill family members, and financial worries.[7] Several other studies suggest that social, geographic, environmental, and genetic factors may contribute to the development of fatigue and depression.[7–9]

Differential Diagnosis

Psychological	***Hematologic***	***Pharmacologic***
Depression	Anemia	Antidepressants
Anxiety	Leukemia or lymphoma	Antihistamines
Substance abuse	***Infectious***	Benzodiazepines
Eating disorder	Endocarditis	Hypnotics
Cardiac	Mononucleosis	Narcotics
Heart failure	Tuberculosis	***Pulmonary***
Endocrine	Human immunodeficiency virus (HIV)	Chronic obstructive pulmonary disease
Addison disease	Hepatitis	Sleep apnea
Diabetes mellitus	Hepatitis	***Rheumatologic***
Thyroid disease	***Neurologic***	Fibromyalgia
Cushing's syndrome	Multiple sclerosis	Lyme disease
Hyperparathyroidism	Myasthenia gravis	Rheumatoid arthritis
Gastrointestinal	Oncologic	Systemic lupus erythematosus
Inflammatory bowel disease	Occult malignancy	
Malabsorption syndromes		
Cirrhosis		

GETTING STARTED WITH THE HISTORY

- Ask the patient to describe his or her fatigue. Fatigue must be distinguished from excessive somnolence (excessive daytime sleepiness),[10] which suggests a primary sleep disturbance. Similarly, generalized fatigue should not be confused with exertional dyspnea or true muscle weakness. Although these symptoms may also result in a decreased ability to perform certain activities, the implications and underlying causes are much different.

- Pay attention to the chronology of the fatigue and any associated symptoms. It is essential to pinpoint the *onset* of fatigue. Usually the onset is insidious, however, patients with CFS often report that the fatigue began just after a viral-type illness.
- Listen for clues to psychosocial issues. The impact of fatigue on the patient's social and occupational function should be ascertained. Associated stressors and recent life events may give clues to the underlying etiology.

Open-Ended Questions	Tips for Effective Interviewing
Tell me about your fatigue. What do you mean when you say you are fatigued?	Distinguish fatigue from other symptoms such as sleepiness or shortness of breath.
Tell me about your energy level. Has the fatigue changed your lifestyle?	Determine the impact of the patient's fatigue on the patient's lifestyle and social and occupational function.
Tell me about any new or unusual circumstances in your life when you first noted the fatigue.	Identify possible precipitating events.

INTERVIEW FRAMEWORK

- Develop a clear picture and story of the patient's fatigue (including the onset, duration, and exacerbating factors).
- Probe for associated symptoms to uncover undiagnosed medical illness.
- Take a thorough medication history.
- Explore social issues.
- Screen for underlying psychiatric disorders (depression, anxiety, substance abuse).

IDENTIFYING ALARM SYMPTOMS

Significant weight loss, night sweats, or fever suggests a systemic illness as a cause of the fatigue. Patients with medical illness are more likely to explain their fatigue in relation to specific activities. In contrast, patients with fatigue of psychogenic origin tend to be "tired all of the time." Patients who have a few organ-specific symptoms (eg, abdominal pain, change in bowel habits) are more likely to have an underlying medical illness, whereas patients with multiple somatic complaints usually have a psychogenic cause.

Serious Diagnoses

Although most cases of fatigue result from anxiety and/or depression, a serious medical condition is sometimes the underlying cause. Serious diagnoses are often apparent at the time of presentation because of associated clinical features. Infections, heart disease, and rheumatologic disorders are suggested by the presence of fever, dyspnea, and joint pain, respectively. Anemia and thyroid disease may be discovered on the basis of laboratory studies. Laboratory studies are of little diagnostic value without suggestive historical or physical examination findings.[11] Occult malignancy is a rare but often feared cause of chronic fatigue and may be suggested by the presence of weight loss, fever, or night sweats.

Alarm Symptoms	Serious Causes	Benign Causes
Fever, night sweats	Infection Lymphoma Occult neoplasm	Viral illness
Weight loss	Infection Malignancy Malabsorption Thyroid disease Depression Eating disorder	

—Continued next page

Continued— Sore throat	Infectious mononucleosis Streptococcal pharyngitis	Viral illness
Lymph node enlargement	HIV Infectious mononucleosis Lymphoma Syphilis	Viral illness
Shortness of breath	Heart failure Chronic obstructive pulmonary disease Anemia	Anxiety
Palpitations	Cardiac arrhythmia Thyrotoxicosis	Anxiety
Joint pain, stiffness	Rheumatoid arthritis Lyme disease	Viral illness
Back pain; diffuse bony pain	Metastatic carcinoma Multiple myeloma	Mechanical low back pain
Excessive thirst, urination	Diabetes mellitus Diabetes insipidus	
Abdominal pain	Peptic ulcer disease Inflammatory bowel disease Intra-abdominal malignancy Mesenteric ischemia	Irritable bowel syndrome Nonulcer dyspepsia
Jaundice	Hepatitis Pancreatic cancer Cirrhosis Drug reaction	Gilbert's syndrome
Chest pain	Coronary artery disease	Anxiety or panic disorder Gastroesophageal reflux disease
Diarrhea	Inflammatory bowel disease Malabsorption Intestinal parasite	Irritable bowel syndrome Laxative abuse
Rectal bleeding	Inflammatory bowel disease Colon cancer	Hemorrhoids
Double vision, difficulty speaking or chewing; pain with chewing	Myasthenia gravis Temporal arteritis Multiple sclerosis	
Sleep disturbance	Depression Sleep apnea	Anxiety disorder

FOCUSED QUESTIONS

After characterizing the patient's fatigue and asking about alarm symptoms, the clinician should proceed to more focused, directed questions. Keep in mind that patients presenting with chronic fatigue often have undiagnosed psychiatric illness.[1,2] Patients may attribute their emotional problem to chronic fatigue. However, in a study of patients with chronic fatigue who were determined to have a psychiatric disorder, either predated or began around the same time as the fatigue in most patients, suggesting the psychiatric disorder was likely to be a primary cause and not merely a complication of fatigue.[12]

QUESTIONS	THINK ABOUT...
Quality	
Has your fatigue affected your ability to perform responsibilities at work or at home?	Chronic fatigue CFS
Have you stopped exercising?	Chronic fatigue CFS
Do you become more weak or tired with exertion?	Muscle or neurologic disease
Do you become short of breath with exercise?	Cardiopulmonary disease Anemia Hyperthyroidism
Time course	
Can you remember exactly when your fatigue started?	The patient with CFS often relates the onset after a viral-type illness.
How long have you been experiencing fatigue?	Fatigue of recent onset may resolve spontaneously.
Do you feel more fatigued in the morning?	Depression
Do you feel tired all day?	Chronic anxiety
Do you feel more fatigued at the end of the day?	Fatigue secondary to medical illness (as opposed to psychogenic)
Did your fatigue begin following surgery?	Postoperative fatigue
Have you ever had radiation therapy?	Postradiotherapy fatigue
Associated symptoms (see Alarm symptoms)	
Modifying factors	
Does your fatigue only happen with exertion?	Muscle weakness Cardiopulmonary disease
Is your fatigue unrelated to physical effort?	Psychogenic fatigue
Do you feel better on the weekends?	Chronic occupational stress
Does your fatigue improve after a good night's rest?	Sleep deprivation
Exploring personal or social issues	
Have you had more stress in your life lately? Have there been any problems in your family? Have you had more pressure at work? Have you experienced a death of a close friend or relative?	Stress-related or psychogenic fatigue

—Continued next page

Continued—

When is the last time you had a vacation?	Overworked patient Lack of balance between work, family, and pleasure
Do you use alcohol? Has anyone suggested that you should reduce the amount of alcohol you drink? Do you need an alcoholic drink first thing in the morning? Have you been annoyed at anyone for suggesting that you cut back on your alcohol consumption? Do you feel guilty about the amount of alcohol you drink?	Alcoholism; the last 4 questions comprise the CAGE screening test. Two or more positive responses have relatively high sensitivity and specificity for alcoholism.[13]
Exploring personal or social issues	
Do you use drugs such as heroin, cocaine, or other illicit drugs?	HIV infection Hepatitis
Do you have more than 1 sexual partner?	HIV infection
Have you recently traveled to developing countries?	Parasitic infections
What medications do you take on a regular basis—both prescribed and over-the-counter? Have you recently started taking any new medications?	Medication-induced fatigue (common causes include antihypertensives, sedative–hypnotics, antidepressants, antihistamines, and narcotics)
Uncovering psychogenic illness	
How would you describe your mood? Have you been feeling sad, blue, or down?	Depression
Have you been more irritable or angry?	Depression
Do you often feel agitated?	Depression Anxiety
Have you lost interest in or avoided social activities? *Have you lost interest in sex?* *Have you had guilty feelings about anything lately?* *Have you had trouble concentrating lately?* *Have you lost interest in things that used to give you pleasure?* *Have you experienced loss of self-esteem?*	Depression
Has your appetite been affected?	Depression (usually decreased)
Have you had more difficulty with sleep?	Depression (often early morning awakening) Anxiety
Do you feel worse in the morning? *Do you feel hopeless?* *Have you thought about suicide?*	Depression
Have you been excessively nervous or anxious? *Are you constantly worried about something?*	Anxiety
Do you experience sudden episodes of intense anxiety? If so, have you experienced chest pain, palpitations, and sweating?	Anxiety Panic attacks
Are you easily distracted?	Anxiety

DIAGNOSTIC APPROACH (INCLUDING ALGORITHM)

In most patients with fatigue, the etiology will be determined by a careful history. If the initial history from the patient does not suggest an organic or medical disorder, the clinician should perform a review of systems focusing on the alarm symptoms, and then guide the interview to probe for concurrent psychiatric disorders. A thorough physical examination should be performed with special attention to those organ systems suggested by the history. Laboratory studies should be directed by the history and physical examination and may not be needed if no concern is raised in the history or examination for an organic cause. Depending on the information gathered, a complete blood cell count, serum chemistries, and thyroid-stimulating hormone measurement may be of assistance to help exclude potentially serious medical illness. An extensive work-up for occult medical illness is generally not warranted.[1] The diagnostic algorithm is shown in Figure 7–1.

CAVEATS

- Testing or further work-up only needs to be obtained if an underlying medical cause is suggested by the patient's history and/or physical examination.

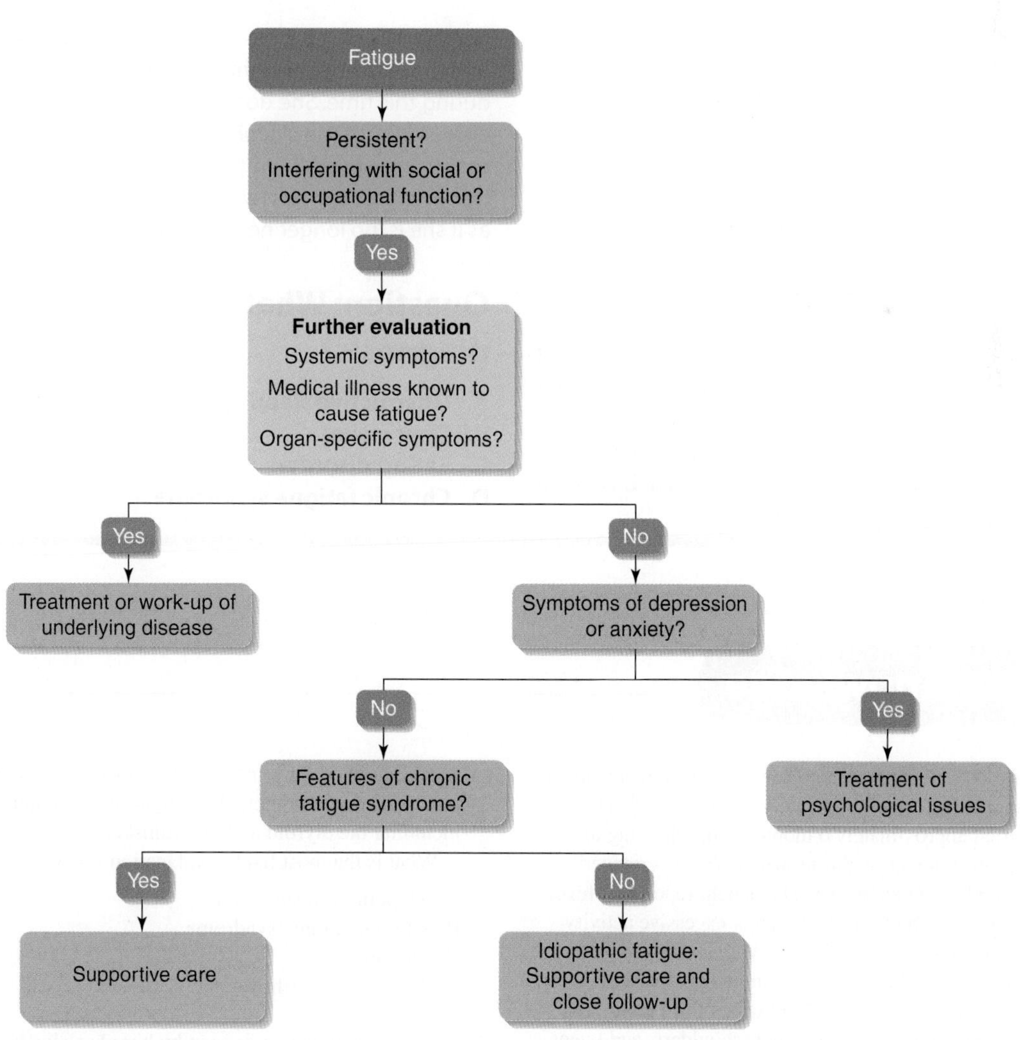

FIGURE 7–1 Diagnostic algorithm: Fatigue.

- Be sensitive to the potential for underlying depression, anxiety, or somatization.
- A significant subset of cases will have no identifiable etiology.

PROGNOSIS

The outcome of patients with chronic fatigue is generally not favorable. In the classic study by Kroenke et al.,[1] only 29 (28%) of 102 patients with chronic fatigue experienced some improvement in their fatigue. However, Elnicki et al.[14] reported that 72% of patients with fatigue (of at least 1 month in duration) improved over the next 6 months. In another study, the outcome was better if the patients had fatigue for less than 3 months and no history of emotional illness.[15] Patients with CFS may have a worse prognosis in terms of improvement or recovery.[16] Even in the nondisabled elderly patient, being "tired" is associated with a greater risk of becoming disabled over the next 5 years.[17] In summary, a long duration of fatigue and presence of an underlying psychiatric disorder seem to predict a poor prognosis. Fortunately, idiopathic fatigue and CFS cause neither death nor organ failure, although the associated fatigue may result in significant morbidity. Prognosis of fatigue caused by underlying medical conditions depends on the disease.

CASE SCENARIO | Resolution

A 45-year-old woman presents to your clinic after suffering from "months" of feeling bad. She feels tired all the time and is finding it difficult to keep up daily activities. Her tiredness is interfering with her ability to play an active role in the lives of her husband and 2 children. She has no significant past medical history and has not seen a physician in several years.

ADDITIONAL HISTORY

Upon further questioning, the patient reports fatigue on and off for the past 3 months. She has no trouble performing her usual level of physical activity; she simply is not interested in working out as she did in the past. She has difficulty concentrating on simple tasks, such as paying bills or balancing her checkbook. At times she feels sad, but denies thoughts of self-harm. Her weight has increased by about 10 lbs during this time. She does not report sleep disturbances or excessive daytime sleepiness. Other than weight gain, she reports no physical symptoms. She does not drink alcohol. Her youngest son has recently started college, and she feels as if she is "no longer needed" by her family.

Question: What is the most likely diagnosis?

A. Obstructive sleep apnea
B. Depression
C. Eating disorder
D. Chronic fatigue syndrome

Test Your Knowledge

1. A 34-year-old woman presents to her primary care physician with a 6-month history of moderately severe fatigue. The fatigue started approximately 6 months ago, following an upper respiratory infection during which she experienced sore throat and head congestion. The patient reports no fever or other systemic symptoms. Exercise or excessive activity seems to worsen the fatigue. The patient has enjoyed good health except for an episode of self-limited postpartum thyroiditis 4 years ago after the birth of her third child. The patient relates discomfort in her hands, shoulders, and knees but no swelling or warmth in any joint. She feels that her fatigue is impacting her ability to care for her 3 children and perform household chores. Her only medication is acetaminophen for joint pain. The review of systems is otherwise unremarkable. Her physical examination is normal, including the thyroid and musculoskeletal examination.

   What is the most likely explanation for her fatigue?

   A. Hypothyroidism
   B. Chronic fatigue syndrome
   C. Depression
   D. Rheumatoid arthritis

2. A 78-year-old woman is seen by her physician because of a 2-month history of progressive fatigue. She has enjoyed good health over the years and maintains a very active lifestyle. She reports an 8-lbs weight loss over the past 6 months and

occasional "dark stools." There is no fever or night sweats. She has a 20-year history of hypertension and hyperlipidemia, which are both well controlled on hydrochlorothiazide and simvastatin. Her mood is generally good, but recently she has become anxious about her current symptoms. There have been no major life-changing events. She is a nonsmoker and drinks an occasional glass of wine with dinner. Her physical examination is remarkable for conjunctival pallor and hemoccult-positive stool on rectal examination.

What is the most likely explanation for her fatigue?

A. Generalized anxiety
B. Apathetic thyrotoxicosis
C. Chronic fatigue syndrome
D. Colon cancer
E. Adverse effect of medication

3. A 55-year-old woman presents to her physician for her annual health maintenance visit. She has a history of osteoporosis and dyslipidemia. She reports that she has felt tired over the past year but has been able to continue to function in her job as a nurse. Her medications include alendronate and atorvastatin. She is married and lives with her husband. She has 2 daughters who live in the area. The patient participates in an aerobics class 3 times weekly but has gained 10 lbs over the last year. She attributes her weight gain to the fact that she often feels rushed when she gets home at the end of the day and her meal selection has not been as "healthy." She has been experiencing more difficulty sleeping and often feels cold. In the summertime, she reports needing a sweater or jacket in air-conditioned rooms and problems with dry skin. She feels her mood is generally good, and she has a good relationship with her husband. Her physical examination is normal.

What is the most likely explanation for her fatigue?

A. Major depression
B. Social stresses
C. Hypothyroidism
D. Generalized anxiety disorder
E. Menopause

References

1. Kroenke K, Wood DR, Mangelsdorf AD, Meier NJ, Powell JB. Chronic fatigue in primary care. Prevalence, patient characteristics and outcome. *JAMA*. 1988;260:929–934.
2. Bates DW, Schmitt W, Buchwald D, et al. Prevalence of fatigue and chronic fatigue syndrome in a primary care practice. *Arch Intern Med*. 1993;153:2759–2765.
3. Reeves WC, Wagner D, Nisenbaum R, et al. Chronic fatigue syndrome: a clinically empirical approach to its definition and study. *BMC Med*. 2005;3:19.
4. Fukuda K, Straus SE, Hickie I, et al. The chronic fatigue syndrome: a comprehensive approach to its definition and study. International Chronic Fatigue Syndrome Study Group. *Ann Intern Med*. 1994;121:953–959.
5. Buchwald D, Umali P, Umali J, Kith P, Pearlman T, Komaroff AL. Chronic fatigue and the chronic fatigue syndrome: prevalence in a Pacific Northwest health care system. *Ann Intern Med*. 1995;123:81–88.
6. Reeves WC, Jones JJ, Maloney E, et al. New study on the prevalence of CFS in metro, urban, and rural Georgia populations. *Pop Health Met*. 2007;5:5.
7. Stewart D, Abbey S, Meana M, Boydell KM. What makes women tired? A community sample. *J Womens Health*. 1998;7:69–76.
8. Ball HA, Siribaddana SH, Sumathipala A, et al. Environmental exposures and their genetic or environmental contribution to depression and fatigue: a twin study in Sri Lanka. *BMC Psychiatry*. 2010;10:13.
9. Van't Leven M, Zielhuis GA, van der Meer JW, Verbeek AL, Bleijenberg G. Fatigue and chronic fatigue syndrome-like complaints in the general population. *Eur J Public Health*. 2010;20:251–257.
10. Pigeon WR, Sateia MJ, Ferguson RJ. Distinguishing between excessive daytime sleepiness and fatigue: toward improve detection and treatment. *J Psychosom Res*. 2003;54:61–69.
11. Lane TJ, Matthews DA, Manu P. The low yield of physical examinations and laboratory investigations of patients with chronic fatigue. *Am J Med Sci*. 1990;299:313–318.
12. Lane TJ, Manu P, Matthews DA. Depression and somatization in the chronic fatigue syndrome. *Am J Med*. 1991;91: 335–344.
13. Mayfield D, McLead G, Hall P. The CAGE questionnaire: validation of a new alcoholism screening instrument. *Am J Psychiatry*. 1974;131:1121–1123.
14. Elnicki DM, Shockcor WT, Brick JE, Beynon D. Evaluating the complaint of fatigue in primary care: diagnoses and outcomes. *Am J Med*. 1992;93:303–306.
15. Ridsdale L, Evans A, Jerrett W, Mandalia S, Osler K, Vora H. Patients with fatigue in general practice: a prospective study. *BMJ*. 1993;307:103–106.
16. Bombardier CH, Buchwald D. Outcome and prognosis of patients with chronic fatigue versus chronic fatigue syndrome. *Arch Intern Med*. 1995;155:2105–2110.
17. Avlund K, Damsgaard MT, Sakari-Rantala R, Laukkanen P, Schroll M. Tiredness in daily activities among non-disabled old people as determinant of onset of disability. *J Clin Epidemiol*. 2002;55:965–973.

Suggested Reading

Goroll AH, May LA, Mulley AG, eds. *Primary Care Medicine: Office Evaluation and Management of the Adult Patient*. 3rd ed. Philadelphia, PA: J.B. Lippincott, 1995:32–38.

Kim E. A brief history of chronic fatigue syndrome. *JAMA*. 1994;272:1070–1071.

Morrison RE, Keating HJ. Fatigue in primary care. *Obstet Gynecol Clin North Am*. 2001;28:225–240.

Stevens DL. Chronic fatigue. *West J Med*. 2001;175:315–319.

Chapter 8

Fever

Anjala V. Tess, MD

CASE SCENARIO

A 29-year-old mother of 3 children presents to your office with "high fever." She was in her usual state of health until 3 days ago when she noticed malaise. The following day, she felt "hot" and noted sharp chest pain when she took a deep breath. That night, her temperature was 102.5°F. She then developed shortness of breath and a dry cough and so presents to you today for evaluation.

- **What additional questions could you ask to try and distinguish between the different major categories of fever?**
- **How might understanding the pattern of fever help you narrow your differential?**
- **What alarm symptoms would indicate the need for an urgent evaluation?**

INTRODUCTION

Temperature regulation in the human body is controlled by hypothalamic nuclei that maintain a set point. Several mechanisms work together to achieve temperature homeostasis. For example, shivering and vasoconstriction generate heat, raising the temperature to the set point. Sweating and cutaneous vasodilation lower the temperature by increasing heat loss. **Fever** occurs when the set point itself is raised to a higher level and the body responds by raising the temperature. Macrophages and monocytes produce cytokines in response to various stimuli, which cause the hypothalamus to raise the set point.

Normal temperature is defined as 98.6°F, although the overall mean oral temperature for healthy persons aged 18 to 40 years is actually 98.2°F ± 0.4°F with a diurnal variation (daily oscillations from 0.9°F to 2.4°F). Temperature can be measured orally or rectally; rectal temperatures measure 1°F greater than oral values.[1]

KEY TERMS

Fever	A rise in body temperature in response to endogenous cytokines. The exact lower cutoff for fever varies from 99.4°F to 100.4°F. A recent study suggests that with modern thermometers, an early morning temperature of greater than 99.0°F or an evening temperature of 100.0°F should be considered abnormal.[1]
Hyperthermia	An elevation in body temperature due to loss of homeostatic mechanisms and inability to increase heat loss in response to environmental heat, as in heat stroke. Can reach levels > 105.8°F.
Fever of unknown origin (FUO)	Fever that lasts 3 weeks or longer with temperatures exceeding 100.9°F with no clear diagnosis despite 1 week of clinical investigation.[2]

ETIOLOGY

Fever is the third most common cause for visits to the emergency department and is listed in the top 20 reasons for visits to the ambulatory clinic.[3,4] Given that many conditions raise the temperature set point, the differential diagnosis of fever is broad.

Most acute febrile illnesses are readily diagnosed based on history, examination, and laboratory testing, and many resolve on their own. Prevalence data are unfortunately limited, but a few studies have addressed the etiology of fever in specific populations, including hospitalized patients and those with FUO.[2,5–7]

Patient Setting	Etiology	Prevalence
Hospitalized patients	Community-acquired infection	51%
	Nosocomial (hospital-acquired) infection	10%
	Possibly infectious	23%
	Noninfectious	31%
FUO	Infection	16%–24.5%
	Malignancy	7%–14.5%
	Inflammatory disorders	22%–26.4%
	Other causes	4%–15.3%
	No diagnosis	25.7%–30%

Differential Diagnosis of Fever

	Prevalence[a]
Infection	
Bacteral Viral Parasitic Fungal Rickettsial	• Prevalence varies by season and geography. • Up to 69% of hospitalized patients may have infectious etiologies including infection of the lungs and pleura, urinary tract, bloodstream, and skin.[5] • Causes of nosocomial infections in one study of hospitalized patients included: bacterial infections (51%), nonbacterial infections (5%), noninfectious etiologies (25%), and unknown source (19%). Among bacterial infections, pneumonia, catheter-related sepsis, Clostridium difficile diarrhea, wound infections, and urinary tract infections were present.[8] • The most common infectious causes of FUO are tuberculosis and intra-abdominal abscesses.[2] • Patients with recent travel abroad may contract bacterial, viral, fungal, or parasitic infections. Malaria and respiratory infections are the most common infections seen, although 25% remain undiagnosed.[9]
Malignancy	
Lymphoma	• Fever can occur in essentially any malignancy as a paraneoplastic feature. ◦ The malignancies most commonly associated with FUO are Hodgkin's disease or non-Hodgkin's lymphoma. ◦ 10%–11% of patients with Hodgkin's disease will have fever and/or night sweats (constitutional symptoms). ◦ Pel-Ebstein fevers, relapsing fever for hours or days followed by days without fever, occur in 16% of cases with Hodgkin's disease.
Leukemia	
Liver metastases	
Hepatocellular cancer	20% of patients have fever.
Renal cell cancer	33% of patients have fever.
Pancreatic cancer	

Inflammatory	
Systemic lupus erythematosus (SLE)	36% of patients with SLE have fever at presentation, and fever develops in up to 52% during evolution of the disease.
Rheumatic fever	
Giant cell arteritis (GCA)	42% of patients with GCA have fever at presentation.
Wegener's granulomatosis	
Rheumatoid arthritis	Up to 25% of patients with rheumatoid arthritis have fever at presentation in addition to a polyarticular arthritis.
Polyarteritis nodosa	
Inflammatory bowel disease (IBD)	42% of patients with IBD will have fever, although fever tends to occur later in course of illness.
Gout	15%–43% of patients with gout have fever as part of the acute attack.
Miscellaneous	
Pulmonary emboli (PE)	Fever develops in 14% of patients.[10]
Drug fever	Fever can be the sole presenting symptom in up to 5% of cases of drug fever. Drug fever accounts for up to 10% of hospitalized patients with new fever.[8]
Factitious fever	Factitious fever may result from manipulation of the thermometer or self-injury, leading to infection or drug fever.
Sarcoidosis	
Adrenal insufficiency	
Hyperthyroidism	
Pancreatitis	

[a]Prevalence estimate is unavailable when not indicated.

Differential Diagnosis of Hyperthermia

Condition	Comment
Heat stroke	May result from central nervous system (CNS) dysfunction or excessive physical exertion in a warm environment. Mortality rate is as high as 10%.
Neuroleptic malignant syndrome (NMS)	An idiosyncratic reaction to antipsychotic medications, such as butyrophenones, phenothiazines, and thioxanthenes. Cumulative data suggest incidence of 0.2% in patients treated with neuroleptic medications. Temperature exceeded 104°F in 39% of patients.[11]
Malignant hyperthermia	A rare genetic abnormality in the muscle membrane that predisposes patients to severe rhabdomyolysis and temperature dysregulation. May occur with certain anesthetics, although can occur with exertion in hot ambient temperatures. Fatality rate is currently 5% compared with 70% in the 1960s.

GETTING STARTED WITH THE HISTORY

- Review vital signs over the preceding days to establish duration and degree of fever.
- Focus your evaluation on associated symptoms. After asking general questions, complete a full review of systems.
- Take a thorough medication history.

- Pattern of fever: Although clinicians often discuss patterns of fever, in small studies, fever patterns have had limited diagnostic value. Sustained fever has been associated with gram-negative rod sepsis and CNS infections.[12] Certain malarial infections are associated with fevers that occur every 48 or 72 hours. Tertian fever is seen in certain malarial infections and occurs every 48 hours. Diurnal fever is defined as a regular rise and fall in temperature, occurring between 4 PM and midnight.

Questions	Remember
How long have you had a fever?	Establish a time course for the symptom.
How and at what site did you measure your temperature?	Determine the method used for measurement.
Describe any new symptoms you have experienced with the fever.	Listen to patient's description of the fever and associated symptoms for diagnostic clues.

INTERVIEW FRAMEWORK

- Ask about alarm symptoms.
- Look for clues that point to the major diagnostic categories: infection, inflammatory, malignancy, or other.
- Remember to ask about recent hospitalizations, travel abroad, new medications, and sick contacts.

IDENTIFYING ALARM SYMPTOMS

Serious Diagnoses

In assessing alarm symptoms, the goal is to identify features suggesting a diagnosis that requires prompt intervention. However, certain alarm symptoms may also suggest that complications from the process causing the fever (eg, septic shock) may be developing.

Alarm Symptoms	If Present, Consider...	However, Benign Causes of This Symptom Include...
High fever (>105.8°F)	CNS infection, NMS, heat stroke	
Rash	Meningitis, bacteremia with septic shock, rickettsial disease, bacterial endocarditis	Viral exanthem, drug fever
Change in mental status and level of sensorium	Meningitis, encephalitis, NMS, heat stroke, bacterial infections with septic shock	
Dizziness or light-headedness	Bacterial infection with septic shock, adrenal insufficiency, PE	Viral infection with labyrinthitis
Recent chemotherapy	Nosocomial infection with neutropenia	
Shortness of breath and chest pain	PE, pneumonia, empyema	

FOCUSED QUESTIONS

Remember that the same associated symptom may occur across major diagnostic categories (eg, diarrhea may suggest a gastroenteritis or inflammatory bowel disease). Seek a constellation of symptoms that suggest a certain diagnosis. For example, diarrhea of several months in duration with associated fever suggests inflammatory bowel disease rather than a viral gastroenteritis.

QUESTIONS	THINK ABOUT...
Have you had any sick contacts? *Have you recently been in the hospital or traveled recently?* *Have you had any recent procedures?*	Infection
Have you lost weight? *Do you have any bony pain?*	Malignancy
Do you have arthritis or a rash? *Do you have a personal or family history of vasculitis or other inflammatory disease?*	Inflammatory disorders
Quality	
How high is your fever? *> 105.8°F*	CNS infections, heat stroke, neuroleptic malignant syndrome
Time course	
How long have you had fevers? *> 3 weeks with a temperature > 100.9°F*	Establishes FUO if initial work-up is negative.
Is there a pattern to the fever?	
• *Continuous/sustained (fluctuation < 0.5°F)*	Suggests CNS disease or gram-negative rod bacteremia.[12]
• *Diurnal (a regular rise and fall in temperature, occurring between 4 PM and midnight)*	Absence of diurnal variation has been associated with, but does not establish, a noninfectious cause.[12]
• *Tertian fever (periodicity of 48 hours)*	Malaria due to *Plasmodium vivax* or *Plasmodium ovale*[9]
• *Quartan fever (periodicity of 72 hours)*	Malaria due to *Plasmodium malariae*[9]
Associated symptoms	
Do you have dry cough, nasal congestion, sinus pain, or a sore throat?	Acute pharyngitis (viral or bacterial), sinusitis, or upper respiratory tract infection
Any redness of your skin?	Cellulitis, phlebitis, fungal infections, drug reaction
Do you have a productive cough or shortness of breath?	Pneumonia (viral, bacterial, fungal), bronchitis, tuberculosis
Do you have any blood in your sputum?	Pneumonia, bronchitis, tuberculosis, PE, lung cancer
Do you have chest pain?	PE, pneumonia, pericarditis, bacterial endocarditis
Do you have burning with urination?	Urinary tract infection, pyelonephritis, renal cell carcinoma, urethritis, prostatitis
Do you have blood in the urine?	Urinary tract infection, pyelonephritis, renal cell carcinoma, Wegener's granulomatosis, SLE, and other vasculitic diseases of the kidney
Have you had nausea or vomiting?	Gastroenteritis (viral or bacterial), cholecystitis, cholangitis, pyelonephritis, hepatitis, pancreatitis
Do you have diarrhea?	Gastroenteritis (viral or bacterial), infectious colitis, parasitic infections, IBD

—Continued next page

Continued—

Do you have any abdominal pain?	Gastroenteritis (viral or bacterial), cholecystitis, cholangitis, pyelonephritis, hepatitis, pancreatic cancer, pancreatitis, liver metastasis, polyarteritis nodosa, IBD
Have you noticed a yellowing of your skin (jaundice)?	Cholecystitis, hepatitis, liver abscesses, malignancy with involvement of the liver
Did you have associated shaking chills?	Bacteremia, endocarditis
Do you have night sweats, weight loss, or malaise?	Hodgkin's disease, non-Hodgkin's lymphoma, renal cell carcinoma
Have you had any stiffness or pain in your joints?	Septic arthritis, SLE, rheumatic fever, GCA, Wegener's granulomatosis, rheumatoid arthritis, polyarteritis nodosa, IBD
Do you have a headache?	GCA, meningitis, encephalitis, sinusitis
Have you had jaw claudication (pain with chewing)?	GCA
Do you have easy bruising or gum bleeding?	Leukemia, lymphoma
Have you had difficulty with speech, double vision, arm or leg weakness, or seizure?	Meningitis, encephalitis, intracerebral hemorrhage, endocarditis with CNS emboli
Have you been confused?	Meningitis, encephalitis, bacterial infection with septic shock
Modifying factors (potential triggers)	
Have you had any recent procedures (eg, dental work)?	Bacterial endocarditis
Have you started any new medications?	Drug fever
Have you recently started any psychiatric medications?	NMS
If you were recently in the hospital, did you have:	
• *Surgery?*	Abscess, wound infection, malignant hyperthermia
• *A urinary or intravenous catheter placed?*	Catheter-associated urinary tract infection or bacteremia
• *Exposure to new antibiotics?*	*C difficile* colitis, drug fever
If you traveled abroad:	
• *Did travel require you to remain immobile for extended periods of time?*	Pulmonary embolus or deep vein thrombosis
• *Did you consume untreated water or dairy products?*	Salmonellosis, shigellosis, hepatitis, amoebiasis, brucellosis
• *Did you eat raw or undercooked meat?*	Enteric infections, cestodiasis, trichinosis
• *Were you exposed to mosquitoes?*	Malaria, dengue fever
• *Were you exposed to ticks?*	Rickettsial disease, tularemia, African trypanosomiasis, Lyme disease
• *Did you take any new prophylactic medications such as antibiotics or antimalarials?*	Drug fever
Have you recently had unprotected sexual intercourse or used intravenous drugs?	Acute HIV, hepatitis B or C infection, syphilis, gonorrhea, or endocarditis
Have you ever lived in a homeless shelter or a prison?	Tuberculosis—either reactivation or disseminated
Have you had recent exertion in the heat?	Heat stroke
Have you ever had heart valve surgery?	Endocarditis

DIAGNOSTIC APPROACH (INCLUDING ALGORITHM)

In evaluating your patient's history, look for clues that point to nosocomial infection, drug fever, or fever in the returning traveler. If these categories seem unlikely, attempt to identify the major category (infectious disease, malignancy, or vasculitis), and then use detailed questions as noted earlier to narrow your differential diagnosis. The diagnostic algorithm is shown in Figure 8–1.

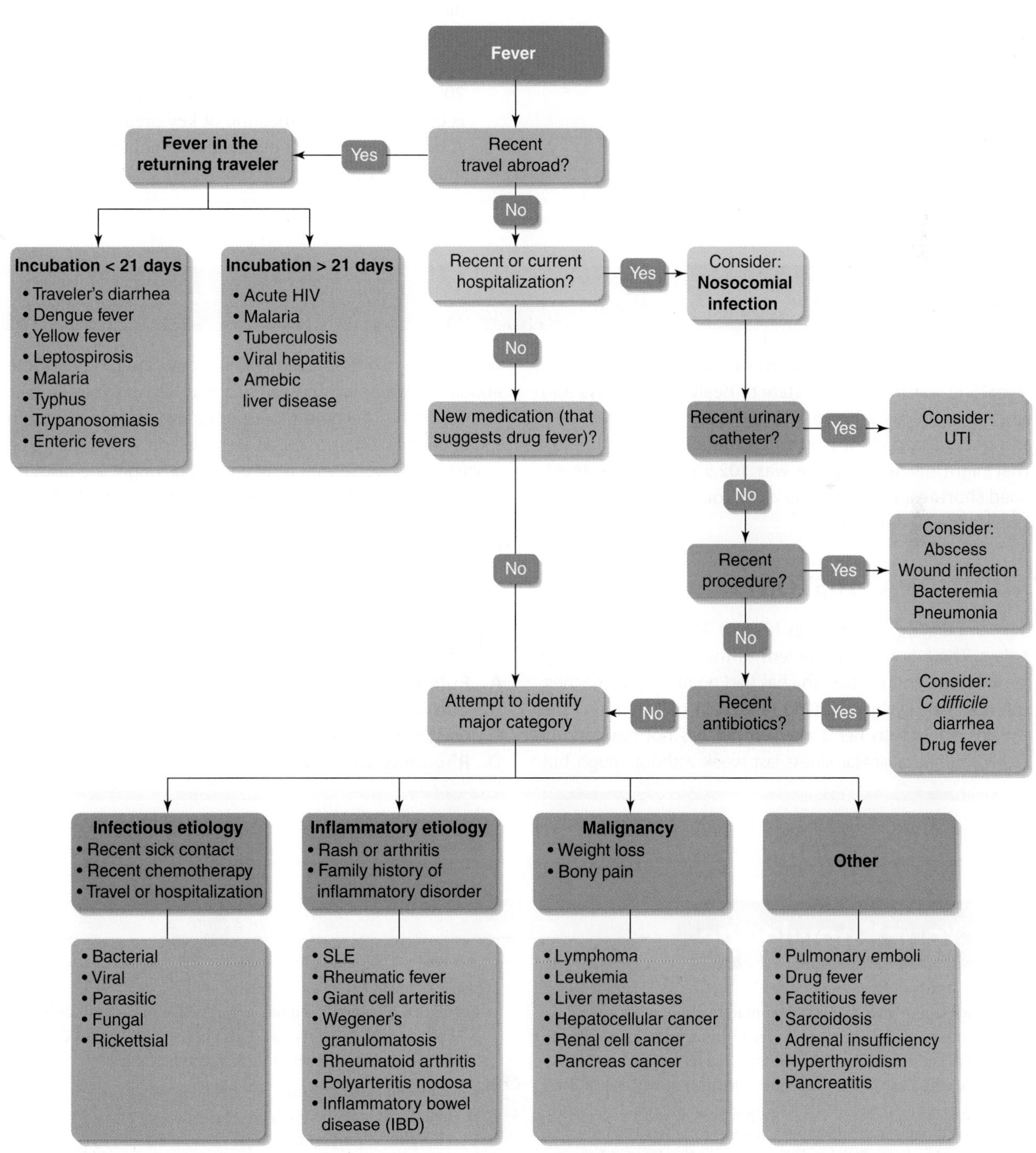

FIGURE 8–1 Diagnostic algorithm: Fever.

CAVEATS

- In general, fever requires prompt evaluation.
- Gather as many associated symptoms and potential triggers to support a unifying diagnosis.
- Elderly and immunosuppressed patients may not mount as high a fever as younger or immunocompetent patients. These patients may present with a lower temperature or no fever at all.
- Never rely on the fever pattern alone to direct your evaluation or laboratory testing.

PROGNOSIS

- Most acute febrile illnesses either resolve or the etiology is quickly identified on the basis of history, examination, and laboratory or radiologic evaluation. The prognosis depends on the underlying diagnosis.
- Among patients with an FUO whose cause remains elusive after several weeks, those without a specific diagnosis have a favorable outcome. Over 50% of patients in whom malignancies are the cause of fever die within 5 years of diagnosis. Mortality is lower (22%) in patients whose fever is a result of infection.[2]
- Mortality rates can reach 10% in heat stroke patients and 20% in those with NMS. Therefore, prompt evaluation is critical with identification of key predisposing factors. A complete list of all medications, including anesthetics, must be reviewed.

CASE SCENARIO | Resolution

A 49-year-old mother of 3 presents to your office with "high fever." She was in her usual state of health until 3 days ago when she noticed malaise. The following day she felt "hot" and noted sharp chest pain when she took a deep breath. That night her temperature was 102.5°F. She then developed shortness of breath and a dry cough and so presents to you today for evaluation.

ADDITIONAL HISTORY

Her temperature has been as high as 103.0°F over the last 3 days. There is no exact pattern to the fever, but it usually resolves with antipyretics. She has had no rash or joint aches. She has had myalgias but no neck pain or confusion. She remains active with her 3 children but has not traveled. All 3 children had a similar illness last week without cough but with a mild rash that faded within a day. She has had some abdominal cramping and diarrhea that were also self-limited. Her cough has become more productive of yellow sputum today, but no blood was noted. Her chest pain continues to be painful and is worse with respiration and cough. She takes no medications other than the over-the-counter analgesics for her fever. Her family history is negative for history of venous thromboembolism or early miscarriage.

Question: What is the most likely diagnosis?

A. Pulmonary embolism
B. Community-acquired pneumonia
C. Gastroenteritis
D. Rheumatoid arthritis

Test Your Knowledge

1. You are seeing an 80-year-old woman in clinic with intermittent fever for 5 weeks. Her fevers have been as high as 102.9°F and respond to antipyretics. She has noted proximal muscle aches as well as some joint stiffness of her hands. Two weeks ago, she developed a left unilateral temporal headache and noted pain in her jaw after chewing for a few minutes. She now has loss of vision in her left eye. She has not been hospitalized recently and has not travelled outside of her state. She has no sick contacts and does not use intravenous drugs.

   What diagnosis do her clinical features suggest?

   A. Pulmonary embolism
   B. Giant cell arteritis (GCA)
   C. Hodgkin's lymphoma
   D. Bacterial endocarditis

2. A 65-year-old diabetic man presents 1 week after hospitalization and surgery for an inflamed appendix. He was hospitalized for 3 days. He underwent intravascular catheter placement and received a urinary catheter and prophylaxis for deep venous thrombosis. He started taking antibiotics with surgery and quickly improved. His catheter was removed, and he was able to ambulate without pain. He was discharged home. He now presents to the emergency room with 3 days of fever, lower abdominal pain, and dysuria. He has no rash, leg pain, dizziness, chest pain, or shortness of breath.

   Which of the following is the most likely iatrogenic cause of his fever?

   A. Placement of urinary catheter
   B. Prophylaxis for deep venous thrombosis
   C. New medications
   D. Anesthesia for his surgery

3. A 21-year-old woman presents to your office 6 months after returning from Mexico. While on her 1-week spring break, she did not travel to rural areas but spent time in a market sampling fresh fruits. She felt well until 2 months ago, when she developed fevers to 101.0°F associated with sweating and pruritus. The fevers last for hours to days and then are quiescent for several days before recurring. She has been seen in a walk-in clinic for these symptoms and underwent a urine test and blood work with no diagnosis. She now comes to you for a second opinion.

   She has no cough, chest pain, joint aches, or rash. She does note anorexia and occasional loose stools. She has lost 25 lbs. She has never lived or worked in an institutionalized setting.

   Which clinical feature is most useful in narrowing the differential diagnosis?

   A. Weight loss
   B. Loose bowel movements
   C. Pattern of fever
   D. Eating fresh fruit

References

1. Mackowiak PA, Wasserman SS, Levine MM. A critical appraisal of 98.6°F, the upper limit of the normal body temperature, and other legacies of Carl Reinhold August Wunderlich. *JAMA.* 1992;268:578–581.
2. Mourad O, Palda V, Detsky AS. A comprehensive evidence-based approach to fever of unknown origin. *Arch Intern Med.* 2003;163:545–551.
3. McCaig L, Burt CW. National Hospital Ambulatory Medical Care Survey: 2001 Emergency Department Summary. Advance data from vital and health statistics; No. 335. Hyattsville, MD: National Center for Health Statistics. 2003. Available at: http://www.cdc.gov/nchs/data/ad/ad335.pdf.
4. Cherry DK, Woodwell DA. National Ambulatory Medical Care Survey: 2000 Summary. Advance data from vital and health statistics; No. 328. Hyattsville, MD: National Center for Health Statistics. 2002. Available at: http://www.cdc.gov/nchs/data/ad/ad328.pdf.
5. McGowan J, Rose RC, Jacobs NF, Schaberg DR, Haley RW. Fever in hospitalized patients. With special reference to the medical service. *Am J Med.* 1987;82:580–586.
6. Zenone T. Fever of unknown origin in adults: evaluation of 144 cases in a non-university hospital. *Scand J Infect Dis.* 2006;38:632–638.
7. Bleeker-Rovers CP, Vis FJ, de Kleijn EMHA, et al. A prospective multicenter study of fever of unknown origin. *Medicine.* 2007;86:26–38.
8. Arbo M, Fine MJ, Hanusa BH, Sefcik T, Kapoor WN. Fever of nosocomial origin: etiology, risk factors, and outcomes. *Am J Med.* 1993;95:505–515.
9. Suh KN, Kozarsky PE, Keystone JS. Evaluation of fever in the returned traveler. *Med Clin North Am.* 1999;83:997–1017.
10. Stein PD, Afzal A, Henry JW, Villareal CG. Fever in acute pulmonary embolism. *Chest.* 2000;117:39–42.
11. Caroff SN, Mann SC. Neuroleptic malignant syndrome. *Psychopharmacol Bull.* 1988;24:25–27.
12. Musher DM, Fainstein V, Young EJ, Pruett TL. Fever patterns. Their lack of clinical significance. *Arch Intern Med.* 1979;139:1225–1228.

Suggested Reading

Bottieau E, Clerinx J, Van den Enden E, et al. Fever after a stay in the tropics. *Medicine.* 2007;8:18–25.

Caroff S, Mann SC. Neuroleptic malignant syndrome. *Med Clin North Am.* 1993;77:185–202.

Cervera R, Khamashta MA, Font J, et al. Systemic lupus erythematosus: clinical and immunologic patterns of disease expression in a cohort of 1,000 patients. The European Working Party on Systemic Lupus Erythematosus. *Medicine (Baltimore).* 1993;72:113–124.

Hunder GG. Giant cell arteritis and polymyalgia rheumatica. *Med Clin North Am.* 1997;81:195–219.

Mackowiak PA. Concepts of fever. *Arch Intern Med.* 1998;158:1870–1881.

Simon HB. Hyperthermia. *N Engl J Med.* 1993;329:483–487.

Weinberger A, Kesler A, Pinkhas J. Fever in various rheumatic diseases. *Clin Rheumatol.* 1985;4:258–266.

Chapter 9

Headache

Gerald W. Smetana, MD

CASE SCENARIO

A 27-year-old woman comes to your office to discuss her "sick headaches," which started during high school. Her mother nudged her to see you. The headaches do not awaken her from sleep but can be disabling and occasionally require her to miss work. Sometimes she vomits during an attack. Over the past 6 months, her headaches have become more severe and frequent, prompting her visit today.

- **What additional questions would you ask to learn more about her headaches?**
- **How do you classify headaches?**
- **How can you determine if this is an old headache or a new headache?**
- **Can you make a definite diagnosis through an open-ended history followed by focused questions?**
- **How can you use the patient history to distinguish between benign headaches and serious ones that require urgent attention?**

INTRODUCTION

Headache is an exceedingly common symptom in primary care and other practice settings, ranking among the top 10 most frequent symptoms that prompt an office visit.[1] Although most patients with headache will prove to have a benign cause, headache may occasionally herald a morbid or life-threatening diagnosis. A careful history will allow clinicians to establish the correct diagnosis in most cases, limit the use of unnecessary and expensive diagnostic testing, and lead to appropriate treatment to reduce suffering and disability. There are 2 general approaches to history taking for headache. The first is to learn the alarm features that should prompt consideration of a serious pathologic cause for headache. The second is to understand the typical features of common benign headache syndromes. This approach allows one to confidently diagnose migraine, tension-type, and cluster headaches based on the presence of characteristic historical features.

KEY TERMS

Primary headache	A chronic, benign, recurring headache without known cause. Examples include migraine and tension-type headache.
Secondary headache	Headache due to underlying pathology.
New headache	A headache of recent onset or a chronic headache that has changed in character. Such headaches are more likely to be pathologic than unchanged chronic headaches.
Aura	Complex neurologic phenomena that precede a headache. Examples include scotoma, aphasia, and hemiparesis.
Photophobia	Pain or increased headache when looking into bright light.
Phonophobia	Pain or increased headache with exposure to loud sounds.
Thunderclap headache	A headache that occurs instantaneously with maximal intensity at its onset.

—Continued next page

Continued—

Cervicogenic headache	Referred headache pain that originates from the neck, often due to muscle tension or cervical degenerative arthritis. Also referred to as occipital neuralgia.
Positive likelihood ratio	The increase in the odds of a diagnosis if a given clinical factor is present.
Negative likelihood ratio	The decrease in the odds of a diagnosis if a given clinical factor is absent.

ETIOLOGY

Most chronic headaches are either migraines or tension-type headaches. The etiology of headache depends on the setting. Patients referred to specialized headache clinics have a disproportionately high frequency of medication-induced headache and chronic daily headache. In a study of unselected individuals in the general population, the prevalence of migraine was approximately 15% among women and 6% among men.[2] The prevalence of tension-type headache was 86% among women and 63% among men. Cluster headache, the remaining primary headache syndrome, is much less common (prevalence of approximately 0.1%).[3] In a study of 872 patients with headache presenting to an emergency department, who would be expected to have a greater likelihood of pathologic headaches, the etiologies were infection (39.3%), tension-type headache (19.3%), posttraumatic (9.3%), hypertension-related (4.8%), migraine (4.5%), subarachnoid hemorrhage (0.9%), meningitis (0.6%), and miscellaneous or no diagnosis (20.9%).[4]

Differential Diagnosis

	Prevalence Among Patients Presenting to Emergency Department With Headache[a]
Primary headaches	
Tension-type headache	12%–19%[4,5]
Migraine with or without aura	3%–5%[4,5]
Cluster headache	
Benign exertional, sexual, or cough headache	
Chronic daily headache	
Secondary headaches (common benign causes)	
Viral syndrome	39%[4]
Medication-induced headache (eg, caffeine, alcohol, analgesics, monosodium glutamate, oral contraceptive pills)	
Temporomandibular joint (TMJ) dysfunction	
Sinusitis	1.0%[5]
Cervicogenic headache	

[a]Empty cells indicate that the prevalence is unknown.

GETTING STARTED WITH THE HISTORY

- Let the patient tell the headache story in his or her own words before asking more directed and focused questions.
- Most headache diagnoses rely *entirely* on the history; the physical examination and laboratory testing only rarely offer diagnostic clues.
- Understand the patient's agenda. Even though most headaches are benign, patients often seek medical care due to concern about a brain tumor or other serious diagnosis.

Questions	Remember
Tell me more about your headaches. *When did these headaches first start?* *Give me an example of your most recent headache; tell me what you experienced from beginning to end.*	Listen to the story. Don't rush the interview by interrupting and focusing the history too soon. Reassure the patient when appropriate.

INTERVIEW FRAMEWORK

- First, correctly classify whether the headache is old or new.
- The differential diagnosis is completely different for old versus new headaches; failure to make this distinction will lead to mistakes in diagnosis, inefficient use of time in the interview, and inappropriate diagnostic testing.
- Inquire about headache characteristics using the cardinal symptom features:
  - Onset
  - Duration
  - Frequency
  - Pain character
  - Location of pain
  - Associated features including aura
  - Precipitating and alleviating factors
  - Change in frequency or character over time

IDENTIFYING ALARM SYMPTOMS

- A recent progression or change in the character of chronic headache raises concern for a pathologic cause of headache.
- Not all secondary headaches are serious (eg, viral syndrome, cervicogenic headache), but headaches that worsen or become associated with new features over a period of weeks to months are more likely to be due to a serious cause and should prompt further evaluation.

Serious Diagnoses

Serious causes for headache are rare, but they are "can't miss" diagnoses due to the morbidity of overlooking these diagnoses. The estimated 1-year prevalence in the general population for selected serious causes is as follows: giant cell arteritis (0.02% among patients > 50 years old),[6] brain tumor (0.02%),[7] metastatic cancer (0.15%),[7] stroke (0.7%), subarachnoid hemorrhage (0.01%), and arteriovenous malformation (0.02%–0.1%).

Diagnosis	Prevalence Among Patients Presenting to Emergency Department With Headache[a]
Posttraumatic headache	9.3%[4]
Hypertensive emergency	4.8%[4]
Subarachnoid hemorrhage	0.9%–1.3%[4,5,8]
Brain tumor	0.8%[8]
Meningitis	0.6%[4,8]
Giant cell arteritis (GCA)	
Benign intracranial hypertension	
Brain abscess	
Carotid or vertebral artery dissection	
Stroke	
Arteriovenous malformation (AVM)	
Carbon monoxide poisoning	

[a]Empty cells indicate that the prevalence is unknown.

After the open-ended questions, ask about the presence of the following alarm symptoms to assess for the possibility of a serious cause and to determine the pace of subsequent evaluation or "triage." Certain symptoms *always* indicate a serious cause for headache, whereas other symptoms increase concern for a pathologic cause but may also occur in benign headache syndromes. The absence of a given alarm symptom generally does *not* substantially reduce the likelihood of a particular serious cause for headache. In other words, the negative likelihood ratio for most of these alarm symptoms approaches unity (1.0).

Alarm Symptoms	If Present, Consider Serious Causes...	Positive Likelihood Ratio for Predicting Any Serious Cause	However, Benign Causes for This Feature Include...
Always indicates a serious cause for headache			
Visual loss	GCA, acute angle-closure glaucoma		
Prolonged visual aura	AVM		
Dysequilibrium	Stroke, brain tumor	49[9]	
Confusion or lethargy	Meningitis, encephalitis, brain tumor, brain abscess	1.5[10]	
New-onset seizure	Stroke, encephalitis, brain tumor	1.36[10]	
May indicate a serious cause for headache			
Fever	Meningitis, encephalitis, brain abscess		Viral syndrome, sinusitis
Weight loss	Brain tumor		
History of malignancy	Brain tumor	2.02[10]	
History of HIV infection	Central nervous system (CNS) lymphoma, toxoplasmosis, cryptococcal meningitis	1.80[10]	Sinusitis
History of neurosurgery or CNS shunt	Hydrocephalus, meningitis		
Eye pain	Acute angle-closure glaucoma		Cluster headache
Thunderclap headache	Subarachnoid hemorrhage	1.9[9]	Cluster headache
New onset after age 50	Brain tumor, stroke, GCA		Cervicogenic headache
Progressive headache over weeks to months	Brain tumor	12[9]	
Diplopia	Brain tumor, GCA, stroke, AVM	3.4 (for diagnosis of GCA)[6]	Ophthalmoplegic migraine
Hemiparesis	Brain tumor, stroke, brain abscess	3.69[10]	Migraine with typical aura
Aphasia	Brain tumor, stroke, brain abscess		Migraine with typical aura

Headache causing awakening from sleep	Brain tumor	1.7–98[9]	Cluster headache
Headache worse at work	Carbon monoxide poisoning		
Headache worse with Valsalva maneuver	Brain tumor	2.3[9]	
Nausea	Brain tumor, hydrocephalus, carbon monoxide poisoning		Migraine
Neck stiffness	Meningitis		Tension-type headache, cervicogenic headache, TMJ dysfunction
Onset of headache with exertion, cough, or sexual activity	Subarachnoid hemorrhage		Benign exertional, cough, or sexual headache

Another way to assess for alarm symptoms is to know which aspects of the history predict a higher likelihood of abnormalities on neuroimaging, which by definition represent a serious cause for headache. In a meta-analysis performed as part of the *Journal of the American Medical Association* Rational Clinical Examination series, the following factors were evaluated as potential predictors of abnormal neuroimaging consistent with a serious cause.[11] Note that the negative likelihood ratio (LR–) for most features is close to 1, indicating that the absence of the finding does not substantially reduce the likelihood of abnormal neuroimaging. An experienced clinician would learn intuitively that features with a high positive LR (LR+), such as abnormal neurologic examination or a headache that is worse with Valsalva, represent indications for neuroimaging.

Feature	LR+ for Serious Cause	LR– for Serious Cause
Cluster type headache[a]	11	0.95
Abnormal neurologic examination	5.3	0.71
Undefined headache[b]	3.8	0.66
Focal neurologic symptoms	3.1	0.79
Worse with exertion or Valsalva	2.3	0.70
Vomiting	1.8	0.47
Worsening headache	1.6	1.0
Quick-onset headache	1.3	0.79
New-onset headache	1.2	0.89
Nausea	1.1	0.86
Increased headache severity	0.83	1.2

[a]See focused questions below for features suggesting cluster headache.

[b]Headache that is difficult to classify and not clearly due to a primary headache disorder such as migraine, tension-type, or cluster headache.

The American Headache Society suggests "SSNOOP" as a mnemonic to identify patients who may have a secondary (serious) cause of headache:

- **S**ystemic symptoms (fever or weight loss)
- **S**ystemic disease (HIV infection, malignancy)
- **N**eurologic symptoms or signs
- **O**nset sudden
- **O**nset after age 40 years
- **P**revious headache history (first, worst, or different headache)

FOCUSED QUESTIONS

After hearing the headache story in the patient's own words and considering possible alarm symptoms, ask the following questions to narrow the differential diagnosis.

QUESTIONS	THINK ABOUT...
Does anyone in your immediate family have migraines?	Migraine
Describe the onset of the headache.	Thunderclap headache must prompt consideration of subarachnoid hemorrhage.
How old were you when you started experiencing these headaches?	The longer a headache has been present, the more likely it is to be benign. Migraine and tension-type headaches usually begin in adolescence.
Is this headache the same as ones you've had before, or is it different in some way?	This question addresses whether the headache is old versus new. Old headaches are usually benign.
Why did you choose to see me for the headache today?	Determine the patient's primary agenda for the visit and the most concerning feature.
Do you have any awareness or warning symptoms that occur before the headache begins?	The presence of a characteristic aura in a recurring headache syndrome establishes a diagnosis of migraine with certainty.
Onset	
Tell me about the onset of a typical headache.	
• *It occurs instantaneously and is severe in the very first second.*	Subarachnoid hemorrhage
• *It develops rapidly over 5–10 minutes.*	Cluster headache
• *It seems to get worse over the first hour or so.*	Tension-type headache Migraine
Duration	
How long does each headache last?	Note that each of the common primary headache syndromes has its own characteristic duration
• *From 4 to 72 hours*	Migraine
• *From 30 minutes to 1 week*	Tension-type headache
• *From 15 minutes to 3 hours*	Cluster headache
Frequency	
If you have recurrent headaches, how often do they occur?	These frequencies may vary substantially from the typical frequencies below.
• *Once or twice per month*	Migraine
• *Once or twice per week*	Tension-type headache
• *1–4 per day*	Cluster headache

What time of the day do your headaches normally occur?	
• *2:00 to 3:00 in the morning*	Cluster headache
• *When I awaken in the morning*	Brain tumor Obstructive sleep apnea TMJ dysfunction
• *Afternoon*	Tension-type headache
• *Weekends*	Migraine Caffeine withdrawal headaches
Pain character	
Is the headache:	
• *Throbbing, like a heartbeat?*	Migraine GCA
• *A band-like tightness or pressure around your head?*	Tension-type headache Cervicogenic headache TMJ dysfunction
• *Piercing or sharp, as in an electric shock feeling?*	Cluster headache Trigeminal neuralgia
Are your headaches:	
• *Severe and disabling?*	Migraine Subarachnoid hemorrhage
• *Mild?*	Tension-type headache GCA Brain tumor (such headaches initially are mild and not disabling; increasing severity over weeks to months is an important clue)
Location of pain	
Where is the pain located in your head?	
• *One side only but can alternate between sides*	Migraine GCA
• *Always on the same side*	Cluster headache Brain tumor AVM GCA Trigeminal neuralgia
• *Both sides of my head*	Tension-type headache GCA
• *Around my eye*	Cluster headache Trigeminal neuralgia Acute angle-closure glaucoma Sinusitis

—Continued next page

Continued—

• *My forehead*	Tension-type headache Cervicogenic headache Sinusitis
• *My temples*	Tension-type headache GCA Cluster headache Migraine
• *The back of my head and neck*	Cervicogenic headache Posterior fossa mass lesion
• *Top of my head (vertex)*	Sphenoid sinusitis Cervicogenic headache
Associated features including aura	
Do you have any warning symptoms that start before your headache?	These may continue once the headache begins (but should last for no more than 1 hour.)
• *Zigzag flashing lights on one side of both eyes for about 20 minutes*	Classic visual aura of migraine
• *Garbled speech*	Aphasia occurs in 11% of all migrainous auras,[3] but one must always consider the possibility of an acute vascular event such as carotid dissection or stroke when such symptoms occur for the first time or last for more than 1 hour.
• *Numbness or tingling on one side of your face or hand*	Hemisensory symptoms occur in 20% of all migrainous auras.[3]
• *Weakness on one side of your body*	Hemiparesis accompanies 4% of migrainous auras[3] but may also represent a stroke or intracranial mass lesion, so it requires urgent evaluation unless it occurs as part of a stable pattern over time.
Do you have any symptoms that occur at the same time as your headache?	For cluster headache, the associated symptoms occur only on the same side as the headache.
• *Red eye*	Acute angle-closure glaucoma Cluster headache
• *Tearing*	Cluster headache
• *Runny nose or nasal congestion*	Cluster headache
• *Forehead or facial sweating*	Cluster headache
• *Eyelid drooping (ptosis)*	Cluster headache
• *Small pupil (miosis)*	Cluster headache
• *Nausea*	Migraine Brain tumor
• *Photophobia*	Migraine Meningitis
• *Phonophobia*	Migraine

Precipitating and alleviating factors (headache triggers)	
Have you found that anything in particular causes your headache to occur?	
• *Certain foods (particularly chocolate, cheese)*	Migraine
• *Alcohol*	Migraine Cluster headache
• *Menses*	Migraine (usually begins immediately before or in the first few days of menses)
• *Caffeine withdrawal*	Migraine
• *Valsalva*	Brain tumor Migraine
• *Physical activity, such as walking up stairs, bending over*	Migraine Brain tumor
• *Turning your head and neck*	Cervicogenic headache
• *Touching your scalp*	GCA
Change in frequency or character over time	
Have you noticed any change in the kind of headaches you experience?	
• *The headaches have changed (eg, from throbbing to nonthrobbing or from temporal to occipital)*	Any new cause of headache
• *More severe over several weeks to months*	Brain tumor

DIAGNOSTIC APPROACH (INCLUDING ALGORITHM)

The first step is to distinguish between old and new headaches. In evaluation of new headaches, clinicians must pay particular attention to the presence of alarm features. While most new headaches are due to viral syndromes and other benign diagnoses, almost all serious or pathologic headaches are new headaches. The diagnostic algorithm is shown in Figure 9–1.

Old headaches are most often due either to migraine or tension-type headache. The above focused questions help to distinguish between these 2 common diagnoses. The presence (LR+) or absence (LR–) of the following features may help distinguish migraine from tension-type headache.[3] A positive LR of 2, for example, means that the likelihood of the diagnosis increases by 2-fold if the particular feature is *present*. A negative LR of 0.5, similarly, indicates that the likelihood of the diagnosis decreases by 2-fold if the factor is *absent*.

Feature	LR+ for the Diagnosis of Migraine Compared to Tension-Type Headache	LR– for the Diagnosis of Migraine Compared to Tension-Type Headache
Nausea	19.2	0.19
Photophobia	5.8	0.25
Phonophobia	5.2	0.38
Exacerbation by physical activity	3.7	0.24

—Continued next page

Continued—		
Unilateral headache	3.7	0.43
Throbbing headache	2.9	0.36
Chocolate as headache trigger	7.1	0.70
Cheese as headache trigger	4.9	0.68

Adapted with permission from Smetana GW. The diagnostic value of historical features in primary headache syndromes. A comprehensive review. *Arch Intern Med.* 2000;160:2729–2737.

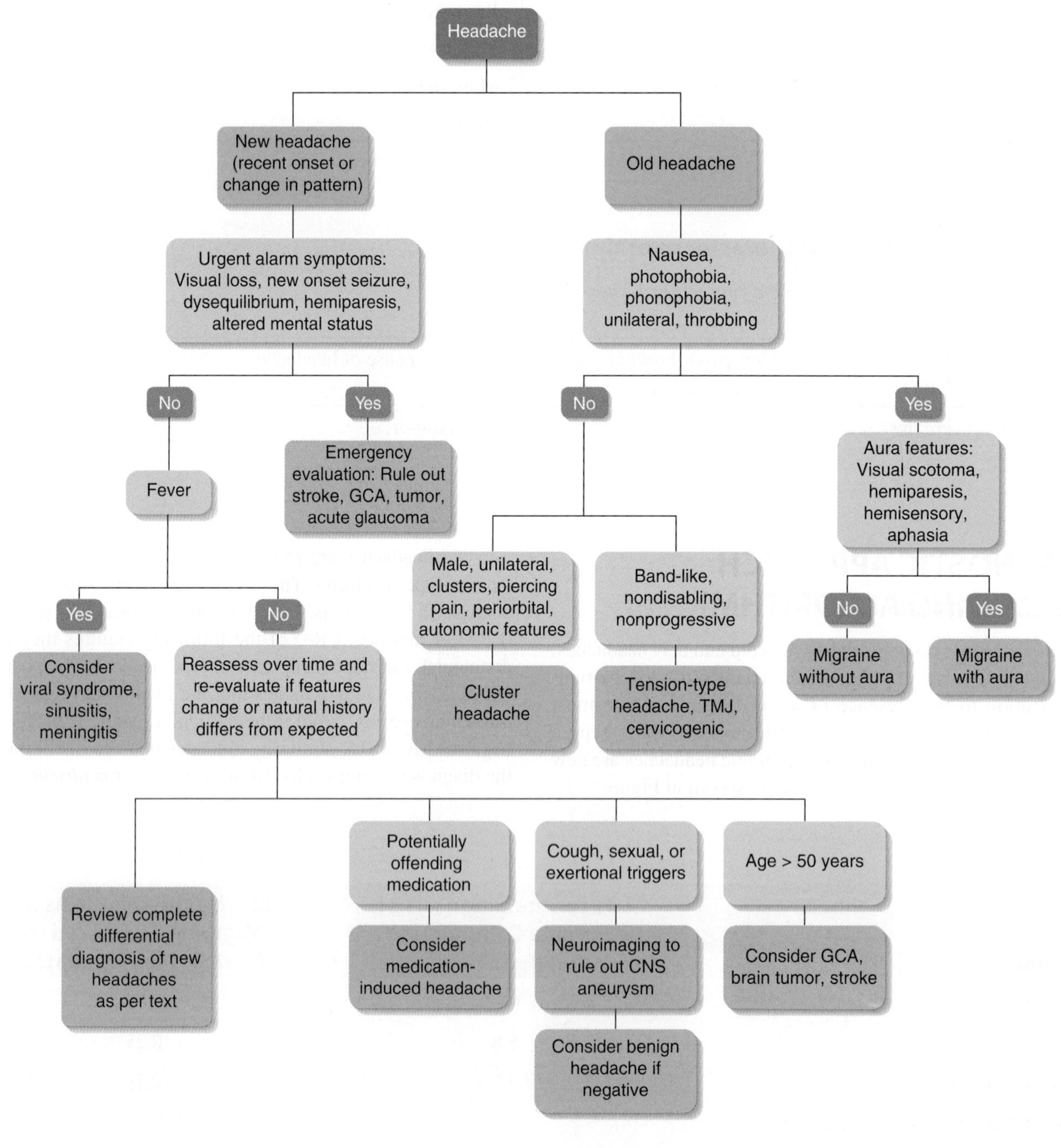

FIGURE 9–1 Algorithm for headache. CNS, central nervous system; GCA, giant cell arteritis; TMJ, temporomandibular joint.

Combinations of these features are particularly helpful to distinguish between migraine and tension-type headache. A helpful mnemonic is POUND[11]:

Mnemonic	
• **P**ulsatile quality	
• 4–72 h**O**urs	
• **U**nilateral location	
• **N**ausea or vomiting	
• **D**isabling intensity	
Total Number of 5 Features Present	**LR+ for Migraine When Compared to Tension Type Headache**
1–2	0.41
3	3.5
4–5	24

CAVEATS

- Remember to first distinguish between old and new headaches in order to correctly move through the diagnostic algorithm.
- Migraine and tension-type headache can only be diagnosed with certainty after a pattern of similar headaches occurs over time. When faced with a patient with a first episode of migraine or tension-type headache, also consider the differential diagnosis for new headaches.
- Reconsider your working diagnosis over time if the time course appears to be too short or too long for your proposed diagnosis. Each headache type has its own characteristic natural history.
- Do not diagnose benign cough, sexual, or exertional headache until neuroimaging has confirmed that no intracranial pathology exists. It is important to exclude CNS aneurysm.
- Gender differences are key considerations in the evaluation of primary headaches. Migraine headache is 3 times more common in women than in men. Cluster headache is 6 times more common in men than in women. Tension-type headache is equally prevalent in women and men.
- Most headache diagnoses are based entirely on history taking. The more typical features that are present, the more confident one can be of the diagnosis. If only a few typical features suggest your working diagnosis, expand the differential diagnosis and consider other diagnostic possibilities.
- Consider benign intracranial hypertension, dural sinus thrombosis, and new-onset migraine in patients with new headaches during pregnancy.

PROGNOSIS

Primary headache syndromes, including migraine, tension-type, and cluster headache, have an excellent prognosis. However, significant disability (lost work and school time) may result from these conditions. The prognosis for new headaches depends on the ultimate diagnosis. Unrecognized and untreated, many causes of new headaches (eg, subarachnoid hemorrhage, GCA, brain tumor, meningitis) may cause significant morbidity or mortality.

CASE SCENARIO | Resolution

A 27-year-old woman comes to your office to discuss her "sick headaches," which started during high school. Her mother nudged her to see you. The headaches do not awaken her from sleep but can be disabling and occasionally require her to miss work. Sometimes she vomits during an attack. Over the past 6 months, her headaches have become more severe and frequent, prompting her visit today.

ADDITIONAL HISTORY

Her headaches are similar in quality to the ones she has had since adolescence. They are now more severe and frequent, but the location, character, and associated symptoms have not changed. They are unilateral, throbbing, and associated with nausea and photophobia. They are usually worse during the first 2 to 3 days of her menses. You determine that this is an "old" headache. She has no alarm symptoms such as fever, dysequilibrium, focal weakness, or neck stiffness. The detail with which she can provide a careful history suggests that her mental status is normal. On some occasions, her headaches are preceded by unusual zigzag flashing lights off to the right side of her visual field lasting 20 minutes or so. On further questioning, she has been under a great deal of stress, and her sleep schedule has been erratic. She has also been drinking up to 5 to 6 cups of coffee per day.

Question: What is the most likely diagnosis?

A. Tension-type headache
B. Migraine
C. Brain tumor
D. Cervicogenic headache

Test Your Knowledge

1. You see a 40-year-old woman with throbbing headaches. She reports that the symptoms began approximately 2 months ago and have gradually worsened. They are always on the right side. On one occasion, she had a prolonged visual aura of zigzag lines that lasted for one day and persisted after the headache had resolved.

   Which of the following features is *not* an alarm symptom that should prompt concern for a serious cause of headache?

   A. New onset of headache at age 40
   B. Throbbing pain
   C. Prolonged visual aura
   D. Worsening pain over 2 months
   E. Pain always on the right side

2. Your patient, a 22-year-old woman with a presumptive diagnosis of migraine headaches, comes to see you for a routine periodic health examination.

   Which of the following locations of head pain would be most consistent with the diagnosis of migraine?

   A. Occipital
   B. Frontal
   C. Temporal
   D. Periorbital
   E. Vertex

3. Mr. Adams, a 66-year-old man, is a long-standing patient of yours. He has never described headache to you before. He schedules an urgent care visit with you to discuss the recent onset of recurring headaches.

   Which of the following features, if present, would be most concerning for a diagnosis of giant cell (temporal) arteritis?

   A. Scalp tenderness
   B. Vertex pain
   C. Unilateral pain
   D. Photophobia
   E. Lacrimation with headache

References

1. Cherry DK, Woodwell DA. National Ambulatory Medical Care Survey: 2000 summary. Advance data from vital and health statistics; No. 328. Hyattsville, MD: National Center for Health Statistics, 2002. Available at: http://www.cdc.gov/nchs/data/ad/ad328.pdf.
2. Rasmussen BK, Jensen R, Schroll M, Olesen J. Epidemiology of headache in a general population. A prevalence study. *J Clin Epidemiol*. 1991;44:1147–1157.
3. Smetana GW. The diagnostic value of historical features in primary headache syndromes. A comprehensive review. *Arch Intern Med*. 2000;160:2729–2737.
4. Dhopseh V, Anwar R, Herring C. A retrospective assessment of emergency department patients with complaint of headache. *Headache*. 1979;19:37–42.
5. Morgenstern LB, Huber JC, Luna-Gonzales H, et al. Headache in the emergency department. *Headache*. 2001;41:537–541.
6. Smetana GW, Shmerling RH. Does this patient have temporal arteritis? *JAMA*. 2002;287:92–101.
7. DeAngelis LM. Brain tumors. *N Engl J Med*. 2001;344:114–123.
8. Ramirez-Lassepas M, Espinosa CE, Cicero JJ, et al. Predictors of intracranial pathologic findings in patients who seek emergency care because of headache. *Arch Neurol*. 1997;54:1506–1509.
9. Frishberg BM, Rosenberg JH, Matchar DB, et al.; for the US Headache Consortium. Evidence-based guidelines in the primary care setting: neuroimaging in patients with nonacute headache, 2000. Available at: http://www.aan.com/professionals/practice/index.cfm.
10. Reinus WR, Erickson KK, Wippold FJ. Unenhanced emergency cranial CT: optimizing patient selection with univariate and multivariate analysis. *Radiology*. 1993;186:763–768.
11. Detsky ME, McDonald DR, Baerlocher MR. Does this patient with headache have a migraine or need neuroimaging? *JAMA*. 2006;296:1274–1283.

Suggested Reading

Edlow JA, Panagos PD, Godwin SA, Thomas TL, Decker WW, American College of Emergency Physicians. Clinical policy: critical issues in the evaluation and management of adult patients presenting to the emergency department with acute headache. *Ann Emerg Med.* 2008;52:407–436.

Frishberg BM, Rosenberg JH, Matchar DB, et al.; for the US Headache Consortium. Evidence-based guidelines in the primary care setting: neuroimaging in patients with nonacute headache. American Academy of Neurology, 2000. Available at: https://www.americanheadachesociety.org/professionalresources/USHeadacheConsortiumGuidelines.asp.

Grimaldi D, Nonino F, Cevoli S, et al. Risk stratification of non-traumatic headache in the emergency department. *J Neurol.* 2009;256:51-57.

Martin V, Elkind A. Diagnosis and classification of primary headache disorders. In: *Standards of Care for Headache Diagnosis and Treatment.* Chicago, IL: National Headache Foundation, 2004:4–18. Available at: http://www.guideline.gov/summary/summary.aspx?doc_id=6111&nbr=003966&string=headache.

Chapter 10

Insomnia

Craig R. Keenan, MD, FACP

CASE SCENARIO

A 52-year-old woman comes to your office complaining of persistent insomnia and requests a prescription for a sleeping pill that she saw on a television advertisement.

- **What are the major diagnostic considerations for this patient with insomnia?**
- **What further information do you need to know about her sleeping problems?**
- **What questions should you ask to determine if the insomnia is related to a serious condition?**

INTRODUCTION

Insomnia is a very common complaint. Between 30% and 50% of adults have insomnia at some time, and it is a persistent problem in about 20% of adults. The prevalence increases with age, and it is more common in women. About 10% of the population has insomnia with significant daytime consequences, including daytime sleepiness or fatigue, diminished energy, poor concentration, memory impairment, irritability, depressed or anxious mood, and interpersonal difficulties.[1]

Although definitions of insomnia vary, most patients describe problems with initiating sleep, frequent or prolonged awakenings, a feeling of nonrestorative sleep, or some combination of these symptoms. Negative impacts on daytime social and/or occupational functioning are present in 20% to 60% of insomnia patients.[2] Insomnia precedes the development of mood disorders in 50% of cases and anxiety disorders in 20% of cases.[2] The risk of developing depression over 1 to 3 years is approximately 5-fold in patients with insomnia.[3] Thus, insomnia can be a harbinger of future psychiatric illness. Lastly, patients with insomnia have an increased risk of industrial accidents (3- to 4-fold risk), road accidents (2- to 3-fold risk), and falls and hip fracture in the elderly population.[2,3]

Insomnia is most often precipitated by other medical or psychiatric disorders, primary sleep disorders, and medication use. This type of insomnia is called **comorbid insomnia**. Insomnia without any identifiable comorbid cause is called idiopathic or **primary insomnia**. The history is the most important diagnostic tool in establishing the underlying comorbid disorders. There are few helpful physical findings, and only rarely are specialized studies (eg, polysomnography or actigraphy) necessary. Because eliminating or mitigating the causes of insomnia remains the cornerstone of treatment, the history is critical to successful treatment.

KEY TERMS

Adjustment sleep disorder	Insomnia associated with acute life events (eg, medical or surgical illnesses, bereavement, divorce, stress).
Advanced sleep phase syndrome	A circadian rhythm disorder in which persons have difficulty with early awakenings but no difficulty initiating sleep early at night, with normal quality and duration of sleep.
Comorbid insomnia	Insomnia resulting from comorbid medical and psychiatric illnesses, medication use, or other primary sleep disorders.

—Continued next page

Continued—

Delayed sleep phase syndrome	A circadian rhythm disorder in which persons have difficulty falling asleep but have normal sleep quality and duration once sleep is initiated.
Insomnia	An experience of inadequate or poor quality sleep characterized by 1 or more of the following: difficulty falling asleep, difficulty maintaining sleep, waking up too early in the morning, or nonrefreshing sleep.
Periodic limb movement disorder (PLMD)	An asleep phenomenon characterized by periodic episodes of repetitive and highly stereotyped limb movements. Such movements may cause insomnia via frequent awakenings. Diagnosed by polysomnography.
Primary insomnia	Insomnia not due to medical, mental, or other disorders.
Psychophysiologic insomnia	Learned or conditioned insomnia. This subtype of primary insomnia usually arises from an episode of acute situational insomnia. The patient then associates the bed with not sleeping and so becomes hyperaroused when he or she would normally be sleeping. When the acute situation resolves, the conditioned insomnia persists.
Restless legs syndrome (RLS)	An awake phenomenon of intense, irresistible urge to move the legs, usually associated with paresthesias or dysesthesias. The discomfort can lead to difficulty falling asleep. Diagnosed by history.
Short sleeper	A person who has decreased total sleep time, but no significant daytime consequences. Considered a normal variant.[3]
Sleep hygiene	The collection of sleep habits that can either cause or ameliorate insomnia including: usual rise time, usual bedtime, regularity of rise and bed times, activities around bedtime (eg, eating, drinking, exercise, sex, work), activities in sleep area (eg, computer, television, or radio that is used in the bedroom), and other daytime activities (eg, daytime naps).

ETIOLOGY

The common precipitants of insomnia and their approximate prevalence are listed in the following Differential Diagnosis box.[2] Many cases are multifactorial.

Over half of insomnia patients have recurrent, persistent, or multiple health problems that contribute to poor sleep.[1,2] Mental disorders are the most common disorders, causing 30% to 40% of cases. Of those, depressive or anxiety disorders are the most common, and nearly 80% of patients with depression have insomnia.[4] Medical or neurologic conditions cause about 4% to 11% of insomnia cases. The most common primary sleep disorders that cause insomnia are RLS, PLMD, and sleep-related breathing disorders. These account for 20% to 30% of insomnia cases. Bed partners are often very helpful in providing evidence of sleep apneas and PLMD by reporting heavy snoring, observed apneas, or limb movements. Medication side effects are also common causes of insomnia. The most common culprits include anticonvulsants, antidepressants, antihypertensives, antineoplastics, bronchodilators, anticholinergics, corticosteroids, decongestants, hormonal therapies, levodopa, stimulants, and nicotine.

The duration of insomnia can help narrow the diagnostic possibilities. **Transient insomnia** lasts less than 1 week; **short-term insomnia** lasts 1 to 3 weeks; and **chronic insomnia** lasts greater than 3 weeks. The causes of transient and short-term insomnia usually involve acute events, including changes in sleep environment, jet lag, changes in a work shift, environmental issues (excessive noise or extremes of temperature), stressful life events, acute medical or surgical illnesses, use of stimulant medications (eg, corticosteroids, decongestants, bronchodilators, amphetamines, or cocaine), or withdrawal from central nervous system depressant substances (eg, alcohol or benzodiazepines). Chronic insomnia often starts with an acute event. When insomnia persists, however, it is generally related to a broader range of problems. The long list of potential causes can be divided into 5 main categories: medical or neurologic disorders, mental disorders, medication and substance effects, lifestyle issues, and sleep disorders.

Some patients with chronic insomnia have no objective evidence of a sleep disorder, a condition called sleep-state misperception. Diagnosis requires specialized studies (polysomnography or actigraphy).

Differential Diagnosis

	Prevalence[a,2]
Mental health disorders	*30%–40%*
Depressive disorders	
Anxiety disorders (eg, posttraumatic stress disorder, generalized anxiety disorder, panic disorder)	
Bipolar disorder	
Other disorders	
Medical or neurologic disorders	*4%–11%*
Chronic pain	
Congestive heart failure (CHF)	
Ischemic heart disease	
Chronic obstructive pulmonary disease (COPD)/asthma	
Peptic ulcer disease (PUD)	
Gastroesophageal reflux disease (GERD)	
Perimenopause	
Chronic fatigue syndrome	
Fibromyalgia, rheumatoid arthritis, other musculoskeletal disorders	
End-stage kidney disease	
Benign prostatic hypertrophy	
Urinary incontinence	
Thyroid disorders	
Diabetes mellitus or insipidus	
Allergic rhinitis	
Stroke	
Dementia	
Neurodegenerative and movement disorders	
Brain tumors	
Posttraumatic insomnia due to brain injury	
Epilepsy	
Headache syndromes	
Fatal familial insomnia	
Medications	*3%–7%*
Side effects of over-the-counter and prescription drugs	
Illicit drug use	
Alcohol abuse	
Caffeine	

—Continued next page

Continued—	
Nicotine	
Withdrawal from central nervous system depressants	
Lifestyle	
Shift work	10%
Poor sleep hygiene or environmental factors (eg, noise, temperature)	
Jet lag	
Stressful life events	
Primary sleep disorders	***12%–16%***
Idiopathic insomnia	
Psychophysiologic insomnia	5%–9%
Sleep apnea syndromes	
Sleep-state misperception	15%
RLS or PLMD	
Circadian rhythm disorders (delayed or advanced sleep phase syndromes)	
Altitude insomnia	

[a]Empty cells indicate that the prevalence is unknown.

GETTING STARTED WITH THE HISTORY

- Review the patient's medical record before the visit. Potential causes of the insomnia (ie, pre-existing medical or psychiatric disorders) should be identified and explored further in the interview.
- If possible, have the patient keep a sleep log for the 2 weeks before the office visit. It provides invaluable information including bed time, arising time, daytime naps, amount of time required to fall asleep, number and duration of nocturnal awakenings, total sleep time, and subjective evaluations of sleep quality (see Sample Sleep Diary).
- If possible, the patient's bed partner should attend the visit to supplement the history.

INTERVIEW FRAMEWORK

- Detail the nature and development of the sleep problem.
  - Determine the chief sleep symptom—difficulty falling asleep, awakenings, or poor or unrefreshing sleep.
  - Determine the chronology of the insomnia including onset, precipitating factors, duration, and frequency.
  - Evaluate the patient's sleep hygiene.
  - Assess effects on daytime functioning and social or occupational function to gauge the severity of insomnia. Validated questionnaires can assist with this, including the Epworth Sleepiness Scale or Insomnia Severity Index, which can be easily found online.
  - Review treatments that the patient has already tried and assess their efficacy.
- Expand the history to cover potentially contributing medical, psychiatric, and sleep disorders.
  - Review past medical and psychiatric history, medications, and substance use history.
  - Perform a review of symptoms that have not been covered by your other questions.
- Get collateral history from a bed partner, whenever possible. They can give information on the quality and quantity of sleep, daytime consequences, and nocturnal events (eg, snoring, apneas, and limb movements).
- Have the patient complete a sleep diary (if not already done). This can help determine an accurate diagnosis and may also be repeated in the future to assess response to treatment.

IDENTIFYING ALARM SYMPTOMS

The alarm symptoms associated with insomnia relate to the severity of the underlying causes.

Alarm Symptoms	Serious Diagnoses	Potential Problems
Heavy snoring, observed apneas, daytime somnolence	Obstructive sleep apnea or central sleep apnea	Untreated hypoxia can lead to right heart failure, pulmonary hypertension Hypersomnolence can lead to motor vehicle or industrial accidents
Suicidal or homicidal thoughts	Severe psychiatric disorders (depression, bipolar disorder, psychosis)	Suicide Homicide
Nocturnal chest pain or pressure	Unstable coronary artery disease	Risk for myocardial infarction or arrhythmia
Nocturnal breathing difficulties	Decompensated pulmonary disease (asthma, COPD) Decompensated CHF Unstable coronary disease Undiagnosed sleep apnea syndromes	Marker for worsening respiratory, cardiac disease Possible chronic hypoxia

FOCUSED QUESTIONS

After initial open-ended questions, it is usually necessary to probe more specifically to explore possible causes of insomnia.

QUESTIONS	THINK ABOUT...
Characterize the sleep complaint	
Describe what you mean by "insomnia."	
Is your main problem:	
• *Falling asleep?*	Anxiety disorders Poor sleep hygiene Delayed sleep phase syndrome RLS Sleep apnea rarely causes problems falling asleep
• *Early awakening?*	Frequently occurs with depression Advanced sleep phase syndrome
• *Frequent awakening?*	Sleep apnea Nocturnal angina or respiratory diseases PLMD Medication effects Environmental factors

—Continued next page

Continued—

• *Nonrefreshing sleep?*	Sleep apnea Fibromyalgia
Determine the chronology	
When did your problems with sleep start?	Childhood onset suggests primary insomnia. Transient or short-term insomnia is often due to an acute life event.
What do you think started the insomnia? Are there any life events that have affected your sleep (births, deaths, job change, move, work stress, new bed partner, financial stress)?	The initial cause of insomnia (it may not be the ongoing cause).
How many nights per week do you have problems with sleep?	Determines severity.
How long does it take you to fall asleep?	
What do you do when you cannot fall asleep?	
Do you wake up at night? If so, how many times and at what time?	
Why do you wake up?	Specific symptoms may suggest medical conditions or medications.
How long do you remain awake?	
What do you think is causing your insomnia now?	May discover environmental factors, stressors, medical or psychiatric problems.
How many hours a night do you sleep?	
Did you use to be a good sleeper?	If long-standing or began in childhood or adolescence, consider primary insomnia.
Are you apprehensive in the evenings about going to sleep?	Preoccupation with insomnia suggests psychophysiologic insomnia.
Assess sleep hygiene	
Describe a usual day and night.	To determine sleep habits. Patterns of sleep at unusual times may help identify circadian rhythm disorders.
What time do you get up on weekdays? On weekends? What time do you go to sleep on weekdays? On weekends?	Erratic bedtime and rise times can lead to insomnia (poor hygiene).
Describe your activities shortly before bedtime? Do you eat after 9 PM? Exercise in the late evening? Have sex? Read or watch TV in bed? Work or pay bills?	All of these activities may cause insomnia.
Do you nap during the day?	Napping can lead to nighttime insomnia.
Does your bed partner adversely affect your sleep?	Bed partner sleep disorders (insomnia, PLMD, sleep apnea, snoring) can cause insomnia.
Do you have a TV or computer in your bedroom?	Nonsleep activities can cause insomnia.

Is your bedroom quiet and dark?	Possible environmental factors (noise, light).
Do you sleep better away from home?	If true, suggests maladaptive conditioning (psychophysiologic insomnia).
Evaluate daytime function to help determine severity of insomnia	
How does your night's sleep affect your day?	
Are you fatigued or sleepy?	Nonspecific; however, excessive daytime sleepiness or falling asleep at inappropriate times suggests sleep apnea or narcolepsy.
Do you have poor concentration?	
Are you irritable?	Irritability may be a consequence of inadequate sleep.
Does it affect your job?	
Does it affect your personal relationships?	
Does it affect your mood during the day?	
Do you nap during the day?	Daytime naps can be a consequence of insomnia or can cause insomnia.
Assess prior treatments	
Are you taking or have you taken anything for your sleep?	Helps in devising treatment plan
What has worked and what has not?	
Have you tried anything else?	Potential nonpharmacologic treatments
Assess for substance, medical, and mental health causes	
What medical problems do you have? Do you have any mental health problems?	
What medications do you take? Do you take any herbal or other over-the-counter medications?	Many herbal preparations and cold or allergy medications contain stimulants. Many prescription drugs cause insomnia.
Do you drink caffeinated beverages or eat chocolate?	Caffeine is a common stimulant often overlooked by patients.
Do you smoke or use tobacco?	Nicotine is a common stimulant.
Do you drink alcohol or use other drugs? How much?	Alcohol and illicit drug use or withdrawal
Do you feel depressed? Do you have feelings of guilt or hopelessness? How is your appetite? Do you find that you don't enjoy things that you used to enjoy? Have you lost or gained weight?	Depressive disorders Bipolar disorder
Do you feel anxious? Have panic attacks?	Anxiety disorders

—Continued next page

Assess nocturnal symptoms	
At night, do you awaken with:	
• *Shortness of breath?*	Uncontrolled asthma COPD Coronary disease CHF Sleep apnea
• *Chest pain or pressure or epigastric pain?*	Coronary artery disease GERD PUD
• *Cough?*	CHF Uncontrolled asthma COPD Other lung disease
Are you a heavy snorer?	Obstructive sleep apnea
Has anyone ever told you that you stop breathing or choke or that you have leg or arm jerking while you are sleeping?	Obstructive or central sleep apnea or PLMD
Do your legs sometimes twitch or can't keep still? Do you get leg pain as you try to go to sleep?	PLMD or RLS
Do you sleep walk or talk?	Parasomnias
Do you feel that you want to sleep at the wrong times?	Circadian rhythm disorders
Do you get up to urinate frequently?	Polyuria due to diuretics Prostate disease Diabetes causes frequent awakenings
Do you have headaches at night?	Headaches (due to any cause) Need further evaluation
Do you have pain at night that keeps you awake?	Any pain syndrome can cause insomnia

DIAGNOSTIC APPROACH (INCLUDING ALGORITHM)

The diagnostic algorithm for insomnia is shown in Figure 10–1.

CAVEATS

- Because insomnia is often multifactorial, it is important to work through all steps in the diagnostic algorithm.
- Insomnia is underrecognized in primary care practice. Less than half of primary care physicians take a sleep history, and physicians are unaware of 60% of severe cases of insomnia.[5–7]
- Insomnia treatment addresses the underlying causes, so multiple modalities are often required. Optimizing treatment of underlying mental, medical, or sleep disorders is the primary treatment, but behavioral therapy to improve sleep hygiene is also a key component. Thus, targets for intervention are readily identified by a thorough history.

PROGNOSIS

Studies show that insomnia is usually very persistent, especially in patients with significant comorbid medical and psychiatric conditions.[8] Recent studies show that 46% to 72% of patients with insomnia continue to have insomnia symptoms 3 years later.[2,8]

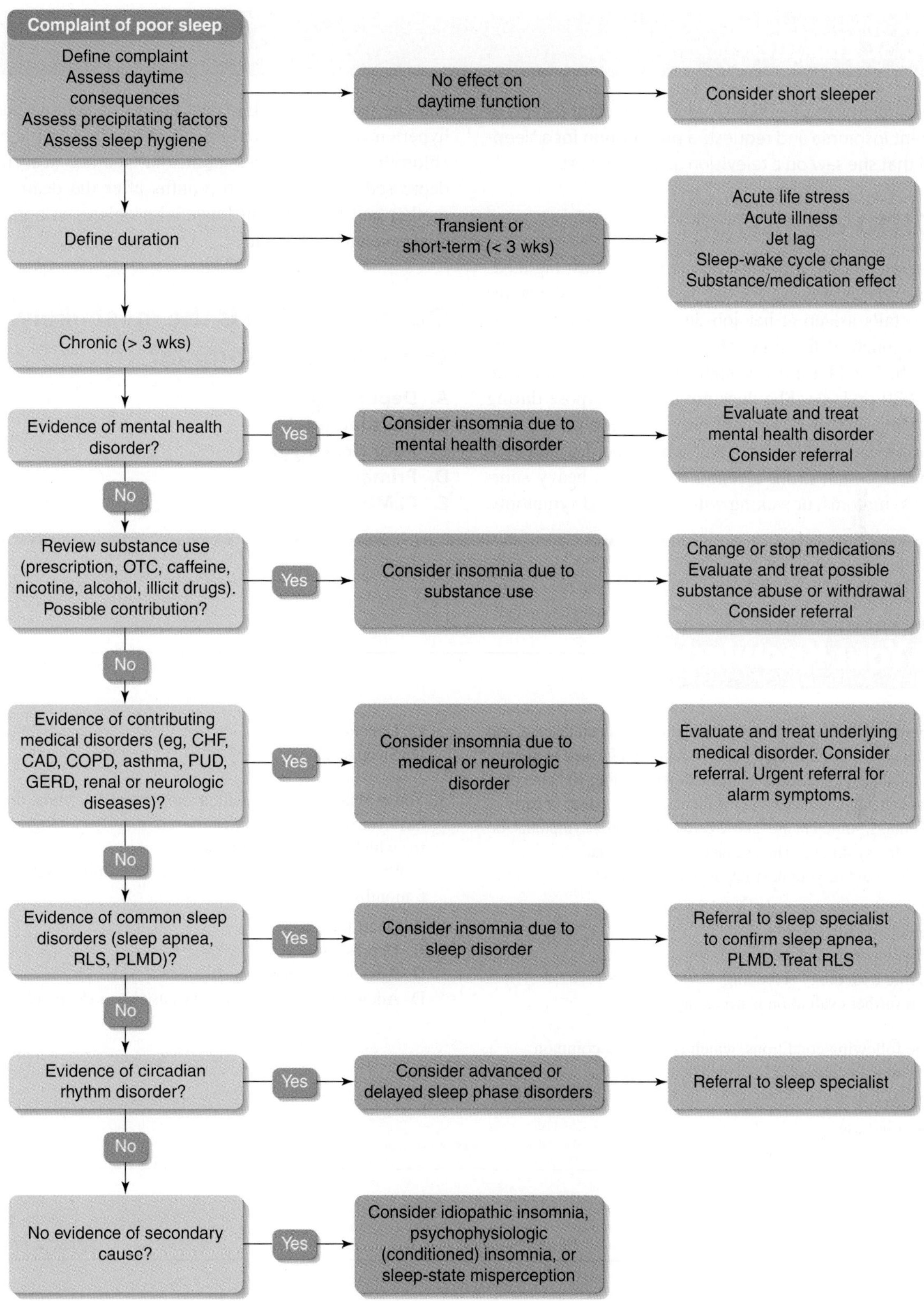

FIGURE 10–1 Diagnostic algorithm: Insomnia. CAD, coronary artery disease; CHF, congestive heart failure; COPD, chronic obstructive pulmonary disease; GERD, gastroesophageal reflux disease; OTC, over the counter; PLMD, periodic limb movement disorder; PUD, peptic ulcer disease; RLS, restless legs syndrome; wks, weeks.

CASE SCENARIO | Resolution

A 52-year-old woman comes to your office complaining of persistent insomnia and requests a prescription for a sleeping pill that she saw on a television advertisement.

ADDITIONAL HISTORY

The patient has had difficulty falling asleep most nights as well as early awakening for the past 6 months. She states that she falls asleep at her job due to this, and she feels fatigued much of the time. Her sleep habits are that she goes to bed at 11 PM every night but does not fall asleep until 12:30 or 1 AM. She does not nap on purpose during the day and uses her bedroom only for sleep or sex. She does drink caffeinated sodas throughout the day and evening but does not drink alcohol. She denies heavy snoring, leg symptoms, or waking with any medical symptoms, and she is not obese. Her past history is notable only for hypertension, and the only medication she takes is hydrochlorothiazide. She does admit that she has been feeling depressed over the past 6 months after the death of her mother and with current financial problems at home. She denies suicidal ideation.

Question: What is the most likely cause of her insomnia?

A. Depression
B. Multifactorial
C. Poor sleep hygiene
D. Primary insomnia
E. PLMD

Test Your Knowledge

1. A 55-year-old man with hypertension, coronary heart disease, and obesity comes in complaining that he feels unrefreshed by sleep with daytime fatigue and sleepiness, despite getting 10 hours of sleep each night. He denies any difficulty falling asleep or early awakenings, stimulant use, active cardiopulmonary symptoms, or psychiatric symptoms. His examination was normal.
   What would be your next step in his evaluation?
   A. Formal polysomnography (sleep study)
   B. Sleep log for 2 weeks
   C. History from bed partner
   D. Urine toxicology screening
   E. No further evaluation is necessary

2. Of the following conditions, which is the most common contributor to comorbid insomnia?
   A. PLMD
   B. Alcohol use
   C. Depression
   D. Sleep apnea

3. You evaluate a patient with insomnia and determine that he has obstructive sleep apnea (based on polysomnography), for which you institute therapy.
   What condition is he at risk for developing over the next 6 months?
   A. Heart failure
   B. Depression
   C. Advanced sleep phase disorder
   D. Addiction to benzodiazepines used as a sleep aid

References

1. Ohayon MM. Epidemiology of insomnia: what we know and what we still need to learn. *Sleep Med Rev.* 2002;6:97–111.
2. Ohayon MM. Observation of the natural evolution of insomnia in the American general population cohort. *Sleep Med Clin.* 2009;4:87–92.
3. Roth T. Insomnia: definition, prevalence, etiology, and consequences. *J Clin Sleep Med.* 2007;3(Suppl):S7–S10.
4. Ohayon MM, Shapiro CM, Kennedy SH. Differentiating DSM-IV anxiety and depressive disorders in the general population: comorbidity and treatment consequences. *Can J Psychiatry.* 2000;45:166–172.
5. Hohagen F, Rink K, Kappler C, et al. Prevalence and treatment of insomnia in general practice. A longitudinal study. *Eur Arch Psychiatry Clin Neurosci.* 1993;242:329–336.

6. Schramm, E, Hohagen F, Kappler C, et al. Mental comorbidity of chronic insomnia in general practice attenders using DSM III-R. *Acta Psychiatr Scand.* 1995;91:10–17.
7. Everitt DE, Avorn J, Baker MW. Clinical decision making in the evaluation and treatment of insomnia. *Am J Med.* 1990;89:357–362.
8. Morin CM, Belanger L, LeBlanc M, et al. The natural history of insomnia: a population-based 3-year longitudinal study. *Arch Intern Med.* 2009;169:447–453.
9. Espie CA, Morin CM, eds. *Insomnia: A Clinical Guide to Assessment and Treatment*. New York, NY: Kluwer Academic/Plenum Publishers, 2003:135–136.
10. Shutte-Rodin S, Broch L, Buysse D, et al. Clinical guideline for the evaluation and management of chronic insomnia in adults. *J Clin Sleep Med.* 2008;4:487–504.

Suggested Reading

Ohayon MM. Observation of the natural evolution of insomnia in the American general population cohort. *Sleep Med Clin.* 2009;4:87–92.

Shutte-Rodin S, Broch L, Buysse D, et al. Clinical guideline for the evaluation and management of chronic insomnia in adults. *J Clin Sleep Med.* 2008;4:487–504.

Sample Sleep Diary [9,10]

Fill out in the morning	Day 1	Day 2	Day 3	Day 4	Day 5	Day 6	Day 7
Rise time today							
Bedtime last night							
Estimated time to fall asleep							
Estimated number of awakenings							
Estimated total time awake during the night							
Estimated amount of sleep							
How restful was your sleep? 0 (not at all) 1 2 3 4 (very)							
Fill out at bedtime							
Rate how you felt today: 0 (very tired) 1 2 3 4 (wide awake)							
Number of naps (time and duration)							
Alcoholic drinks (number and time)							
Caffeinated drinks (number and time)							
Stressors from the day							
Activities this evening (eg, exercise, sex, paying bills)							
Time of evening meal and snacks							

Chapter 11

Lymphadenopathy

Michael H. Zaroukian, MD, PhD, Gina R. Chacon, MD, and Nephertiti Efeovbokhan, MD

CASE SCENARIO

A 19-year-old man comes to your clinic complaining of fever, headache, sore throat, and fatigue that started about 2 weeks ago. He has also noticed multiple swollen lymph glands in the front of his neck. He denies any rhinorrhea or cough. He is concerned because the lymph glands are sore to touch, and his symptoms are not improving.

- **What additional questions are required to learn more about his swollen lymph glands?**
- **How would you classify his lymphadenopathy?**
- **What are the possible causes of enlarged lymph nodes?**
- **How does the interviewer establish a presumptive diagnosis using open-ended questions followed by more focused history taking?**
- **How do you distinguish benign causes of lymphadenopathy from more serious ones that require further evaluation?**

INTRODUCTION

Lymphadenopathy is the enlargement of 1 or more lymph nodes. Patients may be alerted to the presence of enlarged lymph nodes by noticing visible nodular swelling, palpability, pain, or tenderness in 1 or more lymph node regions. It is normal to be able to palpate small lymph nodes in the neck and groin regions but generally not in the supraclavicular fossa, axilla, epitrochlear, or popliteal regions.

Lymphadenopathy generally results from infiltration of lymph nodes by inflammatory or neoplastic cells, proliferation of resident lymphocytes, or expansion due to hemorrhage or abscess formation. In primary care settings, lymphadenopathy is rarely due to malignancy; upper respiratory tract infections or nonspecific conditions account for over two-thirds of cases. However, the risk of malignancy increases with age and other factors.

Careful history taking is important in determining the cause of lymphadenopathy. Patients may be concerned or even anxious that lymphadenopathy may be a manifestation of cancer. The medical interview can assist in excluding malignancy or other serious underlying disease in most patients and inform subsequent evaluation for the remainder.

KEY TERMS

Lymphadenopathy[1]	Abnormal enlargement of 1 or more lymph nodes (> 1.0 cm in adults; > 1.5 cm in children and adolescents).
Generalized lymphadenopathy[2]	Lymph node enlargement affecting multiple body regions.
Localized lymphadenopathy[2]	Lymph node enlargement limited to a single body region (eg, cervical, inguinal).

ETIOLOGY

In primary care practice, more than two-thirds of patients with lymphadenopathy have nonspecific causes or upper respiratory illnesses (viral or bacterial), and less than 1% have a malignancy.[1–4] In one study, 84% of patients referred for evaluation of lymphadenopathy had a "benign" diagnosis. The remaining 16% had a malignancy (lymphoma or metastatic adenocarcinoma). Of the patients with benign lymphadenopathy, 63% had a nonspecific or reactive etiology (no causative agent found), and the remainder had a specific cause demonstrated, most commonly infectious mononucleosis, toxoplasmosis, or tuberculosis. Thus, the vast majority of patients with ***lymphadenopathy*** will have a nonspecific etiology requiring few if any diagnostic tests.[3]

A comprehensive discussion of the myriad agents and diseases associated with lymphadenopathy is beyond the scope of this chapter but can be found elsewhere.[3] The major causes of lymphadenopathy in the United States are listed below using the mnemonic CINEMA DIVITT (**c**ongenital, **i**nfectious, **ne**oplastic, **e**ndocrine, **m**etabolic, **a**llergic, **d**egenerative, **i**nflammatory/immunologic, **v**ascular, **i**diopathic or iatrogenic, **t**raumatic, **t**oxic). Another potentially useful framework for classifying and recalling the myriad causes of lymphadenopathy uses the mnemonic MIAMI (**m**alignancies, **i**nfections, **a**utoimmune disorders, **m**iscellaneous and unusual conditions, and **i**atrogenic causes).[4]

Differential Diagnosis[1,4]

	Prevalence[a] by Category in Primary Care[1,4]
Congenital	
• Congenital syphilis	
Infectious[5]	*18% (upper respiratory infections)*
• Bacteria	
— Actinomycosis	
— Atypical mycobacterial infections	
— Brucellosis	
— Cat-scratch disease (*Bartonella henselae*)	
— Chancroid	
— Chlamydia (lymphogranuloma venereum and trachoma)	
— Diphtheria	
— Leprosy	
— Lyme disease	
— Lymphogranuloma venereum	
— Plague	
— Primary and secondary syphilis	
— Scarlet fever	
— Skin infection (streptococci, staphylococci)	
— Streptococcal pharyngitis	
— Tuberculosis (TB)	
—Tularemia	
— Dental pathology (periodontitis)	
• Viruses	
— Adenovirus	
— Cytomegalovirus (CMV)	
— Epidemic keratoconjunctivitis	
— Epstein-Barr virus (infectious mononucleosis)	
— Hepatitis B and C	
— Herpes simplex	
— Herpesvirus-6	

— Herpesvirus-8	
— Human immunodeficiency virus (HIV)	
— Measles (rubeola)	
— Rubella	
— Mumps	
— Vaccinia (smallpox vaccine)	
— Varicella-zoster virus (chickenpox)	
• Fungi	
— Coccidioidomycosis	
— Cryptococcosis	
— Histoplasmosis	
— Paracoccidioidomycosis	
— Sporotrichosis	
• Parasites	
— Chagas disease	
— Filariasis	
— Kala-azar	
— Leishmaniasis	
— Toxoplasmosis	
— Trypanosomiasis	
• Rickettsiae	
— Q fever	
— Rickettsialpox	
— Scrub typhus	
• Mites	
— Scabies	
Neoplastic	***0.8%–1.1% (4% if age > 40 years)***
• Lymphoma	
• Leukemia	
• Metastatic solid tumors (major primary sites): breast, colon, esophagus, head and neck, kidney, lung, ovary, prostate, skin (melanoma), stomach, testes	
Endocrine	
• Adrenal insufficiency	
• Hyperthyroidism	
• Hypothyroidism	
• Multiple endocrine neoplasia (see Neoplastic)	*—Continued next page*

Continued—	
Metabolic	
• Lipid storage diseases (Gaucher's, Niemann-Pick, Fabry's, Tangier's)	
• Severe hypertriglyceridemia	
Allergic	
• Serum sickness	
Degenerative	
• Amyloidosis (secondary)	
Inflammatory/immunologic	
• Angioimmunoblastic lymphadenopathy	
• Amyloidosis (primary)	
• Dermatomyositis	
• Graft-versus-host disease • Juvenile rheumatoid arthritis	
• Mixed connective tissue disease	
• Primary biliary cirrhosis	
• Rheumatoid arthritis • Serum sickness • Silicone-associated	
• Systemic lupus erythematosus	
• Sarcoidosis	
• Sjögren's syndrome	
Vascular	
• Vasculitis — Churg-Strauss syndrome (adults) — Kawasaki's disease (children)	
Idiopathic or iatrogenic	***29%–64%***
• Nonspecific lymphadenopathy	
• Prescribed medications (see Toxic)	
Traumatic	***32% (including cuts and bites, in which secondary infection causes lymphadenopathy)***
• Abrasions and lacerations	
• Burns	
• Cat-scratch disease (Bartonella henselae)	
• Operations	
Toxic (drugs, chemicals)	
• Antihypertensive medications — Atenolol	

— *Captopril*	
— Hydralazine	
• Antimicrobials	
— Cephalosporins	
— Penicillin	
— Pyrimethamine	
— Sulfonamides	
• Antiseizure medications	
— Carbamazepine	
— Phenytoin	
— Primidone	
• Antirheumatics	
— Allopurinol	
— Gold	
• Sulindac	
• Chemicals	
— Berylliosis	
— Silicosis	

[a]Prevalence estimate is unavailable when not indicated.

GETTING STARTED WITH THE HISTORY

- Before the visit, review the patient's problems and medications as well as his or her past, family, social, sexual, travel, and occupational history for relevant clues.
- Remember that the risk of malignancy increases with age, particularly after age 50.
- Review the anatomy of the lymphatic system and the tissues and organs that drain to each lymph node group.[6]

Open-Ended Questions	Tips for Effective Interviewing
Tell me about the lump(s) you are feeling.	Establish a setting of comfort and trust.
• *Where do you feel it?*	Begin with open-ended questions before focusing.
• *What does it feel like?*	Cover all important question areas not otherwise mentioned by the patient (see mnemonic below: **COLD RAP TAPE**).
• *When did you first notice it?*	
• *Does it seem to be changing with time?*	Character: What is it like?
Have you had any recent illnesses or other symptoms?	Onset: When did it start? Location: Where do you notice it? Duration: How long does it last?

—Continued next page

Continued—

Tell me about your work, hobbies, pets, and travels.	Relieving factors: What makes it better? Aggravating factors: What makes it worse? Precipitating factors: What brings it on? Therapy: What have you tried to make it better? Associated symptoms: Do you have any other symptoms along with this? Past medical history: Have you ever had anything like this before? Emotional impact: What concerns do you have about this and how it may affect your life?
Can you think of any exposures you may have had to infectious agents, chemicals, insects, or people who were ill?	
Have you taken any medications lately?	
Tell me about your current or past use of tobacco and alcohol.	
Have you or any member of your family ever had any type of cancer?	
Tell me about your sexual history.	

INTERVIEW FRAMEWORK

- Establish the onset and course of lymph node enlargement.
- Determine the presence or absence of other symptoms and whether symptoms are localized or generalized.
- Ask about exposures related to work, home, hobbies, habits, pets, travel, sexual activity, and medications.

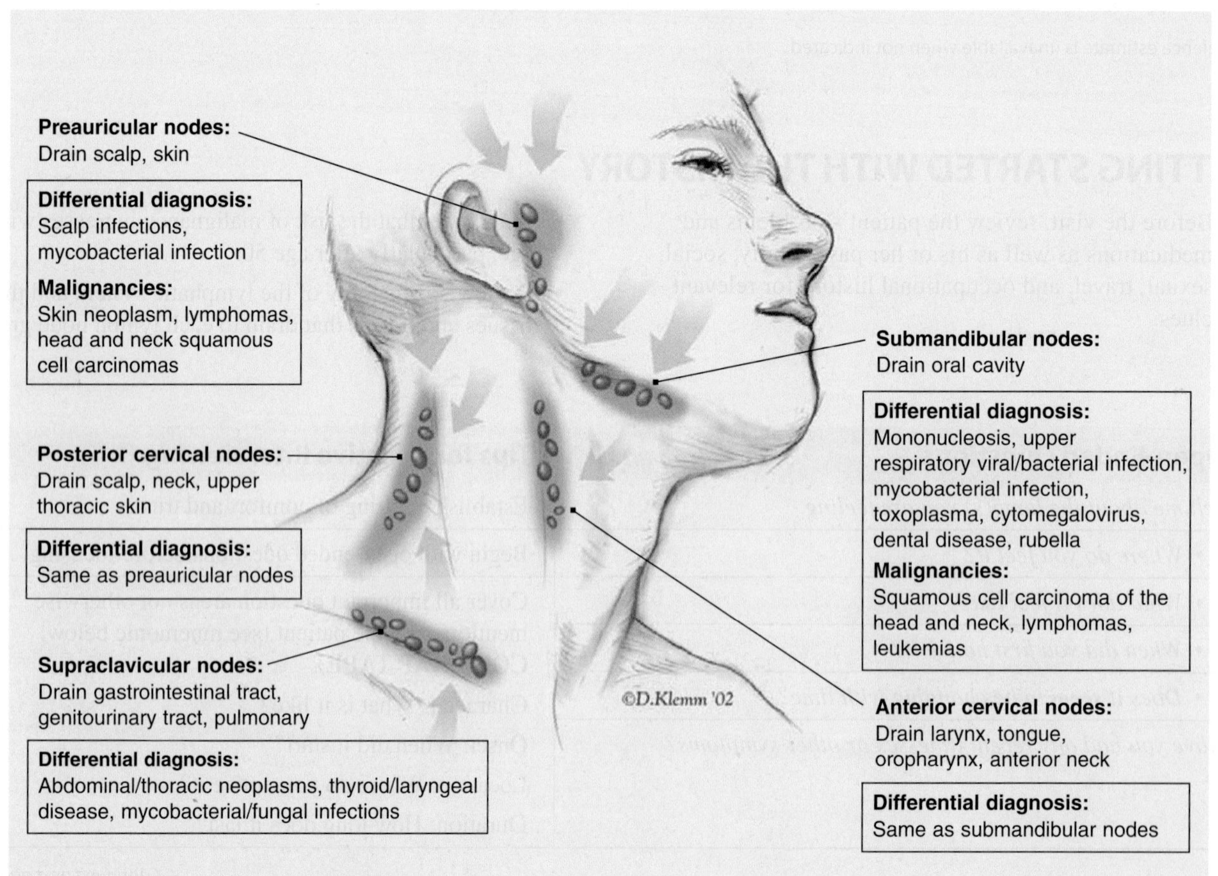

FIGURE 11–1 Lymph nodes of the head and neck, and the regions that they drain. Reprinted with permission from Bazemore AW, Smucker DR. Lymphadenopathy and malignancy. *Am Fam Physician*. 2002;66:2103–2110. Copyright © David Klemm.

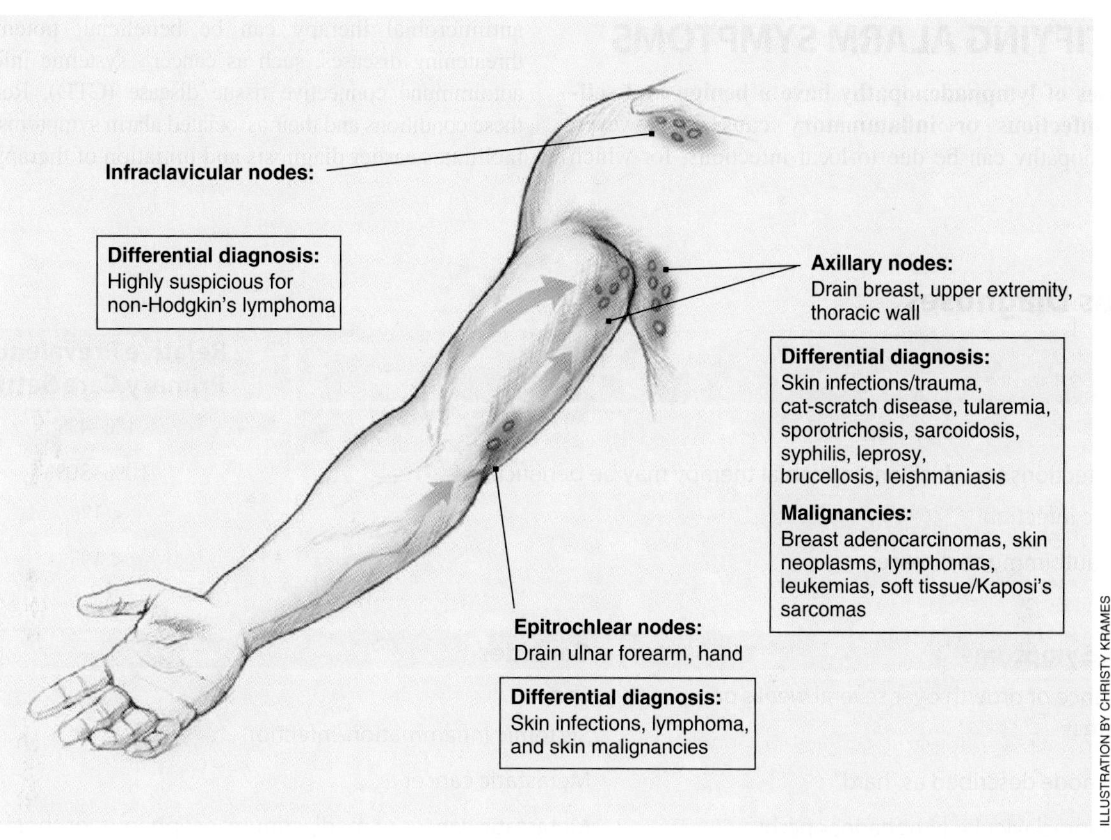

FIGURE 11–2 Axillary lymphatics and the structures that they drain. Reprinted with permission from Bazemore AW, Smucker DR. Lymphadenopathy and malignancy. *Am Fam Physician*. 2002;66:2103–2110. Copyright © Christy Krames.

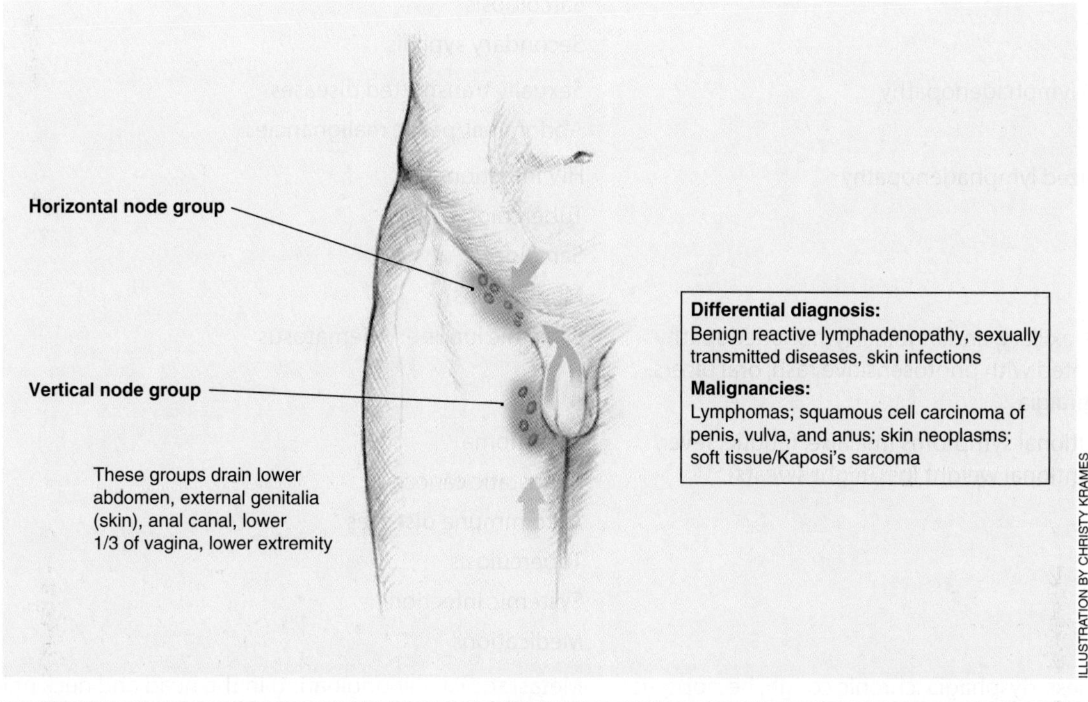

Horizontal node group
Vertical node group
These groups drain lower
abdomen, external genitalia
(skin), anal canal, lower
1/3 of vagina, lower extremity
Differential diagnosis:
Benign reactive lymphadenopathy, sexually
transmitted diseases, skin infections
Malignancies:
Lymphomas; squamous cell carcinoma of
penis, vulva, and anus; skin neoplasms;
soft tissue/Kaposi's sarcoma
ILLUSTRATION BY CHRISTY KRAMES

FIGURE 11–3 Inguinal lymphatics and the structures that they drain. Reprinted with permission from Bazemore AW, Smucker DR. Lymphadenopathy and malignancy. *Am Fam Physician*. 2002;66:2103–2110. Copyright © Christy Krames.

IDENTIFYING ALARM SYMPTOMS

Most cases of lymphadenopathy have a benign and self-limited infectious or inflammatory cause.[7,8] However, lymphadenopathy can be due to local infections, for which antimicrobial therapy can be beneficial; potentially life-threatening diseases, such as cancer[4]; systemic infection; and autoimmune connective tissue disease (CTD). Remembering these conditions and their associated alarm symptoms or features facilitates earlier diagnosis and initiation of therapy.

Serious Diagnoses

	Relative Prevalence in Primary Care Settings
Cancer	1%–4%
Local infections for which antimicrobial therapy may be beneficial	10%–30%
Systemic infection	< 1%
Severe autoimmune disease	< 1%

Alarm Symptoms	Consider
Persistence or growth over several weeks or months	Cancer Systemic inflammation/infection
Lymph node described as "hard"	Metastatic cancer
Right supraclavicular lymphadenopathy	Metastatic cancer of mediastinum, esophagus, or thorax
Left supraclavicular lymphadenopathy	Metastatic cancer originating in thorax, abdomen, or pelvis
Axillary area without local trauma or infection	Breast cancer Other metastatic cancer
Epitrochlear area without local trauma or infection	Lymphoma Sarcoidosis Secondary syphilis
Inguinal lymphadenopathy	Sexually transmitted diseases Abdominal/pelvic malignancies
Generalized lymphadenopathy	HIV infection Tuberculosis Sarcoidosis Medications
Cervical, axillary, and inguinal lymphadenopathy associated with photosensitive rash, oral ulcers, or arthralgia	Systemic lupus erythematosus
Constitutional symptoms (malaise, fatigue, fever, unintentional weight loss, night sweats)	Lymphoma Metastatic cancer Autoimmune diseases Tuberculosis Systemic infection Medications
Hoarseness, dysphagia, chronic cough, hemoptysis	Metastatic cancer originating in the head and neck or lung
Abdominal pain, hematochezia, melena, hematuria	Cancer (gastrointestinal, genitourinary system) Enteric infections

FOCUSED QUESTIONS

After listening to the patient's open-ended description of lymph node enlargement, proceed to focused questions to determine the most likely cause. It is particularly important to inquire about alarm symptoms because their presence greatly influences subsequent diagnostic decision making.

QUESTIONS	THINK ABOUT...
Do you have a history of cancer?	Metastatic cancer
Have you traveled recently?	Infectious causes
Do you have a family history of head and neck (including thyroid, parathyroid) cancer?	Multiple endocrine neoplasia
Do you drink alcohol or use tobacco? If so, how much?	Cancer (head and neck, lung, gastrointestinal)
Have you ever been exposed to radiation?	Cancer
Have you ever had a positive TB skin test? Have you been exposed to anyone with untreated TB?	TB
Have you been exposed to undercooked meats, cat feces, or unpasteurized goat's milk?	Toxoplasmosis
Have you been bitten or scratched by a cat or exposed to a cat with fleas?	Cat-scratch disease (Bartonella henselae)
Do you ever consume unpasteurized milk or cheese?	Brucellosis
Do you hunt, clean, or eat the meat from wild animals?	Tularemia
Do you cut or scratch yourself often?	Repeated minor trauma
Have you had a tick bite or traveled to an area where Lyme disease is endemic (eg, northeast United States)?	Lyme disease
Do you engage in unprotected sexual intercourse?	HIV
Have you ever used injection drugs?	HIV Hepatitis B and C Syphilis
Have you experienced fever, joint pain, or rash with recent medication use?	Medication-associated serum sickness with lymphadenopathy
Do you have a mole that has changed in pigmentation, size, or shape? *Do you have a mole that is bleeding or has become painful, tender, itchy or scaly?*	Melanoma
Have you ever pricked yourself with a thorn from a rose or were you cutting roses?	Sporotrichosis
Do you have blisters in your genital area?	Genital herpes
Do you have a painful blistering rash in a band-like distribution on one side of your body?	Herpes zoster
Quality	
Is the swollen gland:	
• *Painful or tender?*	Infection Inflammatory causes

—Continued next page

Continued—

• *Hard?*	Metastatic cancer
• *Draining?*	Bacterial, mycobacterial infections
Time course	
Tell me how the lymph gland problem has changed over time. Has it:	
• *Been present for over a month?*	Malignancy
• *Continued to increase in size?*	Malignancy
• *Followed use of a new medication?*	Medication
Associated symptoms	
In addition to the lymph gland swelling, have you also had any:	
• *Fevers, chills, or sweats*	Infections Lymphoma Hyperthyroidism
• *Skin rash, redness, bites, insect stings, cuts, or scrapes?*	Bacterial or viral infections Mite infestation Secondary syphilis
• *Sore throat or cold symptoms?*	Viral or streptococcal pharyngitis
• *Genital sores or discharge?*	Sexually transmitted diseases
• *Fatigue?*	Epstein-Barr virus Hepatitis B and C infection CMV Thyroid dysfunction Adrenal insufficiency
• *Unintentional weight loss?*	Malignancy HIV infection TB
• *Breast lumps or discharge?*	Breast cancer
• *Persistent cough, hoarseness, or coughing up blood?*	Head and neck cancer Lung cancer TB Sarcoidosis
• *Difficulty swallowing, abdominal pain, pencil-thin stools, blood in your stool, or pitch black, tarry stool?*	Gastrointestinal malignancy
• *Change in a mole?*	Melanoma
• *Pain or nodule in a testicle?*	Testicular cancer Mumps
• *Blood in your urine?*	Prostate cancer Renal or bladder malignancy
• *Joint pain, mouth ulcers, rashes after sun exposure, dry mouth, or dry eyes?*	Autoimmune CTDs Medication-associated serum sickness

Modifying symptoms	
Does anything seem to make the lymph gland swelling better or worse, such as:	
• *Antibiotic use?*	Better: Infection Worse: Medication-associated lymphadenopathy
• *Aspirin, ibuprofen, naproxen, or other nonsteroidal anti-inflammatory drugs?*	Better: Inflammation Worse: Sulindac-induced

DIAGNOSTIC APPROACH (INCLUDING ALGORITHM)

The diagnostic algorithm for lymphadenopathy is shown in Figure 11–4.

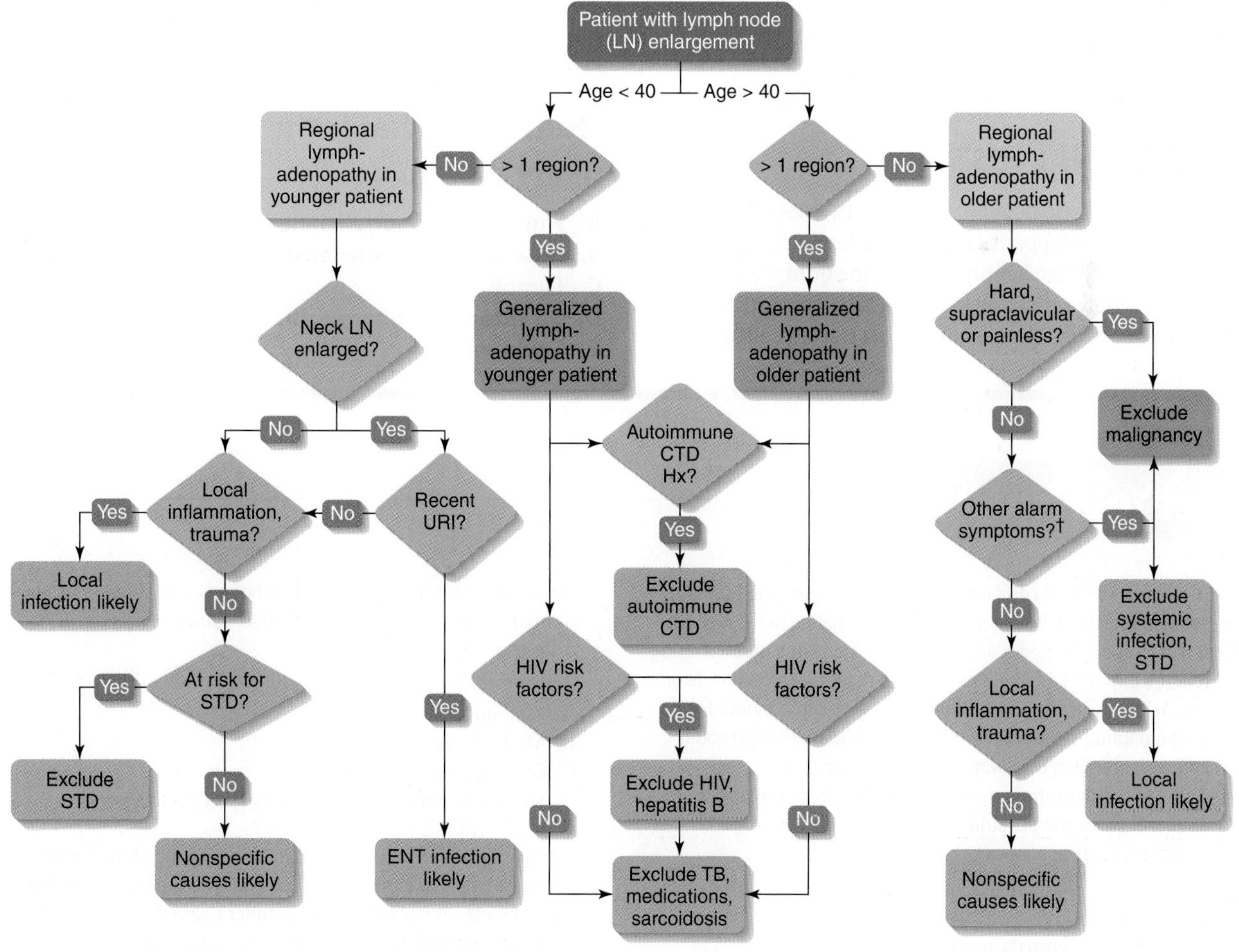

FIGURE 11–4 Diagnostic algorithm: Lymphadenopathy. STD, sexually transmitted disease; CTD, connective tissue disease; Hx, history; TB, tuberculosis; URI, upper respiratory infection; ENT, ear, nose, and throat. †Other alarm symptoms suggestive of malignancy include progressive lymph node enlargement over weeks and months, alcohol and tobacco use, constitutional symptoms (malaise, fatigue, fever, unintentional weight loss, night sweats), hoarseness, dysphagia, chronic cough, hemoptysis, hematuria, hematochezia, melena, abdominal pain, and axillary or epitrochlear adenopathy without local trauma or infection.

CAVEATS

- Remember that what a patient reports as lymph node swelling may actually be another condition (eg, lipoma, sebaceous cyst, abscess, thyroid nodule).
- Lymph node swelling suggestive of a benign, self-limited condition may nevertheless prompt a strongly negative emotional response in patients or family members concerned about the possibility of malignancy.
- Nonspecific lymphadenopathy that is persistent or progressive should prompt repeat evaluation, patient education, and continued shared decision making regarding work-up options and their relative risks, costs, and benefits.

PROGNOSIS

The prognosis of lymphadenopathy in the majority of cases seen in primary care settings is excellent, justifying reassurance and observation when the cause appears to be benign or self-limited, particularly in younger patients.[9] The prognosis of lymphadenopathy due to serious systemic infections (eg, HIV, syphilis, TB) or malignancies depends on a number of factors, including the timeliness of establishing the correct diagnosis, initiation of appropriate therapy, patient-specific immunologic and physiologic responsiveness, and the biologic characteristics of the organism or neoplasm.

CASE SCENARIO | Resolution

A 19-year-old man comes to your clinic complaining of fever, headache, sore throat, and fatigue that started about 2 weeks ago. He has also noticed multiple swollen lymph glands in the front of his neck. He denies any rhinorrhea or cough. He is concerned because the lymph glands are sore to touch and his symptoms are not improving.

ADDITIONAL HISTORY

The patient has also noticed chills, sweats, muscle aches, malaise, and mild left upper quadrant abdominal achiness and fullness. The swollen lymph glands in the front of his neck do not seem to have changed in size since he first noticed them. He does not take any medications. He started college about 3 months ago, and he is in a monogamous relationship with a female partner. He denies injection drug use or unprotected sexual intercourse. He looked in his own throat with a mirror and flashlight and did not notice any white spots or pus. He denies abnormal bruising or bleeding.

Question: What is the most likely diagnosis?

A. Human immunodeficiency virus (HIV) infection
B. Infectious mononucleosis
C. Lymphoma
D. Streptococcal pharyngitis
E. Leukemia

Test Your Knowledge

1. A 30-year-old man comes to your clinic complaining of swollen glands on both sides of his groin that he noticed about 2 weeks ago. The nodes are not painful. He is in a monogamous relationship with a female partner and denies intravenous drug use. You reassure him and tell him to see you in 1 month for re-evaluation. At the follow-up visit, he reports that the nodes appear larger than they were a month earlier.

   Which of the following historical features is most concerning for the possibility of a serious underlying diagnosis such as cancer?

   A. Location of lymph node swelling
   B. Patient age
   C. Progressive growth over time
   D. Painless lymph node enlargement

2. You are seeing a 29-year-old man for a 3-week history of anorexia, muscle aches, and weight loss. He also reports swollen lymph nodes in his neck, axillae, and groin. He has a history of seizures that are controlled with phenytoin. He is not presently sexually active but has had about 6 partners in his lifetime (all women). He also admits to injection drug use.

   Based on his history, what is the most likely diagnosis?

   A. Lymphoma
   B. Medications
   C. Cytomegalovirus infection
   D. Human immunodeficiency virus (HIV) infection

3. A 69-year-old female veterinarian comes to the clinic for her annual medical examination. She feels well but has noticed that the right side of her neck appears fuller than the left.

   Which of the following, if present, would be most concerning for cancer?

   A. Hoarseness and chronic cough
   B. History of exposure to pets
   C. History of multiple sexual partners
   D. Decrease in the size of the lymph nodes with time

References

1. Fletcher RH. Evaluation of peripheral lymphadenopathy in adults. In: Rose BD, ed. *UpToDate.* 17.3 ed., Vol. 2009. Philadelphia, PA: Wolters Kluwer, 2009.
2. Habermann TM, Steensma DP. Lymphadenopathy. *Mayo Clin Proc.* 2000;75:723–732.
3. Henry PH, Longo DL. Enlargement of lymph nodes and spleen. In: Braunwald E, ed. *Harrison's Principles of Internal Medicine.* 17th ed. New York, NY: The McGraw-Hill Companies, Inc., 2008.
4. Bazemore AW, Smucker DR. Lymphadenopathy and malignancy. *Am Fam Physician.* 2002;66:2103–2110.
5. Heitman B, Irizarry A. Infectious disease causes of lymphadenopathy: localized versus diffuse. *Lippincotts Prim Care Pract.* 1999;3:19–38.
6. Ballas ZK. Biology of the immune system. In: Berkow R, ed. *The Merck Manual of Medical Information–Home Edition Online.* Vol. 2003. Whitehouse Station, NJ: Merck & Co., Inc., 2000.
7. Williamson HA Jr. Lymphadenopathy in a family practice: a descriptive study of 249 cases. *J Fam Pract.* 1985;20:449–452.
8. Anthony PP, Knowles SA. Lymphadenopathy as a primary presenting sign: a clinicopathological study of 228 cases. *Br J Surg.* 1983;70:412–414.
9. Slap GB, Connor JL, Wigton RS, Schwartz JS. Validation of a model to identify young patients for lymph node biopsy. *JAMA.* 1986;255:2768–2773.

Suggested Reading

Ferrer R. Lymphadenopathy: differential diagnosis and evaluation. *Am Fam Physician.* 1998;58:1313–1320.

Hurt C, Tammaro D. Diagnostic evaluation of mononucleosis-like illnesses. *Am J Med.* 2007;120:911.e1–e8.

LeBlond RF, Brown DD, DeGowin RL. Non-regional systems and diseases. In: LeBlond RF, Brown DD, DeGowin RL, eds. *DeGowin's Diagnostic Examination.* 9th ed. New York, NY: McGraw-Hill, 2009.

Naeimi M, Sharifi A, Erfanian Y, Velayati A, Izadian S, Golparvar S. Differential diagnosis of cervical malignant lymphadenopathy among Iranian patients. *Saudi Med J.* 2009;30:377–381.

Richner S, Laifer G. Peripheral lymphadenopathy in immunocompetent adults. *Swiss Med Wkly.* 2010;140:98–104.

Chapter 12

Night Sweats

David Feinbloom, MD, and Gerald W. Smetana, MD

CASE SCENARIO

A 48-year-old woman comes to your office to discuss excess sweating. When you inquire further, she states that she often feels flushed and has been waking up from sleep to find that her bedding is wet. The first several times it happened, she did not give it much thought, but now it is happening more frequently, and she is concerned that something may be wrong.

- **How do you distinguish between night sweats and other kinds of sweating?**
- **What conditions are associated with night sweats, and how can the patient history guide you to the right diagnosis?**
- **Can you make a definite diagnosis through an open-ended history followed by focused questions, or is further testing required?**
- **What are the elements of the patient history that can help you to distinguish between benign causes of night sweats and more serious ones that require urgent attention?**

INTRODUCTION

Night sweats are a frequent complaint in the primary care setting. While most often benign, night sweats may be a manifestation of serious systemic disease and should prompt a thorough evaluation to determine the cause. Diagnosis requires a careful medical history, as well as an understanding of the epidemiology and differential diagnosis of this symptom.

Night sweats are drenching sweats that require the patient to change bedclothes. This definition emphasizes the need to distinguish "night sweats" from other conditions that may be associated with increased sweating but do not have the same nocturnal pattern or clinical implications. The causes of night sweats vary, ranging from common, typically benign conditions to serious disorders associated with significant morbidity and mortality.

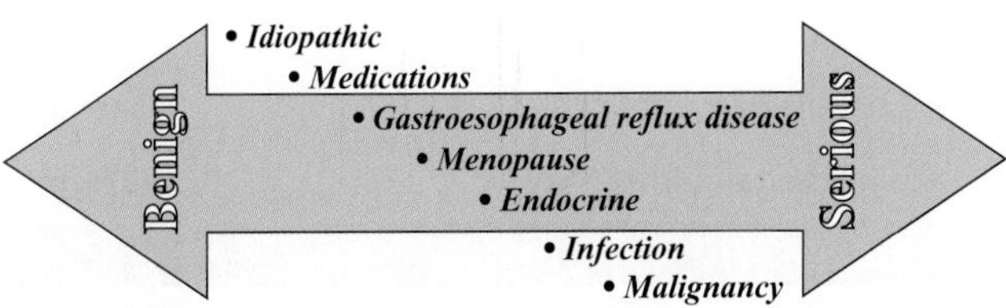

KEY TERMS

Flushing	Acute onset of cutaneous vasodilatation with marked changes in skin color, ranging from bright red to cyanotic. Although it primarily involves the face, neck, and upper chest, it can extend to the whole body including the palms and soles.
Hot flashes	Autonomic symptoms associated with menopause. They are characterized by the sudden onset of intense warmth and redness in the face, chest, and upper back and may include palpitations, profuse sweating, and anxiety. These symptoms typically last only 5–15 minutes.
Hyperhidrosis	Troublesome, benign increase in sweating beyond that necessary to maintain thermal homeostasis.
Night sweats	Drenching sweats that occur during sleep and require the patient to change bedclothes. By definition, the following features must **not** be present: fever, excessive bedding, or increased temperature in the sleeping quarters.

ETIOLOGY

Although numerous causes of night sweats exist, determining a specific etiology can be challenging. Common causes include hormonal changes associated with pregnancy and menopause and medications, particularly antipyretic and antidepressant medications.[1] Unfortunately, the literature on night sweats lacks scope, consistent nomenclature, or rigorous methodology, making an evidence-based approach difficult.

Differential Diagnosis

	Prevalence[a]
Menopause	*14%–80% of women report night sweats associated with menopause.[2,3]*
Infection	
Tuberculosis	29%–62% depending on series.[4] More common in reactivation tuberculosis and in younger patients.
Human immunodeficiency virus (HIV)	9%–70% depending on series.[5] Often seen during the acute retroviral syndrome, during coinfection with an opportunistic pathogen, or with concurrent malignancy (eg, lymphoma).
Endocarditis	17%–25% depending on series[6]
Osteomyelitis	
Abscess (liver, lung, abdomen)	
Bacterial	
• Brucellosis	
Fungal	
• Histoplasmosis	
• Coccidioidomycosis	
• Blastomycosis	
Viral	
• Epstein-Barr virus (EBV)	34% in one series[7]
• Cytomegalovirus (CMV)	60% in one series[8]
Parasites	
Malaria	Up to 91% in one series[9]
Babesiosis	
Malignancy	
Hodgkin's disease	Up to 25%[10]; often seen as part of "B" symptoms
Non-Hodgkin's lymphoma	
Chronic myelogenous leukemia	
Chronic lymphocytic leukemia	
Solid tumors	

• Renal cell carcinoma • Prostate cancer • Medullary thyroid cancer • Germ cell tumors • Metastatic	
Medications[1]	
Antipyretics	
Nonsteroidal anti-inflammatory drugs	
Clozaril	5%
Selective serotonin reuptake inhibitors	5%–10%
Venlafaxine	2%
Donepezil	
Rituximab	15%
Imatinib mesylate	13%–17%
Leuprolide acetate	85%
Danazol	65%
Bicalutamide + luteinizing hormone–releasing hormone	25%
Anastrozole	5%
Raloxifene	2%–3%
Interferon	8%
Saquinavir mesylate	8%
Triptans	1%–3%
Cyclosporine	Up to 4%
Insulin and sulfonylurea	Nocturnal hypoglycemia can manifest as night sweats
Rheumatologic	
Microscopic polyangiitis	71% in one series[11]
Temporal arteritis	Case reports[12]
Miscellaneous	
Obstructive sleep apnea (OSA)	66% in one series[13] but not validated
Chronic fatigue syndrome	30%–40% in one series[14] but complicated by the difficulty in distinguishing this syndrome from coincidental diseases
Dumping syndrome	Reported, but prevalence low
Hyperthyroidism	Increased sweating in 50%–91%,[15] although pure night sweats are less common
Gastroesophageal reflux disease[16]	Reported, but not well characterized

[a]Prevalence is unknown when not indicated.

GETTING STARTED WITH THE HISTORY

- Allow the patient to describe the symptoms in his or her own words without prompting or interrupting.
- Avoid leading questions; leave time at the end to follow up with a few close-ended questions directed at the most likely disorder.
- Patients are often uncomfortable discussing sexual behavior or illegal drug use, and clinicians must be sensitive to these concerns. At the same time, these may be important clues that increase the likelihood of particular infectious etiologies as the cause of night sweats.
- Review medication list before seeing the patient and validate medications during the interview.

Questions	Remember
I understand that you have been having night sweats; can you tell me about them?	Let patients use their own words.
Tell me what you mean by night sweats.	Avoid interrupting.
Can you describe a typical night's sleep, from the time you go to sleep until the time you wake in the morning?	Listen to the patient closely, and try to identify clues that will guide your follow-up questions.
Do you have increased sweating at other times of the day?	Reassurance that night sweats are both common and generally treatable will help the patient to provide a complete history.

INTERVIEW FRAMEWORK

- The first goal is to establish that the complaint of night sweats is consistent with the working medical definition. Therefore, the clinician must first exclude fever, excessive bedding, or elevated room temperature.
- It is best to categorize night sweats into those that are benign in etiology and those that require more thorough testing in order to exclude serious illness. The following characteristics can help to make these distinctions:
  - Onset: Acute, subacute, or chronic
  - Frequency: Isolated, nightly, weekly, monthly
  - Pattern: Escalating, waxing and waning
  - Precipitants: Foods, medications, etc.
  - Associated symptoms: Weight loss, menses, diarrhea, cough, etc.
  - The presence of significant risk factors (eg, travel to areas with endemic infections, unprotected sexual intercourse, injection drug use)

IDENTIFYING ALARM SYMPTOMS

Night sweats may be the sole manifestation of a serious disease. Therefore, distinguishing between benign and serious etiologies is critical. A history of weight loss, lymphadenopathy, cough, hematuria, hemoptysis, hematochezia, rash, arthritis, back pain, diarrhea, high-risk sexual behavior, drug abuse, recent travel, or disease exposure should increase clinical suspicion of a serious disease.

Serious Diagnoses

Serious causes for night sweats are uncommon. Moreover, it is uncommon that a patient will present with night sweats as the sole manifestation of serious illness. Nevertheless, serious causes of night sweats must be ruled out because delay or failure to detect these illnesses can result in significant morbidity and mortality.

Once you have completed the open-ended portion of the medical interview, inquire about symptoms that may suggest a serious diagnosis. Although the following symptoms lack specificity, a positive response should prompt further questions to direct the physical examination and determine the need for diagnostic testing.

Alarm Symptoms	Serious Causes	Benign Causes
Unintentional weight loss	Lymphoma Solid tumors Subacute endocarditis Tuberculosis HIV infection Vasculitis	Change in diet Hyperthyroidism Diabetes mellitus Malabsorption
Loss of appetite or early satiety	Lymphoma Gastrointestinal malignancy	Dyspepsia Depression Medications
Episodic diarrhea	Carcinoid tumor Medullary thyroid carcinoma Inflammatory bowel disease	Viral or bacterial Gastroenteritis Irritable bowel syndrome Medications Hyperthyroidism
Bloody or dark tarry stools	Gastric cancer Colon cancer	Gastritis Peptic ulcer disease Colonic polyps Arteriovenous malformations
Blood in urine	Uroepithelial cancer Renal cell carcinoma Vasculitis	Urinary tract infection Menses Urethritis Renal calculi
Enlarged or tender lymph nodes or glands	Lymphoma Tuberculosis Fungal infections	Viral illness (eg, CMV, EBV) Cellulitis Drug reaction Pharyngitis
Pruritus	Lymphoma Bile duct malignancy Renal failure Polycythemia vera	Dry skin Atopic dermatitis Hypothyroidism
New back pain	Endocarditis Osteomyelitis Malignancy	Degenerative joint disease Sciatica Muscle strain
Testicular swelling or pain	Germ cell tumor Renal cell cancer	Epididymitis Trauma Orchitis Hydrocele/varicocele

—Continued next page

Continued—		
Easy bruising or bleeding?	Leukemia Lymphoma	von Willebrand disease Vitamin C deficiency Steroid-induced purpura
Palpitations	Pheochromocytoma	Atrial or ventricular premature contractions Hyperthyroidism Caffeine Nicotine Medications
New headaches	Pheochromocytoma Central nervous system tumor Giant cell arteritis	Tension headache Migraine headache
Wheezing or shortness of breath	Carcinoid tumor Lung cancer Pericardial or pleural effusion	Asthma Bronchospasm Postnasal drip Medications Allergic reaction
New cough or a cough associated with bloody sputum	Lung cancer Tuberculosis Histoplasmosis Coccidioidomycosis Vasculitis	Bronchitis Sinusitis Cough variant asthma
High blood pressure	Pheochromocytoma Vasculitis	Weight gain Essential hypertension Medications
Recurrent episodes of dizziness or light-headedness	Pheochromocytoma Carcinoid tumor Insulinoma	Hypovolemia/dehydration Benign positional vertigo Vestibular neuritis
Arthritis or arthralgias	HIV infection Rheumatologic disease Endocarditis	Osteoarthritis Posttraumatic
New or recurrent rash	HIV infection Vasculitis Rickettsial disease Syphilis	Viral exanthems Drug eruption Dermatitis

FOCUSED QUESTIONS

After listening to the patient describe his or her night sweats, follow up with a few close-ended questions directed at specific etiologies.

DIAGNOSTIC APPROACH (INCLUDING ALGORITHM)

The first step is to distinguish between night sweats and other situations associated with excess heat or sweating, such as an acute febrile illness, an overheated room, or too many bed coverings. Once you have established that the patient has night sweats, the next step is to identify warning signs or symptoms that suggest a more serious diagnosis. Women of childbearing age should be asked about menopausal symptoms. Because medications are such a common cause of night sweats, it is important to take a thorough medication history, including over-the-counter and herbal supplements. All patients with signs or symptoms of hyperthyroidism should be evaluated.

Less common causes of night sweats include gastroesophageal reflux disease and obstructive sleep apnea, although the latter has recently been called into question.[17]

If the etiology of night sweats remain unknown, it is important that patients be re-evaluated on a periodic basis as new diagnostic symptoms often emerge over time. The diagnostic algorithm for night sweats is shown in Figure 12–1.

CAVEATS

- Night sweats that are new, accompanied by systemic symptoms, or not readily explained by benign processes *are serious until proved otherwise.*
- Be certain to exclude spurious causes of night sweats before embarking on a lengthy evaluation; likewise, fever must be excluded at the outset.
- The presence of weight loss, flushing, diarrhea, hypertension, lymphadenopathy, or cough should raise the clinical suspicion of more serious systemic disease. When unsure, err on the side of caution by ruling out more serious diagnoses.
- The clinical context is crucial in making the correct diagnosis. For example, the common causes of night sweats in a 45-year-old perimenopausal woman are quite different than in a 60-year-old man with weight loss, flank pain, and hematuria. Pay attention to demographics, comorbid illnesses, travel history, and other exposures to narrow the differential diagnosis.
- Always perform a complete review of all prescription, herbal, and over-the-counter medications.
- Re-evaluate your working diagnosis over time, and pay special attention to new or contradictory information.

PROGNOSIS

The prognosis of night sweats depends on the underlying diagnosis. The majority of causes are benign and readily manageable with appropriate treatment. Serious causes of night sweats, including malignancies and infections, are less common. Failure to identify such diseases may result in unnecessary morbidity and mortality and, in the case of HIV infection and tuberculosis, pose a public health risk as well.

CASE SCENARIO | Resolution

A 48-year-old woman comes to your office to discuss excess sweating. When you inquire further, she states that she often feels flushed and has been waking up from sleep to find that her bedding is wet. The first several times it happened, she did not give it much thought, but now it is happening more frequently, and she is concerned that something may be wrong.

ADDITIONAL HISTORY

For the last 3 to 4 months, she has had distinct episodes of intense heat beginning in her face and then spreading to the rest of her body. These episodes are followed by profuse sweating. Recently, these episodes seem to occur more at night and sometimes wake her from sleep. She reports irregular menses and depressed mood but denies history of excess sweating, weight loss, intercurrent illness or exposure, high-risk sexual activity, or constitutional symptoms. She takes no medication, and her physical examination is normal.

Question: What is the most likely diagnosis?

A. Idiopathic hyperhidrosis
B. Hyperthyroidism
C. Menopausal hot flashes
D. Obstructive sleep apnea

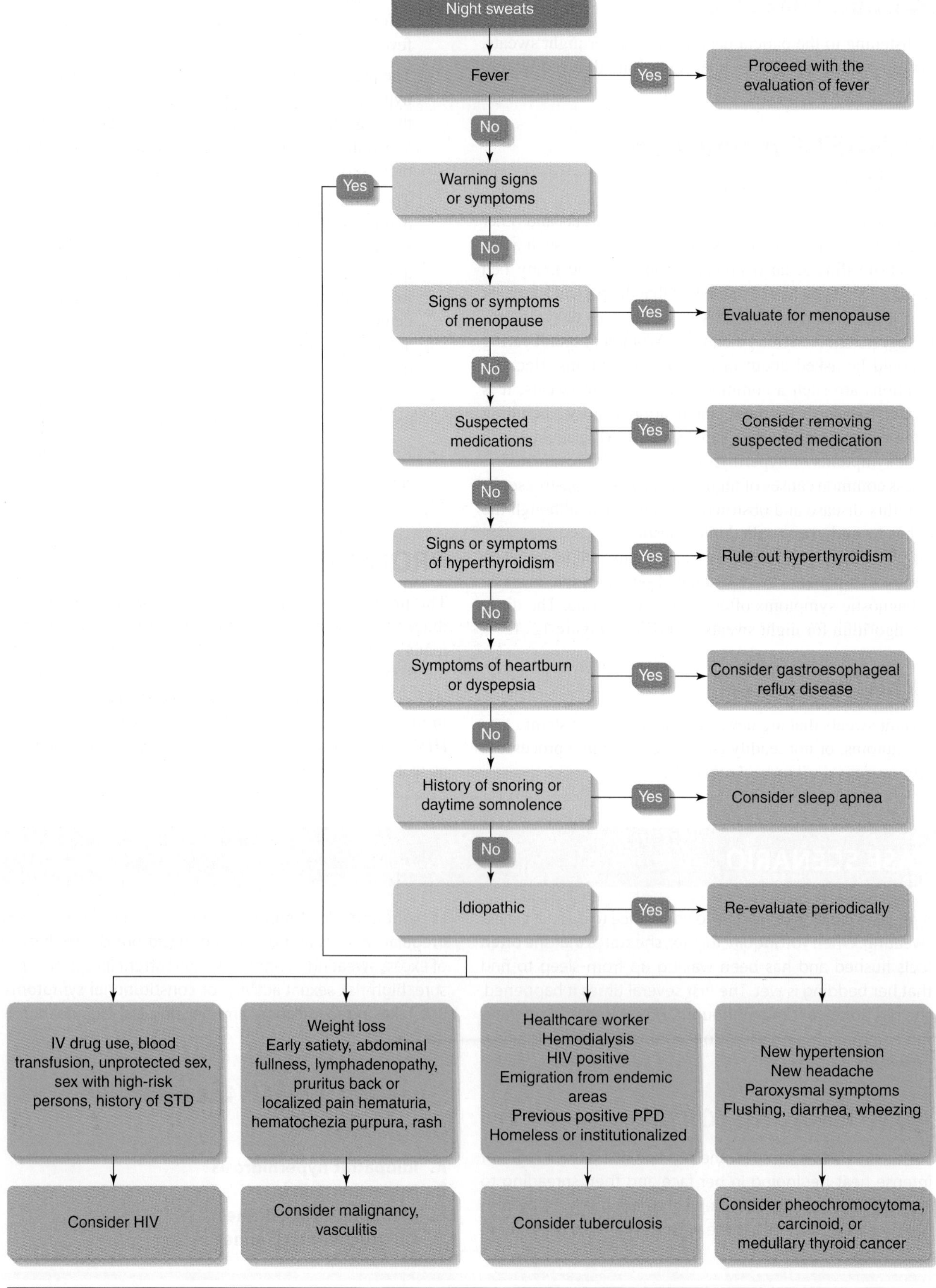

FIGURE 12–1 Diagnostic algorithm: Night sweats. IV, intravenous; PPD, purified protein derivative; STD, sexually transmitted disease.

Test Your Knowledge

1. You see a 29-year-old man with night sweats. He reports that the symptoms began approximately 6 months ago and have gradually worsened.

   Which of the following features is **not** an alarm symptom that should prompt concern for a serious cause of night sweats?

   A. He worked in the Peace Corps when he was 22 years old.
   B. New hypertension
   C. Excessive sweating with exercise
   D. Mild weight loss
   E. Intermittent fevers

2. A 54-year-old nurse presents with night sweats. She cannot remember exactly when they started, but they now occur every night. She reports some mild fatigue and may have lost a few pounds, and has noticed that her urine is sometimes red-tinged. She was taking a selective serotonin reuptake inhibitor (SSRI) antidepressant last year, but takes no medications now. She used marijuana when she was younger, but not anymore, and she confides in you that she had an extramarital affair 8 years ago.

   Which of the following features should prompt concern for a serious cause of night sweats?

   A. Prior drug use
   B. Use of an antidepressant medication
   C. Working as a nurse
   D. Change in her urine
   E. Extramarital affair

References

1. *Physicians' Desk Reference*. 2003 ed. Montvale, NJ: Thompson Healthcare Press, 2003.
2. Danby FW. Management of menopause-related symptoms. *Ann Intern Med*. 2005;143:845–846.
3. von Muhlen DG, Kritz-Silverstein D, Barrett-Connor E. A community-based study of menopause symptoms and estrogen replacement in older women. *Maturitas*. 1995;22:71–78.
4. Aktogu S, Yorgancioglu A, Cirak K, Kose T, Dereli SM. Clinical spectrum of pulmonary and pleural tuberculosis: a report of 5,480 cases. *Eur Respir J*. 1996;9:2031–2035.
5. Cunningham WE, Shapiro MF, Hays RD, et al. Constitutional symptoms and health-related quality of life in patients with symptomatic HIV disease. *Am J Med*. 1998;104:129–136.
6. Jalal S, Khan KA, Alai MS, et al. Clinical spectrum of infective endocarditis: 15 years experience. *Indian Heart J*. 1998;50:516–519.
7. Lambore S, McSherry J, Kraus AS. Acute and chronic symptoms of mononucleosis. *J Fam Pract*. 1991;33:33–37.
8. Wreghitt TG, Teare EL, Sule O, Devi R, Rice P. Cytomegalovirus infection in immunocompetent patients. *Clin Infect Dis*. 2003;37:1603–1606.
9. Jelinek T, Nothdurft HD, Loscher T. Malaria in nonimmune travelers: a synopsis of history, symptoms, and treatment in 160 patients. *J Travel Med*. 1994;1:199–202.
10. Lister T, Crowther D, Sutcliffe S, et al. Report of a committee convened to discuss the evaluation and staging of patients with Hodgkin's disease: Cotwsolds meeting. *J Clin Oncol*. 1989;7:1630–1636.
11. Kirkland GS, Savige J, Wilson D, Heale W, Sinclair RA, Hope RN. Classical polyarteritis nodosa and microscopic polyarteritis with medium vessel involvement—a comparison of the clinical and laboratory features. *Clin Nephrol*. 1997;47: 176–180.
12. Morris GC, Thomas TP. Night sweats—presentation of an often forgotten diagnosis. *Br J Clin Pract*. 1991;45:145.
13. Guilleminault C. Clinical features and evaluation of obstructive sleep apnea. In: Kryger M, Roth T, Dement W, ed. *Principles and Practice of Sleep Medicine*. 2nd ed. Philadelphia, PA: WB Saunders Co., 1994:667–677.
14. Komaroff AL. Clinical presentation of chronic fatigue syndrome. *Ciba Found Symp*. 1993;173:43–54.
15. Spaulding SW, Lippes H. Hyperthyroidism. Causes, clinical features, and diagnosis. *Med Clin North Am*. 1985;69:937–951.
16. Reynolds WA. Are night sweats a sign of esophageal reflux? *J Clin Gastroenterol*. 1989;11:590–591.
17. Mold JW, Goodrich S, Orr W. Associations between subjective night sweats and sleep study findings. *J Am Board Fam Med*. 2008;21:96–100.
18. Rabinovitz M, Pitlik SD, Leifer M, Garty M, Rosenfeld JB. Unintentional weight loss. A retrospective analysis of 154 cases. *Arch Intern Med*. 1986;146:186–187.

Suggested Reading

Chambliss ML. Frequently asked questions from clinical practice. What is the appropriate diagnostic approach for patients who complain of night sweats? *Arch Fam Med.* 1999;8:168–169.

Col NF, Fairfield KM, Ewan-Whyte C, Miller H. In the clinic. Menopause. *Ann Intern Med.* 2009;150:ITC4-1–15.

Eisenach JH, Atkinson JL, Fealey RD. Hyperhidrosis: evolving therapies for a well established phenomenon. *Mayo Clin Proc.* 2005;80:657–666.

Grady D. Management of menopausal symptoms. *N Engl J Med.* 2006;355:2338–2347.

Izikson L, English JC 3rd, Zirwas MJ. The flushing patient: differential diagnosis, workup, and treatment. *J Am Acad Dermatol.* 2006;55:193–208.

Mold JW, Mathew MK, Belgore S, DeHaven M. Prevalence of night sweats in primary care patients: an OKPRN and TAFP-Net collaborative study. *J Fam Pract.* 2002;51:452–456.

Viera AJ, Bond MM, Yates SW. Diagnosing night sweats. *Am Fam Physician.* 2003;67:1019–1024.

Chapter 13

Muscle Weakness

Iris Ma, MD

CASE SCENARIO

A 28-year-old woman presents to the urgent care clinic complaining of weakness. For the past week, she has had weakness and numbness in her right arm and bouts of dizziness. The symptoms became worse 2 days ago but have since stabilized.

- **What additional questions would you ask to learn more about her weakness?**
- **Can you localize her lesion to a specific anatomic site?**
- **How can you use the patient history to determine if the patient requires urgent intervention for weakness?**
- **How do the duration and evolution of symptoms help narrow the differential diagnosis?**

INTRODUCTION

In approaching a patient with a complaint of weakness, the physician must first determine whether the patient has functional or motor weakness. Many patients who complain of weakness are actually suffering from functional weakness due to asthenia, the sensation of exhaustion or lethargy despite normal muscle strength, or increased fatigability, the tiring of muscles with multiple repetitions. Functional weakness may be caused by a variety of conditions including cancer, infection, metabolic derangements, inflammatory diseases, and psychiatric disorders. In these conditions, the patient has trouble completing activities of daily living because of a lack of physical or emotional energy, but has normal muscle strength. Another potential masquerader of weakness is pain that prevents a patient from completing specific activities despite retained muscle strength. Patients with neuromuscular weakness are unable to move their muscles at full strength despite maximum effort and optimization of modifiable factors.

The first step in evaluating any patient complaining of weakness is to distinguish functional weakness from neuromuscular weakness. The history should be completed systematically with a focus on the onset, the evolution of symptoms, and location of the lesion along the motor pathway. Although all patients with weakness warrant a careful evaluation, this chapter focuses on patients whose history suggests true weakness of the muscles. For the remainder of this chapter, the term "weakness" will mean neuromuscular weakness.

KEY TERMS[1]

Ascending paralysis	Motor weakness that begins in the feet and progressively moves up the body.
Bulbar symptoms	Weakness in the muscles of the face and tongue, resulting in difficulty speaking, swallowing, and smiling.
Descending paralysis	Motor weakness that begins in the face and progressively moves down the body.
Distal weakness	Weakness in the distal extremities (eg, foot drop).
Hemiparesis	Weakness on one side of the body.
Monoparesis	Weakness of one limb.

—Continued next page

Continued—	
Paraparesis	Weakness of both legs.
Proximal weakness	Weakness in proximal muscles (eg, shoulder girdle, quadriceps) resulting in difficulty standing up from a seated position or raising arms above head.
Tetraparesis	Weakness of all 4 limbs.
Todd's paralysis	Reversible weakness following a seizure.
Upper motor neuron lesions	Abnormalities of motor pathways that descend from the central nervous system to the alpha motor neurons, resulting in spasticity, hyperreflexia, and increased muscle tone.
Lower motor neuron lesions	Abnormalities of the alpha motor neuron in the brainstem or spinal gray matter, resulting in muscle atrophy, hyporeflexia, and fasciculations.

ETIOLOGY

Thinking about the cause of muscle weakness starts with anatomic localization of the problem. Neuromuscular weakness can be caused by damage or dysfunction at any point between the brain and muscle. Once the source of the weakness is localized, a narrowed differential diagnosis can be explored.

Differential Diagnosis

The differential diagnosis depends on the anatomic localization of the lesion and the duration and evolution of the symptoms. Conditions associated with a sudden loss of muscle function are outlined under alarm conditions. Patients with insidious or episodic development of muscle weakness often delay seeking medical attention.

Anatomic Localization	Diagnosis	Prevalence or Incidence
Central nervous system (CNS) disorders	Dysfunction of the brain:	
	• Stroke or transient ischemic attack (TIA)	Stroke: 3%[2]
	• Intracranial hemorrhage (subarachnoid, subdural, epidural, intraparenchymal)	TIA: 2.3%[2]
	• Neoplasm	
	• Infection	
	• Multiple sclerosis	
	Dysfunction of spinal cord (myelopathy):	
	• Neoplasm	Multiple sclerosis: 0.09%[3]
	• Infection (eg, epidural abscess)	
	• Trauma	
	• Cervical spondylosis	
Motor neuron disease	Diseases affecting primarily lower motor neurons:	
	• Amyotrophic lateral sclerosis (ALS)	4/100,000[3]
Radiculopathies	Dysfunction of spinal nerve roots:	
	• Compression at neural foramina	
	• Impingement from disk herniation	
	• Cervical spondylosis	

Peripheral neuropathies	Mononeuropathy: dysfunction of single peripheral nerve • Radial nerve palsy Polyneuropathy[4,5]: dysfunction of multiple peripheral nerves • Toxic/metabolic: diabetes, alcoholism, vitamin B_{12} deficiency, uremia, heavy metal poisoning • Inflammatory: Guillain-Barré syndrome (GBS), chronic inflammatory demyelinating polyradiculopathy (CIDP), vasculitides (eg, polyarteritis nodosa) • Infiltrative: amyloidosis, sarcoidosis • Infectious: human immunodeficiency virus (HIV), leprosy • Congenital: Charcot-Marie-Tooth disease	Polyneuropathies: 2.4%[4] GBS: incidence 0.6–2.4 cases/ 100,00[6]
Neuromuscular junction disorders	Myasthenia gravis Lambert-Eaton myasthenic syndrome Botulism	Myasthenia gravis: 14/100,00[7]
Myopathies	Genetic: Duchenne muscular dystrophy, Becker muscular dystrophy, mitochondrial myopathies, periodic paralysis, acid maltase deficiency Inflammatory: polymyositis, dermatomyositis, inclusion body myositis Rheumatologic: mixed connective tissue disease Endocrinopathy: hyperthyroidism, hypercortisolism Drug-induced: alcohol, cocaine, statins, glucocorticoids, chloroquine, colchicine (neuromyopathy) Rhabdomyolysis	Duchenne: incidence 2.9/100,00 births[8] Becker: incidence 0.5/100,000 births[8]

GETTING STARTED WITH THE HISTORY

- Let the patient describe the weakness in his/her own words before asking more focused questions.
- The initial interview should be directed at clarifying whether the patient's symptoms suggest true weakness or functional weakness.
- There are few causes of weakness with pathognomonic symptoms or signs. However, investigating the temporal and anatomic pattern of weakness and associated symptoms is instrumental. Narrowing the differential diagnosis for weakness will allow the correct diagnosis to be made efficiently.

Open-Ended Questions	Tips for Effective Interviewing
Tell me about your weakness.	An open-ended question will often yield significant information.
How did your weakness start? When did it start?	The duration and evolution of the patient's symptoms are useful in determining potential etiologies.
Are there specific tasks that are difficult, or do you have difficulty participating in all activities?	Patients who describe weakness with all activities along with fatigue are likely to be suffering from functional weakness.

INTERVIEW FRAMEWORK

- Inquire about the duration and temporal evolution of symptoms.
- Inquire about the distribution of symptoms and localize the problem.
- Inquire about associated signs and symptoms.
- Inquire about risk factors for conditions causing weakness from the past medical, social, and family history.

IDENTIFYING ALARM SYMPTOMS

Weakness developing over hours to days should be evaluated promptly because many of the underlying conditions may cause irreversible neurologic damage or death if diagnosis and therapy are delayed. For example:

- Early thrombolysis can improve the prognosis of stroke; thus, rapid intervention is critical.
- Patients with symptoms and signs of respiratory muscle weakness require prompt endotracheal intubation.
- Early plasmapheresis is vital in the treatment of GBS.

Alarm Symptoms	Serious Causes	Benign Causes
Rapidly progressive descending tetraparesis	Botulism Descending GBS (Miller Fisher syndrome) Organophosphate poisoning Brainstem stroke	
Rapidly progressive ascending paraparesis	GBS	
Rapidly progressive descending paraparesis	Transverse myelitis Spinal cord compression (neoplasm, infection, trauma, disk herniation)	
Sudden-onset hemiparesis	Stroke or TIA Intracranial hemorrhage	Hemiplegic migraine Todd's paralysis Conversion disorder
Sudden-onset monoparesis	Stroke Mononeuropathy	Compressive neuropathy
Localized back pain with paraparesis	GBS Transverse myelitis Spinal cord compression (neoplasm, infection, trauma)	
Others have developed the same weakness	Botulism Organophosphate poisoning	
Tick exposure with tetraparesis	Tick paralysis	
Diplopia, blurry vision, or bulbar symptoms with developing tetraparesis	Botulism Organophosphate poisoning Descending GBS Brainstem stroke Multiple sclerosis	
Radicular pain (electric pain that follows a spinal root distribution) with paraparesis	Transverse myelitis Spinal cord compression (neoplasm, infection, trauma, disk herniation)	

Headache with hemiparesis	Intracranial bleed CNS malignancy Brain abscess	Hemiplegic migraines
Involuntary movements with hemiparesis	Stroke CNS tumor	Todd's paralysis
History of heavy exercise or repetitive activities	Rhabdomyolysis	Compressive neuropathy Exertional fatigue
History of cancer	Metastatic disease Paraneoplastic syndromes	
History of fevers or injection drug use	Epidural abscess	
History of hyperthyroidism (often presents with new-onset atrial fibrillation)	Thyrotoxic periodic paralysis (particularly in Asian men)	

FOCUSED QUESTIONS

If the patient's weakness has developed insidiously, focused questions allow the clinician to clarify the temporal pattern and identify risk factors for associated diseases. The examiner can ascertain the distribution and extent of the weakness before the physical examination is performed. Associated neurologic symptoms (eg, sensory loss, vertigo) and focal weakness commonly represent neurologic causes, whereas proximal weakness suggests a myopathy. Myopathies and myasthenia gravis both affect all striated muscles. However, myasthenia gravis is a disorder of fatiguing and thus affects those muscles that are used most frequently (eg, extraocular muscles). Myopathies proceed irrespective of frequency of use and, therefore, are most noticeable in the larger proximal muscles.

QUESTIONS	IF ANSWERED IN THE AFFIRMATIVE, THINK ABOUT...
Personal and family history and exposures	
Do you have diabetes mellitus?	Mononeuritis Polyneuropathies Stroke
Do you have hypertension, hypercholesterolemia, vascular disease, or history of cigarette smoking or estrogen use?	Stroke
Do you have hyperthyroidism or symptoms of hyperthyroidism?	Thyroid myopathy Myasthenia gravis (occasionally associated with hyperthyroidism)
Are you taking any medications?	Steroid-induced myopathy Statin myopathy Drug-induced myasthenia gravis (penicillamine, aminoglycosides, calcium channel blockers)

—Continued next page

Continued—

Do you drink alcohol? How much?	Alcoholic myopathy Alcoholic polyneuropathy
Do you have kidney disease?	Uremic polyneuropathy
Do you have rheumatoid arthritis? *Have you had a whiplash injury or other history of neck trauma?*	Cervical radiculopathy or myelopathy
Have you ever been treated for a malignancy? Have you had recent weight loss, night sweats, and fatigue?	Lambert-Eaton myasthenic syndrome (particularly small-cell lung cancer) Spinal cord compression
Do you use intravenous drugs or have unprotected sex? *Do you have HIV infection?*	Distal symmetric polyneuropathy Mononeuritis multiplex Toxic polyneuropathies (due to nucleoside reverse transcriptase inhibitors) CIDP Myopathies (polymyositis and zidovudine-related myopathy)
Have you ever had optic neuritis?	Multiple sclerosis
Does heat exacerbate your symptoms?	Multiple sclerosis
Have you lost consciousness in the last week?	Compressive peripheral neuropathy
Do you have a rash or weight loss?	Vasculitis-associated mononeuritis Dermatomyositis Malignancy Hyperthyroidism
Do you have a family history of similar problems?	Charcot-Marie-Tooth disease Familial periodic paralysis Duchenne or Becker muscular dystrophy Mitochondrial myopathy
Time course	
Does your weakness come and go? (episodic weakness)	Myasthenia gravis Multiple sclerosis
Has your weakness steadily worsened? (progressive weakness)	ALS Polymyositis/dermatomyositis Chronic polyneuropathies
Did your weakness appear suddenly and remain constant?	Stroke Compressive neuropathy or radiculopathy
Has your weakness gradually improved?	Compressive neuropathy Multiple sclerosis Mononeuritis

Distribution	
Are you weak on both sides of your body?	Spinal cord compression (neoplasm, infection, degenerative disk disease) Myopathies Myasthenia gravis ALS Multiple sclerosis (transverse myelitis variant)
Is your weakness confined to just one limb or part of one limb?	Peripheral neuropathy or radiculopathy Multiple sclerosis Stroke Todd's paralysis
Does your weakness involve one side of your body or your face?	Stroke or TIA Hemiplegic migraine
Do you have difficulty lifting your head off the bed, standing from a sitting position, or brushing your hair? (proximal muscle weakness)	Polymyositis or dermatomyositis Diabetic amyotrophy (lower extremity proximal muscle weakness) Duchenne and Becker muscular dystrophy
Is it difficult for you to stand on your toes? (distal weakness greater than proximal weakness)	Inclusion body myositis Polyneuropathy or radiculopathy
Has your voice changed? Do you have trouble swallowing?	ALS Polymyositis or dermatomyositis Myasthenia gravis Stroke
Do you have double vision (diplopia)?	Mononeuritis (cranial nerve IV, VI) Myasthenia gravis Multiple sclerosis
Do you have droopy eyelids?	Myasthenia gravis Botulism (acute)
Associated symptoms	
Do you have numbness and tingling in association with your weakness?	Multiple sclerosis Stroke Polyneuropathies Neurologic disorders NOT myopathies
Can you see your muscles twitching? (fasciculations)	ALS
Modifying symptoms	
Does your weakness get worse with exercise?	Myasthenia gravis Mitochondrial myopathies
Does your weakness get better with exercise?	Lambert-Eaton myasthenic syndrome

DIAGNOSTIC APPROACH (INCLUDING ALGORITHM)

The diagnostic algorithm for muscle weakness is shown in Figure 13–1.

CAVEATS

- Although the history can suggest the distribution of weakness and site of localization of the lesion, the physical

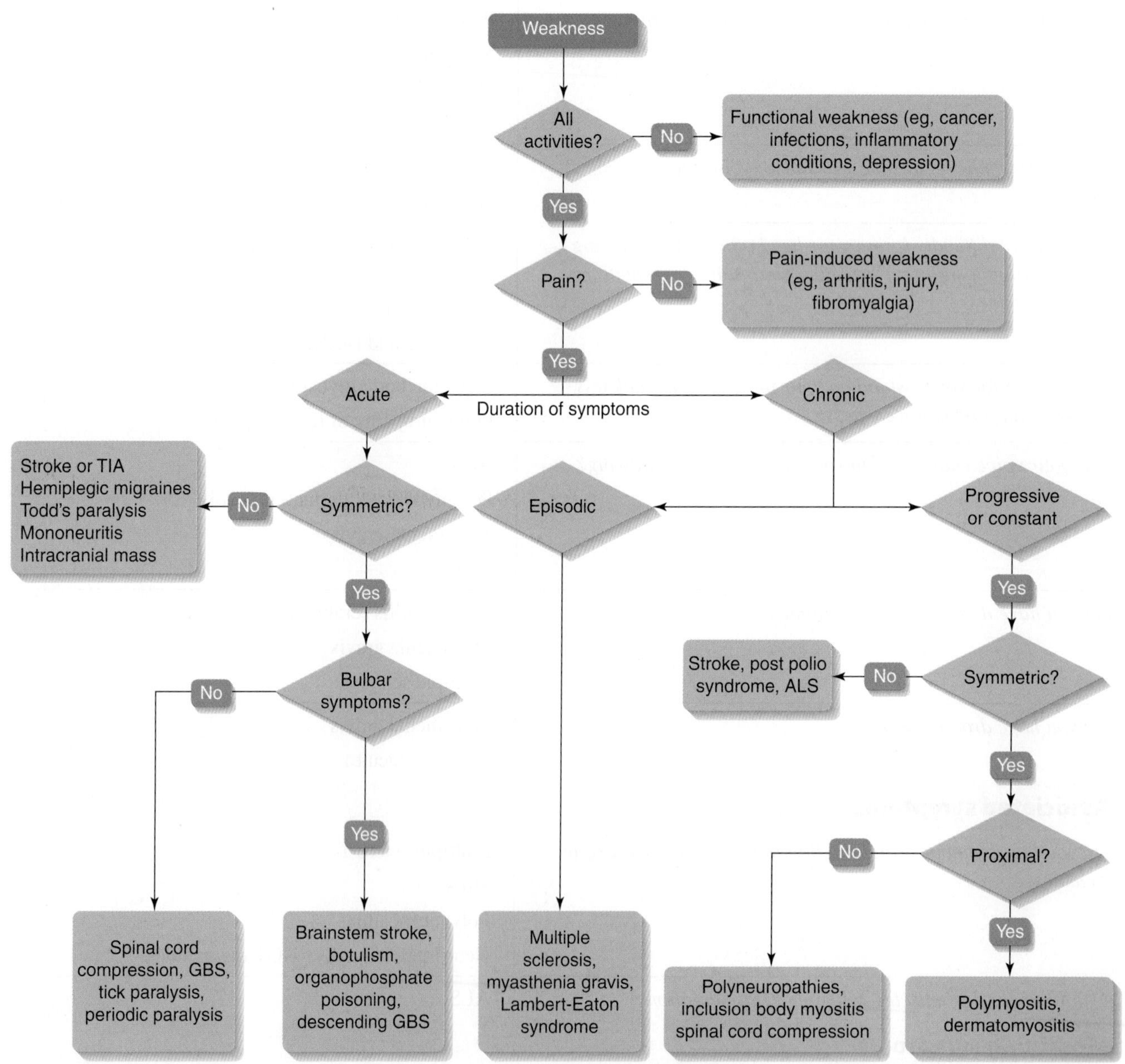

FIGURE 13–1 Diagnostic algorithm: Muscle weakness. ALS, amyotrophic lateral sclerosis; DM, dermatomyositis; GBS, Guillain-Barré syndrome; TIA, transient ischemic attack.

examination is necessary to further refine the differential diagnosis. The clinical evaluation in the hands of experienced neurologists accurately identifies the type and cause of a given neurologic problem approximately 75% of the time.[9]

- When patients have classic symptoms and signs, it may be relatively easy to diagnose the underlying condition. However, many diseases have variable presentations (eg, myasthenia gravis, ALS, multiple sclerosis).
- There may be more than one cause of muscle weakness. For example, a patient with Lambert-Eaton myasthenic syndrome as a paraneoplastic manifestation of small-cell lung cancer may also develop spinal cord compression from metastatic disease.

PROGNOSIS

- The prognosis of acute stroke is improved if the patient receives thrombolysis within 4.5 hours of the onset of symptoms.[10]
- Mononeuritis due to vasculitis of the vasa nervorum may respond to immunosuppressive medications.
- Mononeuropathies due to compression generally resolve over time once the compression is relieved.
- Chronic progressive metabolic polyneuropathies generally do not improve.
- Eighty percent of patients with GBS will recover totally or have only minor residual neurologic dysfunction after treatment with intravenous immune globulin or plasma exchange. Death is generally due to complications of respiratory failure.[6]
- Patients with myasthenia gravis require chronic therapy with immunosuppressants such as prednisone, azathioprine, or cyclosporine.[11]
- Recovery from an acute episode of multiple sclerosis is hastened with the administration of intravenous methylprednisolone. Interferon beta decreases the likelihood of relapse.[12]
- ALS is a uniformly fatal disease.

CASE SCENARIO | Resolution

A 28-year-old woman presents to the urgent care clinic complaining of weakness. For the past week, she has had weakness and numbness in her right arm and bouts of dizziness. The symptoms became worse 2 days ago but have since stabilized.

ADDITIONAL HISTORY

The patient has fatigue and weakness in both legs. Sometimes, paroxysms of severe pain radiate down her spine when she bends her neck. Despite adequate hydration, she feels like the room is "wobbling." Based on the pattern and distribution of symptoms, you determine that she has true neuromuscular weakness. She does not have alarm symptoms of rapidly progressive weakness or sudden-onset hemiplegia, but she does have concerning back pain and paraparesis. Further questioning reveals that her symptoms were initially mild but worsened during a trip to the beach 2 days ago. The patient explains that several months ago she had similar but milder episodes of bilateral leg weakness lasting several days and resolving completely. You probe her further regarding her past medical history, and she describes a painful episode of optic neuritis in her right eye 1 year ago that left her with mild residual vision loss.

Question: What is the most likely diagnosis?

A. Stroke
B. Multiple sclerosis
C. Myasthenia gravis
D. Depression

Test Your Knowledge

1. A 68-year-old man with a history of diabetes, atrial fibrillation, and hyperlipidemia comes to the emergency department complaining of weakness of the right arm and face. He was in his usual state of health until he woke up this morning with right-sided numbness and weakness.
   What is the likely diagnosis?
   A. Stroke
   B. Seizure with Todd's paralysis
   C. Herniated disk
   D. Subdural hematoma
   E. Multiple sclerosis

2. One of your long-time patients, a 60-year-old woman, complains of gradually worsening weakness and fatigue over several months. She has difficulty rising out of bed in the morning and standing up from a seated position. She also describes a 15-pound weight loss. Although she quit smoking last year, she has a 60 pack-year smoking history. After further evaluation, she is diagnosed with small-cell lung cancer and Lambert-Eaton myasthenic syndrome.
   Which of the following symptoms is she likely to have?
   A. Unilateral optic neuritis
   B. Muscle fasciculations
   C. Weakness that gets worse with exercise
   D. Weakness that gets better with exercise
   E. Numbness and paresthesias

3. A 21-year-old man arrives in clinic for his annual physical and complains of generalized weakness for several months. He used to be a track star, but recently quit the team. He has been sleeping more and has a hard time rousing himself from bed in the morning. Since quitting the track team, he has had decreased appetite and the inability to focus in class. He is tired all the time and doesn't seem to enjoy activities that he used to.
   What is the likely diagnosis?
   A. Duchenne muscular dystrophy
   B. Deconditioning
   C. Depression
   D. Myasthenia gravis
   E. Hyperthyroidism

4. A 45-year-old patient is carried into the emergency department with weakness in his legs. The weakness started in his feet, but has spread up his legs over the past few hours. He has numbness and paresthesias in a similar distribution. Until last week, he was in his usual state of health when he contracted an upper respiratory syndrome from one of his children.
   Which of the following diagnoses is most concerning at this time?
   A. Guillain-Barré syndrome
   B. Diabetes mellitus
   C. Polyarteritis nodosa
   D. Charcot-Marie-Tooth disease
   E. Brain abscess

References

1. Hammerstad JP. Strength and reflexes. In: Goetz CG, ed. *Textbook of Clinical Neurology.* 2nd ed. New York, NY: Elsevier, 2003:235–278.
2. Roger VL, Go AS, Lloyd-Jones DM, et al. Heart disease and stroke statistics: 2011 update. *Circulation.* 2011;123:e18–e209.
3. Hirtz D, Thurman DJ, Gwinn-Hardy K, et al. How common are the "common" neurologic disorders? *Neurology.* 2007;68: 326–337.
4. Martyn CN, Hughes RAC. Epidemiology of peripheral neuropathy. *J Neurol Neurosurg Psychiatry.* 1997;62: 310-318.
5. Hughes RA. Peripheral neuropathy. *BMJ.* 2002;324:466–469.
6. Chio A, Cocito D, Leone M, et al. Guillain-Barré syndrome: a prospective, population based incidence and outcome survey. *Neurology.* 2003;60:1146–1150.
7. Phillips LH 2nd, Torner JC, Anderson MS, Cox GM. The epidemiology of myasthenia gravis in central and western Virginia. *Neurology.* 1992;42:1888–1893.
8. Emery AE. Population frequencies of inherited neuromuscular diseases—a world survey. *Neuromuscul Disord.* 1991;1:19–29.
9. Chimowitz MI, Logigian EL, Caplan LR. The accuracy of bedside neurological diagnoses. *Ann Neurol.* 1990;28:78–85.
10. Hacke W, Kaste M, Bluhmki E, et al. Thrombolysis with alteplase 3 to 4.5 hours after acute ischemic stroke. *N Engl J Med.* 2008;359:1317–1329.
11. Drachman DB. Myasthenia gravis. *N Engl J Med.* 1994;330:1797–1810.
12. Noseworthy JH, Lucchinetti C, Rodriguez M, Weinshenker BG. Medical progress: multiple sclerosis. *N Engl J Med.* 2000;343:938–952.

Suggested Reading

Olney RK. Weakness, disorders of movement, and imbalance. In: Kasper DL, Braunwald E, Fauci AS, Hauser S, Longo DL, Jameson JL, eds. *Harrison's Principles of Internal Medicine.* 16th ed. New York, NY: McGraw-Hill, 2005:134–141.

Saguil A. Evaluation of the patient with muscle weakness. *Am Fam Physician.* 2005;71:1327–1336.

Chapter 14

Weight Gain

Timothy S. Loo, MD

CASE SCENARIO

A 35-year-old woman presents to establish care with you. She has no specific concerns. On examination, you observe an obese body habitus and calculate her body mass index (BMI) at 36.5 kg/m^2 based on a weight of 209.5 lb and a height of 63.5 inches. When you raise concern about obesity and potential comorbidities, she reveals that she is unhappy with her current weight and has recently embarked on a diet plan to lose weight. She believes she has been at or near her current weight for the past 4 years. She last felt comfortable with her weight when she was 145 lb.

- **What additional history would help distinguish whether she has primary versus secondary weight gain?**
- **How do you use the history to screen for obesity-related comorbidities?**

INTRODUCTION

Weight gain is an absolute increase in body weight. Weight gain is usually a consequence of accumulation of excess body fat, although processes such as edema and ascites can cause substantial weight gain. Weight gain is common and a significant public health concern. Regardless of baseline weight, weight gain can lead to adverse health consequences and to the development of obesity, a major cause of morbidity and the second leading cause of preventable deaths in the United States. Over the last 2 decades, the prevalence of obesity has risen dramatically; currently, 64% of Americans are overweight, and 30% are obese.

Primary weight gain is the accumulation of adipose tissue that results from an imbalance between caloric intake and energy expenditure. Less commonly, weight gain is due to secondary causes such as endocrine disorders and medication side effects. The patient history serves 3 main goals: (1) to distinguish between weight gain caused by abnormal fluid retention and weight gain caused by body fat accumulation; (2) to identify the contributing factors or secondary causes of excess fat accumulation and; (3) to screen for serious medical complications caused by weight gain or obesity.

KEY TERMS

Body mass index (BMI)	BMI is a measure of relative weight for height. It is defined as weight in kilograms divided by the square of height in meters.[1] It correlates with other measures of body fat and is used as an inexpensive measure of weight-related health risk.
Obesity	A chronic disorder of excessive weight characterized by an excessive accumulation of body fat and a high health risk. It is defined as a BMI ≥ 30 kg/m^2 and further subdivided into class I (BMI 30–34.9 kg/m^2), class II (BMI 35–39.9 kg/m^2), and class III obesity (BMI ≥ 40 kg/m^2).[1]
Overweight	Weight above the established normal range but below the criteria for obesity. It is defined as a BMI between 25 and 29.9 kg/m^2.[1]

ETIOLOGY

Most weight gain is primary weight gain, resulting from excess body fat accumulation due to physiologic or behavioral changes that result in an imbalance between energy intake and expenditure. The natural history of weight change depends on several factors. Weight gain is highest between the ages of 24 and 34 years; after age 55, adults tend to lose weight. Weight gain is also higher among women than men. African American women between 25 and 45 years have slightly higher average weight gain than Caucasians possibly due to differences in socioeconomic status. Furthermore, weight gain can result from a change in the physiology such as during pregnancy or menopause. It can also occur when a cigarette smoker stops smoking because nicotine is a mild stimulant and appetite suppressant.

10-Year Change in BMI and Weight in the United States[2]

Age at Baseline (years)	Change in BMI (kg/m²)		Change in Body Weight (lb)[a]	
	Men	Women	Men	Women
	Mean (95% CI)	Mean (95% CI)	Mean (95% CI)	Mean (95% CI)
25–34	0.9 (0.7, 1.1)	1.3 (1.1, 1.5)	6.1 (4.7, 7.4)	7.6 (6.4, 8.7)
35–44	0.5 (0.3, 0.7)	0.9 (0.7, 1.1)	3.4 (2.0, 4.7)	5.2 (4.1, 6.4)
45–54	0.0 (–0.2, 0.2)	0.3 (0.1, 0.5)	0.0 (–1.4, 1.4)	1.7 (0.6, 2.9)
55–64	–0.3 (–0.5, –0.1)	–0.5 (–0.8, –0.2)	–2.0 (–3.4, –0.7)	–2.9 (–4.7, –1.2)
65–74	–1.1 (–1.3, –0.9)	–1.7 (–1.9, –1.5)	–7.4 (–8.8, –6.1)	–9.9 (–11.1, –8.7)

[a]Change in weight for men at an average height of 5 ft, 9 in and change in weight for women at an average height of 5 ft, 4 in.

Weight gain uncommonly results from secondary causes such as endocrine disorders, genetic syndromes, or medication side effects. Although the prevalence is not well established, secondary weight gain is important because it can be reversed if the underlying cause is addressed. However, secondary causes frequently coexist with primary obesity, so treatment for a specific secondary cause may not entirely reverse weight back to the normal level. Medication side effects are probably the most common secondary cause. Common offenders include glucocorticoids, anticonvulsants, antipsychotics, antidepressants, contraceptives, and diabetic medications. Endocrine disorders causing obesity include hyperinsulinemia, hypercortisolism, hypothyroidism, polycystic ovary syndrome, and hypogonadism. Obesity is also a component of several rare genetic syndromes, including Prader-Willi syndrome, Laurence-Moon syndrome, Cohen syndrome, and Biemond syndrome.

Differential Diagnosis

Physiologic predisposition	*Comments*
Primary weight gain or obesity	Most common cause of weight gain
Menopause[3]	20% of patients gain ≥ 9.9 lb during a 3-year period
Smoking cessation[4]	16%–21% of patients who quit smoking and remain abstinent gain ≥ 33 lb over 10 years
Increase in caloric intake	Alcohol; holiday weight gain
Decrease in physical activity level	
Medications	
Glucocorticoids	Variable weight gain
Diabetic medications[5] (sulfonylurea, insulin)	Sulfonylureas: mean weight gain of 4.0–6.8 lb over 3 years Insulin: Mean weight gain of 6.8 lb over 3 years

Anticonvulsants[6] (gabapentin, valproic acid, carbamazepine)	Valproate: 44%–57% of patients affected with mean weight gain of 46.3 lb
Antipsychotics[7] (phenothiazines, butyrophenones, atypical agents)	Atypical antipsychotics (olanzapine, quetiapine, risperidone, ziprasidone): 9.8%–29% of patients affected with > 7% increase in body weight; mean weight gain: 4.4–26.5 lb
Antidepressants[6,8] (tricyclic antidepressants, monoamine oxidase inhibitors, mirtazapine)	Tricyclics: 13% of patients affected with > 10% increase in body weight; mean weight increase of 1.3–3.1 lb per month Selective serotonin reuptake inhibitors: 4%–26% of patients affected with > 7% increase in body weight; maximum weight gain of 17.0–31.1 lb. Atypical antidepressants (mirtazapine): 10%–13% of patients affected with > 7% increase in body weight.
Injectable or oral contraceptives[9]	18% of patients affected with weight gain > 4.4 lb
Endocrinologic disorders	
Cushing's syndrome Hypothyroidism Hyperinsulinemia Polycystic ovary syndrome Hypogonadism	

GETTING STARTED WITH THE HISTORY

- Allow the patient to describe his or her weight gain.
- Try to understand the patient's concerns about weight gain. A patient may be concerned about acceleration of weight gain or the risk of obesity and its complications or may be seeking assistance to achieve weight control.
- Establish the pace and time course of weight gain and determine whether it is consistent with prior pattern of weight gain.
- Assess for any recent changes in the patient's life such as a recent stressful event, marriage, pregnancy, or recent completion of a weight loss program.
- Be sensitive. Patients may feel embarrassed, stigmatized, or frustrated by their weight gain.

Questions	Remember
Tell me about your weight gain.	Listen to the story.
When did it start?	Avoid interrupting.
How has your weight progressed over time?	Listen to the course of disease and any prior attempts at weight loss for diagnostic clues.

INTERVIEW FRAMEWORK

- Assess for symptoms suggesting weight gain due to excess body fluid accumulation.
- Assess for risk factors contributing to the development of obesity including change in diet or activity level, recent menopause, or mood changes.
- Identify factors that suggest a secondary cause.
- Screen for serious medical complications associated with obesity.

IDENTIFYING ALARM SYMPTOMS

Weight gain due to the accumulation of excess body fluid can occur rapidly, resulting in serious complications. The major causes of abnormal fluid retention are congestive heart failure, renal failure, and chronic liver disease. These conditions can present acutely with pulmonary edema, peripheral edema, ascites, and metabolic derangements.

Serious Diagnoses

	Think about
Accumulation of excess body fluid	Congestive heart failure Renal failure Chronic liver disease
Serious comorbid diseases and their prevalence in the obese population[10]	Impaired glucose tolerance or diabetes (7%–20%) Hypertension (49%–65%) Hyperlipidemia (34%–41%) Coronary heart disease (10%–19%) Sleep apnea (8%–15%) Osteoarthritis (5%–17%)

Alarm Symptoms	Serious Causes	Benign Causes
Accumulation of excess body fluid		
Increased weight over days to weeks	Congestive heart failure Renal failure Chronic liver disease	
Difficulty breathing or coughing at night	Congestive heart failure	Postnasal drip Gastroesophageal reflux Obstructive lung disease
Inability to sleep lying flat	Congestive heart failure	
A recent increase in waist or pant size	Ascites	Constipation Flatulence
Yellowing of the skin or whites of the eyes	Chronic liver disease	
Tea-colored urine	Chronic liver disease	
Prolonged or excessive bleeding	Chronic liver disease Renal failure	Antiplatelet medications Anticoagulants
A decrease in how much you urinate	Renal failure	Benign prostatic hypertrophy
Nausea, vomiting, or generalized itching	Renal failure Chronic liver disease	Thyroid disease Adverse drug reaction
Swelling in the feet, ankles, or legs	Congestive heart failure Renal failure Chronic liver disease	Venous stasis
Development of comorbid diseases		
An increase in thirst or urination	Diabetes	Diuretic use
Blurry vision	Diabetes	Refractive error
Chest tightness or pressure brought on by exertion or emotional stress	Coronary heart disease	Anxiety or panic attack
Snoring or stop breathing during the night	Sleep apnea	
Difficulty staying awake during the day	Sleep apnea	Night shift work Jet lag
Pain or stiffness in weight-bearing joints	Osteoarthritis	Bursitis or muscle or ligament strain

FOCUSED QUESTIONS

After assessing for alarm symptoms, evaluate the factors contributing to the development of obesity.

QUESTIONS	THINK ABOUT...
Chronologic history	
When did the weight gain begin? Is this pattern consistent with previous episodes of weight gain?	Consider patient factors such as age, sex, race, and recent life events to assess whether the weight gain would be considered unusual. Weight gain often occurs with life events such as pregnancy, child rearing, smoking cessation, or a change in marital status or occupation.
Dietary practices	
Describe your typical diet. Have you changed your dietary habits?	A description of dietary practices helps assess how much of the positive energy balance can be attributed to excess caloric intake.
Describe a typical breakfast, lunch, and dinner. Has this changed recently?	Fatty foods predispose to excess caloric intake because they have a higher energy density and greater palatability.
How often do you eat out or eat fast food? Has this changed?	Dining away from home facilitates overeating by providing calorically dense foods in excessively large portion sizes.
Patterns of physical activity	
How often do you engage in planned physical activity? Has this pattern changed?	Sedentary patients are almost twice as likely to gain substantial weight compared with physically active patients. High fitness level has a protective effect with one study showing a lower mortality rate in the fit, overweight group compared with the unfit, normal-weight group.[11]
Weight loss practices	
Are you currently trying to lose weight? When did you start? How much weight did you lose?	Unfortunately, patients who successfully lose weight tend to regain 50% or more of the lost weight after 6 months.
Concurrent psychological conditions	
Have you ever been depressed? How would you describe your mood?	Appetite disturbance can be a vegetative symptom of depression.
Have you been under a lot of stress lately? Do you find yourself eating when you are not hungry to relieve stress?	For some patients, eating is a coping mechanism.
Do you ever go on eating binges? Have you ever taken diuretics or laxatives to help you lose weight? Have you ever made yourself vomit?	Consider eating disorders in patients (especially young women) who admit to binge eating and show excessive concern about body weight or shape.
Medications	
What medication(s) are you taking?	Medications commonly associated with weight gain are listed in the Differential Diagnosis section.

—Continued next page

Family history	
Is there anyone else in your family who is overweight?	Twin, adoption, and family studies suggest that 25%–40% of the variance in BMI can be attributed to genetics.
Endocrine disorders	
	Because no symptom is pathognomonic for these disorders, clinical suspicion relies on the simultaneous development and progression of a constellation of symptoms.
Have you noticed a disproportionate accumulation of fat in the face, trunk, or abdomen?	Cushing's syndrome
Have you noticed any thinning of the skin, reddish purple streaks on the abdomen or flank area, or easy bruising?	
Do you have high blood pressure?	
Do you have elevated blood sugar?	
Do you have an irregular menstrual cycle?	
Have you noticed increasing facial hair or acne?	
Have you been more tired and fatigued?	Hypothyroidism
Do you have dry skin or hair loss?	
Have you been feeling cold?	
Have you been gaining weight despite a poor appetite?	
Have you been constipated?	
Have you been experiencing episodic confusion, headache, seizures, or visual changes when fasting?	Hyperinsulinemia (including insulinoma)
Have you had palpitations, sweating, or tremors when fasting?	
Do you have irregular or infrequent menstrual periods?	Polycystic ovary syndrome
Have you had difficulty becoming pregnant?	
Have you noticed increasing facial hair or acne?	
In men:	
• *Have you had a decrease in libido?*	Hypogonadism
• *Have you had difficulty obtaining erections?*	
• *Have you noted thinning of body and pubic hair?*	
• *Have you been experiencing hot flashes?*	

In women:	
• *Has there been a change in the pattern of your menstrual cycle?*	Hypogonadism
• *Have you been experiencing hot flashes?*	
• *Have you been experiencing insomnia?*	
• *Has your libido decreased?*	
• *Is intercourse uncomfortable or painful?*	

DIAGNOSTIC APPROACH (INCLUDING ALGORITHM)

The diagnostic algorithm for weight gain is shown in Figure 14–1.

CAVEATS

- Weight gain caused by excess body fluid accumulation can occur rapidly over days to weeks, presenting a serious condition that should be evaluated immediately. Weight gain is often not the primary presenting symptom. Because body fat accumulates more gradually, the difference in time course can help distinguish the 2 mechanisms.
- Although the overwhelming majority of cases of weight gain are primary or physiologic, consider secondary causes when the degree of weight gain is inconsistent with the patient's life changes or previous weight gain pattern.

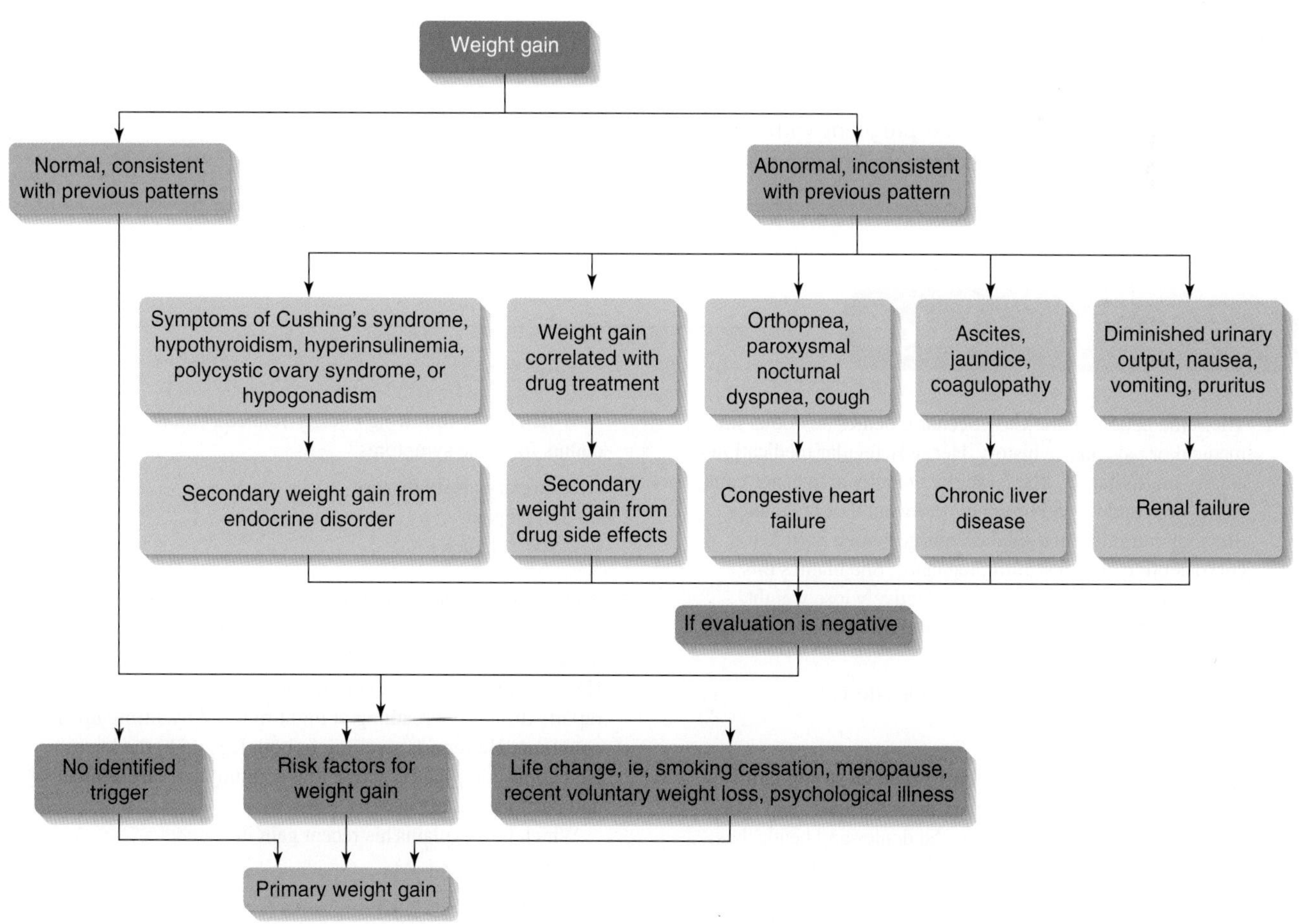

FIGURE 14–1 Diagnostic algorithm: Weight gain.

- Although a secondary cause may contribute to weight gain, it is rarely the sole cause of a patient's obesity.
- Because drug-induced weight gain is probably the most common secondary cause of obesity, always take a thorough medication history.

PROGNOSIS

- Epidemiologic studies show that mortality begins to increase modestly at a BMI above 25 kg/m^2 and that this increase accelerates significantly above a BMI of 30 kg/m^2.[1] This increase in mortality is mostly due to comorbid conditions. Weight loss, even modest amounts, does lead to improvements in the comorbid conditions; whether voluntary weight loss reduces mortality is still unknown.[1]
- Because sustained weight loss is difficult to achieve, more attention should be given to weight gain prevention.

CASE SCENARIO | Resolution

A 35-year-old woman presents to establish care with you. She has no specific concerns. On examination, you observe an obese body habitus and calculate her BMI at 36.5 kg/m^2 based on a weight of 209.5 lb and height of 63.5 inches. When you raise concern about obesity and potential comorbidities, she reveals that she is unhappy with her current weight and has recently embarked on a diet plan to lose weight. She believes she has been at or near her current weight for the past 4 years. She last felt comfortable with her weight when she was 145 lb.

ADDITIONAL HISTORY

She recounts that the last time that she weighed 145 lb was 18 years ago before she became pregnant with her first child. She was able to lose all of the weight gained during the pregnancy after delivery with the first as well as a subsequent pregnancy. However, about 8 years ago, she was unable to lose pregnancy-associated weight after delivery of her third child and subsequently maintained a weight of 176 lb. After her fourth and last pregnancy 4 years ago, she reports losing even less weight after delivery and has maintained a weight just above 200 lb ever since.

Question: Which of the following is this patient's weight gain most likely due to?

A. Primary weight gain
B. Secondary weight gain

Test Your Knowledge

1. The same patient in the Case Scenario denies any other known medical or psychiatric history. Her only regular medication is a daily multivitamin. She is single, sexually active, not using any contraception, and does not desire another pregnancy. She took intramuscular medroxyprogesterone acetate for contraception after her third pregnancy. She blames this medication for not being able to effectively lose weight.
   Which best explains her gain in weight?
   A. Primary
   B. Secondary, from a medication side effect
   C. Both

2. The same patient as in Question 1 reports a strong family history of hypertension, coronary artery disease, and type 2 diabetes. On review of systems, she denies any headaches, exertional chest pain or shortness of breath, orthopnea, paroxysmal nocturnal dyspnea, leg edema, snoring or witnessed apnea at night, or excessive daytime somnolence. She does, however, report some increase in thirst, urination, and visual blurring over the last few months.
   Which of the following obesity-related comorbidities accounts for these symptoms?
   A. Coronary artery disease
   B. Sleep apnea
   C. Type 2 diabetes

3. A 49-year-old man with type 1 diabetes, hypertensive cardiomyopathy, and end-stage renal disease on peritoneal dialysis presents with a 9-lb weight gain over the past month. He had gained 8 lb gradually in the preceding 6 months. He reports difficulty breathing at night relieved by sitting up and coughing. He reports swelling in both legs up to the knees. He claims compliance with a low-sodium diet, furosemide, and peritoneal dialysis.
   Which best explains his recent gain in weight?
   A. Primary weight gain
   B. Secondary weight gain
   C. Excess body fluid accumulation

References

1. Expert Panel on the Identification, Evaluation, and Treatment of Overweight in Adults. Clinical Guidelines on the Identification, Evaluation, and Treatment of Overweight and Obesity in Adults. National Institutes of Health 1998. Available at: http://www.nhlbi.nih.gov/guidelines/obesity/ob_gdlns.htm. Accessed October 11, 2011.
2. Williamson DF, Kahn HS, Remington PL, Anda RF. The 10-year incidence of overweight and major weight gain in US adults. *Arch Intern Med.* 1990;150:665–672.
3. Wing RR, Matthews KA, Kuller LH, Meilahn EN, Plantinga PL. Weight gain at the time of menopause. *Arch Intern Med.* 1991;151:97–102.
4. Flegal KM, Troiano RP, Pamuk ER, Kuczmarski RJ, Campbell SM. The influence of smoking cessation on the prevalence of overweight in the United States. *N Engl J Med.* 1995;333:1165–1170.
5. United Kingdom Prospective Diabetes Study (UKPDS). 13: Relative efficacy of randomly allocated diet, sulphonylurea, insulin, or metformin in patients with newly diagnosed non-insulin dependent diabetes followed for three years. *BMJ.* 1995;310:83–88.
6. Zimmermann U, Kraus T, Himmerich H, Schuld A, Pollmacher T. Epidemiology, implications and mechanisms underlying drug-induced weight gain in psychiatric patients. *J Psychiatr Res.* 2003;37:193–220.
7. Allison DB, Casey DE. Antipsychotic-induced weight gain: a review of the literature. *J Clin Psychiatry.* 2001;62(Suppl 7):22–31.
8. Fava M. Weight gain and antidepressants. *J Clin Psychiatry.* 2000;61(Suppl 11):37–41.
9. Gupta S. Weight gain on the combined pill—is it real? *Hum Reprod.* 2000;6:427–431.
10. Must A, Spadano J, Coakley EH, Field AE, Colditz G, Dietz WH. The disease burden associated with overweight and obesity. *JAMA.* 1999;282:1523–1529.
11. Lee CD, Jackson AS, Blair SN. US weight guidelines: is it also important to consider cardiorespiratory fitness? *Int J Obes Relat Metab Disord.* 1998;22(Suppl 2):S2–S7.

Suggested Reading

Eckel RH. Non-surgical management of obesity in adults. *N Engl J Med.* 2008;358:1941–1950.

Expert Panel on the Identification, Evaluation, and Treatment of Overweight and Obesity in Adults. The Practical Guide—Identification, Evaluation and Treatment of Overweight and Obesity in Adults. National Institutes of Health 2000. Available at: http://www.nhlbi.nih.gov/guidelines/obesity/prctgd_c.pdf. Accessed October 11, 2011.

Lau DCW, Douketis JD, Morrison KM, Hramiak IM, Sharma AM, Ur E. 2006 Canadian clinical practice guidelines on the management and prevention of obesity in adults and children. *CMAJ.* 2007;176(Suppl 8):S1–S13.

Chapter 15

Weight Loss

Thuan Ong, MD, MPH, Miya Allen, MD, and Tonya Fancher MD, MPH

CASE SCENARIO

A 78-year-old Japanese man is brought in for evaluation of a 13-lb weight loss over the course of 6 months. He has moderate Alzheimer's dementia and dependency in all of his activities of daily living and lives in an assisted living facility. He reports a poor appetite and finds food "unappealing." The assisted living facility staff prepare all meals in a Western American cuisine style. The rest of his review of systems is negative with the exception of having discomfort with his dentures. His past medical history is significant for coronary artery disease, hypertension, and hypothyroidism. His medications include aspirin 325 mg daily, lisinopril 20 mg daily, metoprolol 25 mg twice daily, levothyroxine 100 µg daily, and donepezil 10 mg nightly.

- **What additional questions would you ask to learn more about his weight loss?**
- **How would you classify his weight loss?**
- **What are possible causes of his weight loss?**
- **How can you distinguish between etiologies for weight loss?**

INTRODUCTION

Weight loss can be divided into 2 categories: involuntary or voluntary. *Involuntary* weight loss is a manifestation of cachexia associated with many disease states. Population studies have consistently shown increased mortality with involuntary weight loss even after adjusting for pre-existing illnesses and age.[1,2] *Voluntary* weight loss, in the form of healthy dieting, is common among men and women. However, significant voluntary weight loss can herald a psychiatric illness such as an eating disorder, particularly among women. Anorexia is associated with a 12 times higher death rate among women aged 15 to 24 years.[3] A careful history, physical examination, and directed diagnostic testing will suggest an etiology for weight loss in most patients.

KEY TERMS

Anorexia	Loss of the desire to eat.
Anorexia nervosa[4]	Intense fear of gaining weight and refusal to maintain weight at or above a minimally appropriate weight for height and age.
Bulimia nervosa[4]	Recurrent episodes of binge eating followed by recurrent compensatory behavior to prevent weight gain (ie, laxative abuse and self-induced vomiting).
Cachexia	General muscle and/or fat wasting with malnutrition usually associated with chronic disease.
Involuntary weight loss	The unintended loss of weight; sometimes not reported by the patient and only noted upon chart review.
Malnutrition	Poor nutrition due to inadequate or unbalanced intake of nutrients or their impaired utilization.
Voluntary weight loss	The conscious effort to lose weight; frequently not a complaint among those with eating disorders.

ETIOLOGY

Weight loss is a nonspecific sign of many diseases. Most causes of involuntary weight loss belong to 1 of 4 categories: (1) malignancy, (2) psychiatric diseases, (3) chronic inflammation or infectious disease, and (4) metabolic disorders.[5] Cancer is the most common cause of involuntary weight loss, accounting for 16% to 36% of cases. Psychiatric causes of involuntary weight loss (eg, depression) are also common.[6] After healthy dieting, eating disorders (most commonly anorexia nervosa and bulimia nervosa) are the most common cause of voluntary weight loss. Almost 95% of anorexic patients and 80% of bulimics are women. Women in their lifetime have up to 3.7% risk of anorexia and 4.2% risk of bulimia.[7] Involuntary weight loss in older adults is often a syndrome (ie, multifactorial) and related to underlying age-related changes, medical conditions, psychosocial issues, and medication side effects.

Common Causes of Involuntary Weight Loss in Older Adults[6]

Etiology of Weight Loss	Prevalence
Malignancy	16%–36%
Unknown	10%–36%
Psychiatric illness (especially depression)	9%–42%
Gastrointestinal disease	6%–19%
Respiratory disease	~6%
Endocrine disorder (especially hyperthyroidism)	4%–11%
Nutritional disorders due to alcoholism	4%–8%
Renal disease	~4%
Cardiovascular disease	2%–9%
Neurologic disease	2%–7%
Chronic infection	2%–5%
Connective tissue disease	2%–4%
Drug-induced weight loss (medication side effect)	~2%

Differential Diagnosis

Voluntary Weight Loss	
Anorexia nervosa[4]	Diagnostic criteria: • 15% or more below ideal body weight • Fear of weight gain • Body image disturbance • Primary amenorrhea or secondary amenorrhea for 3 consecutive menstrual cycles (in women)
Bulimia nervosa[4]	Diagnostic criteria: • Recurrent binge eating — Large quantity of food in discrete time period AND — A feeling of lack of control over eating • Recurrent compensatory behavior to prevent weight gain • Cycle occurs at least twice weekly for 3 months • Body dissatisfaction

Healthy dieting	Healthy eating plans that reduce calories but do not exclude specific foods or food groups. • Weight loss is slow and steady: three-fourths to 2 lb per week and no more than 3 lb per week. • Includes special diets, such as very-low-calorie diets that require medical supervision. • Includes regular exercise and a plan to maintain weight loss. Healthy dieting should be considered in the context of cultural norms.

GETTING STARTED WITH THE HISTORY

- Review the medical record to confirm weight loss. Clinically significant weight loss is often defined as 10 lb (4.5 kg) or greater *or* more than 5% of the baseline body weight over 6 to 12 months.
- Calculate the body mass index (BMI) = body weight (kg)/height (m^2).
  - A normal BMI is 18.5 to 24.9 kg/m^2.
  - A BMI less than 18.5 is underweight.
- Calculate the ideal body weight (IBW).
  - Males: IBW = 50 kg + 2.3 kg for each inch over 5 ft tall
  - Females: IBW = 45.5 kg + 2.3 kg for each inch over 5 ft tall

INTERVIEW FRAMEWORK

- Involuntary weight loss is usually disturbing to patients. Take time to reassure them that you will work together to find an answer.
- Note the patient's age as this can narrow the differential possibilities.
- Establish whether the weight loss is voluntary or involuntary.
- Assess for anorexia and dietary intake.
- Determine the onset, duration, and amount of weight loss.
- Explore positive responses from the review of symptoms (especially the pulmonary and digestive systems), gender- and age-appropriate cancer screening, and depression and cognitive impairment screening (see Chapter 64, Depressed Mood, for depression screening tools).
- When obtaining the past medical history, ask about chronic inflammatory conditions or exposures.

IDENTIFYING ALARM SYMPTOMS

- With the exception of healthy dieting, significant weight loss itself is an alarm symptom suggesting underlying pathology.
- Cancer accounts for about one-third of patients with involuntary weight loss.[8]
- Eating disorders carry the highest premature mortality rate among all psychiatric illnesses. Eating disorders can lead to electrolyte abnormalities and fatal arrhythmias that may require urgent evaluation.

FOCUSED QUESTIONS

After having the patient tell his or her story, follow-up with a few closed-ended questions to help narrow the differential diagnosis.

QUESTIONS	THINK ABOUT...
Is your appetite increased?	Hyperthyroidism or malabsorption, diabetes, oropharyngeal disorders
Have you lost the desire to eat?	Cancer, psychiatric causes, congestive heart failure, chronic obstructive lung disease, chronic infections, human immunodeficiency virus (HIV)/acquired immunodeficiency syndrome (AIDS), chronic inflammatory or connective tissue disease
Do you have any fevers, chills, or night sweats?	Infection (eg, tuberculosis) or hematologic malignancy

—Continued next page

Continued—

Do you exercise excessively?	Eating disorders
Are you overly concerned about the way you look?	Eating disorders
Are your menstrual periods irregular? (women)	Anorexia nervosa
Have you ever used self-induced vomiting, water pills (diuretics), laxatives, or enemas to control your weight?	Bulimia
Do you have little interest or pleasure in doing things?	Depression
Do you have frequent bowel movements or diarrhea?	Malabsorption
Does fear of abdominal pain make you not want to eat?	Mesenteric ischemia
Are you pregnant?	Hyperemesis gravidarum
Do you have abdominal pain, early satiety, blood in your stool, or trouble swallowing?	Gastrointestinal cancer
Do your symptoms change with different foods?	Malabsorption
Have you ever injected drugs, had unprotected sex, or received blood transfusions?	HIV infection
Do you use cocaine, amphetamines, or over-the-counter medications[a] (eg, ephedra, ephedrine, ma huang, 5-hydroxytryptophan, teas, garcinia [hydroxycitric acid/HCA], herbal fen-phen, phentermine, St. John wort, herbal laxatives, or diuretics, melatonin)?	Drug-induced weight loss
Did the onset of weight loss correlate with starting new medications?	Drug-induced anorexia or increased metabolism (eg, selective serotonin reuptake inhibitors, levodopa, digoxin, metformin, theophylline, opiates, methylphenidate)
Do you feel nervous, sweaty, or warm?	Hyperthyroidism
Do you feel thirsty or that you need to urinate more frequently?	Diabetes mellitus
Do you experience facial flushing or dizziness when you stand (and have high blood pressure)?	Pheochromocytoma
Do you have any new rashes, joint pain, or joint swelling?	Connective tissue disease or autoimmune disorder (eg, rheumatoid arthritis, lupus, sarcoidosis)

[a]A partial list of potential medications; see also http://nccam.nih.gov.

DIAGNOSTIC APPROACH (INCLUDING ALGORITHM)

Patients with medical causes of weight loss usually have signs and symptoms suggesting involvement of a particular organ system. One of the most important tasks is to differentiate malignant or other serious disease from psychiatric causes. Physical examination findings suggest a diagnosis in 55% of patients with involuntary weight loss.[9] Patients with involuntary weight loss who are ultimately diagnosed with cancer all have at least 1 abnormal laboratory test at initial evaluation. Abnormal complete blood cell count, lactate dehydrogenase, albumin, and hepatic enzymes have the highest discriminatory value (Table 15–1).[9,10] All patients with cancer and 94% of those with other organic disease have at least 1 laboratory abnormality.

Table 15–1. Likelihood ratios (LR) of selected laboratory tests for the diagnosis of cancer.[10]

Laboratory Test	LR+ for the Diagnosis of Cancer (95% CI)	LR– for the Diagnosis of Cancer (95% CI)
Abnormal complete blood count[a]	1.5 (1.3–1.9)	0.4 (0.3–0.6)
Albumin < 3.5 mg/dL	2.1 (1.5–2.8)	0.4 (0.3–0.6)
Abnormal hepatic enzymes[b]	2.5 (1.7–3.6)	0.5 (0.3–0.7)
Lactate dehydrogenase > 500 U/L	5.2 (3–11)	0.6 (0.5–0.8)
Any of the above	1.5 (0.9–1.2)	0.2 (0.1–0.4)

CI, confidence interval.

[a] Hemoglobin < 11 g/L for women or < 13 g/L for men, or white blood cell count > 12,000/μL.

[b] Alanine aminotransferase or aspartate aminotransferase > 50 U/L, alkaline phosphatase > 300 U/L, or gamma-glutamyl transferase > 50 U/L.

If the weight loss is unconfirmed by a thorough history and physical examination, delaying further testing may be appropriate. If alarm signs or symptoms develop or weight loss is confirmed at follow-up appointment, diagnostic testing should begin. The diagnostic algorithm for weight loss is shown in Figure 15–1.

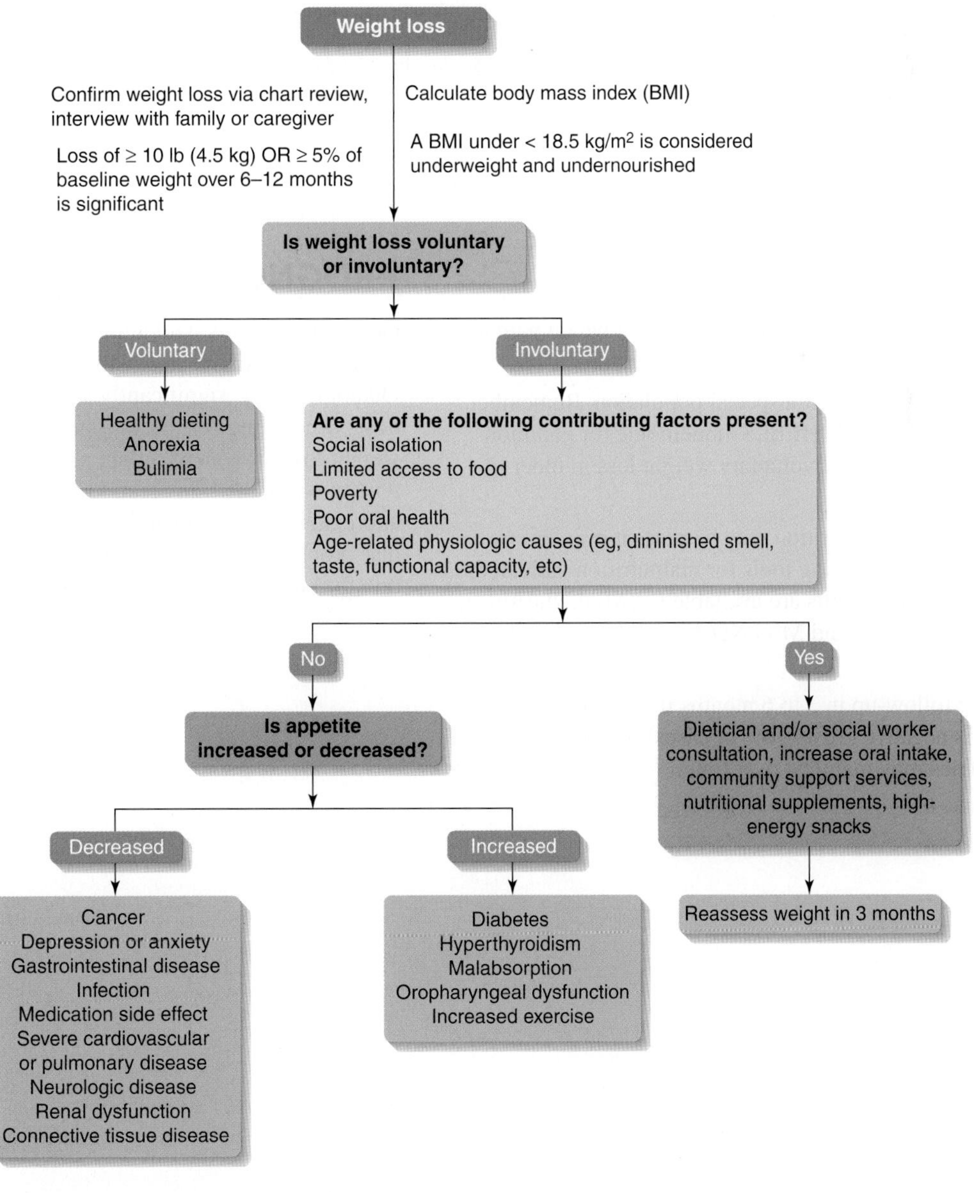

FIGURE 15–1 Diagnostic algorithm: Weight loss.

Common Treatable Causes of Involuntary Weight Loss in Older Adults	
M	**M**edication effects
E	**E**motional problems, especially depression
A	**A**norexia tardive[a] (nervosa), alcoholism
L	**L**ate-life paranoia
S	**S**wallowing disorders
O	**O**ral factors (eg, poorly fitting dentures, cavities)
N	**N**o money
W	**W**andering and other dementia-related behaviors
H	**H**yper-/hypothyroidism, hyperparathyroidism, hypoadrenalism
E	**E**nteric problems (eg, malabsorption)
E	**E**ating problems (eg, inability to feed self)
L	**L**ow-salt, low-cholesterol diets
S	**S**ocial issues (eg, social isolation, inability to obtain preferred foods)

[a] Anorexia tardive is the presence of abnormal attitudes about food intake and body image with severe weight loss in older adults.[12]

CAVEATS

- Do not forget Munchausen syndrome, in which patients may voluntarily lose weight to get attention.
- Older adults represent a special population. Remember the "MEALS ON WHEELS" mnemonic for common treatable causes of involuntary weight loss in older adults[11]:
- Anorexia or malnutrition may be present even before weight loss. Screening tools for malnutrition validated for use in older adults are available (ie, Mini Nutritional Assessment Tool and Mini Nutritional Assessment-Short Form).[13]
- Ensure follow-up in 3 to 6 months if the initial evaluation is negative (10%–36% of cases) because some etiologies may manifest over time.

PROGNOSIS

Generally, patients with unintentional weight loss have higher mortality rates: 9% at 24 months and 38% at 30 months.[8] Outcomes vary significantly according to underlying diagnosis accounting for the weight loss. Patients with idiopathic weight loss have an excellent prognosis: Their survival rate is 95% at 6 months.[8] Eighteen to 20% of patients with untreated anorexia nervosa die within 20 years, most commonly of cardiac problems, renal failure, or suicide. The premature mortality rate for bulimia is 5% at 10 years.[14]

CASE SCENARIO | Resolution

A 78-year-old Japanese man is brought in for evaluation of a 13-lb weight loss over the course of 6 months. He has moderate Alzheimer's dementia and dependency in all of his activities of daily living and lives in an assisted living facility. He reports a poor appetite and finds food "unappealing." The assisted living facility staff prepare all meals in a Western American cuisine style. The rest of his review of systems is negative with the exception of having discomfort with his dentures. His past medical history is also significant for coronary artery disease, hypertension, and hypothyroidism. His medications include aspirin 325 mg daily, lisinopril 20 mg daily, metoprolol 25 mg twice daily, levothyroxine 100 μg daily, and donepezil 10 mg nightly.

ADDITIONAL HISTORY

On examination, he is noted to be thin but not cachectic. His previous BMI 6 months ago was 22 kg/m^2; his current BMI is 20 kg/m^2. He is alert and appropriately responding to questions. He has poorly fitting dentures that have caused an ulceration on his lower left gum line. His screen for depression is negative. The rest of his examination is unremarkable.

Question: What is the most likely explanation for his weight loss?

A. Anorexia from his acetylcholinesterase inhibitor
B. Dysgeusia from his angiotensin-converting enzyme inhibitor
C. Lack of ethnically directed food
D. Poorly fitting dentures
E. All of the above

Test Your Knowledge

1. A 23-year-old woman presents with weight loss of 17 lb over the past 8 months. She reports that she has been trying to lose weight with an increase in daily physical activity and reducing her caloric intake. Her mother was recently diagnosed with diabetes, which has prompted her to be more vigilant about her weight. She denies any other symptoms and has regular menstruation. Her vitals are temperature of 37.0°C, heart rate of 65, blood pressure of 119/72, respiratory rate of 10, and weight of 124 lb with a BMI of 26 kg/m^2 (her previous BMI was 27.5 kg/m^2).

   What is the most likely diagnosis for her weight loss?

   A. Anorexia nervosa
   B. Bulimia nervosa
   C. Healthy dieting
   D. Hyperthyroidism

2. An 84-year-old woman presents with anorexia and involuntary weight loss of 9 lb over the previous 6 months. She has lived in an assisted living facility for 2 years due to her mild to moderate dementia and dependency for all instrumental activities of daily living. She reports that she is feeling tired, does not have an appetite, and has blurry vision that she is unable to characterize further. The staff prepare all her meals and report that there has not been any change in her behavior except that she does not want to eat and pushes food away. Her past medical history is significant for coronary artery disease, atrial fibrillation, hypertension, and Alzheimer's dementia. Her medications include aspirin 325 mg daily, hydrochlorothiazide 25 mg daily, metoprolol 12.5 mg twice daily, donepezil 10 mg nightly, and digoxin 0.250 μg daily (started 7 months earlier for rate control of atrial fibrillation). Her vitals show a temperature of 37.3°C, heart rate of 54, blood pressure of 139/72, respiratory rate of 12, and weight of 99 lb (previous weight, 108 lb). On examination, she is frail and thin and has a visual acuity with Snellen eye chart of 20/50 bilaterally, and an irregularly irregular cardiac rhythm. The rest of her examination is unremarkable.

   What is the most likely cause of her involuntary weight loss?

   A. Cardiac cachexia
   B. Digoxin toxicity
   C. Normal physiologic changes
   D. Worsening dementia

3. A 67-year-old woman presents with involuntary weight loss of 12 lb over the course of 6 months. She reports eating "voraciously." Her review of systems is only pertinent for occasional palpitations and loose stools. Her past medical history includes smoking 1 pack per day for the past 15 years. She takes no medications or supplements. On examination, her vitals are notable for heart rate of 108 and blood pressure of 157/89. She appears thin but well nourished, with thinning eyebrows laterally, warm and smooth skin, and a high-frequency, low-amplitude action tremor in both hands.

   What is the most likely diagnosis causing her weight loss?

   A. Anorexia nervosa
   B. Diabetes
   C. Hyperthyroidism
   D. Lung cancer

References

1. Pamuk ER, Williamson DF, Serdula MK, Madans J, Byers TE. Weight-loss and subsequent death in a cohort of United-States adults. *Ann Intern Med.* 1993;119:744–748.
2. Wallace JI, Schwartz RS, Lacroix AZ, Uhlmann RF, Pearlman RA. Involuntary weight-loss in older outpatients: incidence and clinical significance. *J Am Geriatr Soc.* 1995;43:329–337.
3. Sullivan PF. Mortality in anorexia-nervosa. *Am J Psychiatry.* 1995;152:1073–1074.
4. American Psychiatric Association. *Diagnostic and statistical manual of mental disorders.* Revised 4th ed. Washington, DC: American Psychiatric Association, 2000.
5. Reife CM. Involuntary weight-loss. *Med Clin N Am.* 1995;79:299–313.
6. Alibhai SMH, Greenwood C, Payette H. An approach to the management of unintentional weight loss in elderly people. *Can Med Assoc J.* 2005;172:773–780.
7. Bell C, Bulik C, Clayton P, et al. Practice guideline for the treatment of patients with eating disorders (revision). *Am J Psychiatry.* 2000;157:1–39.
8. Bouras EP, Lange SM, Scolapio JS. Rational approach to patients with unintentional weight loss. *Mayo Clin Proc.* 2001;76:923–929.
9. Metalidis C, Knockaert DC, Bobbaers H, Vanderschueren S. Involuntary weight loss. Does a negative baseline evaluation provide adequate reassurance? *Eur J Intern Med.* 2008;19:345–349.
10. Hernandez JL, Riancho JA, Matorras P, Gonzalez-Macias J. Clinical evaluation for cancer in patients with involuntary weight loss without specific symptoms. *Am J Med.* 2003;114:631–637.
11. Morley JE, Silver AJ. Nutritional issues in nursing-home care. *Ann Intern Med.* 1995;123:850–859.
12. Beers MH, Berkow R, eds. *The Merck Manual of Geriatrics.* 3rd ed. Whitehouse Station, NJ: John Wiley & Sons, 2000.
13. Bauer JM, Kaiser MJ, Anthony P, Guigoz Y, Sieber CC. The Mini Nutritional Assessment: its history, today's practice, and future perspectives. *Nutr Clin Pract.* 2008;23:388–396.
14. Powers PS, Santana CA. Eating disorders: a guide for the primary care physician. *Prim Care.* 2002;29:81–98.

Suggested Reading

Bulik CM, Reba L, Siega-Riz AM, Reichborn-Kjennerud T. Anorexia nervosa: definition, epidemiology, and cycle of risk. *Int J Eat Disord.* 2005;37(Suppl):S2–S9.

Evans WJ, Morley JE, Argilés J, et al. Cachexia: a new definition. *Clin Nutr.* 2008;27:793–799.

Pritts SD, Susman J. Diagnosis of eating disorders in primary care. *Am Fam Physician.* 2003;67:297–304.

Singer P, Attalp-Singer J, Shapiro H. Body mass index and weight change: the sixth vital sign. *Isr Med Assoc J.* 2008;10:523–525.

Steinhausen HC, Weber S. The outcome of bulimia nervosa: findings from one-quarter century of research. *Am J Psychiatry.* 2009;166:1331–1341.

SECTION III

HEAD, EYES, EARS, NOSE, AND THROAT

Chapter 16

Red Eye

David F. Jacobson, MD

CASE SCENARIO

A 41-year-old woman presents to your clinic complaining of a "red eye." The redness is diffuse and has been present for 2 days. She also reports mild, watery discharge and a slight sensation of grittiness. She does not have significant pain and has not noticed any change in her vision.

- **What focused questions can you ask to narrow your diagnostic considerations?**
- **What alarm symptoms should prompt immediate referral to an ophthalmologist?**
- **How would you discern whether her eye complaints signify ocular involvement from a systemic disease?**

INTRODUCTION

Ophthalmologic complaints are very common in clinical practice, accounting for approximately 3% of emergency department visits.[1] Frequently, patients report a "red eye," which generates a broad range of diagnostic possibilities. Most causes of a "red eye" are benign or self-limited and can be managed by a primary care physician. However, some etiologies require urgent referral to an ophthalmologist. While the physical examination is important, a good history is critical in separating the benign causes of a "red eye" from those associated with increased morbidity. See Figure 16–1 for an illustration of the structures of the orbit and eyelid.

KEY TERMS

Conjunctiva	A thin outer membrane lining the inner lids (palpebral conjunctiva) and the globe (bulbar conjunctiva)
Meibomian gland	A modified sweat gland in the tarsal plate of the eyelid
Ciliary body	Part of the eye involved in production of aqueous humor and in accommodation, located between the iris and the choroid
Choroid	A vascular layer in the eye between the sclera and retina
Chemosis	Edema of the conjunctiva
Orbital septum	Also known as the palpebral ligament; serves as the anterior boundary of the orbit
Foreign body sensation	The feeling that something is "stuck" in the eye
Seronegative spondyloarthropathies	Reactive arthritis, psoriatic arthritis, inflammatory bowel disease, ankylosing spondylitis

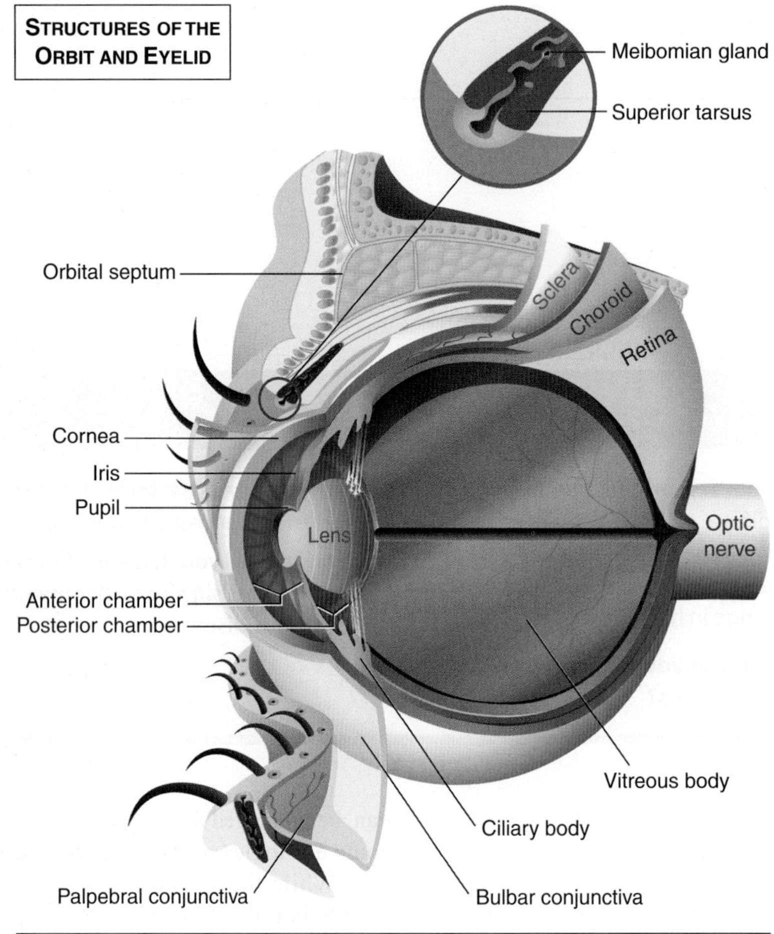

FIGURE 16–1 Structures of the orbit and eyelid. (Illustration by Richard Wong.)

ETIOLOGY

The erythema in a "red eye" is often caused by conjunctival inflammation but also may result from dilated scleral or episcleral vessels or inflammation of the deeper structures of the eye and surrounding tissues. Although the exact incidence of diagnoses presenting as a "red eye" is not well defined, most are benign. In the emergency department, 75% of ophthalmologic complaints are due to conjunctivitis, corneal abrasions, or foreign bodies.[1] In a study of patients presenting to an outpatient clinic with eye symptoms, the most common diagnoses were conjunctivitis and benign disorders of the eyelid such as blepharitis. In the same study, morbid diseases were rare; acute angle-closure glaucoma composed only 1.2% of diagnoses and uveitis composed only 0.6%.[2]

Differential Diagnosis

	Explanation[1,3–5]	Prevalence per 1000 Population (ages 1–74)[a,6]
Ocular diagnoses that do not require ophthalmology referral		
Chalazion	Chronic granulomatous inflammation of the meibomian gland	
Hordeolum ("stye")	Acute suppurative inflammation of glands along the lash line	1

Blepharitis	Acute or chronic inflammation of the eyelid due to seborrheic dermatitis or staphylococcal infection resulting in redness and crusting	26
Pterygium	A benign lesion typically on the nasal aspect of the bulbar conjunctiva that results from prolonged exposure to ultraviolet light	16
Subconjunctival hemorrhage	Bleeding from subconjunctival vessels May be associated with hypertension, bleeding diatheses, or Valsalva (coughing, straining)	
Conjunctivitis	Inflammation of conjunctiva	13
• Viral	Adenovirus is a common cause	
• Bacterial	Staphylococcus aureus, Streptococcus pneumoniae, and Haemophilus influenzae are the most common etiologies; hyperacute conjunctivitis raises concern for gonococcal infection and requires immediate referral to ophthalmology	
• Allergic	Patients may have a history of atopy and usually complain of itching Chemosis may be present	
Foreign body/corneal abrasion	The patient will typically report a history of trauma or something getting into the eye (foreign bodies may be removed by a primary care physician or referred to an ophthalmologist)	
Episcleritis	Dilation of episcleral vessels, most commonly idiopathic	
Ocular diagnoses requiring referral to an ophthalmologist		
Scleritis	Inflammation of the sclera Frequently associated with autoimmune or connective tissue disease such as rheumatoid arthritis and granulomatosis with polyangiitis	
Uveitis	Inflammation of the iris (iritis), ciliary body (cyclitis), or choroid (choroiditis) Anterior uveitis (involvement of the iris and ciliary body) is more common than posterior uveitis (choroiditis) 30%–70% of cases are associated with human leukocyte antigen B27 Often associated with systemic illnesses such as seronegative spondyloarthropathies, sarcoidosis, and many bacterial, viral, parasitic, and fungal infections[5]	

—Continued next page

Continued—		
Acute angle-closure glaucoma	Elevated intraocular pressure due to obstruction of outflow of aqueous humor, more prevalent in an older population	3[b]
Endophthalmitis	Intraocular inflammation/infection May result from local extension from trauma or ocular surgery or from hematogenous spread	
Keratitis	Corneal inflammation Causes may be bacterial (s aureus, s pneumoniae, Pseudomonas aeruginosa [in contact lens wearers]) and viral (herpes simplex and varicella zoster)	2
Extraocular causes of red eye		
Periorbital cellulitis (preseptal)	Bacterial infection of the soft tissues anterior to the orbital septum	
Orbital cellulitis	Bacterial infection involving deeper orbital tissues posterior to the orbital septum Frequently represents extension from underlying sinusitis More serious than periorbital cellulitis	

[a]Empty cells indicate that the prevalence is unknown

[b]This prevalence pertains to glaucoma "causing visual decrease" and does not necessarily reflect only acute angle-closure glaucoma. Acute glaucoma is an uncommon presentation in the outpatient setting.

GETTING STARTED WITH THE HISTORY

- Begin with open-ended questions and allow the patient to provide the history in his or her own words.
- You will then need to ask focused questions to help differentiate between benign causes of a "red eye" and more serious causes that will require referral to an ophthalmologist.
- While taking the history, pay attention to the general appearance of the patient. Patients with more serious diagnoses may be sitting in a darkened examination room, be unable to keep the affected eye open, or appear physically ill.

INTERVIEW FRAMEWORK

- Determine the acuity of the illness.
- Assess whether the patient has had similar episodes before.
- Ask about:
  - Prescription or over-the-counter medications
  - Systemic diseases that may have ocular manifestations (inflammatory bowel disease, connective tissue diseases like rheumatoid arthritis, other autoimmune diseases, or chronic infiltrative or inflammatory diseases like sarcoidosis and tuberculosis)
  - Trauma or recent eye surgery
  - Contact lens use (*this puts patients at increased risk for corneal problems such as infectious keratitis; extended-wear lenses have a higher risk than daily wear lenses*)[7]
- Always assess for alarm symptoms.

IDENTIFYING ALARM SYMPTOMS[1–4]

A priority in history taking is to screen for alarm symptoms that suggest more serious, sight-threatening diseases that require emergent or urgent referral to an ophthalmologist. If the patient was exposed to a caustic agent, the first priority should be immediate irrigation and referral to an emergency department. If there is no exposure history, the examiner should focus on alarm symptoms such as pain, foreign body sensation, decreased visual acuity, and photophobia. Unfortunately, there is little information regarding the positive or negative predictive values of the following alarm symptoms.

Alarm Symptoms	Serious Causes	Benign Causes
Foreign body sensation	Keratitis	Foreign body/corneal abrasion Conjunctivitis (patients typically report a gritty feeling and not a true foreign body sensation)
Nausea and vomiting	Acute angle-closure glaucoma	
Pain	Keratitis Scleritis Uveitis Acute angle-closure glaucoma Endophthalmitis Orbital cellulitis	Episcleritis (may have mild, dull pain)
Photophobia	Keratitis Scleritis Uveitis	Foreign body/corneal abrasion
Decreased visual acuity	Keratitis Uveitis Acute angle-closure glaucoma Endophthalmitis Scleritis (sometimes)	Conjunctivitis (visual acuity is intact but discharge may cause mild visual blurring that clears with blinking)
Diplopia	Orbital cellulitis	

FOCUSED QUESTIONS[1,3–5]

QUESTIONS	THINK ABOUT...
General	
Did something get in your eye?	Foreign body
Is the eye redness localized?	Subconjunctival hemorrhage Inflamed pterygium Episcleritis
Have you had recent sick contacts?	Viral conjunctivitis
Have you had prolonged exposure to ultraviolet light? (outdoor jobs or hobbies)	Pterygium
Were you coughing or straining prior to your eye becoming red?	Subconjunctival hemorrhage
If discharge is present	
Is it watery?	Allergic conjunctivitis Viral conjunctivitis
Are your eyelashes matted together in the morning with purulent crusting?	Bacterial conjunctivitis

—Continued next page

Continued—

Was the onset of purulent discharge hyperacute? (< 24 hours)	Gonococcal conjunctivitis
Have you had a recent upper respiratory infection or sick contact?	Viral conjunctivitis
Are you sexually active?	Gonococcal conjunctivitis Chlamydial conjunctivitis
Is the discharge chronic?	Chlamydial conjunctivitis
If pain or discomfort is present	
Is there a mild burning sensation?	Extraocular processes such as: Blepharitis Conjunctivitis Pterygium Episcleritis
Is the pain sharp?	Keratitis Corneal ulcer/abrasion
Is the pain dull and aching?	Episcleritis Scleritis Uveitis Acute angle-closure glaucoma
Associated symptoms	
Do you see halos around lights?	Acute angle-closure glaucoma
Do you have significant itching?	Allergic conjunctivitis
Do you have diplopia or pain with movement of your eyes?	Orbital cellulitis
Do you have nausea, vomiting, or abdominal pain?	Acute angle-closure glaucoma
Relevant medical history	
Are you taking blood thinners (anticoagulants)?	Subconjunctival hemorrhage
Do you wear contact lenses?	Keratitis Corneal ulcer/abrasion
Do you have rheumatoid arthritis?[a]	Scleritis Episcleritis (less common association than scleritis)
Do you have a history of seronegative spondyloarthropathies?[a]	Uveitis

[a]*Note that there is significant overlap in the systemic diseases that may be associated with episcleritis, scleritis, and uveitis. The above are classic associations.*

DIAGNOSTIC APPROACH (INCLUDING ALGORITHM)

The main focus for the initial evaluation is to screen for alarm symptoms; if present, the patient needs referral not only for prompt and appropriate treatment, but also to further allow diagnostic examination that may only be possible in an ophthalmologist's office. In the absence of alarm symptoms, the history alone will frequently point to a specific diagnosis and allow for selection of appropriate treatment. The diagnostic algorithm for red eye is shown in Figure 16–2.

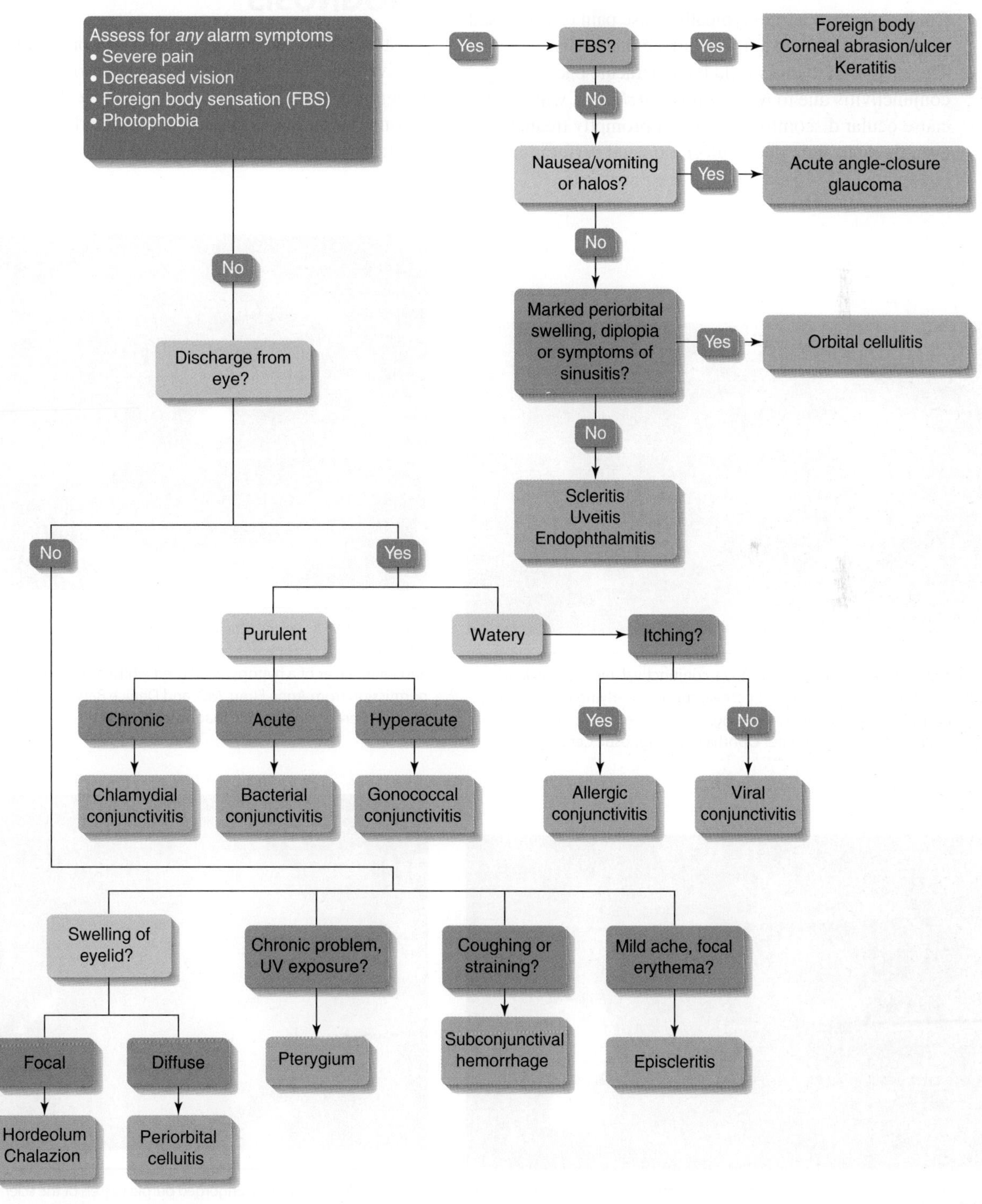

FIGURE 16–2 Diagnostic algorithm: Red eye.

CAVEATS

- It is important to distinguish *foreign body sensation* from the more benign gritty or sand-like sensation that is common in conjunctivitis. A *true* foreign body sensation heralds active corneal involvement resulting in significant discomfort. This may result in the patient having objective difficulty in keeping the affected eye open.
- Conjunctivitis does not typically cause pain or decreased visual acuity beyond a mild blurring due to discharge. The exception to this would be hyperacute bacterial conjunctivitis due to *Neisseria gonorrhoeae*, which can cause ocular discomfort and, if not promptly treated, even threaten sight due to ulceration and perforation.
- Acute angle-closure glaucoma may present as a severe headache rather than eye pain. Other systemic symptoms such as nausea, vomiting, and abdominal pain can further confuse the diagnosis.
- Although episcleritis is usually idiopathic, it may be caused by the systemic diseases associated with scleritis.

PROGNOSIS

Most causes of red eye are self-limited or require simple supportive care such as warm compresses or topical antibiotics. Diagnoses that threaten vision are typically associated with alarm symptoms discussed earlier and require immediate referral to an ophthalmologist. See Figures 16–3 to 16–8.

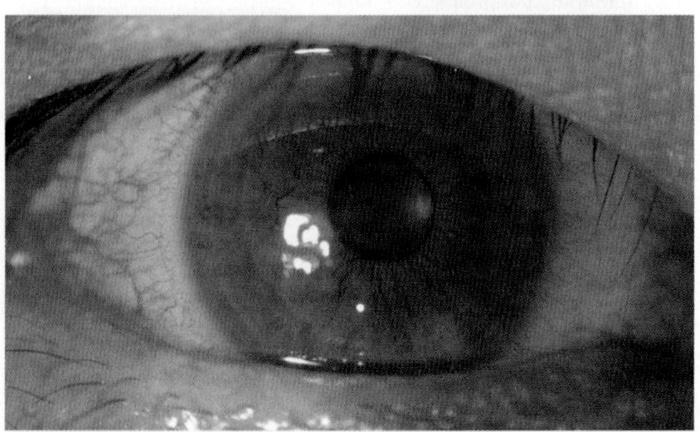

FIGURE 16–3 Herpes keratitis: 1–2+ conjunctival injection, lack of purulent discharge, and irregular corneal surface overlying the dendrite. (Used with permission from Anne Fung, MD, and Denice Barsness, California Pacific Medical Center Ophthalmic Diagnostic Center.)

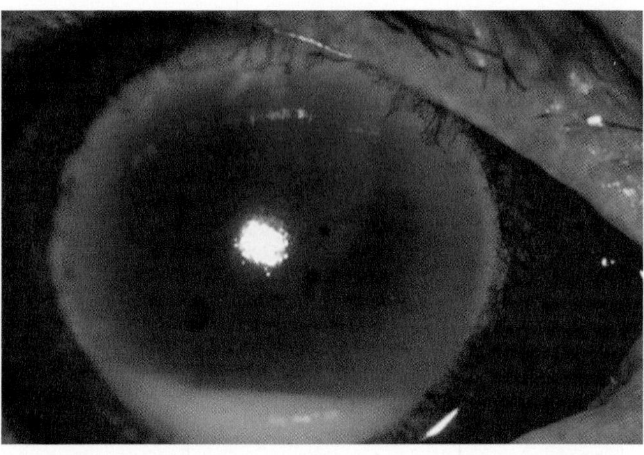

FIGURE 16–5 Endophthalmitis: 3+ conjunctival injection, corneal edema with hazy appearance, pigment on inner surface of cornea, and white layer of a hypopyon (settled white blood cells). (Used with permission from Anne Fung, MD, and Denice Barsness, California Pacific Medical Center Ophthalmic Diagnostic Center.)

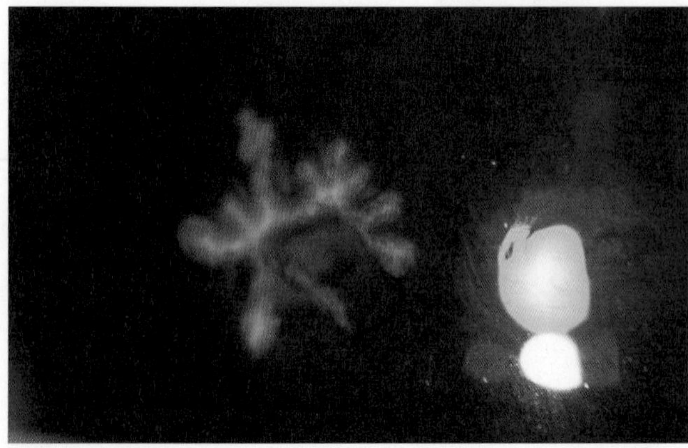

FIGURE 16–4 Herpes dendrite: Close-up of previous eye with fluorescein stain and cobalt blue light showing the branching pattern of the viral dendrite. (Used with permission from Anne Fung, MD, and Denice Barsness, California Pacific Medical Center Ophthalmic Diagnostic Center.)

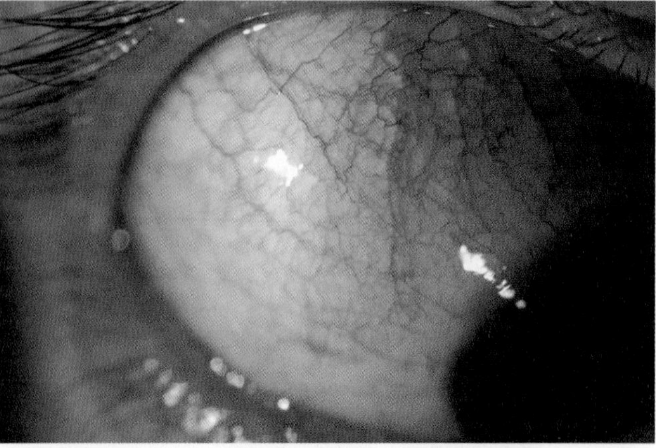

FIGURE 16–6 Scleritis: Engorged purple vessels of the sclera are visible under the 2+ injected conjunctival vessels. Eye is generally tender to the touch in areas of scleritis. It may also develop a blue hue in areas of scleral thinning (not shown). (Used with permission from Anne Fung, MD, and Denice Barsness, California Pacific Medical Center Ophthalmic Diagnostic Center.)

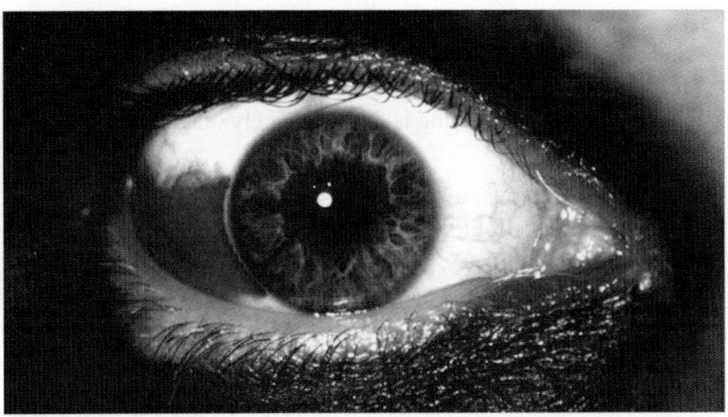

FIGURE 16–7 Subconjunctival hemorrhage: Blood red patch of hemorrhage in area of capillary breakage. It is painless without change in vision and fades in 7 to 10 days. Pain or decreased vision would indicate another problem. (Used with permission from Anne Fung, MD, and Denice Barsness, California Pacific Medical Center Ophthalmic Diagnostic Center.)

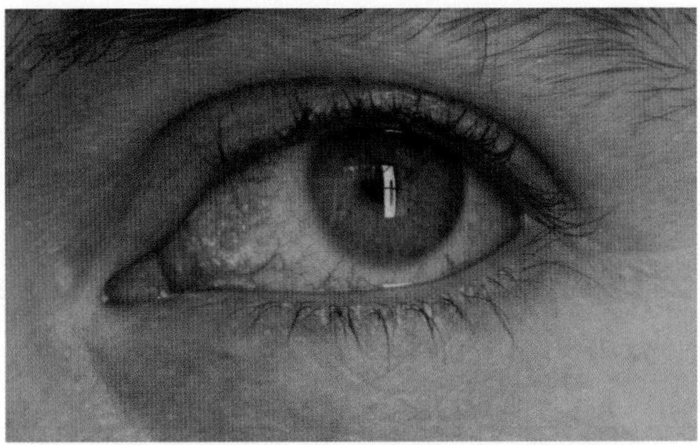

FIGURE 16–8 Viral conjunctivitis: Note 1–2+ conjunctival injection with "glassy" appearance of cornea and conjunctiva and absence of purulent material. If pain present, referral to ophthalmology is required (could be a secondary iritis). (Photo provided by David F. Jacobson, MD.)

CASE SCENARIO | Resolution

A 41-year-old woman presents to your clinic complaining of a "red eye." The redness is diffuse and has been present for 2 days. She also reports mild, watery discharge and a slight sensation of grittiness. She does not have significant pain and has not noticed any change in her vision.

ADDITIONAL HISTORY

You are reassured by the lack of pain or visual changes. Further questioning confirms the absence of photophobia or a foreign body sensation beyond slight grittiness. She does not take any medications, denies previous episodes, and does not have any other systemic complaints. She tells you that her 3-year-old daughter recently had a "cold."

Question: Which of the following is the *most* likely cause of her red eye?

A. Viral conjunctivitis
B. Bacterial conjunctivitis
C. Scleritis
D. Endophthalmitis

Test Your Knowledge

1. While taking a detailed history from a patient with "red eye," which of the following would *not* be considered an alarm symptom (ie, prompting concern for a potentially serious disease requiring referral to an ophthalmologist)?

   A. A gritty feeling in the eye
   B. Decrease in visual acuity
   C. Inability to keep the eye open
   D. Photophobia

2. A 67-year-old woman comes to your office with sudden onset of unilateral headache and decreased visual acuity. The symptoms started the previous evening while she was watching television in a dark room. She describes the headache as a deep throbbing pain behind her right eye. She took ibuprofen and a sleeping pill and went to sleep but awakened early this morning with more pain and noted that her eye was diffusely red. In the waiting room, she developed nausea and had 1 episode of emesis. She describes blurred vision and seeing halos around lights. She denies significant discharge other than tearing of the affected eye. She denies a foreign body sensation, photophobia, or fever.

   Of the following, which diagnosis is most consistent with this patient's presentation?

   A. Subconjunctival hemorrhage
   B. Acute angle-closure glaucoma
   C. Bacterial conjunctivitis
   D. Scleritis

3. A 35-year-old man presents with fever and pain behind his left eye. One week earlier, he had a "cold" with rhinorrhea and nasal congestion that progressed to a "sinus headache." His nasal congestion worsened over the past few days, and he developed left-sided tooth pain and pressure behind his left eye. Over the past 24 hours, he reports swelling around the eye, diffuse redness, fever of 101°F, pain with eye movement, and mild diplopia. He denies discharge, photophobia, or foreign body sensation.

   Which of the following is the most likely diagnosis?

   A. Episcleritis
   B. Bacterial conjunctivitis
   C. Periorbital cellulitis
   D. Orbital cellulitis

References

1. Magauran B. Conditions requiring emergency ophthalmologic consultation. *Emerg Med Clin North Am.* 2008;26:233–238.
2. Dart JK. Eye disease at a community health centre. *BMJ.* 1986;293:1477–1480.
3. Mahmood AR, Narang AT. Diagnosis and management of the acute red eye. *Emerg Med Clin North Am.* 2008;26:35–55.
4. Leibowitz HM. The red eye. *N Engl J Med.* 2000;343:345–351.
5. Wright JL, Wightman JM. Red and painful eye. In: *Rosen's Emergency Medicine*. 7th ed. New York, NY: Mosby, 2009.
6. National Center for Health Statistics, Ganley JP, Roberts J. Eye conditions and related need for medical care among persons 1–74 years of age: United States, 1971–72. *Vital and Health Statistics*. Series 11, No. 228. DHHS Pub. No. (PHS) 83–1678. Public Health Service. Washington, DC: US Government Printing Office, March 1983. Available at: http://www.cdc.gov/nchs/data/series/sr_11/sr11_228.pdf. Accessed October 12, 2011.
7. Robinson B. The prevalence of selected ocular diseases and conditions. *Optom Vis Sci.* 1997;74:79–91.

Suggested Reading

Jacobs DS. Evaluation of the red eye. UpToDate online, 2003. Available at: http://www.uptodateonline.com. Accessed October 12, 2011.

Leibowitz HM. The red eye. *N Engl J Med.* 2000;343:345–351.

Chapter 17

Ear Pain

Daniel J. Sullivan, MD, MPH

CASE SCENARIO

A 45 year-old man comes to your office with a 2-week history of left ear pain. The ear pain began shortly after an upper respiratory infection. He describes the pain as "a pressure" and also notes "crackling" in the ear.

- **What other associated symptoms should you ask about?**
- **How does the time course help to distinguish among different causes of ear pain?**
- **How does the age of the patient help with narrowing the diagnostic possibilities?**

INTRODUCTION

Ear pain is a common complaint in primary care practice, both in pediatric and adult populations. In a random sample of 411 adults in Finland, 7.5% of men and 23.4% of women had experienced ear pain that was not associated with infection in the previous 6 months.[1] The cause of ear pain may be in or near the ear, or it may be referred from a distant site. In most cases, a careful history narrows the possible causes considerably. The physical examination is also essential. Most local causes of ear pain produce specific physical findings, whereas the examination of the ear and its immediately surrounding structures is typically normal in cases of referred pain.

KEY TERMS

Acute otitis media	The presence of infected fluid in the middle ear, caused by bacterial or viral pathogens.
Negative predictive value	The likelihood, given a negative test (or the absence of a symptom), that the condition of interest is absent.
Otalgia	Ear pain.
Otitis externa	An inflammation (usually infectious) of the external auditory canal.
Otorrhea	Discharge from the ear canal.
Pinna	The external ear, including the external acoustic meatus.
Positive predictive value	The likelihood, given a positive test (or the presence of a symptom), that the condition of interest is present.
Sensitivity	How frequently a test (or symptom) is positive (present) in those with the condition of interest.
Serous otitis	The presence of uninfected fluid in the middle ear, usually resulting from the blockage of the eustachian tube from an upper respiratory tract infection or from allergy.
Specificity	How frequently a test (or symptom) is negative (not present) in those without the condition of interest.
Tragus	The tongue-like projection of the cartilage of the ear in front of the external acoustic meatus.

ETIOLOGY

In most cases, the cause of ear pain is localized and can be divided into outer ear problems and inner ear problems. Outer ear problems are located external to the tympanic membrane and include otitis externa, ear canal foreign bodies, earwax, and mastoiditis. Occasionally, a furuncle may cause ear pain. Inner ear problems are located at the tympanic membrane or deep to it and include acute otitis media (OM)—the single most common cause of ear pain—and eustachian tube dysfunction. Injuries to the tympanic membrane, which can occur from barotrauma or from direct trauma to the ear, can also cause ear pain.

In children, acute OM is the most common cause of ear pain. The history is limited in its contribution to making a diagnosis of acute OM.[2] In one study, the positive predictive value of earache for acute OM in children younger than 4 years with upper respiratory tract symptoms was 83%, with the negative predictive value being 78%.[3] Another study found that earache was the symptom that most reliably predicted acute OM in children. However, the sensitivity of earache for OM was only about 60%, with a specificity of about 85%.[4]

Ear pain may originate at a distant site. In such cases, the pain is referred to the ear via a nerve. The sensory innervation of the ear is complex, involving the vagus nerve, the glossopharyngeal nerve, the trigeminal nerve, the facial nerve, and the sensory components of the cervical (C2 and C3) nerve roots. Accordingly, a variety of conditions may cause pain to be referred to the ear, including temporomandibular joint (TMJ) dysfunction; dental processes; pathology of the cranial nerves; and disease at the base of the tongue, larynx, or hypopharynx.

In a series of 615 patients with ear pain and a normal-appearing ear (referred pain), the ultimate diagnoses were dental problem (38%), TMJ dysfunction (35%), cervical spine disorder (8%), neuralgia (5%), aerodigestive disorder (4%), malignancy (3%), and other (6%).[5]

Differential Diagnosis

	Frequency
Outer ear pain	
Furuncle	Relatively uncommon
Otitis externa	Common
Foreign body	Relatively common in children
Mastoiditis	Uncommon
Inner ear pain	
OM	Common
Eustachian tube dysfunction (serous OM)	Common
Barotrauma	Uncommon
Referred pain	***Prevalence[a]***
Dental problems (especially third molar)	38.4%
TMJ dysfunction	35.4%
Cervical spine (especially arthritis)	8.4%
Neuralgias (trigeminal, geniculate, sphenopalatine, glossopharyngeal)	4.9%
Gastrointestinal etiology (including gastroesophageal reflux)	3.7%
Tumors	2.9%
Other (thyroiditis, Eagle syndrome, angina, parotid disease, angina, carotid aneurysm)	6.4%

[a]Among patients referred to a tertiary ear, nose, and throat practice.[5]

GETTING STARTED WITH THE HISTORY

- As always, the initial approach should be open-ended. Let the patient (or parent) tell the story.
- With a young child, the parent or caretaker may be the main source of the history. Ask the caregiver why he or she believes the child is having ear pain.
- Ascertain the time course of the ear pain as well as associated symptoms and aggravating factors because the various causes of ear pain can often be distinguished by these 3 factors.

Questions	Remember
Tell me about your ear pain.	Resist the temptation to interrupt with specific questions before the patient has had a chance to tell you the story.
What other symptoms do you have?	
What makes the pain worse?	
How long have you had the pain?	

INTERVIEW FRAMEWORK

It is important to differentiate relatively acute or subacute ear pain from chronic pain. In general, patients with referred pain have had pain for months or years. An exception to this rule is referred pain from a third molar abscess, which can have an acute onset.

Because several common causes of ear pain are infectious, consider infection early in the interview. The presence of fever narrows the diagnostic possibilities. The presence of other upper respiratory tract infection symptoms (eg, sore throat, nasal congestion, cough) suggests OM or serous otitis. Seasonal allergies may also predispose to serous otitis and OM by compromising the function of the eustachian tubes.

The patient's age is an important consideration in determining the most likely cause of ear pain. Acute OM is by far the most important cause of ear pain in children but is an infrequent cause of ear pain in adults. Referred pain is very uncommon in children, but its relative frequency in adults increases with age.

IDENTIFYING ALARM SYMPTOMS

Serious Diagnoses

Serious causes of ear pain are quite rare. Clinicians should consider and exclude the following 4 serious diagnoses in any patient with ear pain: referred pain from malignancy, necrotizing (malignant) external otitis, temporal arteritis, and mastoiditis.

Referred pain from a malignancy usually has been present for some time. In a series of patients with referred pain, the time between onset of ear pain and tumor diagnosis ranged from 4 to 21 months, with a mean of 7.5 months.[4] These patients are typically older; the mean age at diagnosis in this series was 55.8 years.

Necrotizing (malignant) external otitis is a rare condition in which external otitis progresses to invade the temporal bone and adjacent structures. It is almost exclusively due to infection with *Pseudomonas aeruginosa.* The condition occurs in immunocompromised patients, especially older diabetic patients, and should be considered when the patient does not respond promptly to treatment for otitis externa. In one case series, the average age of the patients was 73.6 years, and 64.2% of the patients had diabetes. Otalgia (97.8%) and otorrhea (91.3%) were common, with facial paralysis being less common (19.6%).[6] Early recognition of this disease is critical because it carries a relatively high mortality (up to 46% in older case series).[7]

Consider temporal arteritis when a patient over the age of 50 reports acute or subacute onset of headache, pain in the temporal area, or scalp tenderness. A relatively specific symptom of temporal arteritis is jaw claudication, which is defined as pain in the proximal jaw near the TMJ, brought on or aggravated by a brief period of chewing and relieved by resting the jaw.[8] A patient may describe this as ear pain, but careful questioning should clarify the location of the pain. Temporal arteritis rarely presents with true ear pain. Prompt diagnosis of temporal arteritis is essential because it can cause sudden and permanent blindness if untreated.

Mastoiditis generally occurs in children when OM spreads to the mastoid air cells behind the ear. A typical presentation is fever with postauricular swelling, tenderness, and erythema, which can sometimes push the ear forward by a mass effect. Patients often report becoming ill several weeks earlier, improving, but then developing fever and signs of local infection. The condition must be promptly recognized and treated because the infection may spread to nearby critical structures such as the temporal bone, meninges, and brain.

Alarm Symptoms	Serious Causes	Positive Likelihood Ratio (LR+)	Benign Causes
Weight loss	Tumors	LR data do not exist but about 25% of all patients with significant weight loss will have no cause found[9]	
Persistent ear pain with discharge, worse at night	Necrotizing (malignant) external otitis		"Ordinary" external otitis
Pain near the ear with chewing in a patient over the age of 50	Temporal arteritis	4.2[8]	TMJ dysfunction
Pain and swelling behind the ear in a child with a recent upper respiratory tract infection or ear infection	Mastoiditis		Lymphadenopathy

FOCUSED QUESTIONS

QUESTIONS	THINK ABOUT...
Do you grind your teeth?	TMJ dysfunction
Do you swim?	Otitis externa
Do you have a skin condition such as psoriasis or seborrheic dermatitis?	Otitis externa
Do you use Q-tips or other objects to clean your ears?	Otitis externa
Have you been struck in the ear?	Barotrauma
Have you recently been scuba diving?	Barotrauma
Are you diabetic? On chemotherapy?	Necrotizing (malignant) external otitis
Are you otherwise immunocompromised?	
Is the pain worse with chewing?	TMJ dysfunction (common) or temporal arteritis (uncommon)
(For a young child) Does the child pull on his or her ear?	Acute OM
Quality	
Is the ear pain	
• *Severe, deep within the ear?*	OM
• *Like pressure or a clogged feeling?*	Eustachian tube dysfunction (serous otitis) Earwax
• *Burning, knife-like, or tingling?*	Neuralgia (trigeminal, geniculate, sphenopalatine, glossopharyngeal, or cervical nerve root)
• *Bilateral?*	Otitis externa Gastroesophageal reflux TMJ dysfunction

Time course	
Was the ear pain preceded by an upper respiratory tract infection?	
• *By 10 days or less?*	OM, eustachian tube dysfunction (serous otitis)
• *By 10 days or more?*	Mastoiditis
Has the pain been present for more than a few weeks?	Referred pain
Was there severe pain at the time of air travel or diving under water?	Barotrauma
Associated symptoms	
Do you have fever?	OM or mastoiditis
Do you have pain and/or swelling behind the ear?	Mastoiditis
Is there a discharge from the ear?	Otitis externa or perforated eardrum from OM
Did the pain decrease dramatically after the discharge began?	Perforated eardrum from OM
Is there a loss of hearing?	OM Eustachian tube dysfunction (serous otitis) Barotrauma
Are there crackling or gurgling sounds in the affected ear?	Eustachian tube dysfunction (serous otitis)
Do you have jaw clicking?	TMJ dysfunction
Do you have itching as well as pain?	Otitis externa Primary dermatitis (psoriasis or seborrhea)
Has there been any weight loss?	Malignancy (referred pain)
Do you have seasonal allergies or hay fever?	Eustachian tube dysfunction (serous otitis)
Modifying symptoms	
Does flexing the neck aggravate the pain?	Arthritis of the neck (referred pain from C2, C3 radiculopathy)
Does pulling on the ear make the pain worse?	Otitis externa
Does the pain worsen with swallowing?	Elongated styloid process (Eagle syndrome)
Is the pain worse in the morning?	TMJ dysfunction Gastroesophageal reflux
Is the pain worse with hot or cold foods?	Infected third molar
Is the pain worse at night?	Necrotizing (malignant) external otitis
Can the pain be provoked by light touch?	Neuralgia

DIAGNOSTIC APPROACH (INCLUDING ALGORITHM)

In approaching the patient with ear pain, the first step is to distinguish between acute or subacute ear pain and chronic ear pain. In acute ear pain, ask about fever and concurrent symptoms of an upper respiratory tract infection. Chronic ear pain is likely to be referred pain. Dental problems, especially TMJ dysfunction, are common causes of chronic ear pain, so they should be considered in any patient with long-standing ear pain.

Pain unresponsive to simple analgesics or that is burning or lancinating in quality should prompt consideration of a process affecting one of the nerves that supplies sensory fibers to the ear or immediate vicinity (eg, trigeminal nerve). The diagnostic algorithm for ear pain is shown in Figure 17–1.

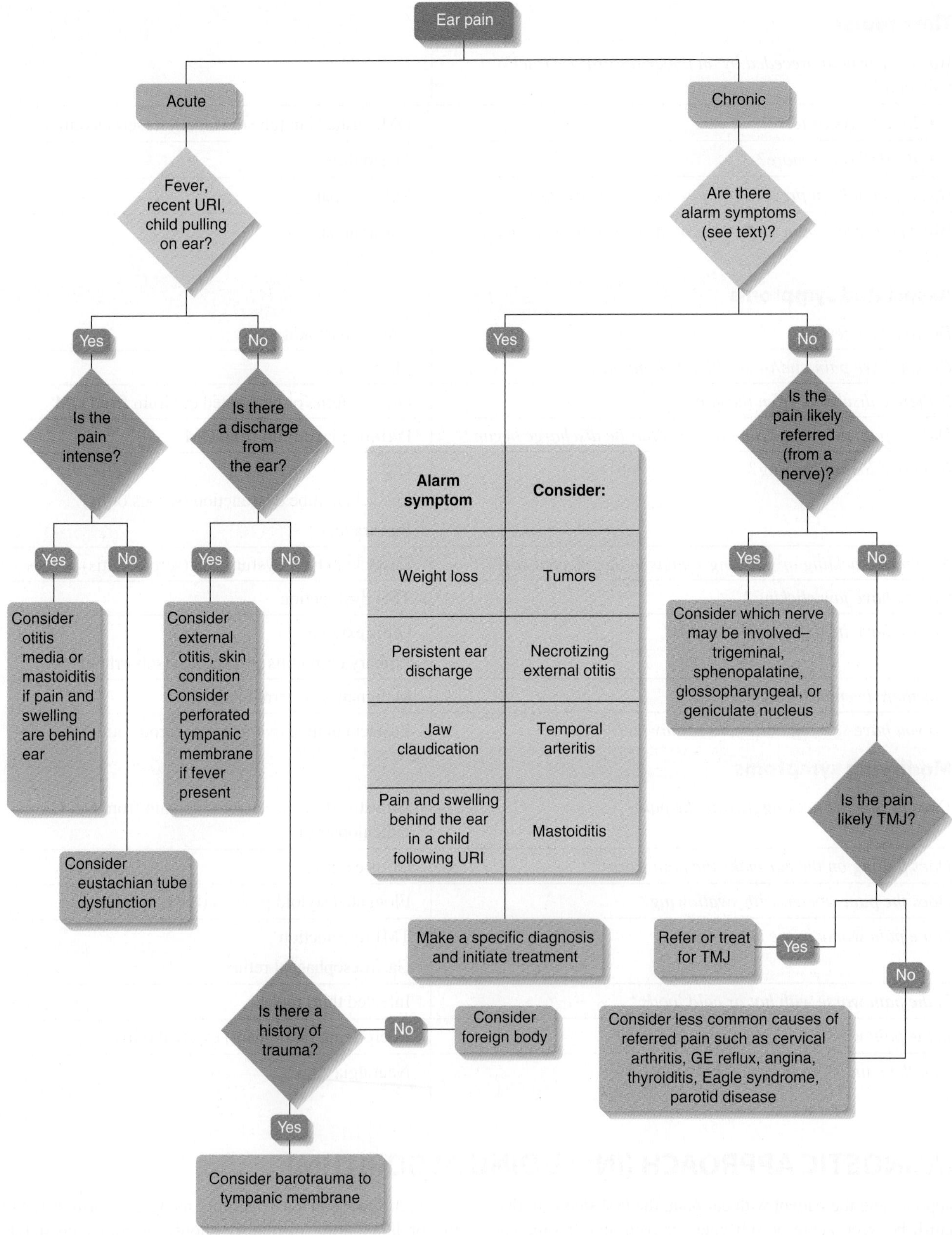

FIGURE 17–1 Diagnostic approach: Ear pain. GE; gastroesophageal; TMJ, temporomandibular joint; URI, upper respiratory infection.

CAVEATS

- The history often only provides a starting point, because the physical examination is frequently critical to making the diagnosis. Most local causes of ear pain have characteristic physical findings, whereas most cases of referred pain will have a normal ear examination.
- The character and severity of pain may be a helpful feature. The pain of acute OM is generally severe, often interfering with sleep. In contrast, the pain of eustachian tube dysfunction is usually modest, often described by a patient as discomfort or fullness. Referred pain from inflammation of a nerve is frequently described by patients as burning, knife-like, or "electric." It may be provoked by light touch.
- Earwax (cerumen) uncommonly causes ear pain. If earwax is present, it must be removed to exclude the possibility that the true pathology lies behind the eardrum (as in OM).

PROGNOSIS

The prognosis of ear pain is generally favorable. In most cases, the pain resolves relatively quickly with appropriate treatment. Some of the disorders causing referred ear pain are more chronic, such as TMJ dysfunction.

CASE SCENARIO | Resolution

A 45-year-old man comes to your office with a 2-week history of left ear pain. The ear pain began shortly after an upper respiratory infection. He describes the pain as "a pressure" and also notes "crackling" in the ear.

ADDITIONAL HISTORY

The patient reports that he cannot hear well with his left ear; he describes sounds as being "muffled" on the left but normal on the right. He has had no fever and feels well, apart from being frustrated by his ear problem. He tried an over-the-counter decongestant and this seemed to help somewhat.

Question: What is the most likely diagnosis?

A. Acute otitis media
B. Serous otitis
C. TMJ dysfunction
D. Temporal arteritis

Test Your Knowledge

1. A 5-year-old boy is brought in to the office by his mother because of 2 days of right ear pain. The mother reports that he has been crying and pulling on the ear. He has a temperature of 39.7°C.
   What is the most likely diagnosis?
   A. Otitis externa
   B. Otitis media
   C. Foreign body in the ear
   D. Malignant otitis externa

2. A 22-year-old college student who is on the swim team reports 1 week of left ear pain. She noted a slightly yellow, watery discharge from the ear on her pillow this morning, which prompted her to make an appointment. She has no fever and mentions that the pain is worse when she pushes on the tragus.
   What is the most likely diagnosis?
   A. Perforated eardrum from otitis media
   B. Temporomandibular joint dysfunction
   C. Otitis externa
   D. Infected upper third molar tooth

3. A 35-year-old male consultant tells you of several months of bilateral ear discomfort that is more pronounced on the left than the right. The pain is worse in the morning and worse when he chews. He has been working long hours recently to meet a deadline.
   What is the most likely diagnosis?
   A. Serous otitis
   B. Temporal arteritis
   C. Temporomandibular joint dysfunction
   A. Referred pain from tight neck muscles

References

1. Kuttila S, Kuttila M, Le Bell Y, et al. Aural symptoms and signs of temporomandibular disorder in association with treatment need and visits to a physician. *Laryngoscope.* 1999:109;1669–1673.
2. Rothman R, Owens T, Simel D. Does this child have acute otitis media? *JAMA.* 2003;290:1633–1640.
3. Heikkinen T, Ruuskanen O. Signs and symptoms predicting acute otitis media. *Arch Pediatr Adolesc Med.* 1995;149:26–29.
4. Kontiokari T, Koivunen P, Neimela M, et al. Symptoms of acute otitis media. *Pediatr Infect Dis J.* 1998;17:676–679.
5. Leonetti JP, Li J, Smith PG. Otalgia. An isolated symptom of malignant infratemporal tumors. *Am J Otol.* 1998;19:496–498.
6. Franco-Vidal V, Blanchet H, Debear C, et al. Necrotizing external otitis: a report of 46 cases. *Otol Neurotol.* 2007;28:771–773.
7. Chandler JR. Malignant external otitis. *Laryngoscope.* 1968;78:1257–1294.
8. Smetana GW, Shmerling RH. Does this patient have temporal arteritis? *JAMA.* 2002;287:92–101.
9. Rabinovitz M, Pitlik SD, Leifer M, Garty M, Rosenfeld JB. Unintentional weight loss: a retrospective analysis of 154 cases. *Arch Intern Med.* 1986;146:186–187.

Suggested Reading

Greenes D. Evaluation of earache in children. In: Barsow DS, ed. *UpToDate*. Waltham, MA: UpToDate, 2010.

Shah R, Blevins N. Otalgia. *Otolaryngol Clin North Am.* 2003;36:1137–1151.

Chapter 18

Hearing Loss

Felipe J. Molina, MD

CASE SCENARIO

A 75-year-old man presents to your office for a routine office visit. During the visit, you inquire about hearing loss. He wasn't planning on discussing this but reports that he has trouble understating the television or when someone speaks in a whisper; his family is concerned that he doesn't hear as well as he used to. He hasn't been attending social events or family gatherings recently because he feels embarrassed having to ask people to repeat words or phrases.

- **What background and historical data can help suggest a certain type of hearing loss?**
- **When does hearing loss require urgent specialist evaluation, and what are the historical clues that help you to identify this?**
- **How can you narrow the differential diagnosis of hearing loss using focused questions after obtaining an open-ended history?**

INTRODUCTION

Hearing loss is the third most common chronic condition in older Americans after hypertension and arthritis.[1] Ten percent of the US population (28 million Americans) have some degree of hearing loss.[2] The prevalence increases significantly with age; between 25% and 40% of patients over the age of 65 are affected.[1] The most common causes of hearing loss—presbycusis and noise-induced hearing loss—develop insidiously and are underreported, underdiagnosed, and undertreated. These benign causes of hearing loss, if unrecognized, can lead to decreased functioning, social isolation, and depression. More dramatic but less common presentations of hearing loss, such as sudden-onset hearing loss or hearing loss with associated symptoms, are more likely to be reported by patients and lead to prompt referral and treatment. A careful history allows the clinician to narrow the diagnosis and take appropriate next steps.

The approach to hearing loss involves 2 key steps. First, determine the presence of hearing loss and its severity by asking screening questions or using a questionnaire. Second, focus on alarm symptoms and determine the etiology through a series of specific questions.

It is important to understand the basic anatomy of the auditory system. The auditory system is divided into the **outer ear**, **middle ear**, and **inner ear**. The **outer ear** is composed of the pinna and external ear canal. Its functions include protection, sound localization, passive augmentation of sound, and transfer of sound waves to the tympanic membrane (eardrum) causing it to vibrate. The **middle ear** includes the tympanic membrane and the ossicular chain of 3 small bones—the malleus, incus, and stapes—in the air-filled cavity behind it. The ossicular chain transmits sound vibrations from the tympanic membrane to the cochlea. The cochlea, which lies in perilymph fluid within the temporal bone, the vestibular apparatus, and the eighth cranial nerve (vestibulocochlear) comprise the **inner ear**. This is where mechanical sound is transduced into an electrical impulse via hair cells as sound travels through endolymph fluid within the cochlea to the auditory nerve.

KEY TERMS

Conductive hearing loss	Caused by disorders of the outer and middle ear whereby mechanical transmission of sound to the inner ear is blocked. Defined by the presence of an air–bone gap on audiometry, the difference between air and bone conduction thresholds.
Sensorineural hearing loss	Caused by disorders of the inner ear (cochlea or auditory nerve) usually from damage to the cochlear hair cells. Defined as an audiogram showing pure-tone threshold of 40 dB or higher at 1 and 2 kHz in 1 ear or at 1 or 2 kHz in both ears.[3] Normal conversation is between 45 and 60 dB.[4]
Mixed hearing loss	The presence of both sensorineural and conductive hearing loss.
Noise-induced hearing loss	Gradual irreversible sensorineural hearing loss due to cochlear hair cell damage as a result of exposure to continuous or intermittent loud noise. Exposure to an average of > 85 dB over 8 hours can cause noise-induced hearing loss.[4]
Ototoxic medications	Medications that cause sensorineural hearing loss from injury to the cochlear hair cells.
Presbycusis	Age-related sensorineural hearing loss due to both genetic and environmental factors. Usually, it is gradual and bilateral; loss of high-frequency sounds occurs first.[5]
Sudden sensorineural hearing loss (SSNHL)	Uncommon condition with unclear etiology. Hearing loss of at least 30 dB in 3 contiguous frequencies over a period not exceeding 3 days.[6] Most cases are unilateral. Possible causes include viral infection, vascular, autoimmune, or migraine. Associated with increased risk for stroke.[7]
Tinnitus	An intrinsic noise heard in the ears, described as ringing (or roaring, crickets, or bells). Usually sensorineural in origin but can also be caused by disorders of the outer and middle ears.

ETIOLOGY

Hearing loss is categorized into 2 major types: **conductive** and **sensorineural**. Most adults with hearing loss in the United States have sensorineural hearing loss (> 90% of cases). Presbycusis is by far the most common cause of sensorineural hearing loss, followed by noise-induced hearing loss. Conductive hearing loss represents less than 10% of hearing loss. The most common causes of conductive hearing loss in adults are cerumen impaction, otosclerosis, cholesteatoma, and tympanic membrane perforation secondary to chronic otitis media.

Differential Diagnosis[2,4,6,8–10]

	Prevalence or Incidence[a]
Conductive hearing loss	
Outer ear	
• Cerumen impaction	< 10% of hearing loss
• Otitis externa, trauma, squamous cell carcinoma, psoriasis	
• Exostosis, osteoma	
Middle ear	
• Chronic otitis media	*18/100,000 per year*[9]
• Otosclerosis	*1.0%*[2]
• Cholesteatoma, barotrauma, tympanic membrane perforation, temporal bone trauma, glomus tumor	

Sensorineural	*> 90% of hearing loss (17 million)*[2]
Presbycusis	37% of adults older than 75 years[2]
Noise-induced	10 million people[2,4]
Acoustic neuroma	1/60,000 adults per year[10]
Ménière's disease	3–5 million people[2] with 300,000 new cases per year[2]
SSNHL	4000 new cases[2] or 1/10,000 per year[6]
Meningitis, ototoxic medications, viral cochleitis, autoimmune disease, multiple sclerosis, perilymphatic fistula, syphilis, cerebrovascular ischemia, penetrating trauma, meningioma, thyrotoxicosis, migrainous, congenital malformations, viral	
Mixed	
Otosclerosis, chronic otitis media, trauma, neoplasm	
Meningitis, ototoxic medications, viral cochleitis, autoimmune disease, multiple sclerosis, perilymphatic fistula, syphilis, cerebrovascular ischemia, penetrating trauma, meningioma, thyrotoxicosis, migrainous, congenital malformations, viral	

[a]Prevalence is unknown when not indicated.

INTERVIEW FRAMEWORK

Before asking specific questions, review background demographic and historical data that are predisposing factors for certain types of hearing loss.

FACTOR	THINK ABOUT...
Age[2,6]	
• *30–60 years old*	Otosclerosis Ménière's disease Acoustic neuroma Autoimmune disease SSNHL
• *> 65 years*	Presbycusis
• *Any age*	Noise-induced
Sex[1,2,6]	
• *Male = female*	Ménière's disease SSNHL
• *Male > female*	Presbycusis

—Continued next page

Continued—	
• *Female > male*	Otosclerosis Vertiginous migraine Autoimmune disease
Other factors	
Past medical history	Autoimmune disease (systemic lupus erythematosus [SLE], rheumatoid arthritis, Wegener's granulomatosis, Sjögren syndrome, antiphospholipid syndrome, polyarteritis nodosa, giant cell arteritis, Behçet disease, Cogan syndrome) Diabetes Cardiovascular disease Stroke Renal insufficiency Hyperlipidemia Recurrent ear infections Multiple sclerosis Syphilis Recent head trauma Migraines Thyrotoxicosis
Medications	Loop diuretics, antibiotics (aminoglycosides, eg, gentamicin), nonsteroidal anti-inflammatory drugs (NSAIDs), aspirin, chemotherapy (cisplatin), antimalarials, minocycline
Family history	Genetic: Alport, Usher, and Waardenburg syndromes; other multifactorial causes Genetically predisposing conditions: presbycusis, otosclerosis (50%–70% of cases have a positive family history[2]), Paget disease, neurofibromatosis type 2, migraine
Social history	Occupational noise exposure: construction, manufacturing, agriculture Loud hobbies: loud music, hunting, motorcycles Smoking Barotrauma: scuba diving, flying Cold water exposure
Risk factors for presbycusis	Smoking Noise exposure Diabetes Cardiovascular disease Ototoxic medications History of recurrent ear infections Family history of presbycusis

GETTING STARTED WITH THE HISTORY

- First ask the patient to describe the hearing loss in his or her own words.
- During the annual visit for either an older patient or a patient with significant noise exposure, ask about hearing loss even if he or she does not report it. A meta-analysis showed that a positive response to this single question has a positive likelihood ratio (LR) of 2.2 and negative LR of 0.45 for subtle hearing impairment and a positive

LR of 2.5 and negative LR of 0.13 for moderate to severe hearing impairment.[11]

- In a recent questionnaire study, patients who felt that they had trouble hearing women's or children's voices or that they would benefit from a hearing aid were highly likely to have hearing loss (specificity, 1.0; negative LR, 0.81–0.98).[12]
- The Hearing Handicap Inventory for the Elderly Screening (HHIE-S) questionnaire is a standard tool developed to identify a hearing handicap and takes 2 to 5 minutes to complete. The total score determines the presence and severity of a hearing handicap. From meta-analysis data, hearing impairment is less likely with a score less than 8 (negative LR, 0.38). A score greater than 8 increases the probability of abnormal audiometry (positive LR, 3.8); higher scores do not appear to significantly increase this likelihood.[11]
- If hearing loss is reported, determine whether the patient indeed has hearing loss and the severity. Next, focus on determining the etiology.

Hearing Handicap in the Elderly Screening Questionnaire (HHIE-S)[3]

Symptom	Yes	No	Sometimes
1. Does a hearing problem cause you to feel embarrassed when meeting new people?	4	0	2
2. Does a hearing problem cause you to feel frustrated when talking to members of your family?	4	0	2
3. Do you have difficulty hearing when someone whispers?	4	0	2
4. Do you feel handicapped by a hearing problem?	4	0	2
5. Does a hearing problem cause you difficulty when visiting friends, relatives, or neighbors?	4	0	2
6. Does a hearing problem cause you to attend religious services less often than you would like?	4	0	2
7. Does a hearing problem cause you to have arguments with family members?	4	0	2
8. Does a hearing problem cause you difficulty when listening to TV or radio?	4	0	2
9. Do you feel that your hearing limits or hampers your personal or social life?	4	0	2
10. Does a hearing problem cause you difficulty when in a restaurant with relatives or friends?	4	0	2

Scores: 0–8 = no handicap; 10–24 = mild to moderate handicap; 26–40 = severe handicap.

IDENTIFYING ALARM SYMPTOMS

- Because most benign causes of hearing loss present gradually and bilaterally, any symptoms that differ from these are alarming.
- Sudden or rapid onset of hearing loss is the most concerning symptom for a serious cause of hearing loss.
- Other concerning symptoms include rapidly progressive, unilateral, or asymmetric hearing loss; a sense of ear fullness; and association with other neurologic symptoms such as tinnitus or vertigo.
- After determining the severity of hearing loss and any predisposing factors, ask specifically about the presence of alarm symptoms. Keep in mind that some benign causes of hearing loss can also present with alarm symptoms.

Serious Diagnoses

Certain uncommon causes of hearing loss require immediate recognition and prompt treatment or referral to an otolaryngologist because early management may prevent progression, complications, and irreversible damage[6]:

- Trauma (eg, tympanic membrane perforation)
- Tumor (eg, acoustic neuroma)
- Autoimmune disease
- Cerebrovascular disease
- Meningitis
- Multiple sclerosis
- Syphilis
- Ménière's disease
- SSNHL

Alarm Symptoms	If Present, Consider Serious Causes…	However, Benign Causes for This Feature Include…
Sudden or rapid onset	SSNHL Vascular embolism or insufficiency Autoimmune disease Trauma (barotrauma, tympanic membrane perforation, perilymphatic fistula, cochlear concussion) Meningitis	Viral cochleitis Migraine Otitis media Ototoxic medications
Rapidly progressive	Autoimmune disease Syphilis	Ototoxic medications
Unilateral or asymmetric	Vascular embolism or insufficiency Acoustic neuroma Ménière's disease SSNHL Autoimmune disease	Cerumen impaction Viral cochleitis
Tinnitus	Ménière's disease Acoustic neuroma Trauma (perilymphatic fistula, barotrauma) SSNHL	Noise-induced Presbycusis Otosclerosis Viral cochleitis Ototoxic medications
Vertigo	Ménière's disease Autoimmune disease Acoustic neuroma Trauma (barotrauma, perilymphatic fistula) Multiple sclerosis Syphilis Meningitis SSNHL	Thyrotoxicosis Genetic Migraine Aminoglycosides
Sense of ear fullness	SSNHL Ménière's disease Autoimmune Acoustic neuroma	Otitis media Migraine TMJ dysfunction Cerumen impaction

FOCUSED QUESTIONS

QUESTIONS	THINK ABOUT...
Quality	
Is your hearing loss	
• *Mild to moderate?*	Presbycusis Aminoglycosides
• *Severe to profound?*	Autoimmune Meningitis Syphilis
Is your hearing loss in 1 or both ears?	
• *Unilateral*	Viral cochleitis SSNHL Acoustic neuroma Vascular Cerumen Ménière's disease Migraine
• *Bilateral symmetric*	Presbycusis Noise-induced Ototoxicity Genetic Otosclerosis Meningitis Syphilis
• *Bilateral asymmetric*	Autoimmune Multiple sclerosis
Time course	
Was the onset of your hearing loss:	
• *Sudden or rapid?*	Viral cochleitis Vascular embolism or insufficiency SSNHL Perilymphatic fistula Barotrauma Otitis media Tympanic membrane perforation Autoimmune Migraine Meningitis
• *Gradual?*	Presbycusis Noise-induced Ototoxicity Acoustic neuroma

—Continued next page

Continued—

Does your hearing loss fluctuate?	Ménière's disease Autoimmune disease Syphilis Genetic Migraine Perilymphatic fistula
Is your hearing loss getting worse over time:	
• *Slowly?*	Presbycusis Noise-induced Otosclerosis Ménière's disease Acoustic neuroma Ototoxicity Multiple sclerosis Trauma Genetic
• *Rapidly?*	Autoimmune Syphilis Ototoxicity
Associated symptoms	
Do you have other symptoms that have occurred with your hearing loss?	
• *Ringing in the ear(s)*	Ménière's disease Acoustic neuroma Noise-induced Presbycusis Ototoxicity SSNHL Migraine Autoimmune Otosclerosis Perilymphatic fistula Viral labyrinthitis
• *Ear pain or drainage*	Infection (otitis externa, otitis media), tumor, trauma, cerumen impaction
• *Itchy ear(s)*	Otitis externa
• *Fullness or pressure in your ear(s)*	Otitis media Ménière's disease Autoimmune Barotrauma Acoustic neuroma Vertiginous migraine Cerumen impaction SSNHL

• *Fever*	Otitis media Meningitis
• *Dizziness*	Ménière's disease Autoimmune Acoustic neuroma Multiple sclerosis Syphilis Meningitis Aminoglycosides Perilymphatic fistula SSNHL Genetic Thyrotoxicosis Migraine Viral labyrinthitis
• *Facial numbness or weakness*	Acoustic neuroma
• *Double vision*	Acoustic neuroma
• *Headache*	Acoustic neuroma Migraine Meningitis
Modifying symptoms	
Is it more difficult for you to hear:	
• *High-pitched sounds?*	Presbycusis Noise-induced Ototoxicity Genetic
• *Low-pitched sounds?*	Ménière's disease Migraine
• *When there is background noise, like in a restaurant?*	Presbycusis Noise-induced
• *The TV or radio compared to others?*	Presbycusis Noise-induced
• *A conversation in a group of people rather than one-on-one?*	Presbycusis Noise-induced
Do loud noises bother you?	Presbycusis Noise-induced Migraine
Is it difficult to tell where sound is coming from?	Multiple sclerosis Noise-induced Presbycusis
Do you ever hear speech but cannot understand it?	Presbycusis Acoustic neuroma Noise-induced
At work, do you need to shout at someone 3 feet or less (an arm's length) away to be heard?	Noise-induced

DIAGNOSTIC APPROACH (INCLUDING ALGORITHM)

In a patient with hearing loss who does not have cerumen impaction, consider the time course of the hearing loss. For sudden-onset hearing loss, historical clues such as the presence of pain or fever or a history of trauma can point to specific etiologies. For gradual-onset hearing loss, whether the deficit is unilateral or bilateral and slowly or rapidly progressive can narrow the differential diagnosis. The diagnostic algorithm for hearing loss is shown in Figure 18–1.

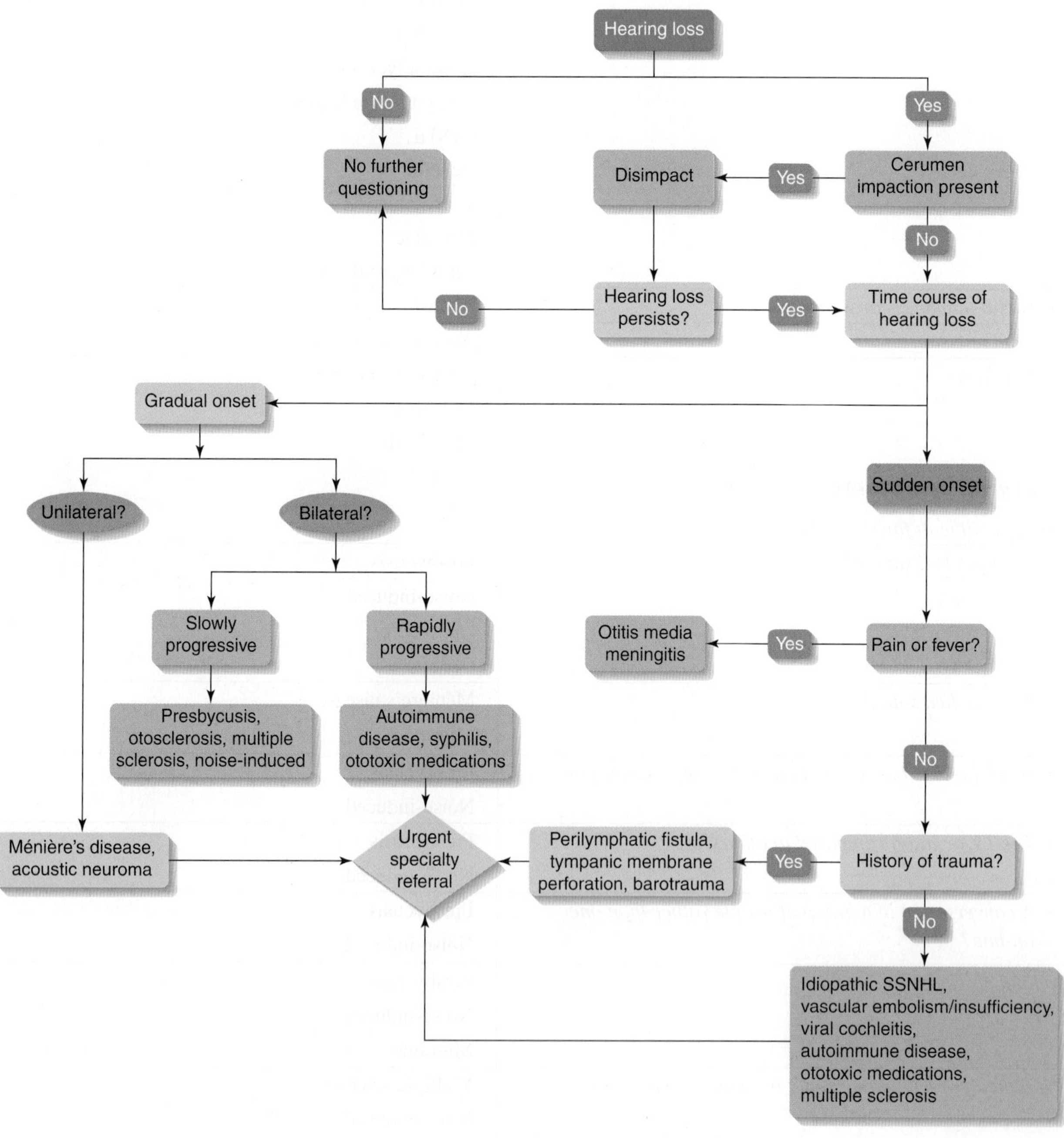

FIGURE 18–1 Diagnostic algorithm: Hearing loss. SSNHL, sudden sensorineural hearing loss.

CAVEATS

- Most hearing loss results from presbycusis. However, prompt evaluation is warranted if the diagnosis is uncertain or if any alarm symptoms are present.
- Because patients with gradual hearing loss often do not report this complaint, healthcare providers should take the initiative to ask about it. Patients often ignore or accept hearing loss; alternatively, they may not be as aware of their problem as those around them. Therefore, always include the patient's family and friends in history taking.
- Because the HHIE-S measures a patient's perceived handicap from hearing loss, it is more likely to detect hearing loss in motivated patients who have already sought medical attention about their hearing loss.
- Many patients will not wear hearing aids. Reasons include embarrassment about cosmetic appearance, the stigma associated with using them, cost, and technical difficulty. However, technologic and cosmetic advances in the hearing aid industry may improve patient compliance.

PROGNOSIS

- Causes of reversible hearing loss include SSNHL (70%–90% experience full recovery, either spontaneously or with prompt initiation of corticosteroid therapy),[6] syphilis, barotrauma, viral labyrinthitis, otitis media, tympanic membrane perforation, cochlear concussion, temporal bone fracture, and ototoxicity from medications such as aspirin, antimalarials, loop diuretics, and NSAIDs.
- Causes of irreversible hearing loss include presbycusis, chronic otitis media, Ménière's disease (after repeated attacks), ototoxicity from antibiotics or chemotherapy, noise-induced hearing loss, and autoimmune hearing loss.
- Because most causes of hearing loss are treatable, screening and early detection are important. Any patient with subjective hearing loss should be referred for further evaluation by an audiologist or otolaryngologist.

CASE SCENARIO | Resolution

A 75-year-old man presents to your office for a routine office visit. During the visit, you inquire about hearing loss. He wasn't planning on discussing this but reports that he has trouble understating the television or when someone speaks in a whisper; his family is concerned that he doesn't hear as well as he used to. He hasn't been attending social events or family gatherings recently because he feels embarrassed having to ask people to repeat words or phrases.

ADDITIONAL HISTORY

The patient's hearing loss has been gradual, and both ears are affected equally. He hasn't noticed ringing in his ears, dizziness, or disequilibrium. He denies a sudden worsening of his symptoms. He has the most trouble hearing in crowded restaurants or large gatherings.

Question: What is the most likely diagnosis?

A. Ménière's disease
B. Presbycusis
C. Acoustic neuroma
D. Multiple sclerosis

Test Your Knowledge

1. Ms. Valenti is a 33-year-old patient of yours without significant medical history. She scheduled an urgent care visit to discuss hearing loss and a sensation of pressure in her ear that began 2 days ago. After further questioning, you are concerned for possible sudden sensorineural hearing loss.

   Which of the following symptoms is NOT usually associated with SSNHL?

   A. Tinnitus
   B. Vertigo
   C. Fever
   D. Unilateral hearing loss
   E. Rapidly progressive hearing loss

2. A 60-year-old man sees you with concerns about hearing loss. On further questioning, he cannot remember an acute onset of hearing loss and believes it has been gradual over time.

   Which of the following features would make you the most concerned for acoustic neuroma?

   A. Fever
   B. Unilateral hearing loss
   C. Rapidly progressive hearing loss
   D. Fluctuating hearing loss
   E. Itchy ears

3. You see a 45-year-old male construction worker for a periodic health examination. On review of symptoms, he reports subjective hearing loss. Concerned about noise-induced hearing loss, you assess for modifying symptoms.

   Which sounds or situation would you expect the patient to be LEAST likely to have difficulty with?

   A. High-pitched sounds
   B. Low-pitched sounds
   C. With background noise
   D. TV or radio
   E. A conversation in a group of people rather than one-on-one

ACKNOWLEDGMENT

The author thanks Mia Marcus, MD, and Eileen Reynolds, MD, for their major contributions to a previous version of this chapter.

References

1. Cruickshanks KJ, Wiley TL, Tweed TS, et al. Prevalence of hearing loss in older adults in Beaver Dam, Wisconsin. The Epidemiology of Hearing Loss Study. *Am J Epidemiol.* 1998;148:879–886.
2. Castrogiovanni A. Incidence and prevalence of hearing loss and hearing aid use in the United States. Available at: http://www.asha.org/research/reports/hearing.htm. Accessed October 12, 2011.
3. Ventry IM, Weinstein BE. Identification of elderly people with hearing problems. *ASHA.* 1983;25:37–42.
4. Rabinowitz PM. Noise-induced hearing loss. *Am Fam Physician.* 2000;61:2749–2756, 2759–2760.
5. Lichtenstein MJ, Bess FH, Logan SA. Validation of screening tools for identifying hearing impaired elderly in Primary Care. *JAMA.* 1988;259:2875–2878.
6. Zadeh MH, Storper IS, Spitzer JB. Diagnosis and treatment of sudden-onset sensorineural hearing loss: a study of 51 patients. *Otolaryngol Head Neck Surg.* 2003;128:92–98.
7. Lin HC, Chao PZ, Lee HC. Sudden sensorineural hearing loss increases the risk of stroke: a 5-year follow-up study. *Stroke.* 2008;39:2744–2748.
8. Lewis-Culinan C, Janken J. Effect of cerumen removal on the hearing ability of geriatric patients. *J Adv Nurs.* 1990;15:594–600.
9. Ruben RJ. The disease in society: evaluation of chronic otitis media in general and cholesteatoma in particular. In: Sade J, ed. *Cholesteatoma and Mastoid Surgery.* Amsterdam: Kugler, 1982:111–116.
10. Harcourt JP, Vijaya-Sekaran S, Loney E, Lennox P. The incidence of symptoms consistent with cerebellopontine angle lesions in a general ENT out-patient clinic. *J Laryngol Otol.* 1999;113:518–522.
11. Bagai A, Thavendiranathan T, Detsy AS. Does this patient have hearing impairment? *JAMA.* 2006;295:416–428.
12. Boatman DF, Miglioretti DL, Eberwein C, Alidoost M, Reich SG. How accurate are bedside hearing tests? *Neurology.* 2007;68:1311–1314.

Suggested Reading

Bagai A, Thavendiranathan T, Detsy AS. Does this patient have hearing impairment? *JAMA*. 2006;295:416–428.

Bogardus ST, Yueh B, Shekelle PG. Screening and management of adult hearing loss in primary care: clinical applications. *JAMA*. 2003;289:1986–1990.

Nadol JB. Hearing loss. *N Engl J Med.* 1993;329:1092–1102.

Rauch SD. Clinical practice. Idiopathic sudden sensorineural hearing loss. *N Engl J Med.* 2008;359:833–840.

Yueh B, Shapiro N, MacLean CH, Shekelle PG. Screening and management of adult hearing loss in primary care: scientific review. *JAMA*. 2003;289:1976–1985.

Chapter 19

Tinnitus

Malathi Srinivasan, MD

CASE SCENARIO

A 75-year-old man is brought in by his daughter for progressive mainly unilateral tinnitus, hearing loss, and dizziness for the past year. About 3 weeks ago, he began experiencing unsteadiness and sustained a fall while walking up the stairs.

- **What additional questions would you ask to further characterize the tinnitus?**
- **How do you classify tinnitus?**
- **What are the alarm symptoms or signs that warrant a rapid assessment, including possible central nervous system (CNS) imaging?**
- **What maneuvers can help distinguish between different types of tinnitus?**
- **Can you make the diagnosis of tinnitus purely from the history?**

INTRODUCTION

Tinnitus is a common symptom in primary care, with great heterogeneity in terms of presentation, severity, and etiology. The term "tinnitus" originates from the Latin word *tinnire*, which means "to ring." Although commonly defined as **ringing in the ears**, a better definition is that "tinnitus is the conscious expression of a sound that originates in an involuntary manner."[1] Tinnitus may be reported by patients as ringing, hissing, buzzing, pulsing, humming, or whistling.[2] Tinnitus may cause insomnia; difficulty hearing in social situations; anxiety; annoyance; frustration; and feelings of inadequacy, social anxiety, or loss of control. Only 4% to 8% of patients with tinnitus report moderate to severe tinnitus that interferes with their daily life.[3] Tinnitus must be distinguished from auditory hallucinations (see Key Terms).

A truly evidence-based approach to tinnitus is handicapped by lack of epidemiologic and observational data. Thus, likelihood ratios for associated tinnitus symptoms cannot be generated. Most studies have included very small numbers of patients.

KEY TERMS

Tinnitus	A person's perception of a simple involuntary sound that is usually not audible to the observer. The monotonous sound may range in pitch, tone, and amplitude. Often described as hissing, buzzing, ringing, whizzing, pulsing, whooshing, or "steam escaping." It may be caused by normal body functions or by dysfunction of the peripheral or central auditory systems. The perception of tinnitus and degree of disability are often influenced by psychological factors. Serious pathology may cause either loud or muted tinnitus.
Auditory hallucination	A person's perception of an involuntary sound, often a complex sound, which may be noisy, musical, or voices. Generally indicates psychiatric disturbance (eg, psychosis).
Hyperacusis	Sound and noise intolerance, usually causing discomfort from sounds that would not bother a healthy individual. Sometimes associated with tinnitus.

—Continued next page

Continued—

Subjective tinnitus	Tinnitus, usually continuous, that only the patient can hear. A "phantom sound" caused by peripheral (middle/inner ear) or central (auditory track to cortex) damage and subsequent reorganization with loss of suppression of neural activity. Ninety-five percent of all tinnitus patients have this form. As in phantom limb pain, symptom control is difficult, but patients often feel better in noisy environments (self-masking).
Objective tinnitus	Tinnitus that is caused by the body and perceived by a normal healthy ear. The physician can often hear this sound. Fewer than 5% of tinnitus patients have this form. Clonic muscular contractions and vascular bruits are common causes.
Pulsatile tinnitus	Tinnitus that pulses in time with the cardiac cycle. Implies a vascular source, mandating a thorough evaluation for potential vascular causes including tumors.[4]
Bilateral tinnitus	Tinnitus perceived in both ears. May be of central origin, in the central auditory pathways, or reflect systemic damage (noise, medications, toxins, infection).
Unilateral tinnitus	Tinnitus localized to 1 ear. Typically of peripheral origin (middle ear, cochlea, acoustic nerve).

ETIOLOGY

The perception of tinnitus is extremely common, and often, no distinct etiology is found. Overall, 9% of the US population reports tinnitus, with prevalence increasing with age.[5] Most tinnitus is subjective, coexisting with conductive (eg, recurrent infections or otosclerosis) or sensorineural (eg, cochlear damage from medications, loud music) hearing loss. A lesion anywhere along the auditory pathway can cause tinnitus (see Chapter 18, Hearing Loss). Physiologically, it is useful to think of the anatomy associated with tinnitus, working from the outer ears to the CNS (Figure 19–1).

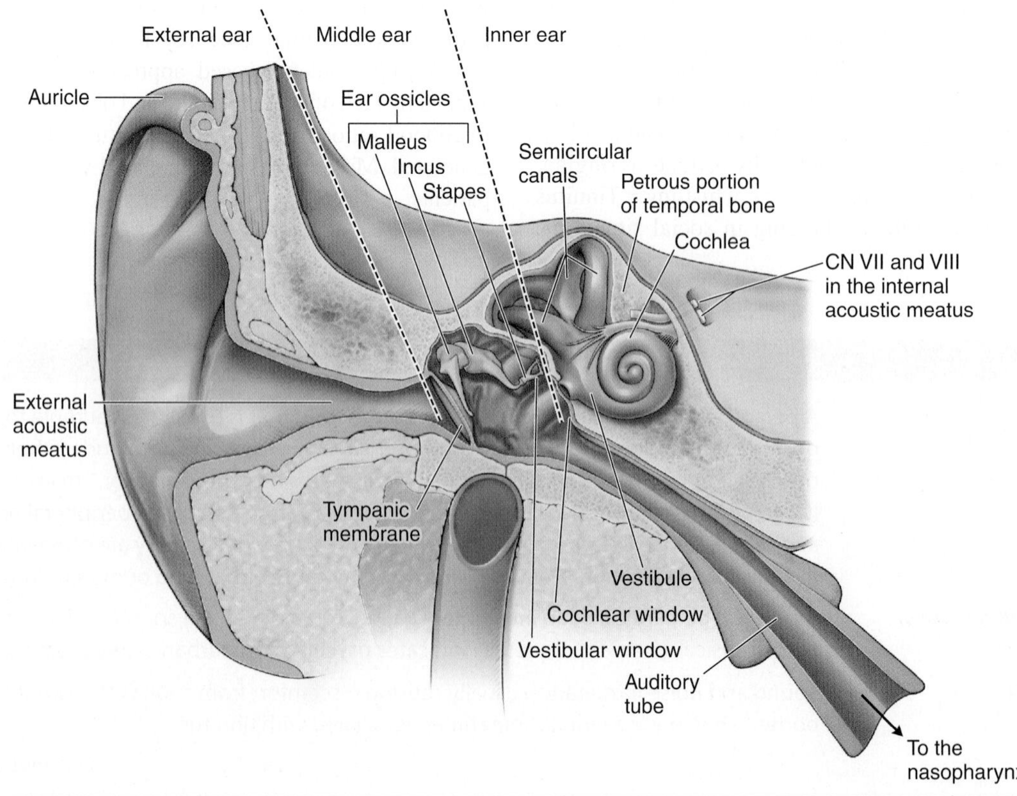

FIGURE 19–1 Coronal section of the temporal bone showing the hearing apparatus.

EPIDEMIOLOGY

Tinnitus is more common with advancing age. Men are 1.4 to 1.8 times more likely to be affected by tinnitus than women. Whites are 2.2 times more likely to be affected than blacks, whereas individuals from poorer families are 1.3 to 2.3 times more likely to report tinnitus. In children, the prevalence of tinnitus ranges from 1% to 13%.[5,6] Tinnitus and hearing loss are highly associated, although hearing loss is 2 to 3 times more common than tinnitus.[5] In a study of 757 patients with subjective (endogenous) tinnitus,[7] the following symptoms were reported: decreased hearing (98%), concurrent nausea (96%), constant tinnitus (87%), decreased performance especially vigilance (68%), concurrent headaches (66%), vertigo-related uncertainty (55%), swaying (51%), and dizziness (51%). In this sample, 80% reported that their tinnitus had lasted for many years. Tinnitus is highly associated with depression, anxiety, and other personality disorders. Perception of tinnitus is altered by the patient's attention to the sounds, level of stress, and ambient noise level. A few key questions can help guide appropriate history taking and diagnosis.[8]

Differential Diagnosis

	Prevalence[a]
Subjective tinnitus (95% of cases)	*Study of 200 patients[9]*
Cochlear origin	75%
CNS	18%
Conductive causes (usually with sensorineural hearing loss)	4%
Vascular causes	3%
Objective tinnitus (5% of cases)	*Study of 84 patients[10]*
Pulsatile tinnitus (intracranial/extracranial)	
• Unknown causes	32%
• Vascular structures	
– Dural arteriovenous malformations	20%
– Carotid narrowing (eg, stenosis, dissection, or fibromuscular dysplasia)	20%
– Carotid-cavernous sinus fistula	7%
– Other vascular sources	2%
– Internal carotid artery aneurysm	1%
• Nonvascular structures	
– Glomus tumor, other tumors, intracranial hypertension, etc	13%
Nonpulsatile tinnitus	
• Impacted cerumen	
• Clonic muscular contractions	
– Palatal myoclonus	
– Stapedius spasm	
– Tensor tympani spasm	
• Patulous eustachian tube (persistently open)	

[a]Prevalence is unknown when not indicated.

Symptom-based differential diagnosis may be enhanced by correlating the tinnitus symptoms to origin of the sensation.

Conductive System (Outer Ear, Tympanic Membrane, Ossicles)

Bilateral tinnitus may occur with damage to the conductive hearing system from environmental (prolonged noise exposure) or systemic (medications that damage the cochlear hairs) causes. Unilateral tinnitus with conductive hearing loss results from tympanic membrane damage, recurrent unilateral ear infections, ossicle damage, or trauma. Blowing tinnitus may be caused by a patulous (persistently open) eustachian tube, as the tympanic membrane moves in time with the respiratory cycle. Pulsatile or clicking tinnitus may be caused by stapedius muscle spasm, sometimes up to 175 to 200 contractions per minute.

Sensorineural Transduction (Cochlea)

Many cochlear disorders are associated with tinnitus, including Ménière's disease and postinfectious cochlear labyrinthitis. In addition, many common medications can damage cochlear stereocilia, often irreversibly. With cochlear disorders, spontaneous otoacoustic emissions (SOAEs) may be heard with a small microphone placed in the patient's ear canal.

Central Auditory Pathways Alteration (Eighth Nerve and Brain)

The closer the focal pathology is to the external ear, the more likely that tinnitus will be unilateral. For instance, unilateral and progressive neurosensory hearing loss may be caused by a tumor that grows out of the myelin sheath of the eighth cranial nerve (called an acoustic neuroma or schwannoma). Alternatively, once the auditory pathways have combined in the auditory cortex, myelin or axonal brain lesions can produce bilateral tinnitus and other neurologic deficits. After head trauma or CNS infections, tinnitus may be caused by nerve sensitivity after cortical reorganization due to auditory disinhibition of normal background sounds. Finally, low serotonin levels may contribute to tinnitus and to depression.

Referred Sounds

Not all tinnitus originates in the ear and CNS. Pulsatile tinnitus may be caused by vascular structures near the ear and high cardiac output states such as pregnancy. Like stapedius myoclonus, palatal myoclonus may also result in a sensation of "clicking" or pulsation.

GETTING STARTED WITH THE HISTORY

- The initial questions should be open-ended.
- Let the patient (or parent) tell the story.
- The degree of functional impairment should be assessed with a validated tinnitus instrument.[11]

Open-Ended Questions	Tips for Effective Interviewing
Tell me about your tinnitus.	Create a comfortable setting.
When did it start? How has it changed?	Give the patient enough time to finish his or her story.
What makes it better or worse? What else have you noticed with your tinnitus?	Whenever possible, do not interrupt the patient.
How does the tinnitus affect your life?	
What do you think is causing this symptom?	

INTERVIEW FRAMEWORK

First characterize the tinnitus as pulsatile or nonpulsatile, as unilateral or bilateral, and as subjective or objective (eg, you can hear it too). Then determine if there is hearing loss.

IDENTIFYING ALARM SYMPTOMS

- The most frequently occurring causes of tinnitus are benign, such as those resulting from cochlear damage or repeated sound exposure.
- It is critical to diagnose any disorder that may result in deafness or life-threatening diseases.

Alarm Symptoms	Serious Causes	Benign Causes
Episodic tinnitus, vertigo, nausea, and hearing loss	Ménière's disease	Labyrinthitis (self-limited)
Pulsatile tinnitus	Vascular tumor Arterial or venous stenosis, aneurysm, or shunt	Pseudotumor cerebri High cardiac output states (pregnancy, hyperthyroidism) Flow murmur
Bilateral progressive conductive hearing loss and tinnitus	Otosclerosis	Tympanic membrane scarring Recurrent infection Chronic noise exposure
Unilateral progressive hearing loss	Acoustic neuroma (eighth nerve tumor)	Conductive hearing loss (eg, recurrent middle ear infection or trauma to ear structures) Sensorineural hearing loss (eg, ototoxic medications)
Bilateral sensorineural hearing loss	Toxin-associated tinnitus	Chronic noise exposure SOAEs
Headaches	Intracranial tumors Glomus tumors Pseudotumor cerebri	Migraine
Focal neurologic symptoms	Multiple sclerosis Stroke or transient ischemic attack Intracranial tumor	
New seizures	Intracranial tumor Intracranial infection	Unrelated causes of seizure (alcohol withdrawal, primary seizure disorder)
Weight loss, fevers, fatigue	Intracranial tumor Giant cell arteritis	

FOCUSED QUESTIONS

The accurate diagnosis of tinnitus is contingent on obtaining an accurate and precise medical history. In addition to the alarm symptoms, the following questions can aid in narrowing the differential diagnosis.

QUALITY	THINK ABOUT...
Does the tinnitus sound like it is blowing, in time with your breathing?	Patulous eustachian tube
Does the tinnitus sound like it is clicking?	Myoclonic muscular contractions (stapedius, palatal muscles, etc)
Does the tinnitus pulse in time with your heartbeat?	Vascular causes of tinnitus High cardiac output states
Is the tinnitus low-pitched, with intermittent sound muffling?	Incomplete cerumen impaction

—Continued next page

Continued—

Associated symptoms and exposures	
Have you sustained any head trauma or been involved in any car accidents that resulted in whiplash?[7]	SOAEs or neuronal disinhibition
Do you play an instrument or in a band? Have you attended loud concerts?	Sound-associated sensorineural damage
Have you been exposed to solvents?	Cochlear stereocilia damage
Have you had a recent viral infection (especially mumps, rubella, cytomegalovirus)?	Labyrinthitis
Do you use Q-tips to clean your ears? Is sound muffled?	Cerumen impaction
Do you become significantly dizzy or feel like you can't keep your balance?	Ménière's disease Labyrinthitis Eighth nerve tumor
Is there any possibility that you are pregnant? Are you sexually active (women)?	Anemia-associated high cardiac output states
Have you recently had heavy or chronic blood loss?	
Do you wear protective ear wear during (acute or chronic) loud noise exposure?	Noise-associated sensorineural damage
Medications	
Does aspirin make the tinnitus better?	SOAEs (a small percentage improve with aspirin)
Have you been taking large amounts of aspirin or nonsteroidal anti-inflammatory drugs (NSAIDs)?	NSAID-associated cochlear and neuronal damage
Are you taking any over-the-counter, herbal, or prescription medications?	Other medication-associated cochlear and neuronal damage
Past medical, family, occupational history	
Anxiety and depression inventories	Anxiety and depression can alter tinnitus perception
Does anyone in your family have early deafness?	Otosclerosis (autosomal dominant) Tympanic membrane scarring
Does anyone in your family have a genetic disorder where they form tumors on their nerves?	Neurofibromatosis
Are you a boxer?	Stereocilia damage or cortical reorganization problems
Have you been involved in a job with chronic loud noise exposure (such as construction or road work)? For how long?	Sound-associated sensorineural damage

DIAGNOSTIC APPROACH (INCLUDING ALGORITHM)

After taking the tinnitus history, a focused physical examination should be performed to look for objective tinnitus diagnoses. It includes careful examination of the head, neck, external auditory meatus, and tympanic membranes. Testing the acoustic reflex and tympanic membrane mobility (office procedures), screening tests for conductive or sensorineural hearing loss (Weber, Renee, and office screening tools for hearing loss), and a full neurologic screening examination are also important.

Patients with mild to moderate tinnitus, no hearing loss, and no signs of neurologic, cardiac, or otologic dysfunction can be monitored at regular intervals. However, patients with subjective or objective hearing loss require a full audiologic examination (see the diagnostic approach in Figure 19–2).

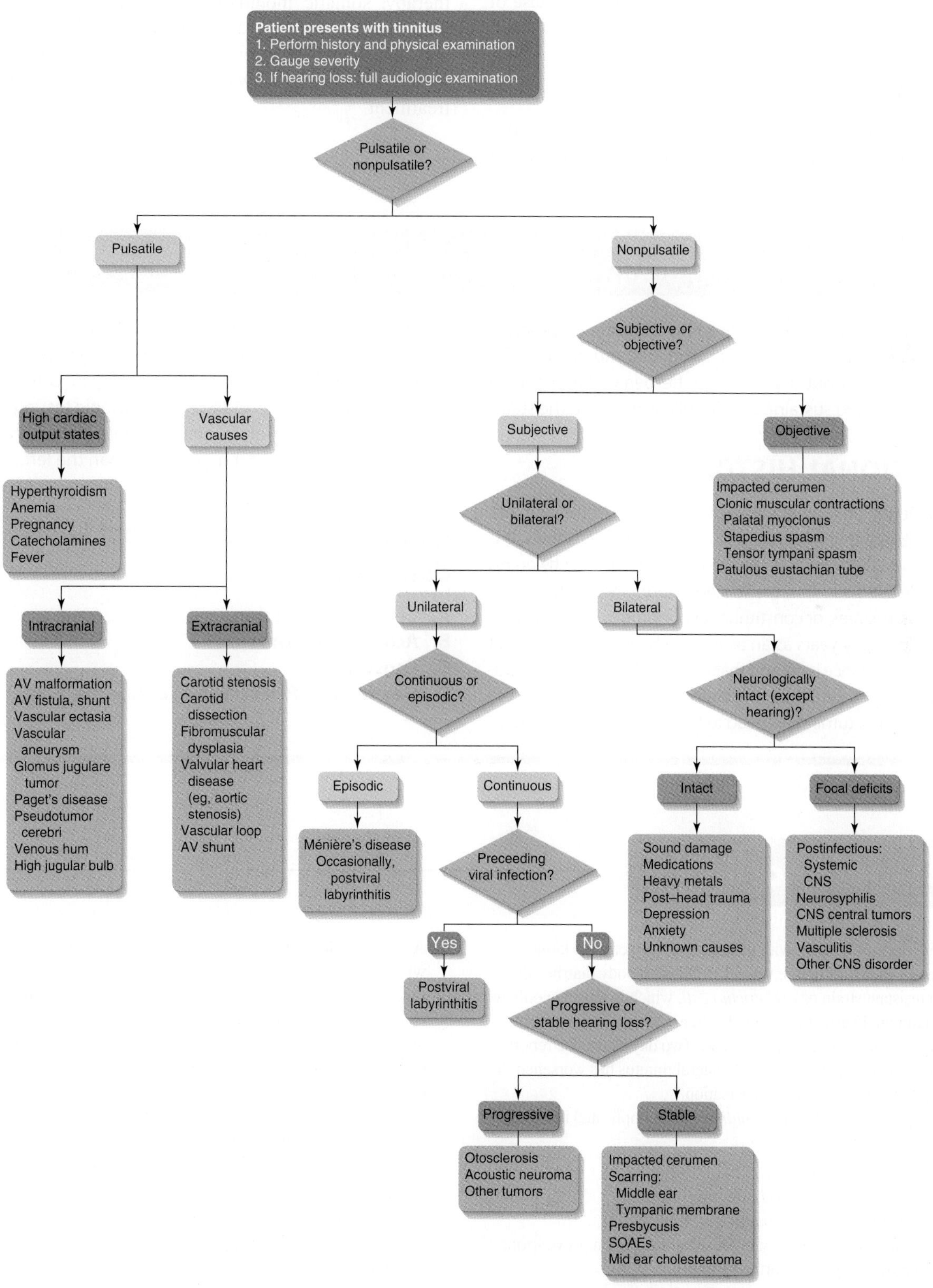

FIGURE 19–2 Diagnostic approach: Tinnitus. AV, arteriovenous; CNS, central nervous system; SOAEs, spontaneous otoacoustic emissions.

ADDITIONAL EVALUATION

If initial evaluation based on history, physical examination, and initial diagnostic testing is unrevealing, consider referring to an otolaryngologist for specialized evaluation.[6,12] Specialized otic and CNS pathway testing may help localize the cause of the patient's symptoms.

PROGNOSIS

Tinnitus is difficult to treat. Multiple clinical trials of tinnitus therapy show no significant, reproducible benefit of medication.[13] Medications (eg, antidepressants, benzodiazepines, pain modulators) and complementary medicines (eg, Ginkgo biloba, ginseng) have only modest success. The placebo effect in most tinnitus studies ranges from 5% to 30%. Other therapies for benign causes include tinnitus retraining therapy, somatic modulation, cognitive retraining therapy, amplification devices, cochlear implantation, pitch matching, and tinnitus maskers. Specific diagnoses such as pseudotumor cerebri or schwannoma may respond to appropriate treatment.

CASE SCENARIO | Resolution

A 75-year-old man is brought in by his daughter for progressive mainly unilateral tinnitus, hearing loss, and dizziness for the past year. About 3 weeks ago, he began experiencing unsteadiness and sustained a fall while walking up the stairs.

ADDITIONAL HISTORY

The patient's tinnitus is constant and nonpulsatile and has been interfering with enjoyment of his favorite TV shows. It is low- to moderate-pitched, fairly loud, and occurs mostly on his right side. He has not experienced nausea, headaches, focal weakness, seizures, or constitutional symptoms. In the past, he worked for many years as an airline mechanic. He reports that his sense of balance is off and that there is a heaviness or "deadness" in his right ear. During the interview, he asks you to repeat your questions, turning his head to the left to hear you better.

The physical examination is essentially normal, including the cardiac examination. There is no nystagmus. Tympanic membrane appears normal, and you cannot hear any additional sounds. Additional audiologic testing shows moderate bilateral high-frequency sensorineural hearing loss affecting the right ear much more than the left.

Question: What is the most likely diagnosis?

A. Cerumen impaction
B. Acoustic neuroma
C. Otosclerosis
D. Hearing loss from trauma (airline mechanic)

Test Your Knowledge

1. A 54-year-old woman with diabetes mellitus, chronic kidney disease, and heart failure was admitted for bloody diarrhea due to a resistant strain of *Escherichia coli*, which is sensitive only to gentamicin. During her hospitalization, she requires increasing doses of diuretics for fluid overload. Two days later, she reports that her low-level nonpulsatile bilateral tinnitus has worsened to the point that it obscures conversation.

   Which of the following is *unlikely* to be implicated in exacerbating her tinnitus?

   A. Furosemide (diuretic)
   B. Gentamicin (for *E coli* infection)
   C. Acetaminophen (for pain)
   D. Aspirin (for secondary myocardial infarction prevention)
   E. Ibuprofen (for osteoarthritis pain)

2. A 15-year-old high school student complains of a loud whooshing noise that worsens when taking tests or running long distances. He recently lost 15 lbs after joining the track team. No one else around him can hear the noise, and his classmates think he is making this up. His mother reports he has been behaving erratically and is worried that he is taking drugs. He feels like the noise is impairing his concentration and that he has a "bucket on his head." He is also upset about losing athletic competitions.

   What is the most likely cause of these sounds?

   A. Auditory hallucinations
   B. Myoclonic stapedius muscle spasm
   C. Patulous eustachian tube
   D. Malingering

3. A 47-year-old construction worker reports intermittent dizziness, occurring twice weekly for 15 to 60 minutes, accompanied by severe, nonpulsatile tinnitus for the past year. He recently lost his job because he injured his back after falling off a ladder. His disability application was denied on the first application because the evaluator was concerned that he was "faking" the severity of his injury. He is upset that he cannot provide for his family but has begun to restrict his driving and is afraid to climb buildings. His wife is threatening to leave him, because he is a changed man. In the office, he denies dizziness or tinnitus. The physical examination and laboratory tests are normal.

   What is the most likely diagnosis?

   A. Otosclerosis
   B. Ménière's disease
   C. Labyrinthitis
   D. Intracranial arteriovenous malformation (AVM)

References

1. McFadden D. Tinnitus: facts, theories and treatments. Report of Working Group 89. Committee on Hearing, Bioacoustics and Biomechanics. National Research Council. Washington, DC: National Academy Press, 1982.
2. Stouffer JL, Tyler RS. Characterization of tinnitus by tinnitus patients. *J Speech Hear Disord.* 1990;55:439–453.
3. Coles RR, Hallam RS. Tinnitus and its management. *Br Med Bull.* 1987;43:983–998.
4. Sismanis A. Pulsatile tinnitus. *Otolaryngol Clin North Am.* 2003;36:389–402.
5. Adams PF, Hendershot GE, Marano MA. Current estimates from the National Health Interview Survey, 1996. Washington, DC: National Center for Health Statistics, Centers for Disease Control and Prevention, 1999.
6. Fritsch MH, Wynne MK, Matt BH, Smith WL, Smith CM. Objective tinnitus in children. *Otol Neurotol.* 2001;22:644–649.
7. Claussen C-F, Pandey A. Neurootologic differentiations in endogenous tinnitus. *Int Tinnitus J.* 2009;15:174–184.
8. Moller AR. Pathophysiology of tinnitus. *Otolaryngol Clin North Am.* 2003;36:249–266.
9. Reed GF. An audiometric study of two hundred cases of subjective tinnitus. *Arch Otolaryngol.* 1960;71:84–94.
10. Waldvogel D, Mattle HP, Sturzenegger M, Schroth G. Pulsatile tinnitus—a review of 84 patients. *J Neurol.* 1998;245:137–142.
11. Newman CW, Jacobson GP, Spitzer JB. Development of the Tinnitus Handicap Inventory. *Arch Otolaryngol Head Neck Surg.* 1996;122:143–148.
12. Van de Heyning P, Meeus O, Blaivie C, Vermeire K, Boudeway A, De Ridder D. Tinnitus: a multidisciplinary clinical approach. *B-ENT.* 2007;3(Suppl 7):3–10.
13. Dobie RA. A review of randomized clinical trials in tinnitus. *Laryngoscope.* 1999;109:1202–1211.

Chapter 20

Sore Throat

Craig R. Keenan, MD, FACP, and Zachary Holt, MD

CASE SCENARIO

A 19-year-old man comes to your office with a complaint of a sore throat. His illness began 3 days ago with a sore throat, followed by persistent fevers of 102°F.

- **What are the common diagnostic considerations for patients with acute sore throat?**
- **What questions are helpful in determining the cause of sore throat?**
- **How do you assess for the presence of potentially serious causes of sore throat?**

INTRODUCTION

Sore throat was the sixth most common reason for seeking outpatient care in 2000, accounting for 2.1% of all ambulatory visits in the United States.[1] Although the term "sore throat" is frequently equated with pharyngitis (inflammation of the pharynx), sore throat often results from other causes. Most cases are benign or self-limited, but sore throat may be the presenting symptom for dangerous and potentially life-threatening conditions. The following discussion covers acute sore throat, which is much more common than chronic sore throat.

The general approach to patients with acute sore throat has been to identify and treat cases of group A β-hemolytic streptococcal (GAS) pharyngitis ("strep throat") in order to prevent acute rheumatic fever (ARF). GAS infections may also cause suppurative sequelae including peritonsillar abscess, severe parapharyngeal infections, or retropharyngeal abscess. Antibiotic treatment of GAS pharyngitis prevents ARF, decreases the transmission of GAS, shortens the illness by 1 to 2 days, and may reduce suppurative complications.[2] However, because ARF is so uncommon in the United States, between 3000 and 4000 cases of GAS pharyngitis would need to be treated to prevent a single case.[3] Even without antibiotics, most cases of GAS pharyngitis resolve uneventfully after 7 to 10 days. Poststreptococcal glomerulonephritis is a very rare complication of GAS pharyngitis, and antibiotics do not reduce its incidence.[3]

The classic history for GAS pharyngitis is the sudden onset of sore throat, odynophagia, fever greater than 101°F, abdominal pain, headache, nausea, and vomiting. Cough, rhinorrhea, and diarrhea are usually absent. The classic physical findings include pharyngeal erythema with tonsillar exudates, palatal petechiae, and anterior cervical adenopathy. Unfortunately, there is broad overlap of clinical manifestations between GAS and nonstreptococcal pharyngitis. Although only 5% to 15% of adults with sore throat have a positive GAS culture, 47% to 75% of such patients receive antibiotics.[3–5] Thus, the desire to treat GAS infections has led to the overprescribing of antibiotics; the proper exclusion of patients without GAS could lead to significant reductions in inappropriate antibiotic use.

Recent evidence suggests that the traditional approach to acute pharyngitis should incorporate consideration of another infectious agent, *Fusobacterium necrophorum*. This bacterium is the causative agent for acute pharyngitis in approximately 10% of patients age 15 to 30 years old, which is equivalent to GAS.[6] *F necrophorum* causes Lemierre syndrome (LS), a potentially life-threatening suppurative thrombophlebitis of the internal jugular vein, which may lead to bacteremia and metastatic infections via septic emboli (usually pulmonary abscesses). The mortality of patients with LS approaches 5%, with significant morbidity in survivors.[6] The incidence of LS appears to be rising,[7] and it develops in 1 in 400 cases of *F necrophorum* pharyngitis, which is much more common than ARF after GAS pharyngitis.[6] Patients with LS typically have sore throat for several days before the syndrome develops, so there may be a window of opportunity to treat with antibiotics and prevent its development, although this assertion remains unproven. Thus, an expert recently recommended treating adolescent and young adult patients (age 15–24) with symptoms of severe acute pharyngitis with antibiotics to prevent LS.[6] This approach is not yet widely accepted.

KEY TERMS

Odynophagia	Pain with swallowing.
Dysphagia	Difficulty initiating the swallowing process (oropharyngeal dysphagia) or difficulty in passage of a bolus from the upper esophagus to the stomach (esophageal dysphagia).
Sore throat	Pain in the throat region. Odynophagia is the usual symptom, but occasionally dysphagia also occurs.
Pharyngitis	Inflammation of the pharynx, including the tonsillar and adenoid lymphoid tissue.
Trismus	Inability to open the jaw. May result from processes affecting the motor branch of the trigeminal nerve and from pressure or infection of the muscles of mastication.
Clinical prediction rule	A clinical tool that quantifies the individual contributions that various components of the history, physical examination, and basic laboratory results make toward the diagnosis, prognosis, or likely response to treatment in a given patient.

ETIOLOGY AND DIFFERENTIAL DIAGNOSIS

The differential diagnosis for sore throat is extensive (Table 20–1). The prevalence for each of the various causes has not been well established. Most patients with acute sore throat will have infectious pharyngitis, usually a viral infection, although bacterial pharyngitis causes up to 40% of cases. Less common causes include herpes simplex, syphilis, and gonorrheal infections. Primary HIV infection often presents with sore throat as a key feature. Group C *Streptococcus* is an increasingly important pathogen that presents much like GAS pharyngitis.[8]

Table **20–1. Differential diagnosis and estimated prevalence of causes of sore throat.**

Differential Diagnosis	Associated Organisms and Conditions	Estimated % of Infectious Pharyngitis[11,12,a]
Infectious		
Bacterial pharyngitis	Group A streptococci	13–30
	Other streptococci	5
	Mycoplasma pneumoniae	< 1
	Moraxella catarrhalis	
	Chlamydia pneumoniae	
	Staphylococcus aureus	
	Neisseria meningitidis	
	F necrophorum	5
Viral pharyngitis	Rhinovirus, coronavirus, adenovirus, parainfluenza	> 32
Herpetic stomatitis, pharyngitis	Herpes simplex virus 1 and 2. May be sexually transmitted or seen in immunocompromised patients.	4
Acute epiglottitis/supraglottitis[b]	*Haemophilus influenzae*	
Gonococcal pharyngitis	Sexually transmitted via oral sexual contact. Often asymptomatic but can cause acute pharyngitis.	< 1
Infectious mononucleosis	Epstein-Barr virus, cytomegalovirus; syndrome of fatigue, fever, pharyngitis, splenomegaly (50%), posterior cervical lymphadenopathy, occasional rash	1
Peritonsillar abscess[b]		

Table 20–1. Differential diagnosis and estimated prevalence of causes of sore throat. (*continued*)

Differential Diagnosis	Associated Organisms and Conditions	Estimated % of Infectious Pharyngitis[11,12,a]
Infectious		
Parapharyngeal infections[b] (Lemierre syndrome)	*F necrophorum*	
Retropharyngeal infections[b]		
Necrotizing ulcerative gingivostomatitis (Vincent angina)[b]	Anaerobes (including *Fusobacterium nucleatum*)	
Primary HIV infection	HIV. Syndrome of sore throat, fever, truncal rash, diffuse lymphadenopathy, weight loss, fatigue, and mucocutaneous ulcers. Usually occurs 2–4 weeks after HIV exposure and lasts 2 weeks.	< 1
Oropharyngeal candidiasis	*Candida albicans*. Seen in immunocompromised persons or users of inhaled corticosteroids.	
Influenza	Influenza viruses. Seasonal syndrome of sudden-onset fever, myalgias, and sore throat. Measures to prevent spread sometimes important.	2
Diphtheria[b]	*Corynebacterium diphtheriae*. Rare due to high vaccination rates. Characteristic pharyngitis with gray pseudomembrane in throat on examination.	< 1
Herpangina	Coxsackievirus	< 1
Secondary syphilis	*Treponema pallidum*. Syndrome of fever, weight loss, sore throat, anorexia, malaise, headache, and rash.	
Toxic shock syndrome[b]	Streptococci or staphylococci	
Noninfectious		
Sinusitis	Postnasal drip, nasal congestion	
Allergic rhinitis	Rhinitis, postnasal drip, conjunctivitis	
Acute/subacute thyroiditis	Symptoms of hyperthyroidism or hypothyroidism	
Head and neck cancer	Laryngeal, tongue, oropharyngeal	
Lymphoma	Adenopathy, fever, night sweats, weight loss	
Gastroesophageal reflux	Heartburn, acid taste	
Esophageal spasm		
Cervical spondylosis		
Postoperative		
Postirradiation		
Burn or irritant injuries	Smoking cocaine, drinking caustic agents	
Coronary artery disease[b]	Angina may present as neck pain	
Glossopharyngeal neuralgia		
Systemic illnesses		
Adult-onset Still's disease[13]	Accompanied by fever, rash, arthritis	
Wegener's granulomatosis		
Sarcoidosis		

[a]Incidence unknown when not indicated.

[b]Potentially life-threatening.

Common noninfectious causes include acid irritation of the pharynx or larynx due to gastroesophageal reflux disease (GERD),[9] postnasal drip (due to sinusitis or allergic rhinitis), thyroiditis, and head and neck malignancies. In addition, 15% to 50% of patients complain of sore throat after surgeries.[10] Sore throat may also be a core symptom of systemic illnesses such as adult-onset Still disease, Wegener's granulomatosis, and sarcoidosis.

Most cases of sore throat are benign, but there are important exceptions. First, the clinician must be aware of several suppurative complications of oropharyngeal infections that present with sore throat. Although rare, such complications may be life-threatening, so prompt recognition is important. There is usually a history of preceding pharyngitis or oral infection, which spreads to the peritonsillar space (peritonsillar abscess), parapharyngeal space (carotid sheath infection causing LS), submandibular space (Ludwig's angina), or retropharyngeal space (retropharyngeal abscess). Finally, the possibility of a head and neck cancer, lymphoma, or acute human immunodeficiency virus (HIV) infection should be considered.

GETTING STARTED WITH THE INTERVIEW

Use open-ended questions to determine the symptoms and chronology of the illness (eg, "Tell me about this illness, starting with the first symptoms that you noticed").

The diagnosis of sore throat also relies heavily on the physical examination. You will need to do a careful examination (eg, throat redness or exudates, swollen lymph nodes) and often laboratory testing, so do not spend too much time elaborating the symptoms.

INTERVIEW FRAMEWORK

- First, determine the duration of the sore throat and whether it is acute or chronic (> 2 weeks in duration). The common causes of sore throat (viral and bacterial infections) usually resolve within 1 to 2 weeks. Chronic symptoms should prompt consideration of less common conditions including atypical infections (eg, infectious mononucleosis), noninfectious etiologies (eg, malignancy, allergic rhinitis, GERD, adult-onset Still's disease, chronic sinusitis), or complications of acute infections (eg, peritonsillar abscess, LS).
- If the patient reports fever, rhinorrhea, lymphadenopathy, malaise, myalgias, or headache, think about an infectious cause. Direct your subsequent questions to determine the specific infectious cause and the severity of the illness:
  - Ask about alarm symptoms (eg, trismus, drooling, shortness of breath) (Table 20–2).
  - Ask the questions to evaluate for GAS pharyngitis (Tables 20–3 and 20–4).
  - Take a detailed sexual history to determine whether the patient is at risk for sexually transmitted causes (herpes, gonorrhea, syphilis, HIV).
- Ask about heartburn, acid brash, or nocturnal cough, which suggest GERD as a potential cause. Also ask about postnasal drip as a possible contributing factor.
- Perform a review of systems to detect other symptoms that may be related to a systemic disease masquerading as an infection (eg, weight loss, chronic cough, chronic fevers), especially if the symptoms are chronic.

Table **20–2. Serious diagnoses and alarm symptoms.**

Symptoms	Serious Diagnoses	Potential Complications
Sore throat, dysphagia, or odynophagia with any of the following: • Drooling • Respiratory distress • Inability to open mouth fully (trismus) • Muffled voice • Stiff neck • Erythema of neck	Acute epiglottitis or supraglottitis Peritonsillar abscess Parapharyngeal space infection Retropharyngeal space infection Submandibular space infection (Ludwig's angina) Superficial jugular thrombophlebitis (Lemierre syndrome).	Airway obstruction; sepsis; spread to parapharyngeal or retropharyngeal spaces, with subsequent spread to pleura, mediastinum, carotid sheath, or jugular vein
History of recent foreign body impaction or oropharyngeal procedure (trauma)	Retropharyngeal abscess	Airway obstruction; sepsis; spread to mediastinum, pleural space, or pericardium
Fever, rash, diffuse adenopathy, sore throat	Primary HIV infection	Transmission of disease
Recent cocaine smoking	Mucosal burn injury to pharynx and larynx	Respiratory obstruction
Weight loss, fevers, night sweats	Lymphoma, head and neck cancers	Advanced malignancy

Table **20–3. Likelihood ratios for GAS infection for common historical and physical examination features.**[2]

Symptom	LR+[a]	LR–[a]
Reported fever	0.75–2.6	0.66–0.94
Absence of cough	1.1–1.7	0.53–0.89
Absence of runny nose	0.86–1.6	0.51–1.4
Presence of myalgias	1.4	0.93
Presence of headache	1.0–1.1	0.55–1.2
Presence of nausea	0.76–3.1	0.91
Duration of symptoms < 3 days	0.72–3.5	0.15–2.2
Streptococcal exposure in previous 2 weeks	1.9	0.92

[a]The range of likelihood ratios from the studies are presented for each variable. If there was agreement among all studies, a single summary likelihood ratio is presented.

- Always review the past medical and social history, including substances, tobacco, and medication use. Patients with heavy alcohol and tobacco use are at increased risk for head and neck cancer. Patients who are immunosuppressed (eg, HIV, active cancer, immunosuppressive medications) are at high risk for suppurative complications.

IDENTIFYING ALARM SYMPTOMS

The alarm symptoms suggest severe infections of the supraglottic, submandibular, peritonsillar, parapharyngeal, or retropharyngeal spaces, which often require prompt surgical intervention.

Table 20–4. Centor Clinical Prediction Rule.[14]

Symptom or Sign	Points
History of fever	1
Absence of cough	1
Tonsillar exudates	1
Anterior cervical adenopathy	1
Total Score	**LR+ for GAS**
4 points	6.3
3 points	2.1
2 points	0.75
1 point	0.3
0 points	0.16

FOCUSED QUESTIONS

If infection is likely and there are no alarm symptoms, focus on determining whether the patient has GAS pharyngitis. Many studies have evaluated the usefulness of historical and physical examination findings in differentiating GAS from other causes of acute pharyngitis. There are no symptoms that reliably predict *F necrophorum* infection, and it shares many features of GAS infection.[6]

Ebell et al.[2] evaluated studies from children and adults to calculate the positive and negative likelihood ratios (LR+ and LR–) for various elements of the history. The LR+ are all below 5, with most between 1 and 2; and LR– are mostly between 0.5 and 2.0 (Table 20–3). Thus, the presence or absence of each element alone is weak evidence for or against GAS pharyngitis and does *not* appreciably change the posttest probability.

Given the poor predictive ability of individual historical elements, clinical prediction rules that incorporate both history and physical examination elements were created. The most widely accepted rule for adults is the Centor Clinical Prediction Rule.[14] Clinicians should apply this clinical prediction rule to help determine the likelihood of GAS pharyngitis. In patients with either 0 to 1 or 4 points, the associated LR considerably alters the probability of GAS infection. Scores of 2 to 3 points do not appreciably affect the probability.

DIAGNOSTIC APPROACH (INCLUDING ALGORITHM)

There is no consensus on the best approach to the diagnosis and treatment of GAS pharyngitis.[15,16] The diagnostic algorithm (Figure 20–1) is adapted from a major clinical practice guideline for adults with acute pharyngitis and incorporates the rising consideration of *F necrophorum* in adolescents and young adults.[6,17]

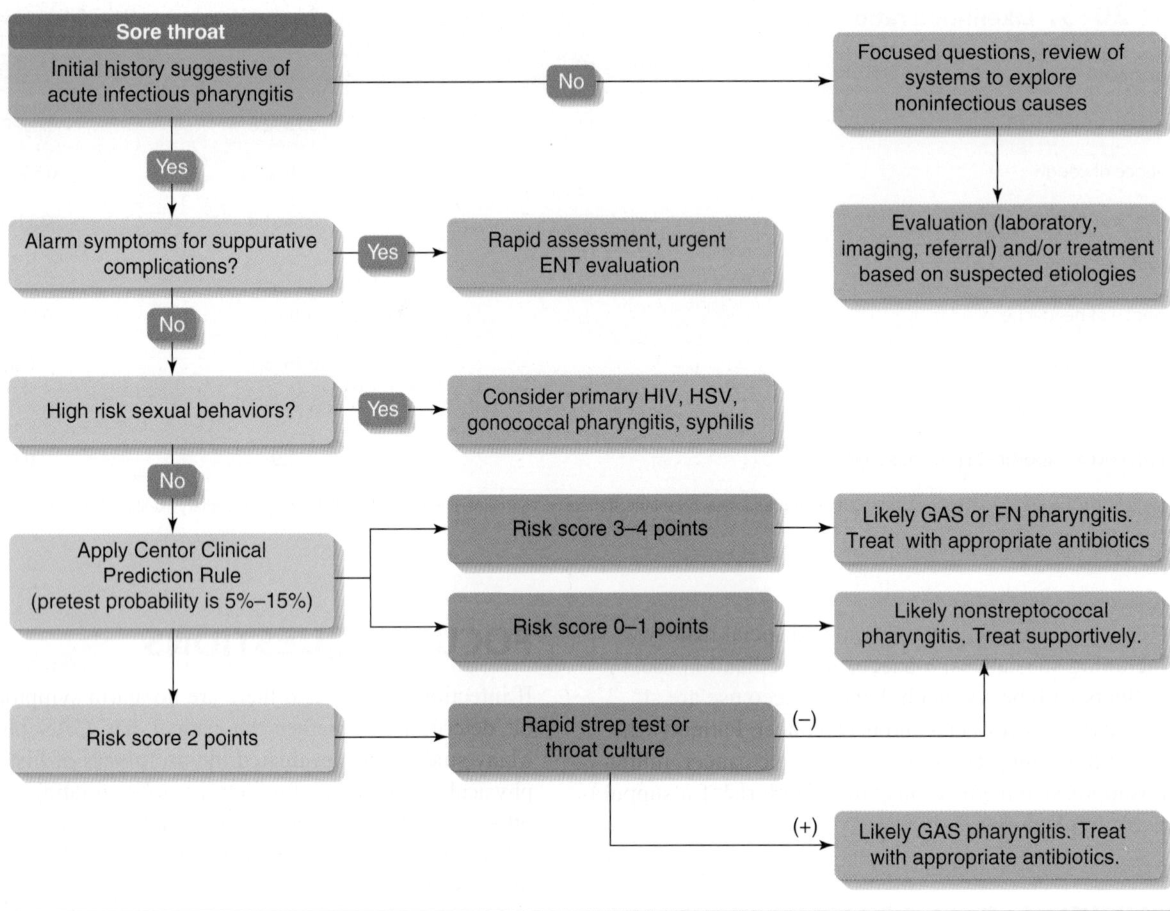

FIGURE 20–1 Diagnostic algorithm: Sore throat. ENT, ear, nose, and throat; FN, *F necrophorum*; GAS, group A *Streptococcus*; HIV, human immunodeficiency virus; HSV, herpes simplex virus.

CAVEATS

- The clinical decision rules and guidelines were developed based on ambulatory, immunocompetent patients in the United States and Canada where the endemic rate of rheumatic fever is low. As such, they cannot be applied to immunosuppressed patients, patients with chronic or recurrent pharyngitis, or those with a history of rheumatic fever. Finally, such tools do not apply when there is a known outbreak or a high endemic rate of rheumatic fever.
- There is controversy about whether empiric antibiotics are warranted in patients with a Centor Clinical Prediction Rule score of 3. Some experts recommend treating only patients with a positive rapid strep test to reduce antibiotic use and antibiotic resistance. Others emphasize empiric treatment of patients with severe pharyngitis, because there is a 10% false-negative rate for rapid GAS strep tests and because group C and G *Streptococcus* infections will also test negative. Thus, failing to treat patients who test negative will deny this group the rapid symptom relief associated with antibiotic therapy.
- Empiric antibiotic treatment of adolescents and young adults with acute pharyngitis for possible *F necrophorum* is recommended by one expert but not yet universally accepted or included in practice guidelines. Penicillin or cephalosporins are first-line therapy, whereas macrolides are not effective.
- Patients with diabetes, recent chemotherapy, or other immunocompromised states are more susceptible to suppurative complications of bacterial pharyngitis.
- Although dangerous conditions are rare in patients with sore throat, the clinician should always consider suppurative complications, head and neck malignancies, and primary HIV infection.
- Patients with sore throats often expect antibiotics. Physicians should take the time to explain to their patients that antibiotics are frequently unnecessary.

CASE SCENARIO | Resolution

A 19-year-old man comes to your office with a complaint of a sore throat. His illness began 3 days ago with a sore throat, followed by persistent fevers of 102°F.

ADDITIONAL HISTORY

He notes that he has a mild cough, some mild nausea, and no rhinorrhea. He reports odynophagia but no drooling, neck swelling, or difficulty breathing. He does not smoke or use drugs. He has not been sexually active for 6 months. His examination reveals a fever of 101.8°F, white exudates on his reddened tonsils, and no cervical lymphadenopathy.

Question: What is the most likely diagnosis?

A. Group A streptococcal pharyngitis
B. *F necrophorum* pharyngitis
C. Laryngeal inflammation from gastroesophageal reflux disease
D. Viral pharyngitis

Test Your Knowledge

1. For the patient in the Case Scenario, what is the next step in his evaluation and treatment?

   A. Symptomatic treatment (only) for presumed viral infection
   B. Antibiotics to cover group A *Streptococcus* and *F necrophorum*
   C. Perform rapid strep testing in the office and treat if positive
   D. Perform throat culture, start antibiotics, and then stop antibiotics if the culture comes back negative

2. A 47-year-old man with a history of hypertension presents with a complaint of a sore throat for 5 months. It is mild and occurs daily. He denies postnasal drip, allergy symptoms, weight loss, and shortness of breath, but notes some mild heartburn and occasional hoarse voice. He has never smoked and does not drink alcohol. His examination shows no abnormalities of the oropharynx and no lymphadenopathy.

   What would be your next step in his evaluation?

   A. Rapid strep test to test for GAS infection
   B. Magnetic resonance imaging (MRI) of the neck
   C. Ear, nose, and throat (ENT) evaluation
   D. Empiric therapy with antiallergy medications

3. A 26-year-old woman presents with sore throat, odynophagia, and fevers for 8 days. Over the last 24 hours, she has been unable to swallow her secretions and is drooling. She has trouble opening her mouth and has noted that her anterior neck seems swollen.

   Which of the following should you consider?

   A. Acute epiglottitis
   B. Retropharyngeal abscess
   C. Lemierre syndrome
   D. All of the above

References

1. Cherry DK, Woodwell DA. National Ambulatory Medical Care Survey: 2000 Summary. Advance Data from Vital and Health Statistics 2002;328. Available at: http://www.cdc.gov/nchs/data/ad/ad328.pdf. Accessed October 13, 2011.
2. Ebell MH, Smith MA, Barry HC, et al. Does this patient have strep throat? In: Simel DL, Drummond R, Keitz SA, eds. *The Rational Clinical Examination: Evidence-Based Clinical Diagnosis*. New York, NY: McGraw Hill Medical, 2009:615–626.
3. Cooper M, Hoffman JR, Bartlett JG, et al. Principles of appropriate antibiotic use for acute pharyngitis in adults: background. *Ann Intern Med.* 2001;134:509–517.
4. Linder JA, Stafford RS. Antibiotic treatment of adults with sore throat by community primary care physicians. A national survey, 1989–1999. *JAMA.* 2001;286:1181–1186.
5. Linder JA, Chan JC, Bates DW. Evaluation and treatment of pharyngitis in primary care practice: the difference between guidelines is largely academic. *Arch Intern Med.* 2006;166:1374–1379.
6. Centor RM. Expand the pharyngitis paradigm for adolescents and young adults. *Ann Intern Med.* 2009;151:812–815.
7. Karkos PD, Asrani S, Karkos CD, et al. Lemierre's syndrome: a systematic review. *Layrngoscope.* 2009;119:1552–1559.

8. Shah M, Centor R, Jennings M. Severe acute pharyngitis caused by group C streptococcus. *J Gen Intern Med.* 2007;22:272–274.
9. Tauber S, Gross M, Issing WJ. Association of laryngopharyngeal symptoms with gastroesophageal reflux disease. *Laryngoscope.* 2002;112:879–886.
10. McHardy FE, Chung F. Postoperative sore throat: cause, prevention, and treatment. *Anaesthesia.* 1999;54:444–453.
11. Amess JA, O'Neill W, Giollariabhaigh CN, et al. A six-month audit of the isolation of *Fusobacterium necrophorum* from patients with sore throat in a district general hospital. *Br J Biomed Sci.* 2007;64:63–65.
12. Bisno AL. Acute pharyngitis. *N Engl J Med.* 2001;344:205–211.
13. Nguyen KH, Weisman MH. Severe sore throat as a presenting symptom of adult onset Still's disease: a case series and review of the literature. *J Rheumatol.* 1997;24:592–597.
14. Centor RM, Witherspoon JM, Dalton HP, et al. The diagnosis of strep throat in adults in the emergency room. *Med Decis Making.* 1981;1:239–246.
15. Bisno AL, Peter GS, Kaplan EL. Diagnosis of strep throat in adults: are clinical criteria really good enough? *Clin Infect Dis.* 2002;35:126–129.
16. Centor RM, Allison JJ, Cohen SJ. Pharyngitis management: defining the controversy. *J Gen Intern Med.* 2007;22:127–130.
17. Snow V, Mottur-Pilson C, Cooper RJ, et al.; American Academy of Family Physicians; American College of Physicians-American Society of Internal Medicine; Centers for Disease Control. Principles of appropriate antibiotic use for acute pharyngitis in adults. *Ann Intern Med.* 2001;134:506–508.

Suggested Reading

Centor RM. Expand the pharyngitis paradigm for adolescents and young adults. *Ann Intern Med.* 2009;151:812–815.

Cooper M, Hoffman JR, Bartlett JG, et al. Principles of appropriate antibiotic use for acute pharyngitis in adults: background. *Ann Intern Med.* 2001;134:509–517.

Ebell MH, Smith MA, Barry HC, et al. Does this patient have strep throat? In: Simel DL, Drummond R, Keitz SA, eds. *The Rational Clinical Examination: Evidence-Based Clinical Diagnosis.* New York, NY: McGraw Hill Medical, 2009:615–626.

SECTION

IV

DERMATOLOGY

Chapter 21

Inflammatory Dermatoses (Rashes)

Mona A. Gohara, MD, Julie V. Schaffer, MD, Naheed R. Abbasi, MD, Melanie M. Kingsley, MD, Jessica M. Sheehan, MD, and Kenneth A. Arndt, MD

CASE SCENARIO

A 23-year-old young woman comes to your office with a rash. The rash started as red, round, pruritic bumps on the abdomen approximately 1 week before presentation and has spread. More recently, 1.5-cm round scaly patches and plaques have developed on the trunk and extremities.

- **What additional questions regarding personal and family history would you ask?**
- **What types of social or occupational exposures may be relevant to this case?**
- **What specific questions about the location of the eruption may help in making a diagnosis?**

INTRODUCTION

Dermatologists are not the only physicians who assess and treat patients with skin disorders. The results of the National Ambulatory Medical Care Survey (1990–1994)[1] showed that US dermatologists saw only 40% of patients with diseases of the skin, hair, or nails. In the primary care setting, 25% of all visits were found to involve skin disorders. Data from both the United States and Canada reveal a continued undersupply of dermatologists, resulting in the need for nondermatology physicians and physician extenders to provide primary care of skin disease.[2,3] These data support the importance of a fundamental understanding of the skin to all healthcare professionals.

As the body's most accessible organ, the skin is too important to be ignored. A close inspection of the skin can afford important insight into the presence and nature of cutaneous and internal disease.

KEY TERMS

Primary lesions

Bulla	A circumscribed, elevated lesion that measures ≥ 1 cm and contains serous or hemorrhagic fluid (ie, a large blister).
Macule	A circumscribed, nonpalpable discoloration of the skin that measures < 1 cm in diameter.
Nodule	A palpable, solid, round or ellipsoidal lesion measuring ≥ 1 cm; it differs from a plaque in that it is more substantive in its vertical dimension compared with its breadth.
Papule	An elevated, solid lesion that measures < 1 cm.
Patch	A circumscribed, nonpalpable discoloration of the skin that measures ≥ 1 cm.
Petechiae	Nonblanching reddish macules representing extravascular deposits of blood, measuring ≤ 0.3 cm (less than the size of a pencil eraser).
Plaque	A palpable, solid lesion that measures ≥ 1 cm.
Purpura	Nonblanching reddish macules or papules representing extravascular deposits of blood, measuring > 0.3 cm.

—Continued next page

Continued—

Pustule	A lesion that contains pus; may be follicular (centered around a hair follicle) or nonfollicular.
Vesicle	A circumscribed, elevated lesion that measures < 1 cm and contains serous or hemorrhagic fluid (ie, a small blister).
Wheal	A round or annular (ring-like), edematous papule or plaque that is characteristically evanescent, disappearing within hours; may be surrounded by a flare of erythema (ie, a hive).
Secondary lesions	
Atrophy	A depression in the skin resulting from thinning of the epidermis, dermis, and/or subcutaneous fat.
Crust	A collection of dried blood, serum, and/or cellular debris.
Erosion	A focal loss of epidermis; does not penetrate below the dermal–epidermal junction and, therefore, can heal without scarring.
Lichenification	Thickening of the epidermis resulting from repeated rubbing, appearing as accentuation of the skin markings.
Scale	Excess dead epidermal cells; scale may be fine, silvery, greasy, desquamative, or adherent.
Scar	Abnormal formation of connective tissue, implying dermal damage.
Ulcer	A focal loss of full-thickness epidermis and partial to full-thickness dermis, which often heals with scarring.
Other	
Nikolsky sign	In the area adjacent to a bulla, application of lateral pressure on normal-appearing epidermis produces further shearing of the skin.

ETIOLOGY

Inflammatory skin eruptions ("rashes") represent a heterogeneous group of disorders with etiologies ranging from drug reactions to infections (viral, bacterial, or fungal) to autoimmune attacks on the skin. The pathogenesis of many primary inflammatory dermatoses (eg, psoriasis) is unknown. A small subset of inflammatory dermatologic conditions is particularly common in clinical practice. For example, cutaneous drug eruptions represent the most frequent reason for inpatient dermatology consultation as well as the most common form of adverse drug reaction.[4] Common chronic inflammatory skin conditions include psoriasis, atopic dermatitis, stasis dermatitis, and acne vulgaris.

Differential Diagnosis

Ask the following questions (with or without a brief examination of the skin) to determine the morphologic pattern of the eruption.

Question	Morphologic Pattern
Do you have a rash consisting of many small red spots and/or bumps?	Exanthematous eruptions
Do you have scaly spots and/or bumps on your skin?	Papulosquamous dermatoses
Do you have red, itchy, oozy, crusty, and scaly skin?	Eczematous dermatoses
Have blisters developed on your skin? Do you ever have bumps on your skin that are filled with fluid?	Vesiculobullous disorders
Do you have "pus bumps" or pimples on your skin?	Pustular dermatoses

Do you have red or purple spots or bumps that do not fade when you press on them? (ie, lesions are nonblanching)	Purpuras
Do you have areas of red, hot skin? Do you have spots on your skin that look like targets?	Erythemas
Do you have hives?	Urticaria
Do you have bumps deep in your skin?	Subcutaneous nodules
Morphologic Pattern	**Possible Diagnoses**
Exanthematous eruptions	• Morbilliform drug eruption (maculopapular eruption; accounts for ~ 70% of exanthematous eruptions in adults) • Drug rash with eosinophilia and systemic symptoms (DRESS) • Acute graft-versus-host disease (GVHD) • Scarlet fever • Viral exanthems, such as measles (rubeola), rubella (German measles), roseola (exanthem subitum), and erythema infectiosum (fifth disease), account for 80%–90% of exanthematous eruptions in children
Papulosquamous dermatoses	• Lichen planus • Pityriasis rosea • Psoriasis • Seborrheic dermatitis • Lupus erythematosus • Dermatomyositis • Tinea corporis/cruris/faciei (ringworm, jock itch) • Secondary syphilis (lues)
Eczematous dermatoses	• Atopic dermatitis • Allergic contact dermatitis (20% of contact dermatitis) • Irritant contact dermatitis (80% of contact dermatitis) • Venous stasis dermatitis • Autosensitization dermatitis (id reaction) • Systemic contact dermatitis
Vesiculobullous disorders	• Stevens-Johnson syndrome/toxic epidermal necrolysis (SJS/TEN) • Bullous pemphigoid • Pemphigus vulgaris • Porphyria cutanea tarda (PCT) • Dermatitis herpetiformis • Phytophotodermatitis • Herpes simplex viral infection (cold sores, fever blisters) • Varicella (chickenpox) • Zoster (shingles) • Staphylococcal scalded skin syndrome (SSSS) • Bullous impetigo *—Continued next page*

Continued— Pustular dermatoses	• Acute generalized exanthematous pustulosis (AGEP) • Generalized pustular psoriasis (von Zumbusch) • Acne vulgaris • Steroid acne • Acne rosacea • Periorificial dermatitis • Folliculitis • Cutaneous candidiasis • Disseminated gonococcal infection
Purpuras	• Thrombocytopenic purpura • Schamberg pigmented purpuric dermatosis • Actinic purpura • Scurvy (vitamin C deficiency) • Leukocytoclastic vasculitis • Polyarteritis nodosa • Cryoglobulinemia, type I (monoclonal) • Cholesterol emboli • Calciphylaxis • Purpura fulminans • Rocky Mountain spotted fever • Acute bacterial endocarditis • Ecthyma gangrenosum
Erythemas and urticaria	• Phototoxic reactions • Urticaria • Erythema multiforme • Sweet syndrome • Erysipelas • Cellulitis • Necrotizing fasciitis ("flesh-eating bacteria" syndrome) • Lyme disease (erythema migrans) • Toxic shock syndrome (TSS)
Subcutaneous nodules	• Erythema nodosum • Nodular vasculitis (erythema induratum) • Lipodermatosclerosis • Pancreatic panniculitis • α_1-Antitrypsin deficiency panniculitis • Lupus panniculitis

GETTING STARTED WITH THE HISTORY

- Due to the unique accessibility of the skin as an organ, the diagnosis of dermatologic diseases is highly dependent on the physical examination. However, the history plays a key role in putting the skin findings in context, understanding the evolution of the disease process, and arriving at the correct diagnosis. The history is especially important when the eruption is in a later stage or not active at the time of the evaluation, or when only secondary lesions are present (eg, bullae have ruptured and left erosions with "collarettes" of scale, or all lesions are excoriated and crusted).

- To elicit the history of a dermatologic condition, start with open-ended questions such as "tell me about what has been going on with your skin," and listen to the patient's story.
- With regard to the physical examination, in addition to recognizing the primary lesion and any secondary changes (see above), several other observations can serve as clues to help further categorize an eruption:
  - Color (eg, pink, red, purple, or violaceous)
  - Palpation (eg, soft, firm, or hard)
  - Margination (well- or ill-defined borders)
  - Shape/configuration of lesions (annular [ring-like], linear, retiform [branching])
  - Location/distribution of lesions (symmetric versus asymmetric, grouped versus scattered)
- A complete skin examination includes inspection of the entire cutaneous surface (including the palms and soles); the nails; the hair/scalp; and the oral, conjunctival, and genital mucosa.

INTERVIEW FRAMEWORK

Gather general information.	• When did you first develop this rash? • Have you had any similar rashes in the past? • On what part of the body did it start? Where did it spread to next? • How long does each individual spot or bump last? • Do you think the rash is getting better or worse? • Is the rash itchy? Is it painful or tender when you touch it? • Is there anything that makes the rash better or worse (eg, sun exposure)? • Have you been putting anything at all on the rash, such as lotions or ointments?
Obtain a drug history. An eruption may be a reaction to a medication (including prescription, nonprescription, and herbal remedies) or to anything else that may have been ingested, inserted, or inhaled.	• Determine the date of onset of the eruption (many occur within 1–2 weeks of starting a drug, but some have a delayed onset or even develop after a drug is discontinued). • Make a "drug chart" including all agents the patient was taking at the time of onset as well as during the prior 3 months, and the date each agent was started and stopped. • Determine whether the patient has any history of reactions to medications and, if so, what these reactions were.

IDENTIFYING ALARM SYMPTOMS

Although the vast majority of skin conditions are not life-threatening, it is extremely important to recognize the warning signs of a potentially serious eruption.

Serious Diagnoses

Morphologic Pattern	Serious Diagnoses
Exanthematous eruptions	DRESS GVHD
Papulosquamous dermatoses	Erythrodermic psoriasis Systemic lupus erythematosus Dermatomyositis

—Continued next page

Continued—	
Eczematous dermatoses	Erythrodermic dermatitis
Vesiculobullous disorders	SJS/TEN Pemphigus vulgaris Disseminated herpes simplex viral infection Disseminated zoster
Pustular dermatoses	Generalized pustular psoriasis Disseminated gonococcal infection
Purpuras	Leukocytoclastic vasculitis with systemic involvement Polyarteritis nodosa Calciphylaxis Purpura fulminans Rocky Mountain spotted fever Acute bacterial endocarditis Ecthyma gangrenosum
Erythemas	Urticaria/angioedema associated with anaphylaxis Erysipelas Necrotizing fasciitis TSS
Subcutaneous nodules	Pancreatic panniculitis

Alarm Signs and Symptoms	Serious Causes	Benign Causes
Painful skin	SJS/TEN Pemphigus vulgaris Pustular psoriasis Calciphylaxis Necrotizing fasciitis	SSSS Phototoxic reaction
Confluent erythema (bright red skin all over)	DRESS Acute GVHD TEN TSS	Severe morbilliform drug eruption SSSS AGEP Scarlet fever
Erythroderma (redness and scaling involving > 90% of the skin)	Drug eruption (20%) Severe psoriasis (20%) Cutaneous T-cell lymphoma (8%) Atopic dermatitis (9%) Contact dermatitis (6%) Autosensitization dermatitis Seborrheic dermatitis (4%)	(Erythroderma in itself is a potentially serious condition.)

Dusky or grayish-purple skin (signals impending necrosis)	SJS/TEN Various causes of retiform purpura (including calciphylaxis, purpura fulminans, and polyarteritis nodosa) Ecthyma gangrenosum Necrotizing fasciitis	
Widespread blistering or sloughing skin	SJS/TEN Severe pemphigus vulgaris	SSSS
Painful erosions of the mucous membranes	SJS/TEN Pemphigus vulgaris	Erythema multiforme Herpes simplex viral infection with primary gingivostomatitis
Palpable purpura (red or purple, nonblanching papules)	Leukocytoclastic vasculitis with systemic involvement Rocky Mountain spotted fever	Leukocytoclastic vasculitis with involvement limited to the skin
Facial swelling	DRESS Acute cutaneous lupus erythematosus Dermatomyositis (particularly if periocular) Angioedema	AGEP
Swollen mouth or tongue, difficulty swallowing, tingling of the top of the mouth, and/or itching of the palms and soles	Anaphylaxis	
High fever (> 40°C)	DRESS SJS/TEN Purpura fulminans Rocky Mountain spotted fever Acute bacterial endocarditis TSS	Scarlet fever Roseola AGEP
Arthritis	Systemic lupus erythematosus Disseminated gonococcal infection Leukocytoclastic vasculitis with systemic involvement Pancreatic panniculitis	Rubella (unless pregnant) Erythema infectiosum psoriasis Leukocytoclastic vasculitis with involvement limited to the skin Erythema nodosum
Shortness of breath or difficulty breathing	Anaphylaxis	
Hypotension	Purpura fulminans Ecthyma gangrenosum Anaphylaxis TSS	

FOCUSED QUESTIONS

QUESTIONS	THINK ABOUT...
Exanthematous eruptions	
Have you started any new medications in the past 2 weeks?	Morbilliform drug eruption
Have you had a bone marrow or peripheral blood stem-cell transplantation within the past 3 months or recently stopped posttransplantation immunosuppressive medications?	GVHD
Have you recently had a sore throat, high fever, and headache?	Scarlet fever
Did you have cough, runny nose, and red eyes just before developing this rash?	Measles
Has your child just had a high fever for several days, during which he or she otherwise looked well?	Roseola
Did your child have bright red cheeks, followed by lacy redness on the arms that is most noticeable when he or she is hot?	Erythema infectiosum
Are your immunizations up to date?	If not, consider measles or rubella
Papulosquamous dermatoses	
Do you have itchy, purple, flat-topped bumps on your wrists or shins that you rub frequently? *Do you have an itchy rash in areas exposed to the sun?*	Lichen planus
Have you started a new medication within the past year?	Lichenoid drug eruption
Did you develop a single scaly pink spot on your trunk, followed by an eruption of multiple similar but smaller spots?	Pityriasis rosea
Do you have well-defined areas of thick, red skin covered with silvery scale on your elbows, knees, or scalp? *Are the joints of your hands swollen and painful?* *Do you have a family history of psoriasis?*	Psoriasis ± psoriatic arthritis
Have you had redness and greasy scaling of your eyebrows, around your nose, and in/around your ears for many years? *Do you have dandruff?*	Seborrheic dermatitis
Are you particularly sensitive to the sun? *Have you noticed redness of your cheeks and the top of your nose in a "butterfly" shape?*	Systemic lupus erythematosus
Do you have difficulty combing your hair or climbing stairs? *Have you ever been diagnosed with any kind of cancer?*	Dermatomyositis
Do you have pets, particularly a kitten?	Tinea corporis
Do you have a history of a genital ulcer in the past 6 months? *Have you had multiple sexual partners in the past year?* *Have you had unprotected sexual intercourse?*	Secondary syphilis
Eczematous dermatoses	
Is your rash extremely itchy? *Have you had itchy rashes since childhood?* *Do you or does anyone in your family have eczema, hay fever, or asthma?*	Atopic dermatitis

Did you do yard work or other outdoor activities a day or 2 before the rash developed? Is the rash extremely itchy?	Allergic contact dermatitis due to poison ivy
Do you have an itchy rash on your lower legs? *Are your legs often swollen at the end of the day?* *Do you have varicose veins?*	Venous stasis dermatitis
Vesiculobullous disorders	
Did your skin suddenly become painful? *Do you have sores in your mouth?* *Have you started a new medication in the past 2 months?*	SJS/TEN
Did you have itchy pink bumps/spots before blisters developed?	Bullous pemphigoid
Did you have sores in your mouth before blisters developed on your skin?	Pemphigus vulgaris
Do you have fragile skin and blistering, particularly on the backs of your hands, which is worse after exposure to the sun?	Porphyria cutanea tarda
Do you have recurrent lesions of the lip or buttock that are preceded by a day of itching/tingling/burning?	Herpes simplex viral infection
Were your lesions preceded by several days of intense pain, pain with slight touch by clothing, or tingling?	Zoster
Is your child febrile, extremely irritable, and complaining that his skin hurts (especially in the folds)?	SSSS
Pustular dermatoses	
Do you have a fever and painful skin? *Do you have a history of psoriasis?*	Pustular psoriasis
Are you taking prednisone or other systemic corticosteroids?	Steroid acne
Do you use corticosteroid creams or ointments on your face?	Steroid rosacea or perioral dermatitis
Does your face flush easily when you drink hot liquids?	Acne rosacea
Have you been in a hot tub in the past week?	Pseudomonas folliculitis
Is your rash extremely itchy? Do you have human immunodeficiency virus (HIV)?	Eosinophilic folliculitis
Do you have diabetes or perspire excessively? *Has the area involved recently been under occlusion?*	Cutaneous candidiasis
Are you taking antibiotics, prednisone, or other systemic corticosteroids?	Cutaneous candidiasis
Have you had multiple sexual partners in the past year? *Have you had unprotected sexual intercourse?* *Do you have painful, swollen joints?*	Disseminated gonococcal infection
Purpuras	
Do you have nosebleeds, bleeding gums, or excessive bleeding with your menses?	Thrombocytopenic purpura
Do you develop bruises and tearing with minimal trauma to your skin? *Are you taking prednisone or other systemic corticosteroids?*	Actinic purpura

—Continued next page

Continued—

Have you had fevers, pain or swelling of your joints, severe spasms of abdominal pain, or bloody stools or urine?	Leukocytoclastic vasculitis/Henoch-Schönlein purpura
Have you started anticoagulant therapy within the past few months? *Have you recently had a cardiac or other arterial catheterization or thrombolytic therapy?*	Cholesterol emboli
Do you have renal failure? Are you on dialysis?	Calciphylaxis
Did you develop a severe headache, fever, and generalized achiness 2–4 days before your rash started?	Rocky Mountain spotted fever
Have you had a tick bite or spent much time outdoors in the past 2 weeks?	
Have you had high fevers and shaking chills? *Have you used injection drugs?*	Acute bacterial endocarditis
Erythemas and urticaria	
Have you recently been out in the sun?	Phototoxic reaction
Are you taking any medications? (Doxycycline and ciprofloxacin are common culprits.)	
Is your rash itchy? How long does each individual spot last?	Urticaria (if individual lesions last < 24 hours)
Have you started any new medications in the past week?	
Have you had a recent cold or sore throat?	
Have you had a recent cold sore/fever blister (ie, herpes simplex viral infection)? Have you ever had spots like this before?	Erythema multiforme
Did you have a sudden onset of fever, chills, and a headache? *Is the red area spreading and extremely tender?*	Erysipelas
Do you have diabetes? How much do you drink? Do you use intravenous drugs? Have you had cellulitis of this area before?	Cellulitis
Was the area extremely tender previously, but now you can't feel when it is touched?	Necrotizing fasciitis
Has the border of the lesion been expanding outward? *Have you had a tick bite or spent much time outdoors in the past 2 weeks?* *Was the tick on your body for > 24 hours?*	Erythema migrans
Have you recently undergone a surgical procedure, given birth, had a skin infection, or used contraceptive sponges or other vaginally inserted devices? *Do you have a fever, muscle aches, a sore throat, vomiting, or diarrhea?*	TSS
Subcutaneous nodules	
Do you have tender bumps on your shins that develop in crops and leave a bruise-like spot when they resolve? *Have you had fevers and joint pains? (These symptoms may be associated with erythema nodosum, particularly in the setting of sarcoidosis.)* *Have you recently had a sore throat or a diagnosis of strep throat?* *Do you take oral contraceptive pills?* *Do you have inflammatory bowel disease or chronic diarrhea?* *Have you recently traveled to the southwestern United States? (Coccidioidomycosis is endemic in this area.)*	Erythema nodosum

DIAGNOSTIC APPROACH (INCLUDING ALGORITHM)

As noted earlier, the first step is to classify the morphologic pattern of the eruption. This entails careful visual inspection and palpation to identify the primary lesion and its distribution, with particular attention to whether or not the lesions blanch with pressure and whether any lesions contain fluid. Recognition of secondary changes, such as the presence of scale or crust, is also important, and clinicians should always pay particular attention to alarm features. Once clues from the history and physical examination have been used to determine the overall pattern of the eruption, the focused questions help highlight distinguishing features of the potential diagnoses within each category. See Figure 21–1 for the diagnostic approach algorithm for inflammatory dermatoses.

CAVEATS

- An early eruption of erythema multiforme that does not yet have obviously targetoid lesions may resemble a morbilliform drug eruption.
- Morbilliform drug eruptions often become purpuric on the lower extremities.
- Tinea corporis or faciei that has been treated with topical corticosteroids may have an atypical appearance and lack scale (tinea incognito).
- Asymmetric linear streaks or bizarre shapes often signal an external insult to the skin as seen in allergic and irritant contact dermatitis.
- Patients with venous stasis dermatitis, particularly those with venous ulcers that have been treated with topical antibiotics, often have a superimposed allergic contact dermatitis and may develop an autosensitization (id) eruption.
- Determination of whether bullae are tense or flaccid and whether the Nikolsky sign is positive can help classify vesiculobullous eruptions (see Figure 21–1).
- Zoster involving the tip of the nose should raise concern about possible ocular involvement.
- Generalized pustular psoriasis may be precipitated by rapid withdrawal of systemic corticosteroids.
- Not all purpura is due to the same process that caused the lesion itself; secondary purpura often results from venous stasis (particularly on the lower legs), trauma (eg, due to scratching pruritic primary lesions), or thrombocytopenia (usually platelet count < 50,000/μL).
- Early lesions of leukocytoclastic vasculitis and Rocky Mountain spotted fever are often partially blanching.
- Tracing the edge of a lesion and noting migration/resolution within a few hours can help confirm the diagnosis of urticaria.
- When evaluating patients with a history of urticaria, it is important to determine whether they develop wheals upon stroking the skin (dermographism, a form of pressure-induced urticaria that could represent the cause of the eruption).
- Acute lipodermatosclerosis may mimic cellulitis; involvement of both legs and localization to the area above the medial malleolus are suggestive of the former diagnosis.

PROGNOSIS

It is not possible to categorically apply a prognosis to such a heterogeneous group of skin diseases. Although the majority of dermatologic disorders have an overall "benign" prognosis, it is important to remember that diseases such as pemphigus vulgaris, TEN, acute GVHD, and Rocky Mountain spotted fever may have a high mortality rate if not identified and treated properly. In addition, the psychological impact of skin disease is often profound.

CASE SCENARIO | Resolution

A 23-year-old young woman comes to your office with a rash. The rash started as red, round, pruritic bumps on the abdomen approximately 1 week before presentation and has spread. More recently, 1.5-cm round scaly patches and plaques have developed on the trunk and extremities.

ADDITIONAL HISTORY

Your patient is a graduate student and has recently begun working out with a personal trainer at the gym. She is sexually active with 1 partner. She does not routinely use condoms but has no history of genital ulceration. She recalls no antecedent sore throat or illness. She has no sun sensitivity or joint pain. She is otherwise healthy and takes no medications. She has no family history of psoriasis or lupus. On further physical examination, you note no unusual findings of the oral mucosa, no involvement of the scalp or hair, no nail changes, and no lymphadenopathy.

Question: What is the most likely diagnosis?

A. Tinea corporis
B. Psoriasis
C. Pityriasis rosea
D. Subacute cutaneous lupus erythematosus
E. Secondary syphilis

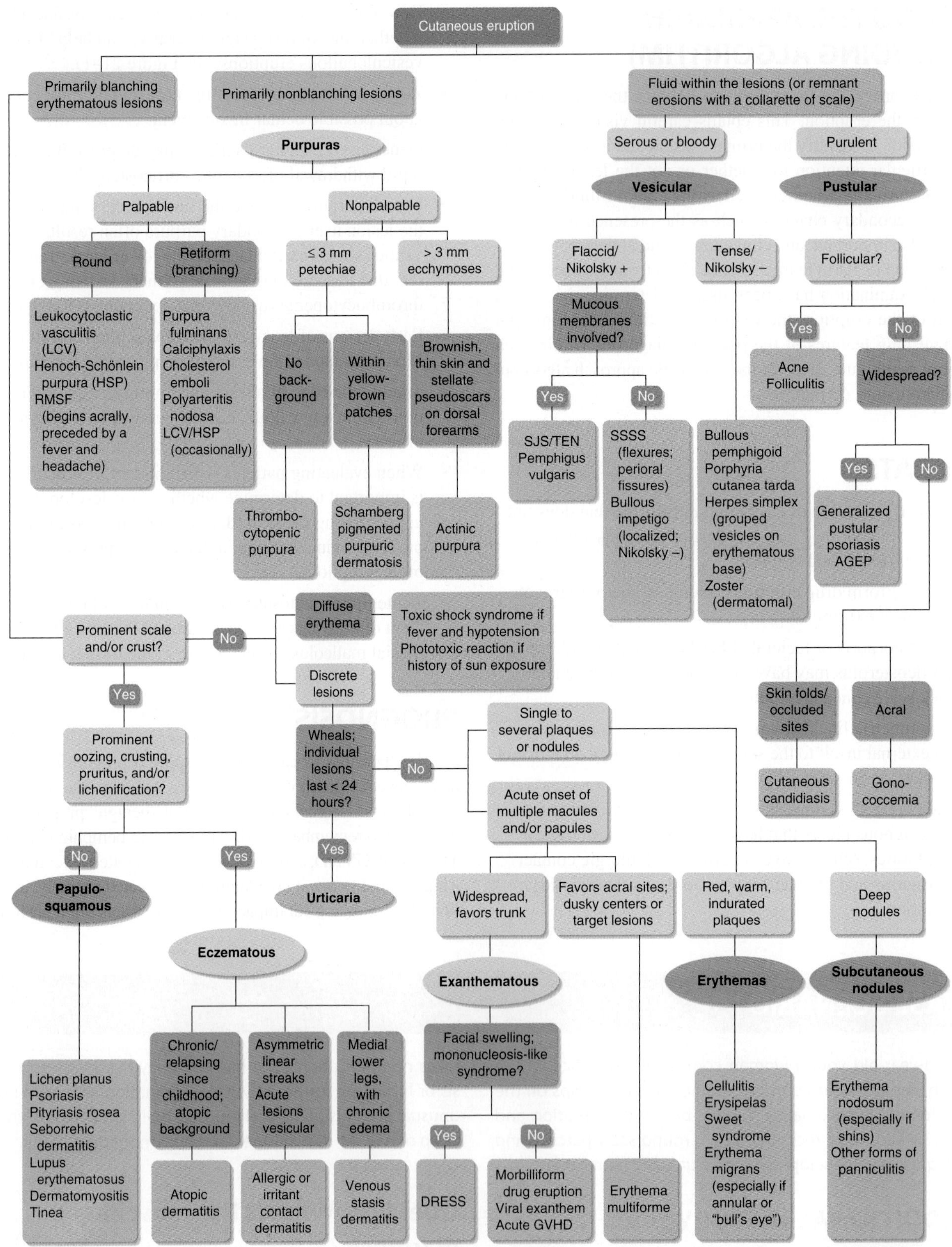

FIGURE 21–1 Diagnostic approach: Inflammatory dermatoses ("rashes"). AGEP, acute generalized exanthematous pustulosis; DRESS, drug rash with eosinophilia and systemic symptoms; GVHD, graft-versus-host disease; RMSF, Rocky Mountain spotted fever; SJS, Stevens-Johnson syndrome; SSSS, staphylococcal scalded skin syndrome; TEN, toxic epidermal necrolysis.

Test Your Knowledge

1. A 10-year-old boy presents with very itchy blisters on his arms and legs. In addition, he woke up this morning with swelling and pruritus around his left eye. He is afebrile. On examination, he has several vesicles in a linear array on his arms and legs as well as redness and swelling of his left upper and lower eyelid.
   What is your diagnosis?
   A. Herpes zoster
   B. Herpes simplex
   C. Drug eruption
   D. Allergic contact dermatitis

2. Your patient presents complaining of chronic scaling and erythema around his nose and eyebrows. Upon further questioning, he also reports dandruff of the scalp and a family history of atopy.
   What is the most likely diagnosis for his facial scaling?
   A. Seborrheic dermatitis
   B. Tinea faciei
   C. Psoriasis
   D. Atopic dermatitis

3. A 16-year-old girl presents to you with painful blisters on her skin and oral and genital mucosa. Her eyes feel very dry and itchy. She has a temperature of 99°F and complains of malaise. One week ago, you prescribed trimethoprim-sulfamethoxazole for a urinary tract infection. On examination, she has large flaccid bullae, and her skin is painful to touch.
   What is your diagnosis?
   A. Bullous pemphigoid
   B. Scarlet fever
   C. Stevens-Johnson syndrome/toxic epidermal necrolysis
   D. Herpes simplex

References

1. Feldman SR, Fleischer AB Jr, Wolford PM, White R, Byington R. Increasing utilization of dermatologists by managed care: an analysis of the National Ambulatory Medical Care Survey, 1990-1994. *J Am Acad Dermatol*. 1997;37:784–788.
2. Kimball AB, Resneck JS. The US dermatology workforce: a specialty remains in shortage. *J Am Acad Dermatol*. 2008; 59:741–745.
3. Maguiness S, Shearles GE, From L, Swiggum S. The Canadian Dermatology Workforce Survey: implications for the future of Canadian dermatology—who will be your skin expert? *J Cutan Med Surg*. 2004;8:141–147.
4. Nigen S, Knowles SR, Shear NH. Drug eruptions: approaching the diagnosis of drug-induced skin diseases. *J Drugs Dermatol*. 2003;2:278–299.

Suggested Reading

Bolognia J, Jorizzo J, Rapini R, eds. *Dermatology*. New York, NY: Mosby, Inc., 2007.

Callen J, Jorizzo J, Bolognia J, Piette W. *Dermatologic Signs of Internal Disease*. Philadelphia, PA: W. B. Saunders Co., 2009.

Wolff K, Goldsmith LA, Paller AS, et al., eds. *Fitzpatrick's Dermatology in General Medicine*. New York, NY: McGraw-Hill, 2007.

Chapter 22

Pruritus

Emmy M. Graber, MD

CASE SCENARIO

A 79-year-old woman comes to your office to discuss her "itching." Although her skin is extremely pruritic all over, she has never noticed a rash. The itching does not wake her from sleep, although it is worse in the evening. She has tried "scrubbing her skin" with antibacterial soap and taking hot showers to get "very clean," but this has not helped the itching.

- **What additional questions would you ask to learn more about her pruritus?**
- **How do you classify pruritus without a rash?**
- **Can you make a definite diagnosis through an open-ended history followed by focused questions?**
- **What laboratory tests may be needed to rule out serious etiologies of pruritus?**

INTRODUCTION

Pruritus, or itching, is the most common dermatologic complaint. Pruritus can occur in the presence or absence of cutaneous findings. For the purpose of this chapter, the focus will be on evaluating pruritus in the absence of any other cutaneous manifestations. Patients with pruritus should be evaluated carefully because it may be the presenting symptom of a serious underlying problem. The prevalence of an underlying systemic illness causing the pruritus ranges from 10% to 50%. Meticulous history taking will determine the extent of work-up that is warranted. Asking appropriate questions will reduce the amount of testing required to discover the etiology of the pruritus.

KEY TERMS

Pruritus with cutaneous findings	Itching that occurs in areas of skin changes. These include urticaria (hives), papules, patches, pustules, plaques, or nodules.
Pruritus without cutaneous findings	Itching that occurs in otherwise normal-appearing skin.
Localized pruritus	Itching that occurs in a confined location on the skin.
Generalized pruritus	Itching that occurs on all skin surfaces and is not localized to a particular body part.
Incidence	The number of new diagnoses in a specific population during a specific period of time.
Prevalence	The total number of cases of a disease in a given population at a specific time.

ETIOLOGY

Pruritus without cutaneous findings is usually generalized. Localized pruritus may be due to postherpetic neuralgia, brachioradial pruritus, notalgia paresthetica, or venous insufficiency. Brachioradial pruritus is an intense itching of the forearms suspected to be due to nerve damage. Notalgia paresthetica is a neuropathic disorder of the infrascapular back area that often presents with pruritus. When pruritus is localized in the perianal or genital areas, it can be due to diabetes and is associated with poor diabetic control. For example, vulvar pruritus occurs in 18.4% of diabetic women.[1]

Generalized itch may be due to an underlying internal disease, psychiatric illness, xerosis (dry skin), or senescence. Systemic diseases associated with generalized pruritus include malignancies, hematologic disease, hepatobiliary disorders, infections, endocrine disturbances, and renal disease.

Retrospective studies estimate the prevalence of underlying malignancy in patients with pruritus to range from 2% to 11%.[2,3] Etiologies include direct tumor invasion, distant metastases, paraneoplastic phenomenon, nerve compression, cholestasis, and side effects of treatment. Toxic metabolites released by cancer cells may also lead to itch. It is believed (although not proven in studies) that paraneoplastic pruritus goes away or decreases after tumor resection. Pruritus recurrence may signify reactivation or progression of a tumor. Up to 30% of patients with Hodgkin's lymphoma and up to 10% of patients with non-Hodgkin's lymphoma experience pruritus.[4] Up to 5% of patients with leukemia suffer from pruritus.[5]

Forty-eight percent of patients with polycythemia vera have pruritus; its presence correlates with a decreased blood cell mean corpuscular volume and a higher leukocyte count.[6] Iron deficiency anemia may also be a cause of pruritus (13.6% of males and 7.4% of females).[7]

Hepatobiliary disorders often coexist with pruritus. Eighty percent to 100% of patients with cholestasis experience pruritus.[8] In 25% to 70% of patients with primary biliary cirrhosis, pruritus is a presenting symptom.[9] Of those with hepatitis C, 15% will have pruritus.[10]

Other infections that can cause pruritus include parasitic infections such as hookworm, onchocerciasis, ascariasis, and trichinosis. Most commonly, these infections are associated with cutaneous findings. Patients with human immunodeficiency virus (HIV) infection often have generalized pruritus (13% of newly diagnosed patients); its presence is a marker of disease progression.[11,12]

Severe generalized pruritus can be a presenting symptom of hyperthyroidism, especially when thyrotoxicosis is present. Hypothyroid patients may also experience pruritus, although it is more often secondary to the hypothyroid-induced xerosis (dry skin). Premenstrual pruritus rarely can be due to recurrent cholestasis from oral contraceptive pills. Although rare, generalized pruritus related to menses has been reported. Perimenopausal patients may also experience generalized pruritus that is relieved by hormone replacement therapy. Pruritus may be a presenting symptom of diabetes (although rarely the sole symptom); it occurs in 2.7% of the diabetic population.[13]

Due to advances in hemodialysis, the frequency of uremic pruritus has decreased in recent years, although it is still quite common. Worldwide, the prevalence of uremic pruritus varies from 10% to 77% of patients on hemodialysis, depending on regional population differences.[14]

Pruritus may also be related to underlying psychiatric problems. For example, in a study of 109 inpatients with generalized pruritus, 70% had a psychiatric comorbidity.[15] In another report, 17.5% of patients with depression had generalized pruritus.[16]

Drug-induced reactions usually cause a cutaneous eruption. However, in 5% of cases, generalized pruritus occurs without cutaneous findings.[17] Examples include morphine, hydroxyethyl starch (12%–42% of patients), and chloroquine (65%–75% of patients). Pruritus due to chloroquine occurs within 24 to 36 hours after drug ingestion.[18,19]

Pruritus without cutaneous findings can be due to mild xerosis, but when the dryness is severe, the skin appears as a dried riverbed, known as eczema craquelé. Aging has been also blamed for generalized pruritus. It has been shown that 19.5% of patients over the age of 85 have generalized pruritus without cutaneous findings.[20]

Differential Diagnosis[a]

	Prevalence Among Patients Presenting With Pruritus (Without Cutaneous Findings)	Prevalence of Pruritus Among Patients With the Selected Diagnosis
Localized pruritus		
Postherpetic neuralgia		58%[21]
Brachioradial pruritus		
Notalgia paresthetica		
Venous insufficiency		66%[22]
Perianal pruritus		
Vulvar pruritus		
Generalized pruritus		
Malignancy	2%–11%[2,3]	
Hodgkin's lymphoma		30%[4]

Non-Hodgkin's lymphoma		10%[4]
Leukemia		5%[5]
Polycythemia vera		48%[6]
Iron deficiency anemia (males)		13.6%[7]
Iron deficiency anemia (females)		7.4%[7]
Cholestasis		80%–100%[8]
Primary biliary cirrhosis		25%–70%[9]
Hepatitis C		15%[10]
Parasitic infections		
HIV		13%[12]
Hyperthyroidism		
Hypothyroidism		
Premenstrual		
Menstrual		
Perimenopausal		
Diabetes		2.7%[13]
Renal failure		10%–77%[14]
Psychiatric comorbidity	70%[15]	
Depression		17.5%[16]
Drug reaction		
Xerosis		
Senescence (aging)		

[a]Empty cells indicate that the prevalence is unknown.

GETTING STARTED WITH THE HISTORY

- Allow the patient to describe the pruritus in his or her own words before asking more directed and focused questions.
- The cause of pruritus is made by taking a thorough history and by running the appropriate laboratory tests.
- A carefully focused history will reduce the number of required laboratory tests.

Questions	Remember
Tell me more about your pruritus. *When did the pruritus first start?* *Is the pruritus localized to a single area of the body, or is it widespread?*	Listen to the story. Don't rush the interview by interrupting and focusing the history too soon. Reassure the patient when appropriate.

INTERVIEW FRAMEWORK

- Inquire about pruritus characteristics:
  - Location
  - Onset
  - Frequency
- Inquire about other systemic problems.

IDENTIFYING ALARM SYMPTOMS

- Recent unexplained weight loss and fatigue prompt concern for an underlying malignancy or infection.
- A history of high-risk behaviors such as unprotected intercourse or intravenous drug use may raise suspicion for HIV or hepatitis C.

- Increased urination and increased fluid intake may signify underlying diabetes mellitus.
- A history of chronic kidney disease or end-stage renal disease requiring dialysis treatment may point to uremic pruritus.
- Cold or heat intolerance should prompt further questioning regarding hypothyroidism or hyperthyroidism, respectively.
- Mood changes, suicidal thoughts, and obsessive patterns may point to a psychiatric cause.

Serious Diagnoses

Pruritus may be the first clinical presentation of an underlying systemic disease. The estimated 1-year incidence rates in the US general population for selected serious causes are as follows: malignancy, 1.9%[23]; HIV, 0.018%[24]; hepatitis C, 0.06%[25]; diabetes mellitus over the age of 20 years, 0.53%[26]; and renal failure, 0.04%.[27]

FOCUSED QUESTIONS

After listening to the pruritus history in the patient's own words and considering possible alarm symptoms, ask the following questions to narrow the differential diagnosis.

QUESTIONS	THINK ABOUT...
Have you had any recent unexplained weight loss and/or fatigue?	Malignancy
Have you had a persistent cough, shortness of breath, or chest pain?	Pulmonary malignancy
Have you had a change in your bowel movement frequency or the quality of your stools (eg, blood in the stools)?	Gastrointestinal malignancy
Have you had easy bruising, fever, or lymphadenopathy?	Hematologic malignancy
Have you had pelvic pain, heavy periods, or painful periods?	Gynecologic malignancy
Is your pruritus worse when you get out of a warm shower?	Polycythemia vera
Do you experience light-headedness?	Iron deficiency anemia
Is your diet low in iron?	Iron deficiency anemia
Do you have right upper quadrant stomach pain?	Cholestasis or primary biliary cirrhosis
Have you ever noticed a yellow color to your sclera?	Cholestasis, primary biliary cirrhosis, or hepatitis C
Have you noticed dark urine or clay-colored stools?	Cholestasis
Have you engaged in intravenous drug use or unprotected sexual intercourse?	Hepatitis C or HIV
Have you noticed palpitations, nervousness, and/or heat intolerance?	Hyperthyroidism
Have you noticed weight gain, fatigue, dry skin and hair, depression, and/or cold intolerance?	Hypothyroidism
Is your itching worse just before you menstruate, and are you on an oral contraceptive pill?	Premenstrual pruritus
Does your itching only occur while you are menstruating?	Menstrual pruritus
Have your menstrual periods ceased or become irregular, or are you having hot flashes?	Perimenopausal pruritus
Have you had increased thirst and urination?	Diabetes mellitus

Have you had a decreased urine production?	Renal failure
Have you experienced sadness, suicidal thoughts, manic behavior, obsessive thoughts or activities, or anxiety?	Psychiatric illness
Have you started any new medications such as hydroxyethyl starch, morphine, or chloroquine?	Drug reaction
What kind of soap do you wash with? (Concern with harsh alkaline soaps rather than syndet cleansers with a more neutral pH) Do you omit a body moisturizer from you daily routine? Are you often in a dry, cold climate?	Xerosis

DIAGNOSTIC APPROACH (INCLUDING ALGORITHM)

The first step is to distinguish between localized and generalized pruritus. If the pruritus is generalized (as is most often the case), first one must rule out xerosis as a cause of pruritus. If there are no risk factors for or evidence of xerosis, then the clinician must begin to question about possible underlying etiologies. Figures 22–1 and 22–2 show the diagnostic approaches to generalized and localized pruritus, respectively.

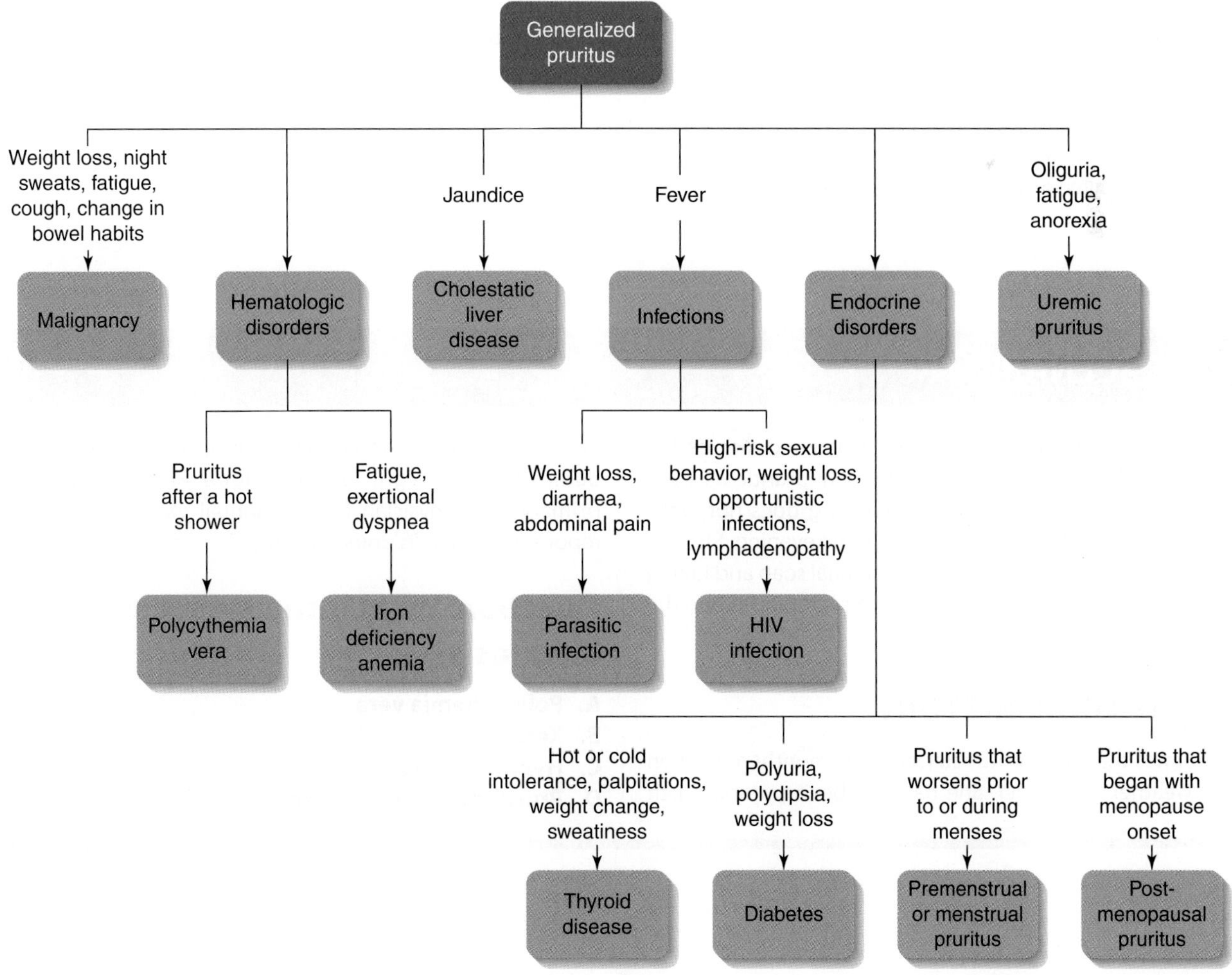

FIGURE 22–1 Diagnostic algorithm: Generalized pruritus.

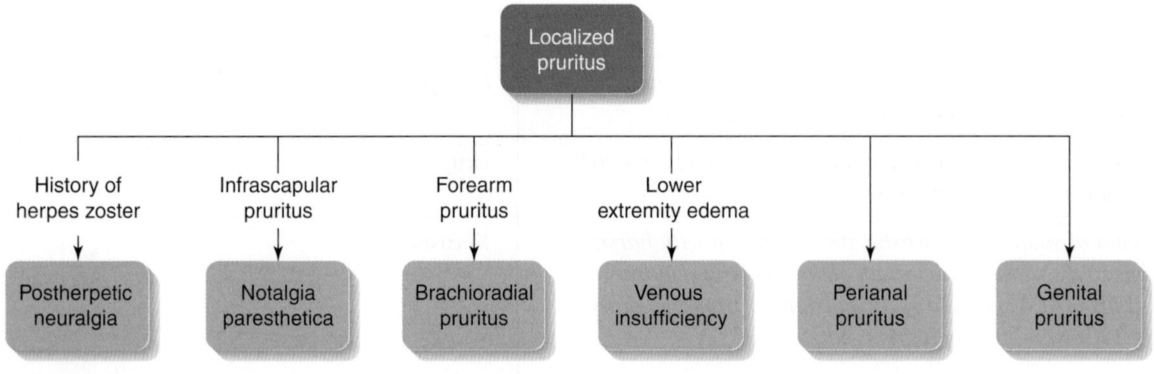

FIGURE 22–2 Diagnostic algorithm: Localized pruritus.

CAVEATS

- First distinguish between localized and generalized pruritus in order to correctly move through the diagnostic algorithm.
- If the patient has generalized pruritus, xerosis must be ruled out as an etiology before considering underlying causes.
- If other symptoms suggest systemic disease, additional physical examination and potentially laboratory tests will establish the diagnosis.
- Do not perform an overabundance of laboratory tests unless indicated after asking directed questions.

PROGNOSIS

Pruritus due to xerosis can have an excellent prognosis once the skin is treated properly. Pruritus due to internal causes may be more difficult to treat. Improving the pruritus often requires treating the underlying cause. Topical creams and anti-itch medications may make the pruritus more tolerable, but its ultimate resolution depends on the treatment of the root etiology.

CASE SCENARIO | Resolution

A 79-year-old woman comes to your office to discuss her "itching." Although her skin is extremely pruritic all over, she has never noticed a rash. The itching does not wake her from sleep, although it is worse in the evening. She has tried "scrubbing her skin" with antibacterial soap and taking hot showers to get "very clean," but this has not helped the itching.

ADDITIONAL HISTORY

She states that her pruritus started a few months ago when the weather got cooler. She has also been putting witch hazel on her skin in an attempt to reduce the itching. She denies recent weight loss or fatigue. She just saw her primary care physician for her annual examination who reported that she "is doing just fine."

Question: What is the most likely diagnosis?

A. Polycythemia vera
B. Xerosis
C. Hypothyroidism
D. Pruritus due to senescence

Test Your Knowledge

1. You see a 69-year-old man with a history of congestive heart failure. He has localized pruritus on his lower legs that is most likely due to which of the following?
   A. Diabetes mellitus
   B. Renal failure
   C. Drug reaction
   D. Venous insufficiency
   E. Postherpetic neuralgia

2. A 32-year-old patient comes to see you complaining of intense pruritus after taking a warm shower. She denies any systemic complaints but states that her hands are also red.
   She most likely has which of the following?
   A. Polycythemia vera
   B. Hepatitis C
   C. Xerosis
   D. HIV
   E. Hodgkin's lymphoma

3. A 46-year-old woman comes to see you complaining of generalized pruritus. Upon questioning, she is sometimes light-headed and follows a strict vegan diet.
   Her pruritus is most likely due to:
   A. Perimenopause
   B. Iron deficiency anemia
   C. Cholestasis
   D. Polycythemia vera
   E. Renal failure

References

1. Weisshaar E, Dalgard F, Weisshaar E, Dalgard F. Epidemiology of itch: adding to the burden of skin morbidity. *Acta Derm Venereol.* 2009;89:339–350.
2. Sommer F, Hensen P, Bockenholt B, Metze D, Luger TA, Stander S. Underlying diseases and co-factors in patients with severe chronic pruritus: a 3-year retrospective study. *Acta Derm Venereol.* 2007;87:510–516.
3. Kantor GR, Lookingbill DP. Generalized pruritus and systemic disease. *J Am Acad Dermatol.* 1983;9:375–382.
4. Stefanato CM, Reyes-Mugica M. Masked Hodgkin's disease: the pruriginous disguise. *Pediatr Hematol Oncol.* 1996;13:293–294.
5. Robak E, Robak T. Skin lesions in chronic lymphocytic leukemia. *Leuk Lymphoma.* 2007;48:855–865.
6. Diehn F, Tefferi A. Pruritus in polycythemia vera: prevalence, laboratory correlates and management. *Br J Haematol.* 2001;115:619–621.
7. Takkunen H. Iron deficiency anemia in the Finnish adult population. *Scand J Haematol Suppl.* 1976;25:1–91.
8. Bergasa NV, Mehlman JK, Jones EA. Pruritus and fatigue in primary biliary cirrhosis. *Baillieres Best Pract Res Clin Gastroenterol.* 2000;14:643–655.
9. Talwalkar JA, Souto E, Jorgensen RA, Lindor KD. Natural history of pruritus in primary biliary cirrhosis. *Gastroenterol Hepatol.* 2003;1:297–302.
10. Cacoub P, Poynard T, Ghillani P, Charlotte F, Olivi M, Piette JC. Extrahepatic manifestations of chronic hepatitis C. *Arthritis Rheum.* 1999;42:2204–2212.
11. Akolo C, Ukoli CO, Ladep GN, Idoko JA. The clinical features of HIV/AIDS at presentation at the Jos University Teaching Hospital. *Niger J Med.* 2008;17:83–87.
12. Dlova NC, Mosam A. Inflammatory noninfectious dermastoses of HIV. *Dermatol Clin.* 2006;24:439–448.
13. Neilly JB, Martin A, Simpson N, MacCuish AC. Pruritus in diabetes mellitus: investigation of prevalence and correlation with diabetes control. *Diabetes Care.* 1986;9:273–275.
14. Murtagh FE, Addington-Hall J, Higgins IJ. The prevalence of symptoms in end-stage renal disease: a systematic review. *Adv Chronic Kidney Dis.* 2007;14:82–99.
15. Schneider G, Driesch G, Heuft G, Evers S, Luger TA, Stander S. Psychosomatic cofactors and psychiatric co-morbidity in patients with chronic itch. *Clin Exp Dermatol.* 2006;154:762–767.
16. Pacan P, Grezesiak M, Reich A, Szepietowski JC. Is pruritus in depression a rare phenomenon? *Acta Derm Venereol.* 2009;89:109–110.
17. Bigby M, Jick S, Jick H, Arndt K. Drug-induced cutaneous reactions. A report from the Boston Collaborative Drug Surveillance Program on 15,438 consecutive inpatients, 1975 to 1982. *JAMA.* 1986;256:3358–3363.
18. Bork K. Pruritus precipitated by hydroxyethyl starch: a review. *Br J Dermatol.* 2005;152:3–12.
19. Olayemi O, Fehintola FA, Osungbade A, Aimakhu CO, Udoh ES, Adeniji AR. Pattern of chloroquine-induced pruritus in antenatal patients at the University College Hospital, Ibadan. *J Obstet Gynaecol.* 2003;23:490–495.
20. Yalcin B, Tamer E, Toy GG, Oztas P, Hayran M, Alli N. The presence of skin diseases in the elderly: analysis of 4099 geriatric patients. *Int J Dermatol.* 2006;45:672–676.
21. Oaklander A, Bowsher D, Galer B, Haanpaa M, Jensen M. Herpes zoster itch: preliminary epidemiologic data. *J Pain.* 2003;4:338–343.

22. Duque MI, Yosipovitch G, Chan YH, Smith R, Levy PI. Itch, pain, and burning sensation are common symptoms in mild to moderate chronic venous insufficiency with an impact on quality of life. *J Am Acad Dermatol.* 2005;53:504–508.
23. American Cancer Society. Cancer prevalence: how many people have cancer? Available at: http://www.cancer.org/docroot/cri/content/cri_2_6x_cancer_prevalence_how_many_people_have_cancer.asp. Accessed October 15, 2011.
24. Hall HI, Ruiguang S, Rhodes P. Estimation of HIV incidence in the United States. *JAMA.* 2008;300:520–529.
25. Everhart JE. *Digestive Diseases in the United States: Epidemiology and Impact.* Darby, PA: Diane Publishing Co., 1994.
26. National Institutes of Health. National Diabetes Information Clearinghouse. Available at: http://diabetes.niddk.nih.gov/. Accessed October 15, 2011.
27. United States Renal Data System. Available at: http://www.usrds.org/qtr/default.html. Accessed October 15, 2011.

Suggested Reading

Weisshaar E, Dalgard F, Weisshaar E, Dalgard F. Epidemiology of itch: adding to the burden of skin morbidity. *Acta Derm Venereol.* 2009;89:339–350.

Zirwas MJ, Seraly MP. Pruritus of unknown origin: a retrospective study. *J Am Acad Dermatol.* 2001;45:892–896.

Chapter 23

Hair Loss

Erika E. Reid, MD, and Peter A. Lio, MD

CASE SCENARIO

A 24-year-old woman comes to your office to discuss hair loss that began several months ago. She initially noticed a small patch of hair missing near the top of her scalp, but then found several other round patches of loss. These areas are not painful or itchy. She has noticed little "dents" in her nails recently. She is very concerned that she will lose all of her hair.

- **What additional questions would you ask to learn more about her hair loss?**
- **How do you classify hair loss?**
- **How can you make a definitive diagnosis through an open-ended history followed by focused questions?**
- **How does the patient history distinguish between nonpermanent (nonscarring) hair loss and permanent (scarring) hair loss that requires timely intervention?**

INTRODUCTION

Hair loss affects nearly 50% of people throughout their lives and often has a profound psychosocial impact.[1,2] Hair loss may be due to primary disease of the hair follicle, systemic disease, hormonal changes, or vitamin deficiencies. A careful history may provide the diagnosis and will often guide a directed physical examination and laboratory testing. The history should be guided by a consideration of the patient's demographics and the characteristics of the hair loss.

KEY TERMS

Nonscarring (noncicatricial) alopecia	Potentially reversible causes of hair loss.
Scarring (cicatricial) alopecia	Irreversible hair loss associated with destruction of the stem-cell reservoir in the middle of the follicle.
Alopecia areata (AA)	An inflammatory process around the follicle that causes isolated or recurrent patches of hair loss.
Telogen effluvium (TE)	The most common type of diffuse hair loss, often triggered by a physically or emotionally stressful event 3–6 months before diffuse shedding begins.
Androgenetic alopecia (AGA)	The pattern of hair thinning and loss related to hormones, aging, and genetics.
Trichotillomania	A condition characterized by the compulsion to pull out one's hair.
Central centrifugal cicatricial alopecia (CCCA)	A scarring alopecia, most common in African American females, that begins at the vertex of the scalp and progresses outward.

ETIOLOGY

There are 2 principal types of hair loss: those associated with hair follicle destruction and those where the follicle is preserved. Alopecia with destruction of the hair follicle is referred to as "scarring" alopecia, whereas alopecia with preserved follicles is "nonscarring." This is an important distinction because scarring and nonscarring alopecias have different differential diagnoses and prognoses. Scarring alopecias necessitate early intervention in order to minimize the amount of permanent hair loss. Nonscarring alopecias are more common than scarring ones, but the prevalence of specific types of alopecias varies with age.

In children, tinea capitis and alopecia areata are the most common causes, followed by telogen effluvium and trichotillomania. Tinea capitis occurs in 4% to 13% of the general population of children; it is very rarely observed in adults.[3–5] Alopecia areata may develop in both children and adults and has a lifetime prevalence of 1% to 2%.[2,6] Trichotillomania is a relatively rare condition, with a lifetime prevalence of about 0.6%.[7] Androgenetic alopecia is very common among adults, and although reported prevalence rates vary widely, most studies estimate that over 50% of Caucasian males over 30 years old and 30% of women over 70 are affected.[6,8] The prevalence of TE and scarring alopecias in individuals of any age has not been well studied.

Differential Diagnosis

	Prevalence Among People in the General Population
Nonscarring alopecias	
Alopecia areata	1%–2%[2,6]
Androgenetic alopecia	50%[9]
Telogen effluvium	
Tinea capitis	4%–13% in children; rare in adults[3–5]
Trichotillomania	0.6% (lifetime prevalence)[7]
Systemic illness (Table 23–1)	
Drug-related hair loss	
Scarring alopecias	
Inflammatory alopecias • Discoid lupus • Lichen planopilaris • Autoimmune blistering disorders	
Traction alopecia	
Central centrifugal cicatricial alopecia (CCCA)	
Severe fungal or bacterial infection	
Injury or burn	

GETTING STARTED WITH THE HISTORY

- Remember that hair loss is often very traumatic and upsetting for patients; taking concerns seriously is imperative to establishing good rapport.
- Consider the patient's age and sex because these demographic features will focus the differential diagnosis.
- Although the final diagnosis of the cause for hair loss requires a careful physical examination and often laboratory testing or skin biopsy, the history will narrow the differential diagnosis and guide further evaluation.

INTERVIEW FRAMEWORK

- The first goal is to determine whether the alopecia is scarring or nonscarring.
- Ask the patient to precisely describe the hair loss.
- Inquire about hair loss characteristics including:
  - Duration
  - Onset
  - Pattern
  - Whole hairs falling out or hair breakage

Table 23–1. Systemic illnesses associated with alopecia.

Iron deficiency anemia
Vitamin B_{12} deficiency
Anorexia nervosa
Menopause
Postpartum state
Human immunodeficiency virus infection
Hyper-/hypothyroidism
Secondary syphilis
Systemic lupus erythematosus
Systemic amyloidosis
Inflammatory bowel disease
Lymphoproliferative disorders
Hepatic failure
Renal failure

- Precipitating factors
- Hair care routine
- Associated symptoms

IDENTIFYING ALARM SYMPTOMS

- The following symptoms raise concern for scarring alopecia. Scarring alopecia may be irreversible and therefore require immediate intervention to prevent progression.
  - Itching
  - Pain
  - Crusting
  - Bleeding
  - Pustulation
  - Scaling of the scalp

FOCUSED QUESTIONS

QUESTIONS	THINK ABOUT...
What is the duration of the hair loss?	If < 1 year and diffuse, TE is likely[10]; if > 1 year and diffuse, AGA is likely
Onset	
Was the onset sudden or gradual?	
• *Sudden*	TE, AA
• *Gradual*	AGA
Pattern	
What is the pattern of the hair loss?	
• *Diffuse*	TE, AGA
• *Focal*	AA, tinea capitis, CCCA
• *Frontal recession and temporal thinning*	AGA in men
• *Midline part widening and central thinning*	AGA in women
Is your hair coming out by the roots, or is it breaking? *Coming out by the roots:*	
• *Increased shedding (hair on pillow, in shower, or coming out in clumps)*	TE
• *Progressive thinning*	AGA
Breaking:	
• *Frequent brushing? Perm/dyes?*	Traction alopecia, CCCA-induced
• *Patchy loss?*	Tinea capitis

—Continued next page

Continued—

Precipitating factors	
What medications do you take?	Drug-induced (Table 23–2)
Have your recently been pregnant?	TE
Are you postmenopausal?	AGA
Have you ever been diagnosed with thyroid problems, autoimmune disease, or anemia?	Systemic illness, AA
Is there a family history of hair loss?	AGA
Do you routinely use straightening or relaxing hair products?	Traction alopecia, CCCA
Any diets, weight loss, or vitamin supplements added in the last 6 months?	TE, vitamin deficiencies
Have you had any illnesses or stressors in the last 6 months?	TE
Do you have any anxiety disorders or obsessive-compulsive tendencies?	Trichotillomania
Do you have a large family size, crowded living conditions, or low socioeconomic status?	Risk factors for tinea capitis[11]
Symptoms	
Have you noticed scaling or pustules?	Scarring alopecia, tinea capitis
Are your eyebrows or eyelash involved?	AA, trichotillomania
Are the spots itchy?	Inflammatory alopecias, tinea capitis, AA (less commonly)
Have you noticed nail pitting?	AA

A careful history of medication use serves 2 purposes. First, it can be used to determine if the patient is taking a medication that may cause alopecia. Second, each medication implies a particular chronic medical condition, some of which may be associated with hair loss. Table 23–2 lists medications that commonly cause alopecia.

Table **23–2. Drugs that commonly cause alopecia.**

Antithyroid agents
Anticonvulsants
Hormonal therapy
β-Blockers
Angiotensin-converting enzyme inhibitors
Lithium

DIAGNOSTIC APPROACH (INCLUDING ALGORITHM)

First, consider the age of the patient. In children, the most common forms of hair loss are tinea capitis and alopecia areata.[10] Next, consider the duration and pattern of the hair loss. If the duration is less than 1 year, consider new drugs or hair care products or new-onset systemic illness. Hair loss of more than 1 year in duration is most likely androgenic alopecia.[10]

The next step is to determine the pattern of hair loss. Diffuse hair loss commonly results from telogen effluvium, whereas focal, patchy loss is typical of alopecia areata and tinea capitis. Androgenic alopecia has a different distribution in men and women: frontal hairline recession and temporal thinning in men versus widening of the midline part and central thinning in women. Hair breakage, as opposed to hair coming out by the roots, suggests an external process such as traction alopecia or trichotillomania. Alarm features that suggest

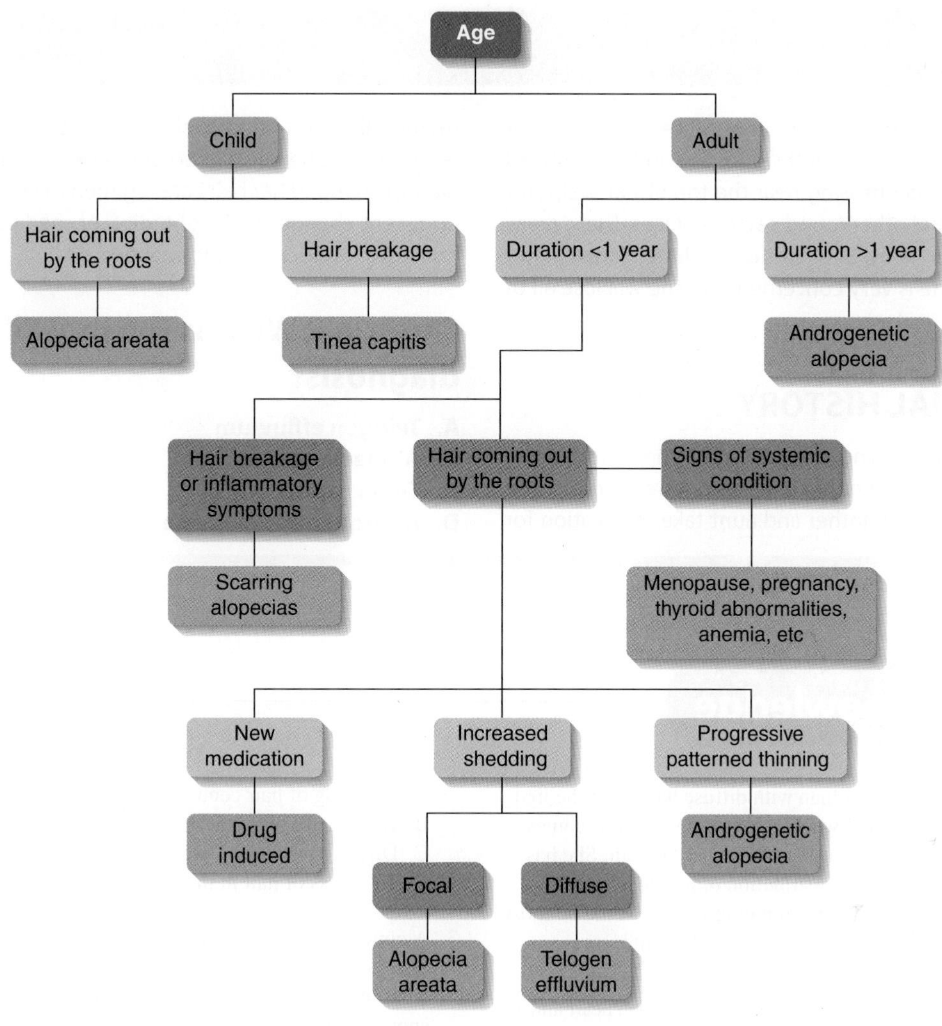

FIGURE 23–1 Diagnostic algorithm: Hair loss.

scarring alopecia include a painful or pruritic scalp, sores, redness, scaling, and bleeding. Scarring alopecia is more serious than nonscarring alopecia and necessitates physical examination, laboratory testing, and scalp biopsy for definitive diagnosis. Figure 23–1 shows the diagnostic algorithm for hair loss.

CAVEATS

- Remember first to consider the age of the patient and the duration of hair loss before asking specific questions.
- Although the duration of hair loss is useful for distinguishing between types of alopecia, patients with any of the classically long-term causes of alopecia may present for evaluation early in the course of disease.
- AGA and AA are common causes of hair loss in all adults, but the prevalence depends highly on age, sex, and ethnicity.
- While the history is a key part of the evaluation of hair loss, the physical examination is generally necessary to distinguish scarring from nonscarring alopecias and to describe the pattern more precisely.
- Laboratory studies are often necessary to rule out endocrine or nutritional causes.

PROGNOSIS

TE has an excellent prognosis and usually resolves spontaneously within 1 year. Tinea capitis is reversible if treated appropriately. The prognosis for AA and AGA is variable; the irreversible destruction of the hair follicle implies a poor prognosis.

CASE SCENARIO | Resolution

A 24-year-old woman comes to your office to discuss hair loss that began several months ago. She initially noticed a small patch of hair missing near the top of her scalp but then found several other round patches of loss. These areas are not painful or itchy. She has noticed little "dents" in her nails recently. She is very concerned that she will lose all of her hair.

ADDITIONAL HISTORY

Upon further questioning, the patient has noticed that the hair is not breaking but rather is falling out by the roots. She recalls that her grandmother and aunt take medication for thyroid disease, although she has never had thyroid problems herself. She has had no prior episodes of hair loss and has not changed her hair care regimen recently. She reports no recent changes in weight, diet, or medications and has no known endocrine abnormalities.

Question: What is the most likely diagnosis?

A. Telogen effluvium
B. Alopecia areata
C. Tinea capitis
D. Androgenetic alopecia

Test Your Knowledge

1. You see a 40-year-old woman with diffuse hair loss. She first noticed hair falling out 3 weeks ago in the shower. It comes out in clumps when she washes or brushes her hair. She has not noticed any particular distribution of hair loss.
   Which of the following precipitating factors would be most consistent with a diagnosis of telogen effluvium?
   A. Thyroid hormone abnormality diagnosed 1 month ago
   B. Death of her father 3 months ago from a sudden heart attack
   C. Initiation of a new type of hair dye 1 month ago
   D. Pain and itching of the scalp prior to hair loss

2. A 73-year-old woman reports a 5-year history of progressive, mild hair loss. She has a strong family history of hair loss in aging individuals of both sexes. She has not experienced any recent changes in weight or diet, takes no medications, and has no history of hair loss prior to the last 5 years.
   Which of the following patterns of hair loss distribution would be most likely?
   A. Thinning of hair centrally and widening of the part
   B. Hair breakage on the top of the head
   C. Discrete patches of hair loss in the frontal region
   D. Total loss of hair at the occipital area

3. A concerned mother brings her 5-year-old son to see you. She states that her son is "going bald." She has noticed small patches of hair breaking off from at least 3 different spots on his head over the last 2 months. He has also been scratching his head recently. The patient's mother has not noticed any rash but feels that there are more "dandruff" flakes. There is no history of anxiety disorders or autoimmune disease.
   Which of the following is the most likely diagnosis?
   A. Telogen effluvium
   B. Alopecia areata
   C. Childhood-onset scarring alopecia
   D. Tinea capitis

References

1. Price VH. Treatment of hair loss. *N Engl J Med.* 1999;341:964–973.
2. Hunt N, McHale S. The psychological impact of alopecia. *BMJ.* 2005;331:951–953.
3. Ghannoum M, Isham N, Hajjeh R, et al. Tinea capitis in Cleveland: survey of elementary school students. *J Am Acad Dermatol.* 2003;48:189–193.
4. Sharma V, Hall JC, Knapp JF, Sarai S, Galloway D, Babel DE. Scalp colonization by *Trichophyton tonsurans* in an urban pediatric clinic. Asymptomatic carrier state. *Arch Dermatol.* 1988;124:1511–1513.
5. Seebacher C, Bouchara JP, Mignon B. Updates on the epidemiology of dermatophyte infections. *Mycopathologia.* 2008;166:335–352.
6. Kos L, Conlon J. An update on alopecia areata. *Curr Opin Pediatr.* 2009;21:475–480.
7. Christenson GA, Pyle RL, Mitchell JE. Estimated lifetime prevalence of trichotillomania in college students. *J Clin Psychiatry.* 1991;52:415–417.
8. Birch MP, Lalla SC, Messenger AG. Female pattern hair loss. *Clin Exp Dermatol.* 2002;27:383–388.

9. Otberg N, Finner AM, Shapiro J. Androgenetic alopecia. *Endocrinol Metab Clin North Am*. 2007;36:379–398.

10. Rietschel RL. A simplified approach to the diagnosis of alopecia. *Dermatol Clin*. 1996;14:691–695.

11. Babel DE, Baughman SA. Evaluation of the adult carrier state in juvenile tinea capitis caused by *Trichophyton tonsurans*. *J Am Acad Dermatol*. 1989;21:1209–1212.

Suggested Readings

Lio PA. What's missing from this picture? An approach to alopecia in children. *Arch Dis Child Educ Pract Ed.* 2007;92:193–198.

Mounsey AL, Reed SW. Diagnosing and treating hair loss. *Am Fam Physician*. 2009;80:356–362.

Springer K, Brown M, Stulberg DL. Common hair loss disorders. *Am Fam Physician*. 2003;68:93–102.

SECTION

V

RESPIRATORY SYSTEM

Chapter 24

Cough

Diego Maselli, MD, and Antonio Anzueto, MD

CASE SCENARIO

A 36-year-old man comes to your office because of a persistent cough that has been bothering him for the past 3 months. His cough is dry and is more frequent during the evenings. He also notes frequent nasal congestion, especially when he is exposed to dusts and cold weather. He reports no hemoptysis, weight loss, wheezing, fever, or changes in his appetite.

- **What additional questions would you ask to learn more about his cough?**
- **How would you classify his cough based on the duration to help with the diagnosis?**
- **Can you make a definite diagnosis through an open-ended history followed by focused questions?**
- **What are the alarm features when evaluating a patient with cough?**

INTRODUCTION

Cough is the most common complaint encountered by office-based healthcare practitioners in the United States.[1] It is important in the clearance of excessive secretions and foreign objects from the airways and is a contributing factor in the spread of infection from person to person. Cough is a mechanical reflex that involves a deep inspiration, which increases lung volume, followed by muscle contraction against a closed glottis, and then sudden opening of the glottis. Although cough may often only be a minor annoyance, it can also be a sign of severe underlying disease.

The clinician faced with a patient with an unexplained cough needs a systematic, integrated approach to this problem.[2] This will limit unnecessary testing and will lead to the proper diagnosis and treatment. History and physical examination are paramount in the diagnosis of cough. First, seek potential alarm features that could represent serious illness. Second, determine the duration of the cough to narrow the differential diagnosis.

Based on duration, cough can be divided into the following 3 categories: acute, lasting less than 3 weeks; subacute, lasting between 3 and 8 weeks; and chronic, lasting greater than 8 weeks.[3]

KEY TERMS

Acute cough	Episodes of cough lasting < 3 weeks.
Asthma	Disease characterized by episodic bronchospasm (reactive airways) and thick mucous secretions most frequently related to an allergic condition.
Bronchiectasis	Disorder characterized by dilated bronchial walls with chronic excessive sputum production.
Chronic bronchitis	Included in the spectrum of chronic obstructive pulmonary disease. Presence of chronic productive cough for 3 months in each of 2 successive years.
Chronic cough	Persistent cough lasting longer than 8 weeks.

—Continued next page

Continued—	
Chronic obstructive pulmonary disease (COPD)	Disease state characterized by airflow limitation that is not fully reversible. The airflow limitation is usually both progressive and associated with an abnormal inflammatory response of the lungs to noxious particles or gases.
Gastroesophageal reflux disease (GERD)	Reflux of the gastric contents into the esophagus, upper airway, and tracheobronchial tree (lung).
Hemoptysis	Cough with expectoration of bloody sputum or blood.
Upper airway cough syndrome (UACS)	Previously known as "postnasal drip syndrome"; characterized by abundant secretions from the upper respiratory tract that drip into the oropharynx and tracheobronchial tree, causing cough.

ETIOLOGY

The most frequent causes of **acute cough** include upper respiratory tract infections (ie, common cold, acute viral or bacterial sinusitis, *Bordetella pertussis* infection); lower respiratory tract infections (ie, acute viral or bacterial bronchitis, community-acquired pneumonia); acute exacerbation of chronic obstructive pulmonary disease (COPD) and asthma; allergic rhinitis; rhinitis due to environmental irritants; and irritation to the bronchial tree by cigarette smoke, fumes, or other chemical products such as house cleaners. In elderly patients, acute cough may be the manifestation of left ventricular failure (chronic heart failure) or aspiration. Less common causes of acute cough include pulmonary embolism, foreign bodies, and bronchiectasis.

Although acute cough usually results from a benign cause, **chronic cough** may occasionally be a symptom of a life-threatening disease. The most common causes of chronic cough are upper airway cough syndrome (UACS; previously referred to as *postnasal drip syndrome*), asthma, and gastroesophageal reflux disease (GERD).[4] The new designation of UACS was established by the American College of Chest Physicians to better describe the constellation of symptoms and rhinosinus diseases that cause cough.[5]

Chronic cough may also be due to a patient's occupation or habits. Up to 25% of smokers have chronic cough related to the irritant effects of cigarette smoke, so-called "smoker's cough." Patients with heavy exposure to pollutants (eg, sulfur dioxide, nitrous oxide, particulate matter) and dusts may also have this type of cough. When the cause is not readily apparent, consider cancer, medications (ie, angiotensin-converting enzyme [ACE] inhibitors), chronic infections (ie, tuberculosis and fungal infections), parenchymal lung disease, and immunosuppression (ie, human immunodeficiency virus).[4]

Differential Diagnosis

	Prevalence[a]
Chronic allergic rhinitis or postnasal drip syndrome	41%
Asthma	24%
GERD[6]	21%
COPD including chronic bronchitis	5%
Bronchiectasis	4%
Lung cancer	< 2%
Related to medication use (ACE inhibitors, β-blockers)	5%–25%
Idiopathic and/or psychological cough	< 5%

[a]Among patients with chronic cough in the ambulatory setting.[6,7]

GETTING STARTED WITH THE HISTORY

- The history is the most important aspect of the evaluation of cough.
- Let the patient talk about the cough in his or her own words.
- One quarter of patients with chronic cough may have more than one cause identified.
- Perform a complete history even after a presumed cause is suggested.

INTERVIEW FRAMEWORK

- The first goal is to seek alarm symptoms that require immediate attention.
- Next, determine whether the cough is acute or chronic.
- In the review of systems, pay special attention to the upper and lower respiratory tract, cardiovascular system, and digestive tract (esophagus).
- Ask about smoking habits and environmental and occupational exposures.
- Take a detailed list of current and prior medications.
- Review the past medical history including history of previous allergies, asthma, sinusitis, recent respiratory infections, tuberculosis exposure, coronary artery disease, and esophageal disease.
- Inquire about cough characteristics using the following cardinal symptom features:
  - Onset
  - Duration
  - Frequency
  - Associated symptoms
  - Precipitating and/or alleviating factors
  - Change in frequency over time

Open-Ended Questions	Tips for Effective Interviewing
Why did you come to see me today for the cough?	Determine the patient's agenda for the visit.
Tell me when and how the cough began.	Listen to the story and do not interrupt.
Have you noticed any other symptoms associated with the cough?	Consider several etiologies for cough during the interview.
	Reassure patients when possible.

IDENTIFYING ALARM SYMPTOMS

- Serious causes of cough are rare.
- After the open-ended portion of the history, ask about alarm symptoms to assess for the possibility of a serious cause and to determine the speed of subsequent evaluation.
- No published data allow a calculation of likelihood ratios for predicting serious causes for the symptoms listed below.

Alarm Symptoms	If Present, Consider Serious Causes...	However, Benign Causes for This Feature Include...
Cough with hemoptysis	Lung cancer Tuberculosis Pulmonary embolism Pneumonia	Acute viral or bacterial bronchitis, COPD exacerbation, bronchiectasis
Cough, fever, and purulent sputum production	Pneumonia Lung abscess	Acute sinusitis
Cough with wheezing and shortness of breath	Asthma COPD exacerbation Heart failure	Acute bronchitis
Cough with chest pain	Pulmonary embolism Acute coronary syndrome (angina pectoris)	COPD exacerbation

—Continued next page

Continued—		
Cough with excessive chronic sputum production	Bronchiectasis Lung abscess Lung cancer	Chronic bronchitis Chronic sinusitis
Cough and unintentional weight loss	Lung cancer Tuberculosis Lung abscess	COPD
Cough, dyspnea, and lower extremity edema	Congestive heart failure Pulmonary embolism	

FOCUSED QUESTIONS

After hearing the patient's story and considering potential alarm symptoms, ask the following questions to narrow the differential diagnosis.

QUESTIONS	THINK ABOUT...
Does mucous drip in the back of your throat?	Allergic, vasomotor, or nonallergic rhinitis Acute nasopharyngitis Acute or chronic sinusitis UACS
Do you have wheezing at rest or during exertion?	Asthma (cough-variant asthma presents as episodes of cough with or without wheezing), congestive heart failure, pulmonary embolism
Do you have heartburn? Have you noticed a food or acid/bitter taste in your mouth? Does overeating or eating particular foods make you cough?	Chronic cough is the only symptom in 75% of patients with GERD. Gastric acid reflux to the lower third of the esophagus may trigger cough.
Have you had recent flu-like symptoms with significant cough?	Consider postinfectious cough if persistent symptoms after a viral infection (ie, the flu).
When did you start your ACE inhibitor? Have you taken another ACE inhibitor in the past?	ACE inhibitor–induced cough is more common in females, is not dose-related, may occur months after starting the medication, and can be produced by any formulation. It occurs in approximately 5%–30% of patients. Cough usually improves after a drug holiday of 1–4 days, based on the half-life of the compound.
Are you under severe stress? Do you know if your cough is present during sleep?	Idiopathic or psychogenic cough is a diagnosis of exclusion. Usually occurs in adolescents.
Quality	
Do you have dry cough?	GERD Irritant cough Postviral infection Interstitial lung disease (pulmonary fibrosis)
Do you need to clear your throat frequently?	UACS Allergic, vasomotor, or nonallergic rhinitis

Time course	
Is this cough worsening over time?	Bronchitis Asthma Congestive heart failure Lung cancer Bronchiectasis
Is your cough worse during a particular season?	UACS Asthma
Has your cough lingered after a recent cold or flu?	Postinfectious cough UACS
Associated symptoms	
Do you cough up any sputum?	Pneumonia Asthma Bronchitis UACS Bronchiectasis Sinusitis Smoker's cough Congestive heart failure
Does your sputum look purulent or yellow-green?	Bronchitis Sinusitis Pneumonia Bronchiectasis COPD exacerbation Tuberculosis UACS
Is your sputum clear or whitish?	Asthma UACS Smoker's cough Bronchitis
Do you cough up large quantities of purulent sputum or sputum with foul odor?	Bronchiectasis Pneumonia Lung abscess
Do you get short of breath with exertion?	Asthma Congestive heart failure COPD Pneumonitis
Is your cough associated with wheezing?	Asthma Congestive heart failure

—Continued next page

Continued—

Do you have associated hoarseness?	GERD Chronic laryngitis Laryngeal nodules/polyps UACS
Do you have a burning feeling in your throat at night or early in the morning?	GERD Allergic rhinitis (with mouth breathing)
Do you have frequent heartburn or a sour taste in your mouth?	GERD
Do you feel frequent secretions in the back of your throat?	UACS Sinusitis
Is your cough seasonal?	Asthma UACS Allergic rhinitis
Have you ever been diagnosed with nasal allergies or allergic rhinitis?	UACS
Do you have chronic bad breath or halitosis?	Chronic sinusitis
Do you have chronic pain in the sinuses over your cheeks or forehead?	Chronic sinusitis
Do you sleep with more than one pillow (orthopnea) or do you wake up choking or short of breath (paroxysmal nocturnal dyspnea)?	Congestive heart failure Obstructive sleep apnea GERD COPD
Modifying factors	
Do you cough during or after exercising?	Asthma UACS Allergic or vasomotor rhinitis
Do you cough when exposed to cold air or cold weather?	Asthma UACS Allergic or vasomotor rhinitis
Does your cough worsen when you lie down?	UACS GERD Congestive heart failure Bronchiectasis Acute bronchitis
Does your cough worsen at night?	Asthma GERD Congestive heart failure
Is your cough precipitated by changes in position?	Bronchiectasis Congestive heart failure
Does your cough improve with over-the-counter antihistamines?	Allergic rhinitis UACS

DIAGNOSTIC APPROACH (INCLUDING ALGORITHM)

The first step is to assess for alarm symptoms. Next, define the duration of the symptoms. Although most cases of acute cough are due to viral infections and other benign diagnoses, serious causes of cough may also present acutely.

Chronic cough (lasting longer than 8 weeks) is usually due to UACS, allergic rhinitis, asthma, GERD, chronic bronchitis, or drugs. Additional diagnostic procedures may be required to identify the cause of chronic cough.

When the diagnosis is in doubt after history and physical examination, potential studies to identify the cause include chest radiography, sinus radiography, pulmonary function tests, barium esophagography, 24-hour esophageal pH monitoring, differential white blood cell count, and occasionally direct laryngoscopy or fiberoptic bronchoscopy. See Figure 24–1 for the diagnostic algorithm for cough.

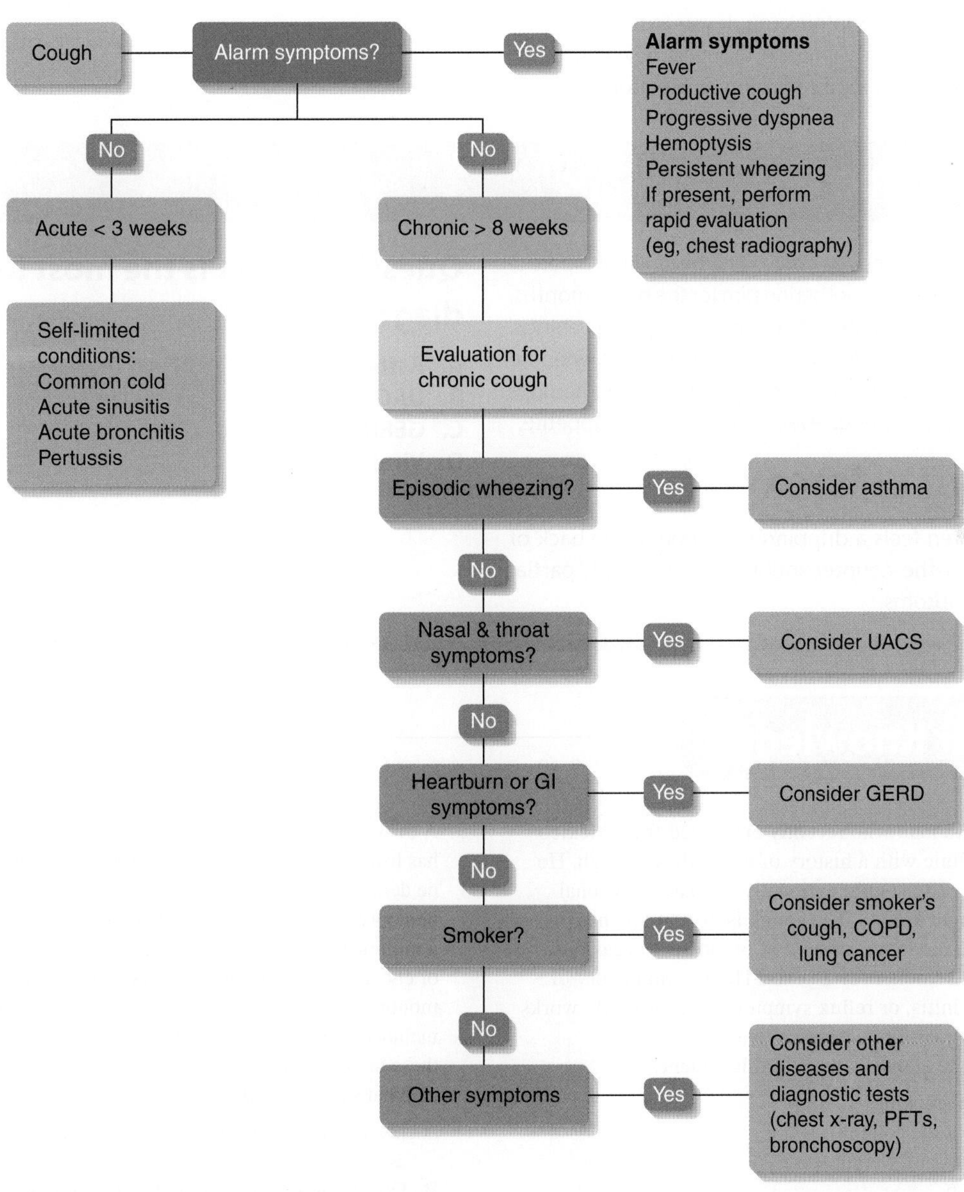

FIGURE 24–1 Diagnostic approach: Cough. COPD, chronic obstructive pulmonary disease; GERD, gastroesophageal reflux disease; GI, gastrointestinal; PFTs, pulmonary function tests; UACS, upper airway cough syndrome.

CAVEATS

- Keep an open mind while obtaining the history; chronic cough is often caused by multiple and simultaneously contributing causes.
- Two of the most common causes of chronic cough are nonpulmonary diseases (GERD and UACS).
- GERD, UACS, and asthma account for 90% of chronic cough in nonsmoking patients with normal chest radiographs.
- Chronic cough occurs in 5% to 25% of patients taking ACE inhibitors. In these patients, cough is not related to the dosage or duration of therapy, and it can present at anytime.
- Patients with alarm symptoms (eg, lower extremity swelling, progressive dyspnea, orthopnea, wheezing, hemoptysis, or fever) require prompt evaluation.

PROGNOSIS

- Specific therapy is successful in eliminating chronic cough in most patients with asthma, UACS, and GERD. On occasions, therapy for more than one disorder may be necessary to control the symptoms.
- Satisfactory treatment of chronic cough due to other etiologies depends on the therapy and prognosis of the underlying disease.
- Complications of chronic cough include headache, pneumothorax, pneumomediastinum, syncope, urinary incontinence, trauma to chest muscles, rib fractures, and psychological fear of public appearances.

CASE SCENARIO | Resolution

A 36-year-old man comes to your office because of a persistent cough that has been bothering him for the past 3 months. His cough is dry and is more frequent during the evenings. He also notes frequent nasal congestion, especially when he is exposed to dusts and cold weather. He reports no hemoptysis, weight loss, wheezing, fever, or changes in his appetite.

ADDITIONAL HISTORY

The patient often feels a dripping sensation in the back of this throat. Over-the-counter antihistamines provide partial relief of his symptoms.

Question: What is the most likely diagnosis?

A. Asthma
B. UACS
C. GERD
D. Viral infection

Test Your Knowledge

1. A 28-year-old man who recently emigrated from Mexico visits your clinic with a history of 4 months of cough. He has lost 15 to 20 lbs unintentionally and has occasional fevers and night sweats. The cough is dry, and he has coughed up a moderate amount of blood on 3 occasions. He has been a smoker for 2 years. There is no history of wheezing, rhinitis, or reflux symptoms. He currently works as a security guard in a chemical plant.

   What are the alarm features in this patient?

   A. History of smoking
   B. Duration of the cough
   C. Hemoptysis and weight loss
   D. Type of job

2. In the patient in Question 1, what is the most likely diagnosis?

   A. Lung cancer
   B. Acute bronchitis
   C. Tuberculosis
   D. Chronic obstructive pulmonary disease

3. A 56-year-old man sees you for a long-standing cough. He has had a cough for at least 6 months. On a review of systems, he denies wheezing, nasal congestion, weight loss, fevers, or hemoptysis. He has occasional heartburn characterized by a midline retrosternal burning, especially after heavy meals or chocolate. He has had frequent hoarseness over the past month. Another physician did a preliminary work-up that included a chest x-ray and blood and urine studies. All of these tests were normal.

   What should you do next?

   A. Do additional questioning/testing for possible bronchial asthma
   B. Do additional questioning/testing for possible GERD
   C. Do additional questioning/testing for possible infectious causes of cough
   D. Follow his symptoms and schedule a follow-up in 1 month

References

1. Cherry DK, Hing E, Woodwell DA, Rechtsteiner EA. National Ambulatory Medical Care Survey: 2006 summary. *Natl Health Stat Report*. 2008;3:1–39.
2. Pratter MR, Brightling CE, Boulet LP, Irwin RS. An empiric integrative approach to the management of cough: ACCP evidence-based clinical practice guidelines. *Chest*. 2006;129(Suppl 1):222S–231S.
3. Irwin RS, Madison M. The diagnosis and treatment of cough. *N Engl J Med*. 2000;343:1715–1721.
4. Pratter MR. Overview of common causes of chronic cough: ACCP evidence-based clinical practice guidelines. *Chest*. 2006;129(Suppl 1):59S–62S.
5. Pratter MR. Chronic upper airway cough syndrome secondary to rhinosinus diseases (previously referred to as postnasal drip syndrome): ACCP evidence-based clinical practice guidelines. *Chest*. 2006;129(Suppl 1):63S–71S.
6. Mello CJ, Irwin RS, Curley FJ. Predictive values of the character, timing and complications of chronic cough in diagnosing its cause. *Arch Intern Med*. 1996;156:997–1003.
7. Smyrnios NA, Irwin RS, Curley FJ, French CL. From a prospective study of chronic cough: diagnostic and therapeutic aspects in older adults. *Arch Intern Med*. 1998;158:1222–1228.

Suggested Reading

Irwin RS, Baumann MH, Bolser DC, et al. Diagnosis and management of cough executive summary: ACCP evidence-based clinical practice guidelines. *Chest*. 2006;129(Suppl 1):1S–23S.

Irwin RS, Gutterman DD. American College of Chest Physicians' cough guidelines. *Lancet*. 2006;367:981.

Taichman D, Fishman AP. Fishman's pulmonary diseases and disorders. In: *Approach to the Patient with Respiratory Symptoms*. 4th ed. New York, NY: The McGraw-Hill Companies, 2008:405–410.

Chapter 25

Dyspnea

Iris Ma, MD, and Catherine R. Lucey, MD

CASE SCENARIO

A 67-year-old man comes to your clinic for his annual appointment concerned about increasing shortness of breath. A year ago he was able to walk up the stairs to his apartment without difficulty, but now he has difficulty walking one block. He has a 70 pack-year smoking history, and several previous attempts to stop smoking have been unsuccessful.

- **Does the patient require urgent intervention?**
- **Is the shortness of breath acute or chronic?**
- **What additional questions would you ask to learn more about his shortness of breath?**
- **What is the organ system involved in the patient's shortness of breath (cardiac, pulmonary, hematologic, or psychiatric)?**

INTRODUCTION

Shortness of breath, or dyspnea, is the sensation of uncomfortable breathing. This feeling of discomfort may reflect an increased awareness of breathing or the perception that breathing is difficult or inadequate. Dyspnea usually indicates pulmonary or cardiac disease, but can also be the presenting symptom of metabolic derangements, hematologic disorders, toxic ingestions, psychiatric conditions, or simple deconditioning. Dyspnea is the second most common reason for emergency department visits in the United States.[1]

Dyspnea can be classified based on the primary physiologic derangement:

- Pulmonary
- Cardiac
- Hematologic (eg, anemia)
- Chest wall or neuromuscular disease
- Metabolic (eg, acidosis)
- Functional (eg, panic disorders)
- Deconditioning

KEY TERMS

Cardiomyopathies	Conditions that damage heart muscle and may cause heart failure. Etiologies are diverse. Common causes include ischemic heart disease, valvular disease, hypertension, infections, toxins, and genetic disorders.
Dyspnea	Abnormally increased awareness of breathing or sensation of difficulty breathing.
Interstitial lung disease	A heterogeneous set of conditions characterized by hypoxia and interstitial (pulmonary vessels, bronchi, connective tissue) abnormalities on chest radiographs. Examples include sarcoidosis, idiopathic pulmonary fibrosis, rheumatoid lung, and pneumoconioses.

—Continued next page

Continued—	
Orthopnea	Dyspnea when lying flat. Typically described in terms of the number of pillows the patient uses to breathe comfortably to sleep.
Paroxysmal nocturnal dyspnea (PND)	Dyspnea that wakes the patient from sleep. The patient may report waking up gasping for air, and classically finds relief by sitting by an open window.
Platypnea	Dyspnea that improves when the patient lies down.
Trepopnea	Dyspnea that occurs in the lateral decubitus position on one side, but not the other.

ETIOLOGY

The purpose of breathing is to meet the metabolic demands of the body. Thus, any condition that increases the work of breathing (eg, airway obstruction, changes in lung compliance, or respiratory muscle weakness) or increases respiratory drive (eg, hypoxia or acidosis) may result in dyspnea.[2] In addition, dyspnea may result from or be exacerbated by primary psychological conditions (eg, anxiety disorders).

The differential diagnosis of dyspnea depends on the duration of the symptom and the clinical setting. Conditions associated with acute dyspnea (developing over hours to a few days) are outlined under alarm conditions.

Conditions associated with insidious development of dyspnea are outlined below. In an analysis of patients referred to a pulmonary clinic for evaluation of chronic, unexplained dyspnea, 67% suffered from asthma, chronic obstructive pulmonary disease (COPD), interstitial lung disease, or myocardial dysfunction.[3]

Differential Diagnosis

Chronic Dyspnea	
Cardiovascular	***Miscellaneous***
Muscle (cardiomyopathies)	Anemia
Vessels (ischemia, pulmonary hypertension)	Chest wall abnormalities (kyphoscoliosis, pectus excavatum)
Valves (regurgitation, stenosis, infection)	Deconditioning
	Metabolic acidosis
Pericardium (effusion, inflammation)	Neuromuscular disease
Pulmonary	***Psychiatric***
Bronchi (mass, foreign body)	Panic attack, anxiety disorders
Bronchioles (asthma, chronic bronchitis)	
Interstitial lung diseases	
Alveoli (emphysema, chronic pneumonia)	
Vessels (chronic pulmonary emboli)	
Pleura (effusions)	
Lung cancer (may occur in any of the above locations)	

GETTING STARTED WITH THE HISTORY

- Begin by assessing the patient's airway, breathing, and circulation. If the patient is unable to complete a full sentence without pausing for a deep breath, move quickly to stabilize the patient. Return to the interview after the patient is more comfortable.
- Start with an open-ended question that lets the patient describe the dyspnea before asking more focused questions.

Open-Ended Questions	Tips for Effective Interviewing
Tell me about your problem with breathing.	Allow the patient to tell the story in his or her own words. Ask focused questions later.
How long has this shortness of breath been going on?	The differential diagnosis varies dramatically depending on the time course.

INTERVIEW FRAMEWORK

- First, classify the duration of symptoms as acute or chronic.
- Listen to the patient's description of dyspnea, particularly exacerbating and alleviating factors and associated signs and symptoms.
- Ask about risk factors for conditions causing dyspnea from the past medical, social, and family histories.

IDENTIFYING ALARM SYMPTOMS

- Acute onset and rapid progression of dyspnea are concerning for impending respiratory failure.
- Always carefully monitor for changes in symptoms because the patient's respiratory status can deteriorate quickly.

Serious Diagnoses

Many causes of dyspnea are serious. Patients with acute or severe dyspnea require rapid diagnostic evaluation as they can develop complete respiratory failure. In these cases urgent intubation and mechanical ventilation should be pursued. Fortunately, in the majority of cases, patients are stable enough to provide a comprehensive history. Patients with chronic dyspnea who are able to talk comfortably may have serious underlying disease, but the clinician has more time to evaluate the patient.

Causes of Acute Dyspnea	Comment
Flash pulmonary edema	Flash pulmonary edema is commonly due to congestive heart failure associated with ischemic heart disease. Almost 50% of patients will require revascularization for coronary artery disease. Other causes include acute valvular insufficiency and severe hypertension.[4]
Pulmonary embolism (PE)	Ninety percent of patients with PE have dyspnea or tachypnea; 20% have dyspnea alone.[5]
Anaphylaxis	Up to 15% of residents in the United States may be susceptible to anaphylaxis.[6] Fifty percent of patients with anaphylaxis will have dyspnea.[7]
Aspiration	Dyspnea due to aspiration generally begins abruptly within hours of the event.
Cardiac tamponade	Tamponade refers to pericardial effusion causing hemodynamic compromise resulting in symptoms of dyspnea and light-headedness.
COPD exacerbation	Bacterial infections underlie over 1/3 of COPD exacerbations, and viral infections may be at the root of another 1/3 of exacerbations.
Acute pneumonia	The prevalence of pneumonia in healthy patients presenting with acute cough is approximately 6%–7%.[8] The prevalence is higher in populations with comorbid illness.
Respiratory muscle weakness	Approximately 40% of patients with acute Guillain-Barré syndrome will require assisted ventilation because of muscular weakness.[9]
Spontaneous pneumothorax	The lifetime risk of spontaneous pneumothorax in men is 12% for heavy smokers and < 0.001% for nonsmokers.[10]
Metabolic acidosis (diabetic ketoacidosis, aspirin overdose, lactic acidosis)	Patients with severe metabolic acidosis compensate by hyperventilating. The tachypnea is not always accompanied by dyspnea.

Alarm Symptoms	If Present, Consider Serious Causes...	Frequency or Positive Likelihood Ratio (LR+)	However, Benign Causes for This Feature Include...
Pleuritic chest pain (sharp, unilateral chest pain that increases with respiration)	PE Pneumothorax Pneumococcal pneumonia	66% of patients with PE will have pleuritic pain[5]	Tietze's syndrome (chest wall joint swelling) Rib fracture
Lip swelling, hives, and wheezing	Anaphylaxis or angioedema	88% of patients with anaphylaxis will have hives; 50% will have wheezing or dyspnea[7]	
Substernal chest pressure	Acute myocardial ischemia or infarction		Esophageal spasm
Pink, frothy sputum	Cardiogenic pulmonary edema		
Fever and sputum production	Acute pneumonia	If febrile, LR+ 1.7–2.1 for pneumonia[11]	Bronchitis
Fever and signs of serious infection or shock	Acute respiratory distress syndrome		
Fever, progressive sore throat, dysphagia, and hoarseness	Epiglottitis		Pharyngitis
Ascending weakness	Guillain-Barré syndrome		
Generalized weakness	Myasthenia gravis		
Known or suspected diabetes or renal failure	Diabetic ketoacidosis or metabolic acidosis		
Suicidality or chronic pain	Aspirin overdose		Panic disorder Primary hyperventilation

FOCUSED QUESTIONS

To narrow the differential diagnosis of dyspnea, the physician should attempt to characterize the patient's dyspnea-related illness. The following questions can be used to outline the time course, precisely describe the dyspnea, and identify predisposing conditions and associated symptoms.

QUESTIONS	IF ANSWERED IN THE AFFIRMATIVE...
Risk factors and associated diseases	**Think about**
Do you have a history of cardiac problems?	CHF
• *Past history of CHF?*	• LR+ 5.8, LR– 0.45[12]
• *Past history of myocardial infarction?*	• LR+ 3.1, LR– 0.69[12]
• *Past history of coronary artery disease?*	• LR+ 1.8, LR– 0.68[12]

Do you smoke?	COPD Desquamative interstitial pneumonia Coronary artery disease Lung cancer • Smoking is a major risk factor for COPD with LR+ of 8.0–11.6.[13,14]
What is your occupation?	Occupational exposure to lung toxins (eg, asbestos), organic material (causing hypersensitivity pneumonitis), or chemicals associated with asthma may explain chronic dyspnea.
Have you had a recent period of prolonged immobilization?	PE
Do you have a history of cancer or lower extremity weakness?	PE
Are you taking birth control pills or estrogen?	PE
Do you have diabetes, high blood pressure, high cholesterol, or heart disease?	Coronary artery disease, cardiomyopathy
Has anyone in your immediate family had a serious heart condition? At what age?	A family history of premature coronary disease is significant when a first-degree relative has had significant coronary heart disease before age 50 if male or age 60 if female.
Have you had unintentional weight loss, night sweats, or fatigue?	Primary lung cancer is the number one cause of cancer-related mortality. The lung parenchyma and pleura are also common sites of metastasis. Chemotherapy can cause pulmonary fibrosis (bleomycin), heart failure (doxorubicin), and anemia. Radiation therapy to the chest can cause constrictive pericarditis and accelerated coronary artery disease. Heart disease may result in arrhythmias.
Do you have any other medical problems?	Many rheumatic diseases (eg, rheumatoid arthritis, systemic lupus erythematosus, polymyositis) cause chronic interstitial lung disease. Neuromuscular diseases may predispose the patient to aspiration or weaken respiratory muscles. Methotrexate (for rheumatologic disease) and nitrofurantoin (for urinary tract infections) can cause interstitial lung disease.
Have you traveled in the past year? Have you travelled to foreign countries?	Histoplasmosis Coccidioidomycosis Blastomycosis Tuberculosis
Do you have any known allergies to foods, insects, or latex?	Anaphylaxis (patients may know that they are allergic to insects, nuts, or shellfish but be unaware that recently ingested food contained these allergens)

—Continued next page

Continued—

Have you been taking your prescribed medications, and in the proper doses?	Nonadherence with CHF or COPD medications often leads to an exacerbation. Conversely, toxic overdoses may also occur. Methotrexate (for rheumatologic disease) and nitrofurantoin (for urinary tract infections) can cause interstitial lung disease.
Have you recently started taking any new medications (eg, β-lactam antibiotics, angiotensin-converting enzyme inhibitors)?	Allergic reactions Angioedema
Quality	**Think about**
Is your chest tight, or does it take an increased amount of effort to breathe?	Asthma Ischemic heart disease
Do you feel that your breathing is rapid and/or shallow?	Interstitial lung disease
Does your breathing only get heavy with activity?	Deconditioning Anemia Pulmonary disease
Do you feel as if your throat is closing or that air can't get all of the way in to your lungs?	Panic disorder
Modifying symptoms	**Think about**
Do you have shortness of breath when lying flat?	Orthopnea (LR+ 2.2, LR– 0.68)[12] and PND (LR+ 2.6, LR– 0.70)[12] are seen in patients with CHF.
Does lying on one side or the other cause increasing shortness of breath?	Trepopnea can occur with unilateral pleural effusion (on the recumbent side) or chronic heart failure (prefer lying on left side).
Can you exercise for some time before getting short of breath?	Exercise-induced asthma; symptoms begin after exercising for some time. Cardiomyopathy; symptoms begin after a short period of exercise (eg, 50–100 ft).
Associated symptoms	**Think about**
Do you have chest pain?	Myocardial infarction: a heaviness, pressure, or crushing substernal pain radiating to the jaw or left arm Spontaneous pneumothorax: unilateral pleuritic pain PE: unilateral or bilateral pleuritic pain Cardiac tamponade: central chest heaviness Pericarditis: pleuritic pain radiating to back with positional improvement
Do you have any itching or hives? Are your lips or tongue swelling?	Anaphylaxis
Have you had a fever?	Acute pneumonia: 80% have fever[5] Acute PE: 20% have fever[11] Chronic pneumonia Inflammatory interstitial lung disease

Have you been coughing?	Asthma: nonproductive cough Acute pneumonia Aspiration Gastroesophageal reflux disease PE: nonproductive cough with occasional scant hemoptysis Flash pulmonary edema: cough with pink frothy sputum COPD: chronic bronchitis: 3 months of productive cough per year for 2 consecutive years Interstitial lung disease
Do you have swelling in your legs or abdomen?	Deep venous thrombosis with PE: unilateral leg edema Cardiomyopathy: bilateral edema (LR+ 2.3, LR– 0.64 for CHF)[12] Pericardial disease: bilateral edema with abdominal swelling Severe right heart failure due to chronic lung disease with pulmonary hypertension: bilateral edema with abdominal swelling
Have you lost weight?	Primary or metastatic lung cancer Chronic pneumonia
Have you had fainting spells?	Primary or secondary pulmonary hypertension
Do you have rashes or joint pains?	Interstitial lung diseases associated with systemic inflammatory conditions (eg, sarcoidosis)
Do you have weakness in your arms or legs or difficulty speaking or swallowing?	Aspiration (stroke, Guillain-Barré syndrome, myasthenia gravis, amyotrophic lateral sclerosis)
Do you have any numbness or tingling in your fingertips? *Did you feel a sense of impending doom or extreme fear?*	Panic attack or anxiety disorder

CAVEATS

- The history and physical examination identify the etiology of dyspnea in nearly 70% of cases. The remainder will require more specific testing, such as chest radiographs or pulmonary function tests.[3]
- The causes of dyspnea are often multifactorial. For example, heavy smoking is a risk factor for both COPD and coronary artery disease. Patients with chronic lung or heart disease may also suffer from deconditioning. Adequate treatment of the patient requires identification of all causes of dyspnea because the therapies may differ.
- Platypnea is encountered with right-to-left shunts in the atria or pulmonary vasculature (eg, hepatopulmonary syndrome) and in emphysema.
- Be particularly cautious about assuming anxiety is the cause of acute or chronic dyspnea because patients with dyspnea caused by organic disease are often anxious.

PROGNOSIS

The prognosis of dyspnea depends on the etiology and severity of the underlying disease. Acute dyspnea is often reversible. Myocardial infarctions, pulmonary emboli, aspiration pneumonia, pneumothoraces, and asthma can generally be successfully treated once diagnosed. In contrast, chronic dyspnea may reflect disease that has progressed to an irreversible stage. Dyspnea associated with chronic pulmonary or cardiac disease may improve if the patient stops smoking and participates in cardiopulmonary exercise training/rehabilitation.

DIAGNOSTIC APPROACH (INCLUDING ALGORITHM)

See Figure 25–1 for the diagnostic approach algorithm to dyspnea.

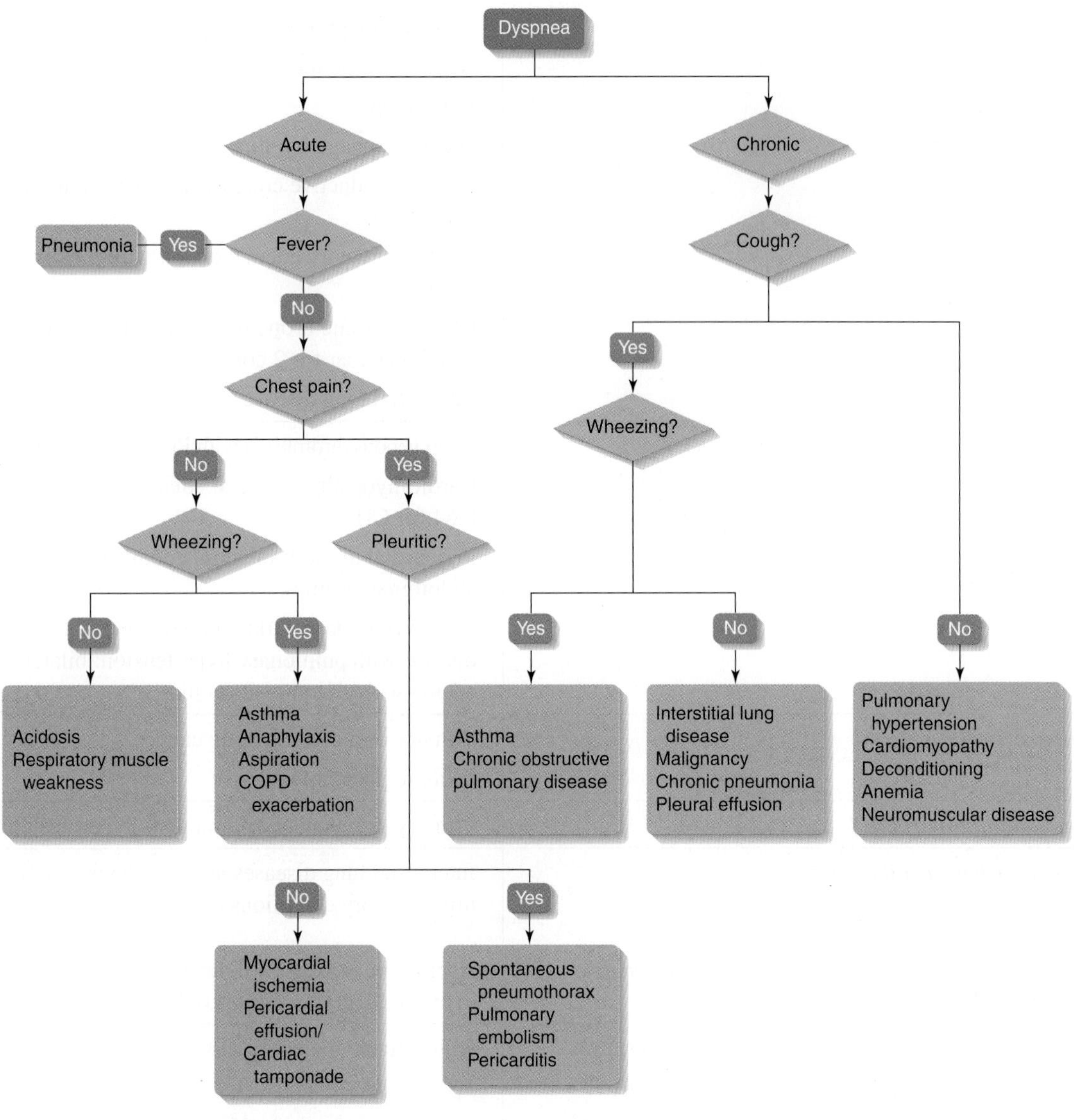

FIGURE 25–1 Diagnostic approach: Dyspnea.

CASE SCENARIO | Resolution

A 67-year-old man comes to your clinic for his annual appointment concerned about increasing shortness of breath. A year ago he was able to walk up the stairs to his apartment without difficulty, but now he has a hard time walking one block. He has a 70 pack-year smoking history, and several previous attempts to stop smoking have been unsuccessful.

ADDITIONAL HISTORY

This patient has had slowly progressive dyspnea with exercise but no symptoms at rest. The chronicity of the patient's symptoms and his ability to engage in conversation reassure you that he does not require urgent intervention. He expresses frustration that he is unable to get a full breath when simply walking around his home. The dyspnea often worsens when he has a "cold," but he denies an acute increase in symptoms. There are no other triggers. When you ask about related symptoms, he describes a persistent cough productive of thick green sputum. The cough has been an irritating presence for the past several months. He denies fevers, chest pain, chest tightness, or orthopnea.

Question: What is the most likely diagnosis?

A. Asthma
B. Chronic obstructive pulmonary disease
C. Congestive heart failure
D. Pneumonia

Test Your Knowledge

1. A 67-year-old hospitalized man complains of shortness of breath for the past hour. Although lying in the bed, he is breathing quickly and appears nervous. He was admitted 4 days earlier after being hit by a car and was found to have a displaced tibial fracture, which required immediate operative intervention. Chest radiograph at admission showed a 5-cm lung mass suspicious for cancer. The patient has a 60 pack-year smoking history. He has had a persistent nonproductive cough for the past several months but denies any other symptoms.

   What is the most likely cause of his dyspnea?

   A. Lung mass
   B. Pulmonary embolism
   C. Rib fracture
   D. Anxiety
   E. Deconditioning

2. The captain of the high school cheerleading team presents to clinic with a chief complaint of several months of shortness of breath upon exertion. She is unable to identify any triggering symptoms. She denies hormonal contraceptive use.

   Which of the following is the most important aspect of the history to elicit?

   A. Recent bee sting
   B. Menorrhagia
   C. Recent immobilization
   D. Exposure to asbestos

3. A 67-year-old man with a 40 pack-year smoking history complains of shortness of breath for the past 6 months and swelling in his legs. He often wakes up at night gasping for breath and feels most comfortable sleeping on 3 pillows. He has no past history of COPD or CHF, but he has diabetes and hypertension.

   What is the most likely diagnosis?

   A. Congestive heart failure
   B. Chronic obstructive pulmonary disease
   C. Asthma
   D. Lung cancer
   E. Pulmonary embolism

References

1. Niska R, Bhuiya F, Xu J. National Hospital Ambulatory Medical Care Survey: 2007 Emergency Department Summary. National Health Statistics Reports No. 26. Hyattsville, MD: National Center for Health Statistics, 2010.
2. American Thoracic Society. Dyspnea. Mechanisms, assessment, and management: a consensus statement. *Am J Respir Crit Care Med.* 1999;159:321–340.
3. Pratter MR, Curley FJ, Dubois J, Irwin RS. Cause and evaluation of chronic dyspnea in a pulmonary disease clinic. *Arch Intern Med.* 1989;149:2277–2282.
4. Kramer K, Kirkman P, Kitzman D, Little WC. Flash pulmonary edema: association with hypertension and reoccurrence despite coronary revascularization. *Am Heart J.* 2000;140:451–455.
5. Stein PD, Terrin ML, Hales CA, et al. Clinical, laboratory, roentgenographic, and electrocardiographic findings in patients with acute pulmonary embolism and no preexisting cardiac or pulmonary disease. *Chest.* 1991;100:598–603.
6. Neugut AI, Ghatak AT, Miller RL. Anaphylaxis in the United States: an investigation into its epidemiology. *Arch Intern Med.* 2001;161:15–21.
7. Zweiman B, O'Dowd LC. Anaphylaxis. UpToDate. 2004. Available at: http://www.uptodate.com. Accessed October 16, 2011.
8. Emerman CL, Dawson N, Speroff T, et al. Comparison of physician judgment and decision aids for ordering chest radiographs for pneumonia in outpatients. *Ann Emerg Med.* 1991;20:1215–1219.
9. Sharshar T, Chevret S, Bourdain F, Raphael JC. Early predictors of mechanical ventilation in Guillain-Barré syndrome. *Crit Care Med.* 2003;31:278–283.
10. Bense L, Eklund G, Wiman LG. Smoking and the increased risk of contracting spontaneous pneumothorax. *Chest.* 1987;92:1009–1012.
11. Metlay JP, Kapoor WN, Fine MJ. Does this patient have community-acquired pneumonia? Diagnosing pneumonia by history and physical examination. *JAMA.* 1997;278:1440–1445.
12. Wang CS, Fitzgerald JM, Schulzer M, Mak E, Ayas NT. Does this dyspneic patient in the emergency department have congestive heart failure? *JAMA.* 2005;294:1944–1956.
13. Straus SE, McAlister FA, Sackett DL, Deeks JJ; for the CARE-COAD1 Group. The accuracy of patient history, wheezing and laryngeal measurements in diagnosing obstructive airway disease. *JAMA.* 2000;283:1853–1857.
14. Dawson JK, Graham DR, Kenny J, Lynch MP. Accuracy of history, examination, pulmonary function tests and chest radiographs in predicting high-resolution computed tomography-diagnosed interstitial lung disease. *Br J Rheumatol.* 1997;36:1342–1343.

Suggested Reading

American Thoracic Society. Dyspnea. Mechanisms, assessment, and management: a consensus statement. *Am J Respir Crit Care Med*. 1999;159:321–340.

Azeemuddin A, Graber MA, Dickson EW. Evaluation of the adult with dyspnea in the emergency department. UpToDate. 2010. Available at: http://www.uptodate.com. Accessed October 16, 2011.

van Belle A, Buller HR, Huisman MV, et al. Effectiveness of managing suspected pulmonary embolism using an algorithm combining clinical probability, D-dimer testing, and computed tomography. *JAMA*. 2006;295:172–179.

Chapter 26

Hemoptysis

Diego Maselli, MD, Jay I. Peters, MD, and Sandra Adams, MD, MS

CASE SCENARIO

A 35-year-old man with history of chronic cough comes to your office and is very concerned after having 2 episodes of prolonged coughing that produced blood-streaked sputum. He also reports subjective fever for 4 days and cough productive of yellow sputum. This is the first time he has experienced this constellation of symptoms.

- **What additional questions would you ask to learn more about his hemoptysis?**
- **How would you classify his hemoptysis in terms of quantity?**
- **Can you make a definite diagnosis through an open-ended history followed by focused questions?**
- **What are the alarm features when evaluating a patient with hemoptysis?**

INTRODUCTION

Hemoptysis is the expectoration of blood or blood-stained sputum. It implies that the blood originates from the lungs or bronchial tubes as a result of pulmonary or bronchial hemorrhage.[1] The blood supply to the lungs is derived from the pulmonary and bronchial arterial systems. The low-pressure pulmonary arterial system tends to produce small-volume hemoptysis, whereas bleeding from the bronchial arterial system, which is more common, tends to be profuse. However, it may be difficult to differentiate hemoptysis from bleeding from the upper gastrointestinal tract or upper airway. Based on the amount of blood expectorated, hemoptysis can be classified as scant or mild, submassive or moderate, and massive or severe.[2–4]

KEY TERMS[1–4]

Scant (mild) hemoptysis	Less than 20 mL (less than a tablespoon) in 24 hours. Blood streaks usually noted with expectorated phlegm.
Submassive (moderate) hemoptysis	Between 20 and 250 mL (less than a cup) in 24 hours.
Massive (severe) hemoptysis	More than 250 mL (more than a cup) in 24 hours.
Cryptogenic or idiopathic hemoptysis	No cause is found after extensive diagnostic evaluation.

ETIOLOGY

There are more than 100 causes of hemoptysis. In the primary care setting, the most common causes of hemoptysis are acute and chronic bronchitis, pneumonia, tuberculosis, and lung cancer.[4] Other important causes include bronchiectasis, pulmonary embolism, trauma, fungal infections, foreign bodies, and rheumatologic diseases such as systemic lupus erythematosus, Goodpasture's syndrome, and antineutrophil cytoplasmic antibody (ANCA)–associated vasculitis. Bronchitis is still considered the most common cause of hemoptysis, but it rarely causes massive hemoptysis. Although massive hemoptysis accounts for only 5% to 15% of episodes, it is a true medical emergency that requires intensive care with immediate evaluation for the underlying cause.[5]

Differential Diagnosis[1–4]

	Prevalence
Bronchitis	20%–40%
Lung cancer	15%–30%
Bronchiectasis	10%–20%
Cryptogenic	10%–20%
Pneumonia	5%–10%
Tuberculosis	5%–15%

GETTING STARTED WITH THE HISTORY

- To determine the likely etiology of hemoptysis, consider the amount of blood expectorated, duration of symptoms, and the patient's age, smoking history, and past medical history.
- Differentiate between true hemoptysis versus bleeding from the upper airway or gastrointestinal tract.
- Review medications known to cause or exacerbate bleeding including aspirin and nonsteroidal anti-inflammatory drugs, anticoagulants (warfarin and heparin), and chemotherapeutic agents (which may cause thrombocytopenia).

Distinguishing Between Hemoptysis and Hematemesis

Hemoptysis	Hematemesis
Episode preceded by tingling of throat or chest and then a desire to cough	Coughing usually not reported
Nausea/vomiting absent	Nausea/vomiting present
Frothy sputum	Sputum not frothy (low pH)
Blood-tinged sputum persists for days	No blood-tinged sputum
History of lung disease	History of gastric or liver disease
Symptoms related to significant blood loss (eg, orthostasis) uncommon	Symptoms related to significant blood loss common (eg, orthostatic dizziness)
Asphyxia possible	Asphyxia unusual

INTERVIEW FRAMEWORK

The most important step is to assess for alarm symptoms. Some patients with massive hemoptysis will be unable to give an adequate history.

IDENTIFYING ALARM SYMPTOMS

Massive or severe hemoptysis is considered a life-threatening emergency that requires immediate admission for observation and diagnostic evaluation. Respiratory distress may be related to the amount of hemoptysis, but can also result from poor pulmonary reserve due to comorbid medical conditions. Weight loss, advanced age, and a history of smoking are alarm features concerning for malignancy.[6]

Serious Diagnoses

	Approximate Prevalence[a]
Cancer	40%[b]
Infections • Lung abscess • Pneumonia • Tuberculosis • Fungal infections (Aspergillus is associated with massive hemoptysis)	20% (most commonly tuberculosis or lung abscess)

Alveolar hemorrhage syndrome (ANCA-associated vasculitis, microscopic polyangiitis, systemic lupus erythematosus [SLE], Behçet's syndrome, Goodpasture's syndrome, crack cocaine inhalation, etc.)	< 5%

[a]Prevalence may vary with geographic location and patient population, especially among patients with massive hemoptysis.

[b]Bronchiectasis is less serious but accounts for 30% to 40% of cases.

FOCUSED QUESTIONS

QUESTIONS	THINK ABOUT...
History of present illness (HPI)	
Do you have scant to moderate hemoptysis with increased sputum production?	Bronchitis
Do you have hoarseness? *Do you have a personal history of cancer?* *Do you smoke? If so, how much?*	Cancer
Have you had severe or recurrent pneumonia (including tuberculosis)? *Do you chronically produce large amounts of purulent sputum?*	Bronchiectasis
Do you have fever?	Pneumonia, lung abscess
Have your symptoms lasted a few days or less? *Are you producing purulent sputum?*	Pneumonia
Do you have cough, fever, dyspnea, arthralgias, or skin rash?	SLE, other collagen vascular disease
Do you have hematuria, sinusitis, otitis, or skin lesions?	ANCA-associated vasculitis
Have you had tuberculosis in the past? *Have you been exposed to patients with active tuberculosis?* *Are you human immunodeficiency virus (HIV) positive?*	Tuberculosis
Do you have acute chest pain with dyspnea? *Do you have a recent history of immobilization or surgery?*	Pulmonary embolism or infarct
Past medical and surgical histories	
Do you have a history of	
• *Cancer?*	Primary or metastatic lung cancer
• *Deep venous thrombosis or pulmonary embolism?*	Anticoagulant-related bleeding Pulmonary embolism or infarct
• *Cardiovascular disease (arrhythmias, valvular heart disease, ischemic heart disease, congestive heart failure)?*	Anticoagulant-related bleeding

—Continued next page

Continued—

• *Hemoptysis with exertion?*	Mitral stenosis
• *Chronic liver disease?*	Coagulopathy Thrombocytopenia Upper gastrointestinal bleeding
• *Peptic ulcer disease?*	Upper gastrointestinal bleeding
• *Renal disease?*	ANCA-associated vasculitis Goodpasture's syndrome, SLE
• *Transplantation?*	Bacterial, fungal, or mycobacterial pulmonary infections
• *HIV infection?*	Bacterial, fungal, or mycobacterial pulmonary infections Kaposi sarcoma
• *Vascular surgeries or tracheotomy?*	Aortoenteric fistula
• *Bleeding tendencies?*	Hemophilia, other coagulation disorders Medications
• *Chronic obstructive pulmonary disease?*	Lung cancer
Other	
Have you recently traveled to areas or countries where tuberculosis is endemic (Latin America, South Asia, India, Russia, New York)?	Tuberculosis
Do you use injection drugs?	Infections (endocarditis) Cocaine-induced alveolar hemorrhage Cocaine-induced pulmonary infarct
Do you have any occupational exposures?	Possible exposure to toxic inhalants Cancer
Have you had a recent bronchoscopy or pulmonary surgery?	Iatrogenic

DIAGNOSTIC APPROACH (INCLUDING ALGORITHM)

See Figure 26–1 for the diagnostic algorithm for hemoptysis.

CAVEATS

- Every patient with hemoptysis should have chest radiography and, in many cases, computed tomography of the chest. On occasion, small lesions can be missed with a chest radiograph that may change the diagnostic approach (eg, arteriovenous malformations, mediastinal lymphadenopathy).
- No cause will be found after extensive investigation in up to 20% of cases.
- Consider the possibility that some patients may be malingering.
- Bronchoscopy should be considered in patients with the following characteristics: age over 40, tobacco use, prior history of cancer, and hemoptysis lasting more than 1 week. Bronchoscopy should be considered even if the imaging is unrevealing (see Figure 26–1).[7]
- If the chest imaging and/or bronchoscopy is negative, consider ear, nose, and throat evaluation to look for an upper airway bleeding source.

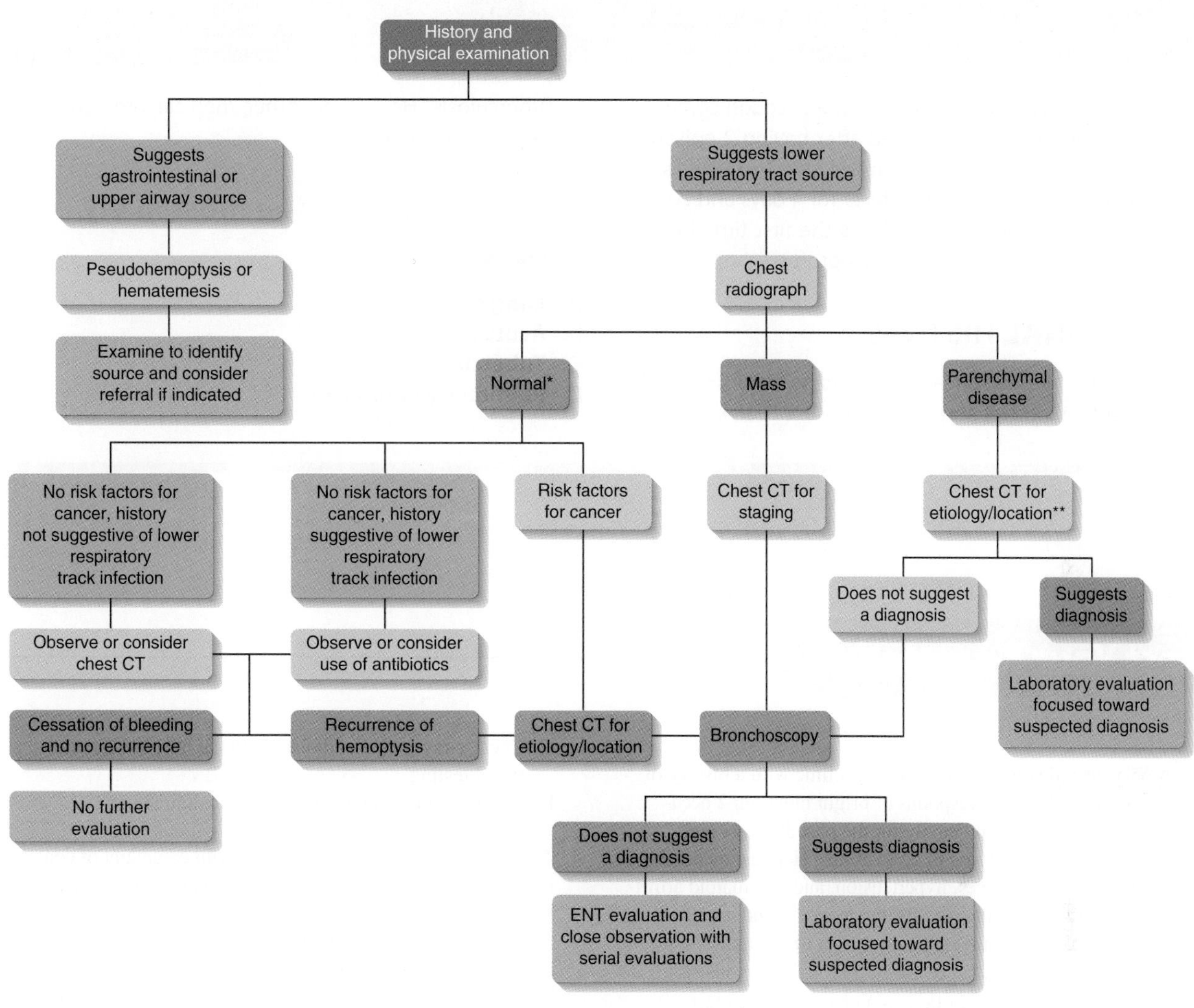

FIGURE 26–1 Diagnostic algorithm: Hemoptysis. CT, computed tomography; ENT, ear, nose, and throat. (Modified from Wineberg SE, Lipson DA. Cough and hemoptysis. In: *Harrison's Principles of Internal Medicine*. 17th ed. New York, NY: McGraw-Hill, 2008:225–228).

PROGNOSIS

The prognosis depends on the amount of hemoptysis, the underlying etiology, and the patient's comorbid conditions. Hemoptysis due to bronchitis has a favorable prognosis and is usually self-limited but may recur. Hemoptysis due to lung cancer, opportunistic infections, and alveolar hemorrhage syndromes has a worse prognosis. Early mortality for the various alveolar hemorrhage syndromes ranges from 25% to 50%.[8] Massive hemoptysis carries a mortality rate of 13% to 58%.[9-12]

CASE SCENARIO | Resolution

A 35-year-old man with history of chronic cough comes to your office and is very concerned after having 2 episodes of prolonged coughing that produced blood-streaked sputum. He also reports subjective fever for 4 days and cough productive of yellow sputum. This is the first time he has experienced this constellation of symptoms.

ADDITIONAL HISTORY

The patient denies dyspnea. He reports no history of smoking, weight loss, travel abroad, or exposure to sick contacts or tuberculosis. He has no other medical problems and takes no medications.

Question: What is the most likely diagnosis?

A. Lung cancer
B. Acute bronchitis
C. Tuberculosis
E. Pulmonary embolism

Test Your Knowledge

1. A 65-year-old woman comes to your clinic with a history of coughing up 1 to 2 tablespoons of bright blood on 2 occasions. She has smoked heavily for the past 30 years and reports recent weight loss of 25 to 30 lbs. Her past medical history includes diabetes, hypertension, and rheumatoid arthritis. Her medications include insulin, atenolol, and ibuprofen.
   What are the alarm features present in this patient?
   A. Quantity of hemoptysis
   B. Advanced age, weight loss, and history of smoking
   C. History of diabetes, hypertension. and rheumatoid arthritis
   D. Current medications

2. In the patient in Question 1, what is the most likely diagnosis?
   A. Bronchitis
   B. Bronchiectasis
   C. Lung cancer
   D. Tuberculosis

3. A 50-year-old woman comes to your office with a history of 2 episodes of coughing blood. The quantity is estimated to be 2 to 3 tablespoons of bright blood on each occasion. She has mild shortness of breath, but she feels comfortable at rest. She has never smoked, denies weight loss or fever, and has no other medical problems.
   What would be the next step in her management?
   A. Referral to a pulmonologist for bronchoscopy
   B. Return to your clinic in the next several weeks to monitor her symptoms
   C. Chest x-ray with an admission to the hospital for additional testing
   D. Complete vital signs and physical examination

4. A 28-year-old man visits your clinic with complaint of coughing up small amounts of blood over the past 2 to 3 weeks and low-grade intermittent fevers for the past 2 months. He smoked for 8 years but stopped 2 to 3 years ago. He reports weight loss of 10 to 15 lbs that he attributes to diet. His laboratory data are unremarkable with the exception of a leukopenia and a positive HIV test.
   What is his most likely diagnosis?
   A. Bronchitis
   B. Bronchiectasis
   C. Lung cancer
   D. Tuberculosis

5. A 30-year-old man comes to the emergency room complaining of mild dyspnea and diffuse chest pain that started suddenly 3 hours ago and worsens with inspiration. While sitting in the waiting room, he has an episode of prolonged coughing that produces small amounts of bright red blood. The physical examination reveals tachycardia and a testicular mass. He has no other medical problems and takes no medications. He just returned from a 12-hour drive to visit his family.
   What is the most likely diagnosis?
   A. Bronchitis
   B. Pulmonary embolism
   C. Pneumonia
   D. Tuberculosis

References

1. Corder R. Hemoptysis. *Emerg Med Clin North Am.* 2003;21:421–435.
2. Lenner R, Schilero G, Lesser M. Hemoptysis: diagnosis and management. *Comp Ther.* 2002;28:7–13.
3. Hirshberg B, Biran I, Glazer M, Kramer MR. Hemoptysis: etiology, evaluation, and outcome in a tertiary referral hospital. *Chest.* 1997;112:440–444.
4. Bidwell JL, Pachner RW. Hemoptysis: diagnosis and management. *Am Fam Physician.* 2005;72:1253–1260.
5. Sakr L, Dutau H. Massive hemoptysis: an update on the role of bronchoscopy in diagnosis and management. *Respiration.* 2010;80:38–58.
6. Jones R, Charlton J, Latinovic R, Gulliford MC. Alarm symptoms and identification of non-cancer diagnoses in primary care: cohort study. *BMJ.* 2009;339:b3094.
7. Thirumaran M, Sundar R, Sutcliffe IM, Currie DC. Is investigation of patients with haemoptysis and normal chest radiograph justified? *Thorax.* 2009;64:854–856.
8. de Prost N, Parrot A, Picard C, et al. Diffuse alveolar hemorrhage: factors associated with in-hospital and long-term mortality. *Eur Respir J.* 2010;35:1303–1311.
9. Ong T, Eng P. Massive hemoptysis requiring intensive care. *Intens Care Med.* 2003;29:317–320.
10. Endo S, Otani S, Saito N, et al. Management of massive hemoptysis in a thoracic surgical unit. *Eur J Cardiothorac Surg.* 2003;23:467–472.
11. Johnson J. Manifestations of hemoptysis. *Postgrad Med.* 2002;112:101–113.
12. Fartoukh M, Khalil A, Louis L, et al. An integrated approach to diagnosis and management of severe haemoptysis in patients admitted to the intensive care unit: a case series from a referral centre. *Respir Res.* 2007;8:11.

Suggested Reading

Corder R. Hemoptysis. *Emerg Med Clin North Am.* 2003;21: 421–435.

Taichman D, Fishman AP. Approach to the patient with respiratory symptoms. In: *Fishman's Pulmonary Diseases and Disorders.* 4th ed. New York, NY: The McGraw-Hill Companies, 2008: 387–425.

SECTION

VI

CARDIOVASCULAR SYSTEM

Chapter 27

Chest Pain

Sumanth D. Prabhu, MD

CASE SCENARIO

A 56-year-old man presents to the emergency department (ED) with a complaint of chest pain that began 60 minutes earlier and has not resolved. He states he has never had a heart attack before. He is a current smoker and has smoked 1 pack per day for 30 years. He has been having intermittent episodes of chest pain off and on for the last 4 months, but today was the first time that the chest pain persisted prompting him to visit the ED.

- **What additional questions would you ask to characterize the chest pain?**
- **What associated features would suggest that chest pain is due to a serious underlying cause?**
- **What associated features would indicate a benign cause for the patient's symptoms?**
- **With additional history, can you reasonably determine the underlying probability of coronary artery disease in this patient?**
- **Can you arrive at a diagnosis to guide further management?**

INTRODUCTION

Chest pain is a commonly encountered symptom in both the emergency department (ED) and the outpatient clinic, resulting from a spectrum of etiologies from minor illness to life-threatening disease. Perhaps the most pressing determination is whether chest pain is due to acute cardiac ischemia or to nonischemic cardiovascular or noncardiac causes. Each of these categories encompasses etiologies that are potentially serious. The initial evaluation, consisting of the history, physical examination, and electrocardiogram (ECG), is exceedingly important for determining the severity and acuity of the clinical presentation and for guiding the proper selection of additional diagnostic and therapeutic modalities. Of these, the history remains the cornerstone of patient assessment.

KEY TERMS[1]

Angina pectoris	Discomfort in the chest and/or adjacent areas (jaw, shoulder, back, arm), usually, but not always, due to myocardial ischemia.
Typical angina	Substernal chest discomfort with the following features: • Characteristic oppressive quality (described as "pressure," "squeezing," or "heaviness," but almost never sharp or stabbing) and duration (typically minutes). • Provoked by exertion or emotional stress. • Relieved by rest or nitroglycerin (within several minutes).
Atypical angina	Chest discomfort that meets 2 of the typical angina characteristics.
Noncardiac chest pain	Chest pain that meets 1 or none of the typical angina characteristics.
Pleuritic chest pain	Sharp chest pain that increases with inspiration or cough.

—Continued next page

Continued—	
Canadian Cardiovascular Society (CCS) Angina Classification System	Clinical grading system based on degree of limitation of ordinary physical activity: Class I: No limitation Class II: Slight limitation Class III: Marked limitation Class IV: Angina occurs with any physical activity or at rest
Myocardial infarction (MI)	Prolonged severe anginal discomfort associated with myocardial necrosis.
Unstable angina (UA)	Angina presenting as rest angina, severe new-onset angina (CCS class III or IV), or acceleration of previously diagnosed effort angina (to at least CCS class III).
Acute coronary syndrome (ACS)	Any clinical presentation compatible with acute myocardial ischemia (encompassing MI and UA).

ETIOLOGY

Chest pain may arise from cardiac, noncardiac, or psychogenic causes. Cardiovascular causes may be subdivided into ischemic and nonischemic etiologies. Myocardial ischemia results from an imbalance between myocardial oxygen supply and demand, such that demand exceeds supply. Ischemic chest pain or angina is most often secondary to obstructive atherosclerotic coronary artery disease (CAD). However, angina may also result from critical aortic stenosis, severe hypertension, hypertrophic cardiomyopathy, severe pulmonary hypertension (with right ventricular ischemia), and coronary spasm. Angina may also be precipitated by extracardiac conditions, such as severe anemia, hypoxia, hyperthyroidism, and hyperviscosity. In all of these conditions, chest pain occurs due to a perturbation of the normal oxygen supply/demand relationship (ie, increased demand and/or decreased supply), even in the absence of CAD. Nonischemic cardiovascular chest pain may accompany aortic dissection, pericarditis, or mitral valve prolapse. Noncardiac chest pain may occur with esophageal and other gastrointestinal (GI) conditions, pulmonary disease, and musculoskeletal and psychiatric disorders. Esophageal pain often resembles angina in quality and frequently is challenging to distinguish from cardiac ischemia. Given the diversity of etiologies for chest pain and the extent of testing required to exclude each possibility, it is difficult to determine the prevalence of every cause.

The prevalence of various disorders is highly dependent on the patient care setting (eg, ED, primary care physician [PCP] office, chest pain observation unit) and the inclusion criteria of the relevant study. In patients presenting to the ED with chest pain, the reported frequency of acute ischemia ranges from 8% to 45%.[2–6] In patients discharged from the ED without a clear diagnosis (ie, acute undifferentiated chest pain), 8% were ultimately found to have ACS.[5] In patients discharged from the coronary care unit with noncardiac chest pain, more than 75% had evidence of esophageal disorders.[7]

Differential Diagnosis

	Prevalence in ED	Prevalence in PCP Office
Cardiovascular		*16%[8]*
Ischemic		
ACS (UA, MI)	8%–45%[2–6]	
Coronary atherosclerosis		
Coronary artery spasm		
Aortic stenosis		
Hypertrophic cardiomyopathy		
Dilated cardiomyopathy		
Tachycardia (ventricular/supraventricular)		
Sympathomimetic toxicity (eg, cocaine)		

Severe hypertension		
Severe pulmonary hypertension		
Severe anemia, hypoxia, hyperviscosity		
Hyperthyroidism, hyperthermia		
Nonischemic		
Aortic dissection	0.003%[9]	
Pericarditis		
Mitral valve prolapse		
Noncardiovascular	*55%–92%*[2–6]	
Gastrointestinal (GI)		8%[8]
Esophageal (spasm, reflux, esophagitis)		
Biliary disease (cholecystitis, choledocholithiasis)		
Peptic ulcer		
Pancreatitis		
Pulmonary		*10%*[8]
Pulmonary embolism (PE)		
Pneumothorax		
Pneumonia		
Pleuritis		
Musculoskeletal		*51%*[8]
Sternoclavicular arthritis		
Costochondritis		
Cervical spine disorders		
Herpes zoster		
Psychogenic		*11%*[8]
Anxiety disorders (hyperventilation, panic attacks)		
Depression		
Somatoform disorders		
Secondary gain		
No diagnosis (undifferentiated)	*23%*[5]	*4%*[8]

GETTING STARTED WITH THE HISTORY

- Remember, acute chest pain may result from potentially life-threatening conditions. Thus, obtain the history in a targeted and expeditious fashion.
- With stable, intermittent chest pain, assess the bedside predictors that distinguish chest pain secondary to cardiovascular disorders versus noncardiovascular disorders.
- Initially, ask open-ended questions so the patient can describe the chest pain. Once a primary description is obtained, quickly move on to more focused questioning for possible underlying etiologies.
- Definitive diagnosis often requires a physical examination, ECG, and additional laboratory testing. However, the history serves as the primary guide for medical decision making.

Questions	Remember
Are you having chest pain right now? If not, when was the last time you had it? How long has this been going on?	Determine whether symptoms are acute or chronic and recurring.
Describe your current chest pain (or a typical prior episode) to me.	Listen to the patient's description.
Does the chest pain prevent you from doing things you would normally do?	Assess the impact of chest pain on the patient's physical activity.

INTERVIEW FRAMEWORK

- Determine whether symptoms represent an ongoing acute episode, which is more likely to be unstable disease, or chronic and recurring episodes, which more often reflect stable disease.
- Characterize the chest pain using the following components:
  - Quality
  - Location
  - Radiation
  - Duration
  - Time course
  - Precipitating/relieving factors
  - Associated symptoms
- Ascertain the presence of associated conditions and risk factors for CAD:
  - Diabetes
  - Smoking
  - Hypertension
  - Hyperlipidemia
  - Family history of premature CAD
  - Postmenopausal status
  - Peripheral vascular disease
  - Cocaine abuse
- Predict the probability of underlying CAD using pain type, age, gender, and risk factors (see below).

IDENTIFYING ALARM SYMPTOMS

Chest pain by itself is an alarm symptom because it can be due to serious causes that require prompt attention. By far, the most common serious cause is acute cardiac ischemia, which includes stable angina, UA, and MI. Albeit less common, other serious conditions to be considered include aortic dissection, PE, spontaneous pneumothorax, pneumonia, and acute GI processes (eg, cholecystitis, pancreatitis) with referred pain.

In general, the suspicion for these serious diagnoses is raised by the results of careful questioning regarding the character and pattern of the pain, associated symptoms, and associated medical conditions. A primary distinction is the differentiation of anginal pain from noncardiac chest pain.

Serious Diagnoses

	Prevalence in ED[a]	Prevalence in PCP Office[a]
Acute myocardial ischemia	8%–45%[2–6]	
• MI	5%–17%[2,4–6]	
• UA	9%–24%[2,4–6]	
• Stable angina and other cardiac conditions	2%–34%[2,4,5]	16%[8]
Aortic dissection	0.003%[9]	
PE		
Spontaneous pneumothorax		
Pneumonia		
Acute GI pathology		

[a]Prevalence is unknown when not indicated.

Alarm Symptoms	If Present, Consider Serious Causes...	Likelihood Ratio (LR)[a]	However, Other Causes for This Feature Include...
Typical angina that is prolonged or occurs at rest OR atypical angina that is prolonged or occurs at rest, with high probability of CAD (see below)	MI UA	1.8–5.8[6,10,11]	Esophageal disease Musculoskeletal chest pain, nonischemic chest pain (eg, mitral valve prolapse), psychogenic chest pain
New-onset or acceleration of effort chest pain (to at least CCS III), typical or atypical with high CAD probability	UA		Esophageal disease Musculoskeletal chest pain Nonischemic chest pain Psychogenic chest pain
Chest pain with prior history of MI	MI UA	2.3–3.8[10,11]	Nonischemic chest pain
Chest pain with diaphoresis (especially profuse diaphoresis)	MI UA PE Aortic dissection	2.0–2.9[6,10]	
Chest pain with nausea/ vomiting	MI UA	1.4–3.5[5,6,10]	Acute GI pathology
Burning chest pain/ indigestion	MI UA	2.3[5]	Gastroesophageal disease
Chest pain radiation to left arm/shoulder	MI UA	1.5–2.3[6,10]	Pericarditis Cervical spine disorders
Chest pain radiation to right arm/shoulder	MI UA	2.4–3.8[5,6,10]	Pericarditis Biliary colic Cervical spine disorders
Chest pain radiation to both arms	MI UA	2.4–7.1[6,10]	Pericarditis Cervical spine disorders
Sudden-onset chest pain and acute dyspnea	PE MI Spontaneous pneumothorax	3.6[12]	Pleuritis Musculoskeletal chest pain
Chest pain with hemoptysis	PE Pneumonia	2.4[12]	Tracheobronchitis
Chest pain with fever	Pneumonia Acute GI pathology		Pleuritis Tracheobronchitis Pericarditis

—Continued next page

Continued—			
Chest pain with syncope (hypotension)	MI PE Arrhythmia Pericardial tamponade	3.1[10]	Vasovagal syncope
Chest pain with palpitations	MI Tachyarrhythmia		
Chest pain with history of Marfan syndrome	Aortic dissection	4.1[9]	
Sudden onset of severe "tearing" or "ripping" chest pain	Aortic dissection	10.8[9]	
Severe persistent chest pain radiating to the back	Aortic dissection Aortic aneurysm		Pericarditis Pancreatitis Peptic ulcer
Severe migrating chest and back pain	Aortic dissection	7.6[9]	

[a]Each LR applies to the adjacent serious cause.

The following features significantly *decrease* the likelihood of MI[6,10,11]:

- Pleuritic chest pain (LR, 0.2)
- Chest pain reproduced by palpation (LR, 0.2–0.4)
- Sharp or stabbing chest pain (LR, 0.3)
- Positional chest pain (LR, 0.3)

The *absence* of sudden-onset chest pain *decreases* the likelihood of acute aortic dissection (LR, 0.3).[13]

As evident from these data, CAD prevalence increases with age. Men with typical angina generally have a high likelihood of CAD, even without risk factors in the older age groups. Women with nonanginal chest pain generally have a low prevalence of CAD.

	Estimating the Pretest Probability (%) of CAD[1,14]					
	Nonanginal Chest Pain		**Atypical Angina**		**Typical Angina**	
Age	**Men**	**Women**	**Men**	**Women**	**Men**	**Women**
30–39 years	3–35	1–19	8–59	2–39	30–88	10–78
40–49 years	9–47	2–22	21–70	5–43	51–92	20–79
50–59 years	23–59	4–25	45–79	10–47	80–95	38–82
60–69 years	49–69	9–29	71–86	20–51	93–97	56–84

NOTE. First number within each range is the probability or prevalence of CAD in patients without risk factors (diabetes, smoking, and hyperlipidemia). Second number is the probability with risk factors. All groups have normal ECGs.

FOCUSED QUESTIONS

Chest pain should be characterized according to the components listed below, and alarm symptoms should be assessed. The pain can be labeled as typical or atypical angina or as noncardiac chest pain. The pain type and the patient's age, gender, and cardiac risk factors allow a reasonable estimation of the probability of underlying CAD.

QUESTIONS	THINK ABOUT...
Quality	
Does it feel like:	
• *Pressure, squeezing, burning, or strangling?*	Myocardial ischemia
• *Tightness or heaviness, "a band across the chest"?*	Esophageal disease (spasm, reflux) (Pulmonary hypertension [with right ventricular ischemia] can present with chest pressure.)
• *Deep, heavy aching (visceral pain)?*	Herpes zoster (prior to rash) can present as a tight band around chest.
• *Indigestion, a need to belch?*	Myocardial ischemia Esophageal disease, peptic ulcer
• *Severe tearing or ripping pain?*	Aortic dissection
• *Sharp and stabbing?*	Pericarditis, pleuritis PE, pneumothorax Musculoskeletal pain Psychogenic pain
• *Dull, persistent ache lasting hours or days localized (< 3 cm) to cardiac apex (inframammary area)?*	Psychogenic pain
Location	
Is the pain diffuse, poorly localized, or retrosternal?	Myocardial ischemia PE
Is pain localized over skin or superficial structures, such as costochondral joints, and reproduced by palpation?	Musculoskeletal pain Costochondritis, chest wall syndrome
Is pain localized (< 3 cm) in the region of the left nipple (circumscribed by 1 finger)?	Noncardiac pain (musculoskeletal, psychogenic, gaseous distention of the stomach)
Radiation	
Does pain radiate to the medial aspect of the left shoulder/arm, right shoulder/arm, or both arms?	Myocardial ischemia Pericarditis Cervical spine disease Cholecystitis (to right shoulder)
Does pain radiate to the lower jaw, neck, or teeth?	Myocardial ischemia
Does pain radiate to the interscapular region or back?	Aortic dissection Thoracic aortic aneurysm Pericarditis Esophageal disease Pancreatitis Peptic ulcer Myocardial ischemia

—Continued next page

Continued—

Does pain radiate to the epigastrium?	Esophageal disease Pancreatitis Peptic ulcer Biliary tract disease Myocardial ischemia
Duration and time course	
How long does it last?	
• *Brief (2–20 minutes)*	Angina pectoris Esophageal disease Musculoskeletal pain Psychogenic pain
• *Very brief (< 15 seconds)*	Noncardiac pain Musculoskeletal pain Hiatal hernia Psychogenic pain
• *Prolonged (> 20 minutes to hours)*	UA/MI Esophageal disease Pulmonary disorders Pericarditis Aortic dissection Musculoskeletal disease Herpes zoster Acute GI pathology Psychogenic pain
Precipitating factors	
What brings the pain on?	
• *Exertion (classically in the cold or against a wind, especially after a heavy meal)*	Angina pectoris
• *Emotional stress or fright*	Angina pectoris Psychogenic pain
• *Eating, meals*	Esophageal pain Peptic ulcer Angina pectoris
• *Lying down or bending after meals*	Esophageal reflux
• *Bending or moving the neck*	Cervical/upper thoracic spine disease
• *Respiration or cough (pleuritic pain)*	PE Pneumothorax Pericarditis, pleuritis Musculoskeletal pain
• *Changes in body position (positional pain)*	Pericarditis Musculoskeletal pain Pancreatitis

Relieving factors	
What relieves the pain?	
• *Rest or sublingual nitroglycerin (usually within 1–5 minutes)*	Angina pectoris Esophageal spasm
• *Sitting up and leaning forward*	Pericarditis Pancreatitis
• *Antacids or food*	Esophagitis, peptic ulcer
• *Holding the breath at deep expiration*	Pleuritis
Associated symptoms	
Do you have any of the following symptoms?	
• *Nausea and vomiting*	Acute myocardial ischemia or MI Acute GI pathology
• *Diaphoresis*	Acute myocardial ischemia or MI PE Aortic dissection
• *Dyspnea*	Acute myocardial ischemia or MI PE Pneumothorax Pneumonia
• *Syncope/hypotension*	Acute myocardial ischemia or MI Massive PE Aortic stenosis Arrhythmia
• *Waterbrash (acid reflux into the mouth)*	Esophageal disease
• *Hemoptysis*	PE, pneumonia
• *Fever*	Pneumonia Pleuritis Pericarditis

DIAGNOSTIC APPROACH (INCLUDING ALGORITHM)

The first step is to determine the acuity of the symptoms. Although there may be overlap, chronic and recurring episodes without any change in symptom pattern are less likely to be emergent and may be evaluated in the outpatient setting. Such diagnoses will include stable angina, GI pain, and musculoskeletal pain. In contrast, an acute or ongoing chest pain episode is more likely to represent an urgent situation and should be evaluated in the ED or inpatient setting. These diagnoses will include UA, MI, aortic dissection, PE, pericarditis, and pneumothorax. In both situations, it is important to assess for alarm symptoms and the probability of underlying CAD. Keep in mind, however, that in addition to the history, proper decision making will also necessitate a targeted physical examination, ECG, and other laboratory testing, as appropriate. See Figure 27–1 for the diagnostic algorithm for chest pain.

CAVEATS

- Angina is often precipitated by effort or physical activity. Thus, it is important to determine whether functional limitations preclude proper assessment of effort-related chest pain or, conversely, whether effort-related chest pain is limiting the patient's physical activity.

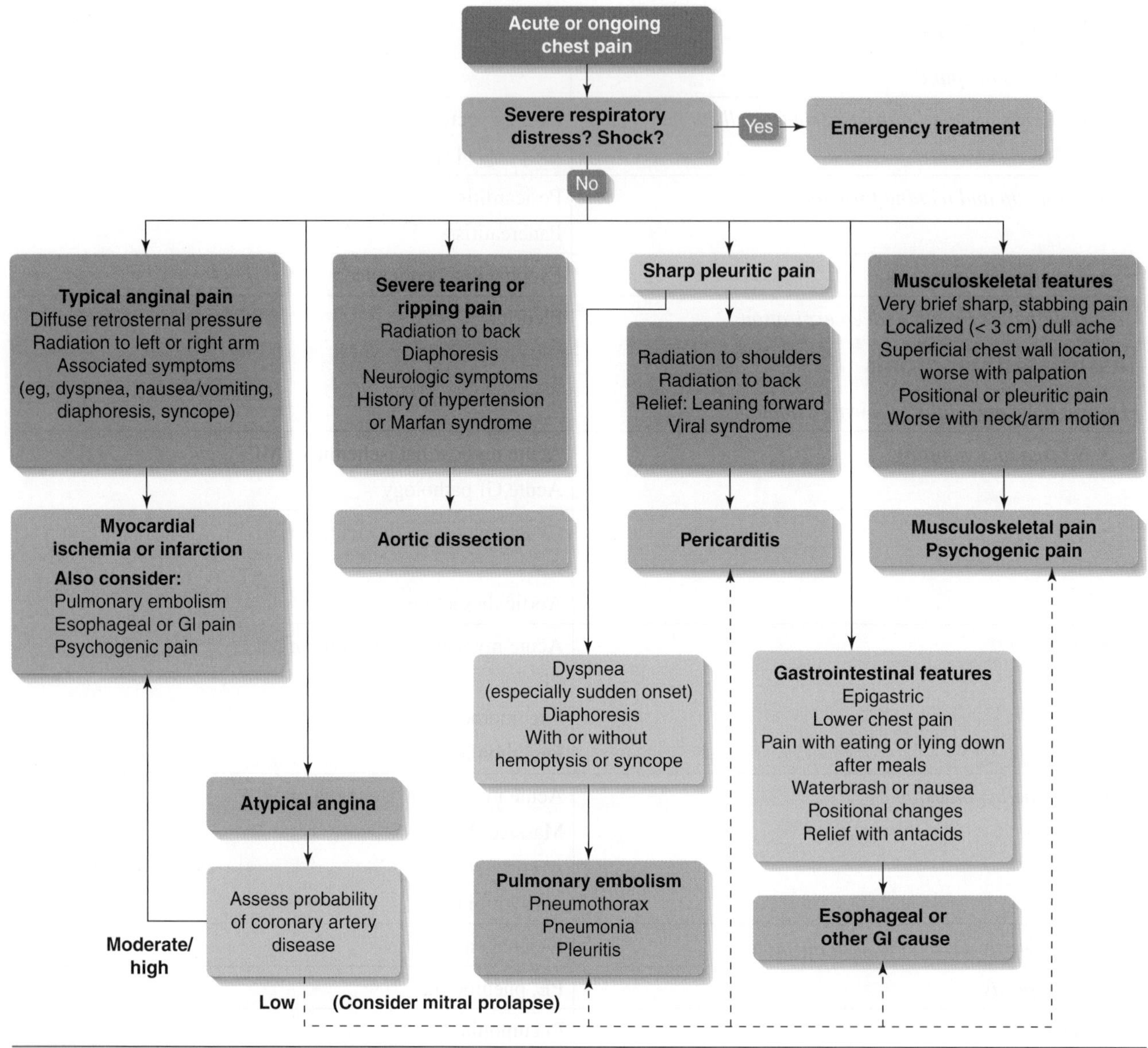

FIGURE 27–1 Diagnostic algorithm: Chest pain. GI, gastrointestinal.

- In clinical practice, myocardial ischemia is the most common serious cause of chest pain encountered. In the majority of patients, this is due to obstructive epicardial CAD.
- Angina is almost never sharp or stabbing, pleuritic, or positional. The following features suggest causes other than angina: (1) very brief pain lasting less than 15 seconds; (2) dull, localized (< 3 cm) pain, especially in the inframammary region; (3) localized, superficial chest pain reproduced by palpation; and (4) radiation to the upper jaw or below the umbilicus.
- In patients with typical angina but low probability of CAD, consider conditions that can produce myocardial ischemia in the absence of significant CAD (eg, systemic or pulmonary hypertension, aortic stenosis, hypertrophic cardiomyopathy, severe anemia, hyperthyroidism).
- Typical angina in an otherwise healthy athlete should raise the possibility of hypertrophic cardiomyopathy, especially if associated with dizziness or presyncope.
- Chest pain associated with PE, although typically pleuritic, may resemble angina due to associated pulmonary hypertension and attendant right ventricular ischemia.
- Be aware of gender differences in chest pain presentation. Atypical angina is more common in women than men. Women with chronic stable angina are more likely to have pain at rest, at sleep, or during mental stress than men.

PROGNOSIS

The prognosis of the patient with chest pain is highly variable and depends on the underlying etiology. Obviously, patients with chest pain due to potentially life-threatening illnesses such as MI, PE, and aortic dissection have a much more guarded prognosis than do patients with esophageal, musculoskeletal, or psychogenic pain. Thus, prompt and targeted evaluation of all patients presenting with chest pain is essential. Specialized chest pain centers with protocol-driven assessment and short-stay observation units can help risk-stratify such patients and efficiently identify those with acute myocardial ischemia versus patients with nonischemic causes.

CASE SCENARIO | Resolution

A 56-year-old man presents to the emergency department (ED) with a complaint of chest pain that began 60 minutes earlier and has not resolved. He states he has never had a heart attack before. He is a current smoker and has smoked 1 pack per day for 30 years. He has been having intermittent episodes of chest pain off and on for the last 4 months, but today was the first time that the chest pain persisted prompting him to visit the ED.

ADDITIONAL HISTORY

The patient initially noticed the chest pain a few months ago while walking or climbing stairs. These episodes would resolve a few minutes after stopping and resting. In the last month, he has noticed that less effort would bring on the pain and has even noticed it while sitting watching television. Today, he awoke from sleep with chest pain that did not go away and so he came to the ED. Today's pain is a diffuse precordial burning and pressure that radiates to both shoulders and arms. Prior episodes have been felt in his lower jaw. Right now he feels nauseous and as if he cannot quite catch his breath; this is something he has never felt previously. On further questioning, some time ago, he was told his cholesterol was high but he never sought further follow-up. He has been under a great deal of stress at work during the last few months.

Question: What is the most likely diagnosis?

A. Acute coronary syndrome
B. Pericarditis
C. Pulmonary embolism
D. Gastroesophageal reflux

Test Your Knowledge

1. You see a 55-year-old woman in the office who reports intermittent chest pain for the last 3 months. She has continued to work as a medical coder but has stopped exercising since she noticed these pains.
   Which of the following features would suggest that her chest pain is not related to myocardial ischemia?
   A. Relationship to effort
   B. Squeezing quality
   C. Association with dyspnea
   D. Pain is sharp and increases with inspiration

2. A 60-year-old male smoker was brought to the ED after passing out while standing up. He regained consciousness a few minutes later but offered complaints of chest pain and dyspnea. The chest pain is right-sided and sharp and worsens with inspiration and cough. His cough is mildly productive and at times blood-tinged. On further questioning, he had felt generally well prior to this episode, although he had knee surgery 6 weeks ago.
   What is the most important diagnostic consideration?
   A. Pericarditis
   B. Pneumonia
   C. Pulmonary embolism
   D. Myocardial infarction
   E. Pneumothorax

3. A 65-year-old man with a prior myocardial infarction presents to your office with intermittent chest pain for the last 10 days. The pain is diffuse and precordial, increases with inspiration or lying down, and is relieved by sitting up and leaning forward. Sometimes the pain can last for hours at a time. It is somewhat different from his prior heart attack pain, but bothers him nonetheless and can bring on a sensation of shortness of breath when it is severe. Three weeks ago, he had what felt like the flu, but this resolved after a few days. The pain is not clearly related to exertion.
   What is the most likely diagnosis?
   A. Pericarditis
   B. Unstable angina
   C. Musculoskeletal chest pain
   D. Pulmonary embolism

References

1. Gibbons RJ, Chatterjee K, Daley J, et al. ACC/AHA/ACP-ASIM guidelines for the management of patients with chronic stable angina: a report of the American College of Cardiology/American Heart Association Task Force on Practice Guidelines (Committee on Management of Patients With Chronic Stable Angina). *J Am Coll Cardiol.* 1999;33:2092–2197.
2. Baxt WG, Shofer FS, Sites FD, Hollander JE. A neural network aid for the early diagnosis of cardiac ischemia in patients presenting to the emergency department with chest pain. *Ann Emerg Med.* 2002;40:575–583.
3. Pozen MW, D'Agostino RB, Selker HP, Sytkowski PA, Hood WB Jr. A predictive instrument to improve coronary-care-unit admission practices in acute ischemic heart disease. A prospective multicenter clinical trial. *N Engl J Med.* 1984;310:1273–1278.
4. Tatum JL, Jesse RL, Kontos MC, et al. Comprehensive strategy for the evaluation and triage of the chest pain patient. *Ann Emerg Med.* 1997;29:116–125.
5. Goodacre SW, Angelini K, Arnold J, Revill S, Morris F. Clinical predictors of acute coronary syndromes in patients with undifferentiated chest pain. *Q J Med.* 2003;96:893–898.
6. Bruyninckx R, Aertgeerts B, Bruyninckx P, Buntinx F. Signs and symptoms in diagnosing acute myocardial infarction and acute coronary syndrome: a diagnostic meta-analysis. *Br J Gen Pract.* 2008;58:105–111.
7. Panju A, Farkouh ME, Sackett DL, et al. Outcome of patients discharged from a coronary care unit with a diagnosis of "chest pain not yet diagnosed." *CMAJ.* 1996;155:541–546.
8. Verdon F, Burnand B, Herzig L, Junod M, Pécoud A, Favrat B. Chest wall syndrome among primary care patients: a cohort study. *BMC Fam Pract.* 2007;8:51.
9. von Kodolitsch Y, Schwartz AG, Nienaber CA. Clinical prediction of acute aortic dissection. *Arch Intern Med.* 2000;160:2977–2982.
10. Panju AA, Hemmelgarn BR, Guyatt GH, Simel DL. The rational clinical examination. Is this patient having a myocardial infarction? *JAMA.* 1998;280:1256–1263.
11. Chun AA, McGee SR. Bedside diagnosis of coronary artery disease: a systematic review. *Am J Med.* 2004;117:334–343.
12. Miniati M, Monti S, Bottai M. A structured clinical model for predicting the probability of pulmonary embolism. *Am J Med.* 2003;114:173–179.
13. Klompas M. Does this patient have an acute thoracic aortic dissection? *JAMA.* 2002;287:2262–2272.
14. Pryor DB, Shaw L, McCants CB, et al. Value of the history and physical in identifying patients at increased risk for coronary artery disease. *Ann Intern Med.* 1993;118:81–90.

Suggested Reading

American College of Emergency Physicians. Clinical policy for the initial approach to adults presenting with a chief complaint of chest pain, with no history of trauma. *Ann Emerg Med.* 1995;25: 274–299.

Douglas PS, Ginsburg GS. The evaluation of chest pain in women. *N Engl J Med.* 1996;334:1311–1315.

Gencer B, Vaucher P, Herzig L, et al. Ruling out coronary heart disease in primary care patients with chest pain: a clinical prediction score. *BMC Med.* 2010;8:9.

Han JH, Lindsell CJ, Hornung RW, et al; Emergency Medicine Cardiac Research and Education Group Internet Tracking Registry for Acute Coronary Syndromes (i*trACS) Investigators. The elder patient with suspected acute coronary syndromes in the emergency department. *Acad Emerg Med.* 2007;14:732–739.

Mant J, McManus RJ, Oakes RA, et al. Systematic review and modelling of the investigation of acute and chronic chest pain presenting in primary care. *Health Technol Assess.* 2004;8:1–158.

Paterson WG. Canadian Association of Gastroenterology Practice Guidelines: management of noncardiac chest pain. *Can J Gastroenterol.* 1998;12:401–407.

Chapter 28

Palpitations

Zachary B. Holt, MD, and Craig R. Keenan, MD

CASE SCENARIO

A 25-year-old man with a history of panic disorder complains of an intermittent rapid heartbeat accompanied by chest pain, a sense of impending doom, and dizziness. He has had these symptoms for 6 months, but they have become more frequent over the past 2 weeks. He "may have blacked out for a few seconds" during an episode a few days ago. He is worried about a possible fatal arrhythmia.

- **Which aspect of the history is most concerning?**
- **Using the history, how does one determine the etiology of palpitations?**
- **Does a history of panic disorder exclude a serious underlying etiology?**

INTRODUCTION

Palpitations are defined as the awareness of one's own heartbeats. Palpitations are a frequent reason for visits to both primary care and cardiology practices, reported in up to 16% of medical outpatients.[1] Although many patients with palpitations have a psychiatric disorder or other benign condition, potentially morbid or mortal arrhythmias must also be considered. Investigation may include expensive and sometimes invasive diagnostic testing, underscoring the importance of a thoughtful clinical evaluation. Because many patients have intermittent symptoms that do not occur during the clinician's examination, the history plays a key role.

KEY TERMS

Palpitations	An awareness of one's own heartbeats.
Arrhythmia	A heart rhythm that results from abnormal or disorganized cardiac conduction.
Supraventricular tachycardia (SVT)	An arrhythmia originating in the atria or the atrioventricular node.
Ventricular tachycardia (VT)	An arrhythmia originating from the ventricles, usually denoting serious cardiac pathology.
Syncope	Transient loss of consciousness with spontaneous recovery (see Chapter 29).
Presyncope	Sensation that one may lose consciousness.
Panic disorder	A psychiatric disorder characterized by episodic panic attacks about which there may be persistent concern or anxiety.
Somatization	A dysfunctional psychological process characterized by the generation of physical symptoms as a result of psychological distress.

ETIOLOGY

Palpitations may result from an abnormal cardiac rhythm, sinus tachycardia associated with a medical condition or psychiatric disorder, or heightened awareness of normal sinus rhythm (Table 28–1). The literature on palpitations generally distinguishes between *any* cardiac rhythm disturbance such as sinus tachycardia or ectopy (ie, premature atrial or ventricular contractions) and a *serious* rhythm disturbance such as supraventricular tachycardia (SVT) or ventricular tachycardia (VT). In a widely cited study, Weber and Kapoor[2] followed 190 patients with palpitations presenting to the emergency department (ED), to a clinic, or for hospital admission. They found a cardiac etiology in 43.2% (68% were serious arrhythmias and 25% were premature atrial or ventricular beats), whereas psychiatric causes constituted 30.5%. In outpatient subjects (28% of the sample), the etiology of palpitations was psychiatric in 45% of patients and cardiac in only 21%. This finding suggests that ED patients have a higher pretest probability of cardiac etiology, although presentation to the ED was not an independent predictor of cardiac etiology.[2] A more recent study of 127 outpatients with palpitations reported an arrhythmia prevalence of 65%, but after excluding subjects with sinus tachycardia or premature beats, this number dropped to 19%.[3] Lastly, a United Kingdom study of 184 cardiology clinic patients found a clinically significant arrhythmia in 34%, premature ectopic beats in 41%, and an awareness of sinus rhythm in the remainder.[4] However, follow-up was limited to 3 months. Thus, although some patients with palpitations have a serious underlying cardiac disorder, most have a benign etiology.

Table **28-1.** **Differential diagnosis of palpitations (prevalence listed where available).**[2,3]

Cardiac	*Arrhythmia* Atrial fibrillation (8%–10%) Atrial flutter (6%) Sick sinus syndrome (1%) *Other SVT* (9%–10%) • Atrioventricular nodal re-entry tachycardia • Atrioventricular re-entry tachycardia • Paroxysmal atrial tachycardia • Multifocal atrial tachycardia Ventricular tachycardia (2%) Premature atrial or ventricular contractions (11%–31%) *Other* Mitral valve prolapse (1.1%) Aortic regurgitation (1.1%) Atrial myxoma (0.5%)
Psychiatric	Panic disorder or panic attack (27%) Agoraphobia Any other phobia Generalized anxiety disorder Somatization disorder Depression
Sinus tachycardia	Hyperthyroidism (2.6%) Hypoglycemia Fever Sepsis Hypovolemia Anemia (1.1%) Stimulants (3.2%) Medications (2.6%) Pheochromocytoma Mastocytosis Idiopathic
Normal sinus rhythm	Cause of palpitations unclear (16%–33%)

Palpitations often reflect an underlying psychiatric illness. Many patients referred for work-up of palpitations have current or past anxiety, depressive, or somatization disorders, constituting 45% of patients referred for Holter monitoring in one series.[5] Patients with high indices of somatization and hypochondriasis are less likely to have symptoms that correlate with an electrocardiographic rhythm disturbance and are no more accurate than controls at perceiving normal cardiac activity.[6,7]

Although it is a common practice to attribute palpitations to panic disorder, there is substantial overlap in the clinical features of panic disorder and arrhythmia. The diagnosis of one does not preclude the presence of the other. In a retrospective study of 107 subjects with known SVT, 67% met *Diagnostic and Statistical Manual of Mental Disorders* (DSM) criteria for panic disorder. Only 45% of subjects were correctly diagnosed with an SVT during initial evaluation. The remaining 55% did not have their SVT recognized for a median of 3.3 years, an unfortunate error particularly prominent in young female patients.[8]

INTERVIEW FRAMEWORK AND GETTING STARTED WITH THE HISTORY

- Let patients describe the symptoms in their own words before asking any closed-ended questions.
- The focus of the interview is to identify patients who require diagnostic testing for serious arrhythmia.
- Identification of a psychiatric disorder will benefit the patient even if unrelated to the palpitations.

ALARM SYMPTOMS

Unfortunately, most studies on the diagnostic accuracy of the history in evaluating palpitations fail to distinguish between benign arrhythmias (ie, those that require no further management; eg, ectopic beats) and arrhythmias requiring further action (eg, atrial fibrillation or VT). Historical features that warrant further investigation for a potential serious arrhythmia include:

- Palpitations associated with syncope or presyncope: Syncope or presyncope symptoms suggest VT or SVT that is sufficiently rapid to reduce effective cardiac output.[9]
- A family history of sudden cardiac death or known arrhythmia: This raises concern for idiopathic VT arising from the right ventricular outflow tract, Brugada syndrome, Wolf-Parkinson-White syndrome, or the prolonged QT syndrome.
- Use of any medications known to prolong the QT interval, such as methadone, antiarrhythmic agents, or antipsychotics[10]: Acquired prolongation of the QT interval can lead to serious ventricular arrhythmias.
- A personal history of heart disease, including coronary artery disease, congenital or valvular heart disease, hypertrophic cardiomyopathy, or dilated cardiomyopathy: This is a predictor of serious arrhythmia.[10] In the absence of a personal history of heart disease symptoms such as chest pain or dyspnea are less helpful because these are often present in panic disorder.[11]

FOCUSED QUESTIONS

- Note the patient's age and gender. Older patients are more likely to have arrhythmias associated with structural heart disease, such as atrial fibrillation or VT. Women constitute a higher proportion of patients with atrioventricular nodal re-entrant tachycardia (AVNRT).
- Elicit a detailed description of the palpitations. In addition, ask the patient to tap out the rhythm of the perceived heartbeats to differentiate between regular and irregular rhythms and fast versus slow rhythms. The sensation of skipped beats or "flip-flopping" in the chest suggests a premature systole with a subsequent pause and forceful contraction. "Fluttering" is nonspecific but may indicate a rhythm disturbance with a fast rate. A rapid and regular pounding sensation in the neck, sometimes associated with witnessed neck pulsations (the "frog sign"), suggests atrioventricular dissociation, the result of simultaneous atrial and ventricular contraction. AVNRT is a common cause of atrioventricular dissociation, but one must also consider premature ventricular contractions and VT.[9]
- Elicit the circumstances in which the palpitations occur. Palpitations in younger patients associated with high-catecholamine states such as exercise or extreme fear may indicate VT, including torsades de pointes due to long QT syndrome (although sinus tachycardia is a far more common cause). Palpitations that occur after termination of exercise in young and middle-aged men may be from SVT, particularly atrial fibrillation, due to relatively increased vagal tone. Palpitations on standing suggest AVNRT.[9]
- Ask about associated symptoms.
  - Syncope or presyncope (alarm symptom) (see Chapter 29 on syncope)
  - Chest pain
  - Shortness of breath
  - Stroke symptoms
  - Vagal symptoms such as diaphoresis
  - Polyuria (atrial stretch causes release of natriuretic peptide, which causes diuresis)
- Take a detailed medication history, concentrating on:
  - Recreational or prescription stimulant use
  - Street drugs such as cocaine or methamphetamines
  - Caffeine

Table **28-2.** **Specific elements of history and suggested etiology.**

Historical Feature	Suggested Diagnosis
Man	Any cardiac etiology
Woman	AVNRT
Younger	Panic disorder Arrhythmia due to bypass tract
Older	Arrhythmia associated with structural heart disease, such as atrial fibrillation or ventricular tachycardia
Fast rate	Arrhythmia
History of panic disorder, anxiety, or hypochondriasis	Sinus tachycardia or perception of sinus rhythm
Description of irregular beat	Arrhythmia
History of heart disease, including hypertension	Arrhythmia
Episodes exceed 5 minutes	Arrhythmia
Perception of neck fullness or regular pounding sensation in neck ("frog throat")	AVNRT
Vagal symptoms (diaphoresis, light-headedness, nausea)	Arrhythmia
Onset associated with excess catecholamine state (exercise, extreme fear)	Ventricular tachycardia or sinus tachycardia
Onset associated with termination of catecholamine state	Atrial fibrillation
Polyuria	SVT
Use of stimulant	Sinus tachycardia
Use of QT-prolonging medication	Torsades de pointes, ventricular tachycardia

- Alcohol
- Tobacco
- β-Agonists
- Theophylline

Table **28-3.** **Selected likelihood ratios (LR) for presence of any arrhythmia.**[10]

Regular rapid pounding in neck	LR+ 177 (CI, 25–1251) [for AVNRT]
Palpitations affecting sleep	LR+ 2.29
Palpitations while at work	LR+ 2.17
History of cardiac disease	LR+ 2.03
Male gender	LR+ 1.73
Description of regular beat	LR+ 1.66
Description of irregular beat	LR+ 1.65
Episode duration < 5 minutes	LR+ 0.38
History of panic disorder	LR+ 0.26 (CI includes 1.0)

CI, confidence interval.

- Medications that can prolong the QT interval or cause arrhythmias.[12] Below are some of the better known offenders; a far more comprehensive list may be found at www.torsades.org:
  - Antiarrhythmics
  - Methadone
  - Antipsychotics (phenothiazines, risperidone)
  - Antibiotics (clarithromycin, erythromycin, sparfloxacin)
  - Antiemetics (droperidol, domperidone)
  - Protease inhibitors
  - Diuretics (by way of electrolyte abnormalities)
- Take a detailed psychiatric history, including history of anxiety, depression, bipolar disorder, posttraumatic stress disorder, panic disorder, and somatization.

DIAGNOSTIC APPROACH (INCLUDING ALGORITHM)

The clinician's first task is to assess for associated syncope, presyncope, and other alarm symptoms. The remainder of the interview should be tailored to the individual patient and generally include a psychiatric history. A careful physical

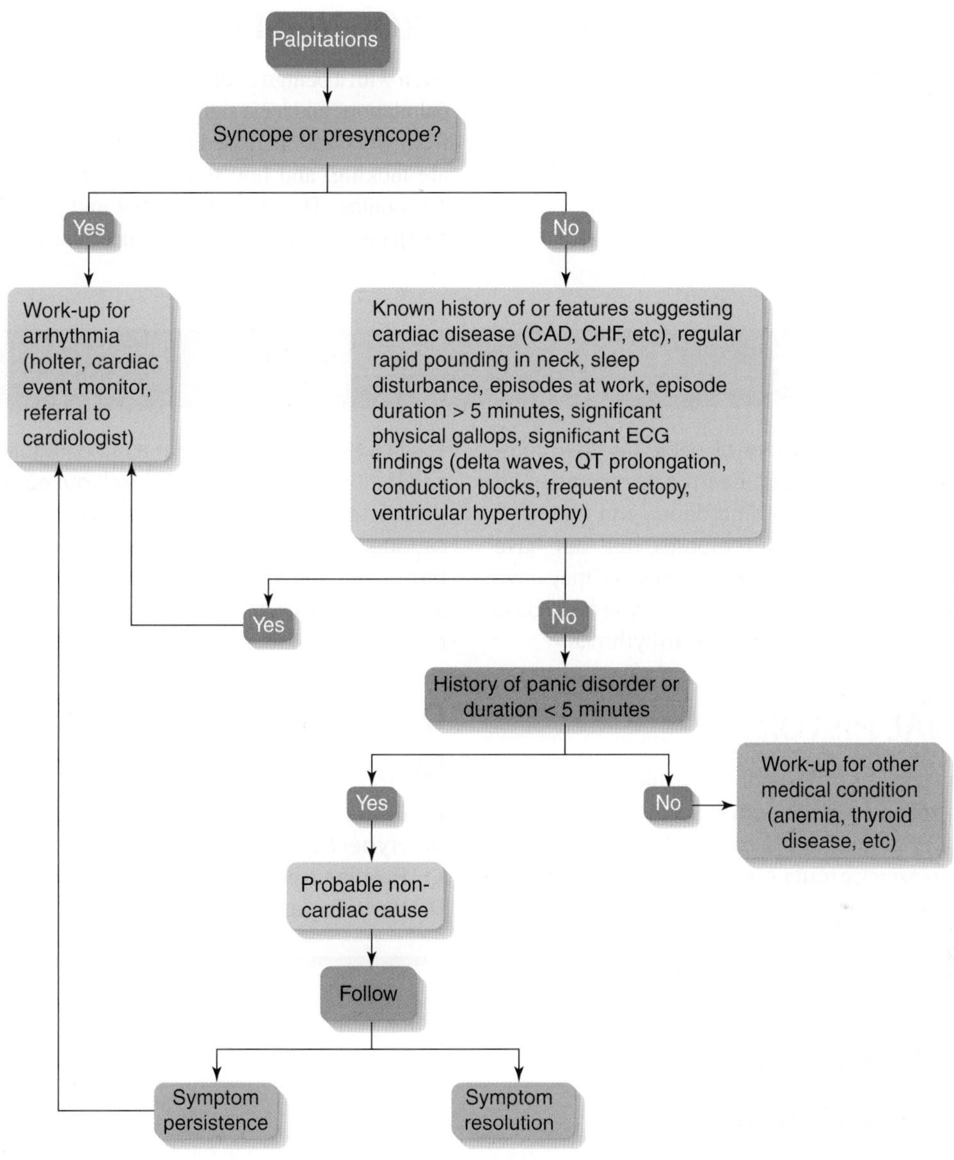

FIGURE 28–1 Diagnostic algorithm: Palpitations. CAD, coronary artery disease; CHF, congestive heart failure; ECG, electrocardiogram.

examination, particularly the cardiac examination, is done to look for evidence of arrhythmia or structural heart disease (eg, cardiomegaly, heart murmurs, gallops). Electrocardiography is generally required to look for evidence of arrhythmia (eg, premature contractions, SVT), structural heart disease (eg, left ventricular hypertrophy, Q waves from prior myocardial infarction, delta waves of Wolff-Parkinson-White syndrome), or conduction abnormalities (eg, QT prolongation). If the patient has abnormalities on history, examination, or electrocardiogram, the clinician should pursue further testing. This often entails prolonged electrocardiographic monitoring or occasionally electrophysiologic study. Consultation with a cardiologist may be helpful if the diagnosis remains unclear or if arrhythmia is highly suspected. See Figure 28–1 for the diagnostic algorithm for palpitations.

CAVEATS

- No single element of the history can reliably distinguish between arrhythmic and nonarrhythmic causes of palpitations.
- Palpitations in and of themselves are neither sensitive nor specific for arrhythmia.
- Many arrhythmias are asymptomatic and will not correlate with symptoms reported during ambulatory electrocardiographic monitoring.
- Most outpatients with palpitations do not have an arrhythmia and unreliably perceive their own cardiac activity.

- Syncope in association with palpitations should prompt a work-up for serious arrhythmia.
- Physicians tend to underdiagnose arrhythmias in patients with psychiatric disorders and palpitations.
- The diagnosis of an anxiety disorder does not preclude the diagnosis of an arrhythmia.

PROGNOSIS

Even with a benign etiology, most patients continue to experience palpitations and have significant disability, including time missed from work and increased medical utilization.[2] Data on mortality are lacking, and few studies follow subjects for longer than 12 months. The study by Weber and Kapoor[2] had 3 deaths in 190 patients at 1 year of follow-up, none related to arrhythmia.

CASE SCENARIO | Resolution

A 25-year-old man with a history of panic disorder complains of an intermittent rapid heartbeat accompanied by chest pain, a sense of impending doom, and dizziness. He has had these symptoms for 6 months, but they have become more frequent over the past 2 weeks. He "may have blacked out for a few seconds" during an episode a few days ago. He is worried about a possible fatal arrhythmia.

ADDITIONAL HISTORY

On further questioning, the patient's panic disorder has been well controlled for years with psychotherapy. He has no known history of heart disease. Over the last 6 months, he has begun an exercise routine, and his palpitations, when they occur, have been consistently associated with this activity. He is able to tap out a rapid, regular pattern to the palpitations. He describes his black-out episode as a perception of tunnel vision near the conclusion of his morning jog, causing him to stop and sit down on the sidewalk, where he passed out and awoke after an unknown length of time. He elaborates on his fear of "dropping dead" and explains that an aunt died suddenly while swimming 5 years ago.

Question: What is the most likely diagnosis?

A. Panic disorder
B. Hyperthyroidism
C. Premature atrial contractions
D. Ventricular tachycardia

Test Your Knowledge

1. A 29-year-old man reports episodic palpitations for the last 2 months. He has recently taken a job as a construction worker and is working on a new high-rise building. He has the episodes whenever he is working on the roof. He reports associated diaphoresis and shortness of breath but denies personal history of cardiac disease, family history of arrhythmia, or dizziness.

   Which of the following points in the history would be *most* reassuring?

   A. Polyuria
   B. A personal history of panic disorder and multiple unexplained symptoms
   C. A family history of long QT syndrome
   D. Use of diphenhydramine for seasonal allergies

2. A 67-year-old woman reports intermittent fluttering in her chest that is not associated with any activity or circumstance. She also has chronic dyspnea with exertion and a history of generalized anxiety. When asked to tap out the rhythm, it is irregular. She was prescribed a diuretic 2 weeks ago for chronic lower extremity edema, which incidentally has improved her difficulty breathing.

   What is the most likely diagnosis?

   A. Atrioventricular node re-entry tachycardia
   B. Panic disorder
   C. Atrial fibrillation

3. A 22-year-old woman presents to your clinic with a 1-year history of a frequent "flip-flopping" sensation in her chest. She has no personal or family history of heart disease and notices her symptoms most after her morning coffee. Two days ago, she got very light-headed during an episode and had to sit down because she thought she was very close to passing out. She was recently put on erythromycin for sinusitis.

   Which of the following statements is most accurate?

   A. She requires no further work-up
   B. An electrocardiogram should be performed to look for QT prolongation
   C. Her symptoms are certain to resolve if she stops ingesting caffeine

References

1. Barsky A, Ahern D, Delamater A. Predictors of persistent palpitations and continued medical utilization. *J Fam Pract.* 1996;42:465–472.
2. Weber BE, Kapoor WN. Evaluation and outcomes of patients with palpitations. *Am J Med.* 1996;100:138–148.
3. Hoefman E, Boer KR, van Weert HCPM, Reitsma JB, Koster RW, Bindels PJE. Predictive value of a history taking and physical examination in diagnosing arrhythmias in general practice. *Fam Pract.* 2007;24:636–641.
4. Mayou R, Sprigings D, Birkhead J, Price J. Characteristics of patients presenting at a cardiac clinic with palpitation. *Q J Med.* 2003;96:115–123.
5. Barsky A, Cleary P, Coeytaux R, Ruskin J. Psychiatric disorders in medical outpatients complaining of palpitations. *J Gen Intern Med.* 1994;9:306–313.
6. Barsky A, Cleary P, Barnett M, Christiansen C, Ruskin J. The accuracy of symptom reporting by patients complaining of palpitations. *Am J Med.* 1994;97:214–221.
7. Barsky A, Cleary P, Sarnie M, Ruskin J. Panic disorder, palpitations, and the awareness of cardiac activity. *J Nerv Ment Dis.* 1994;182:63–71.
8. Lessmier T, Gamperling D, Johnosn-Liddon V, et al. Unrecognized paroxysmal supraventricular tachycardia: potential for misdiagnosis as panic disorder. *Arch Intern Med.* 1997;157:537–543.
9. Zimetbaum P, Josephson ME. Evaluation of patients with palpitations. *N Engl J Med.* 1998;338:1369–1373.
10. Thavendiranathan P, Bagai A, Khoo C, et al. Does this patient with palpitations have a cardiac arrhythmia? *JAMA.* 2009;302:2135–2143.
11. Brugada P, Gursoy S, Brugada J, Andries E. Investigation of palpitations. *Lancet.* 1993;341:1254–1258
12. Roden D. Drug-induced prolongation of the QT interval. *N Engl J Med.* 2004;350:1013–1022.

Suggested Reading

Barsky A. Palpitations, arrhythmias, and awareness of cardiac activity. *Ann Intern Med.* 2001;134:832–837.

Center for Education and Research on Therapeutics. Available at: http://www.azcert.org/medical-pros/qt-registry/step01a-sign-in.asp.

Thavendiranathan P, Bagai A, Khoo C, et al. Does this patient with palpitations have a cardiac arrhythmia? *JAMA.* 2009;302:2135-2143.

Chapter 29

Syncope

John Wolfe Blotzer, MD, and Mark C. Henderson, MD

CASE SCENARIO

A 20-year-old college wrestler comes to your office with his mother because she is concerned that he has "passed out" in church. While attending Sunday services during the summer, he has twice become dizzy while standing and slumped to the floor. He was briefly "out of it" but revived quickly when taken outside. On each occasion, he insisted on completing the religious service.

- **What questions would you ask to further define these episodes?**
- **How would you classify these episodes to determine their likely cause?**
- **Can you make a definite diagnosis based on history?**
- **What questions help distinguish benign episodes from life-threatening ones?**

INTRODUCTION

Syncope is a syndrome of sudden, brief loss of consciousness and postural tone with spontaneous, complete recovery resulting from transient global cerebral hypoperfusion. Syncope may be associated with injury due to loss of consciousness or sudden death from an underlying cardiac cause. It is very common, accounting for up to 3% of emergency department visits and 6% of hospital admissions.[1] Syncope is usually benign and most often caused by a vasovagal episode. Patients typically complain of "fainting," "passing out," falling out," a "dizzy spell," "blackout," "fall," or "collapse." The historian must distinguish syncope from other forms of dizziness such as presyncope, vertigo, disequilibrium, and vaguely described "light-headedness" or "giddiness" (see Chapter 6, Dizziness). Seizures, metabolic disturbances (eg, hypoglycemia), and concussion must be distinguished from syncope and do not result from temporary global cerebral hypoperfusion.

KEY TERMS

Neurally mediated syncope, neural reflex syncope, vasodepressor syncope, neurocardiogenic syncope	Interchangeable terms for syncope primarily involving neural or reflex mechanisms. Examples include vasovagal, situational, and carotid sinus syncope.
Situational syncope	Syncope associated with specific activities (eg, micturition, defecation, coughing, and swallowing).
Vasovagal syncope	The common faint, the most common neural reflex disorder causing syncope.
Syncope mimics	Disorders characterized by loss of consciousness (LOC) that is either prolonged (ie, not transient) or does **not** result from cerebral hypoperfusion (eg, seizures, hypoxia, hypercapnia, intoxications, etc).
Pseudosyncope	Psychogenic (syncope associated with psychiatric disease)

ETIOLOGY[1–7]

Most patients with a simple fainting spell, or vasovagal syncope, do not seek medical attention. Etiologies of syncope vary depending on the clinical setting, study population, definition of syncope, and rigor of the diagnostic evaluation. For instance, psychiatric disease generally causes "pseudosyncope," not true syncope; nevertheless, it is classified as syncope in a number of studies. In general, syncope is classified into the following major categories:

- Reflex (neurally) mediated syncope
- Orthostatic hypotension
- Cerebrovascular disease (a rare cause of syncope)
- Medication-induced syncope
- Cardiac syncope (due to organic heart disease and arrhythmias)
- Syncope due to an unknown cause

Recent studies have classified fewer patients with syncope as having an unknown cause, probably due to more extensive diagnostic evaluation. In a Swiss study of patients with syncope presenting to an emergency department, the causes were as follows: vasodepressor (37%), orthostatic hypotension (24%), carotid sinus hypersensitivity (1%), neurologic (5%), arrhythmias (7%), pulmonary embolism (1%), acute coronary syndromes (1%), aortic stenosis (1%), psychiatric (1.5%), unknown (14%), and miscellaneous (1.5%).[2] A recent study of patients evaluated by electrophysiology demonstrated the following causes: vasovagal (47%), situational (0.7%), carotid sinus hypersensitivity (7.9%), autonomic dysfunction/orthostatic hypotension (5.6%), cerebrovascular disease (1.9%), bradyarrhythmias (13.6%), supraventricular tachyarrhythmias (9.8%), ventricular tachyarrhythmias (12.1%), long QT or hypertrophic cardiomyopathy (1.1%), and unknown (19.8%). Furthermore, 18.4% of patients were considered to have multiple potential causes.[7] The institutionalized elderly are especially apt to have multifactorial syncope.[8]

Differential Diagnosis

	Prevalence
Reflex-mediated	
• Vasovagal syncope	8%–47%
• Situational syncope	1%–8%
• Carotid sinus syncope	0%–8%
Orthostatic hypotension (including volume loss, autonomic insufficiency, adrenal insufficiency, pheochromocytoma, medications)	4%–24%
Neurologic disease (including vertebrobasilar transient ischemic attack, basilar migraine, subclavian steal, and glossopharyngeal neuralgia)	0%–5%
Medications	1%–7%
Cardiac syncope	
• Organic heart disease (including aortic stenosis, hypertrophic cardiomyopathy, pulmonary embolism, pulmonary hypertension, atrial myxoma, myocardial infarction, critical coronary artery disease [left main coronary artery or equivalent], pericardial tamponade, and aortic dissection)	1%–8%
• Arrhythmias (sinus node disease, second- or third-degree heart block, pacemaker malfunction, ventricular tachycardia, torsades de pointes, and supraventricular tachycardia; may also be due to medications that prolong the QT interval)	4%–38%
Unknown	13%–41%
Psychiatric	0%–5%
Miscellaneous (including hypoglycemia, hyperventilation, etc)	0%–7%

GETTING STARTED WITH THE HISTORY

- In addition to the patient, interview any observers of the episode.
- Remember that *syncope* is a medical term. The patient will often report *fainting, falling out, passing out, dizziness,* a *spell,* or *blacking out.*
- Take a thorough family history, past medical history, and current medication history.

Questions	Tips for Effective Interviewing
Please describe for me everything you remember about your (most recent) episode.	Allow the patient to tell the entire story in his or her own words.
Has this ever happened before?	Avoid interrupting.
Describe exactly what you were doing prior to the episode.	Acknowledge the patient's emotions, as losing consciousness can be very frightening.
Describe everything you remember witnesses telling you they observed during the episode.	Respond to the patient's concerns.

INTERVIEW FRAMEWORK

- Determine whether the patient experienced true syncope (abrupt loss of consciousness, loss of postural reflexes, and spontaneous and complete return to consciousness without intervention) rather than another type of "dizziness" or seizure (see Chapter 6).
- If the episode was observed, interview the witness(es).
- Determine the circumstances surrounding the episode, such as body position (standing, sitting, or supine), activity, and environment.
- Determine whether there were any premonitory symptoms before the loss of consciousness (especially important for vasovagal syncope).
- Determine features common to all episodes.
- Assess for alarm symptoms (see below).
- Determine whether there is underlying heart disease (confers a worse prognosis).
- Classify syncope into one of the following subtypes:
  - **Reflex-mediated syncope**, which is suggested by the following: (1) absence of cardiac disease or family history of sudden death; (2) previous history of syncope or family history of syncope (a parental history of fainting increases the relative probability of fainting in offspring, particular if both parents are affected [hazard ratio of 3.35 for the daughter and 11.82 for the son[9]]); (3) occurs after pain or sudden unexpected sight (eg, blood), smell, or sound; (4) prolonged standing in a close, hot environment (eg, crowded assembly); (5) "graying out," loss of hearing, nausea, or vomiting; (6) occurs during or after eating; (7) occurs after exertion; and (8) occurs with pressure on carotid sinus (eg, tight collar, shaving, tumor) or head turning.
  - **Orthostatic hypotension**, which is suggested by the following: (1) occurs after standing up; (2) recent start or change in medication or alcohol use; (3) volume loss (eg, dehydration, occult blood loss); (4) prolonged standing in a close, hot environment (eg, crowded assembly); (5) history of parkinsonism or autonomic neuropathy; and (6) occurs after exertion or with weight lifting or brass instrument use.
  - **Cerebrovascular**, which is suggested by the following: (1) occurrence with arm exercise; (2) blood pressure or pulse differences between the right and left arm; (3) known subclavian steal syndrome; (4) focal neurologic features suggestive of vertebrobasilar transient ischemic attack; or (5) history of migraine.
  - **Medication-induced**, which is suggested by the following: history of a new or increased dose of a vasoactive medication associated with orthostatic hypotension (eg, antihypertensives, anticholinergics), diuretics (via volume loss), or antiarrhythmic agents.
  - **Cardiac syncope**, which is suggested by the following: (1) a family history of sudden death or heart disease; (2) history of organic heart disease (positive likelihood ratio [LR+], 1.7; negative likelihood ratio [LR–], 0.11; absence of a cardiac history has a 97% negative predictive value for cardiac syncope[10]); (3) history of palpitations or arrhythmias; (4) syncope in the supine position; (5) and syncope during exercise.

IDENTIFYING ALARM SYMPTOMS

- Although the etiology of most syncope is vasovagal and has an excellent prognosis, syncope may herald sudden death or be the presenting manifestation of a life-threatening illness such as myocardial infarction, aortic dissection, pulmonary embolism, ventricular tachyarrhythmias, or complete heart block. Patients with cardiac syncope are at increased risk for death, which is related to the underlying heart disease (not the syncope per se). For instance, exertional syncope from aortic stenosis suggests very advanced disease (with mean survival of 2 years unless the valve is replaced).
- In a preliminary, single-center study of emergency department patients with syncope or near syncope, the presence of 1 of 5 clinical variables predicted serious short-term outcomes.[11] Of these, 2 risk factors were historical: shortness of breath and history of congestive heart failure (the other 3 risk factors were abnormal electrocardiogram, systolic blood pressure < 90 mm Hg, or hematocrit < 30%).

Serious Diagnoses

	Prevalence[a]
Structural cardiovascular disease (valvular stenosis, pericardial tamponade, acute coronary syndromes, left atrial myxoma, hypertrophic cardiomyopathy, aortic dissection, arrhythmogenic right ventricular dysplasia)	
Arrhythmias (tachyarrhythmias, bradyarrhythmias, heart block)	In a study of ambulatory patients who died while being monitored, the causative arrhythmia was ventricular tachycardia in 62%, ventricular fibrillation in 8%, torsades de pointes in 13%, and bradycardia in 17%.[10]
Pulmonary hypertension Pulmonary embolism Major volume loss (acute gastrointestinal hemorrhage, massive diarrhea, dehydration) Vertebrobasilar transient ischemic attack Severe autonomic insufficiency	

[a]Prevalence is unknown when not indicated.

Alarm Symptoms	Serious Causes	Benign Causes
Age > 45 years	Cardiac syncope	
History of heart disease	Cardiac syncope[10] LR+ 1.7 LR– 0.11	
Family history of heart disease or sudden death	Long QT syndromes Hypertrophic cardiomyopathy	
Chest pain or dyspnea	Myocardial infarction Unstable angina (left main coronary artery disease or equivalent) Aortic dissection Pericardial tamponade Pulmonary embolism	Panic disorder

Syncope with exertion	Aortic stenosis Pulmonic stenosis Hypertrophic cardiomyopathy Pulmonary hypertension Ventricular fibrillation or tachycardia Severe coronary artery disease	
Absence of nausea or vomiting	Arrhythmia	
Absence of prodrome[11] (especially in patients with heart disease)	Arrhythmia	
Palpitations	Arrhythmia	
Syncope in the supine position	Arrhythmia	
Diplopia, dysarthria, vertigo, or facial numbness	Vertebrobasilar (brainstem) transient ischemic attack	
Syncope with arm exercise	Subclavian steal	

FOCUSED QUESTIONS[10,12–15]

See Chapter 6 for examples of questions to evaluate light-headedness, disequilibrium, presyncope, or vertigo. See Figure 29–1 for the diagnostic approach algorithm for suspected syncope.

A common clinical conundrum is the differentiation between syncope and seizure.

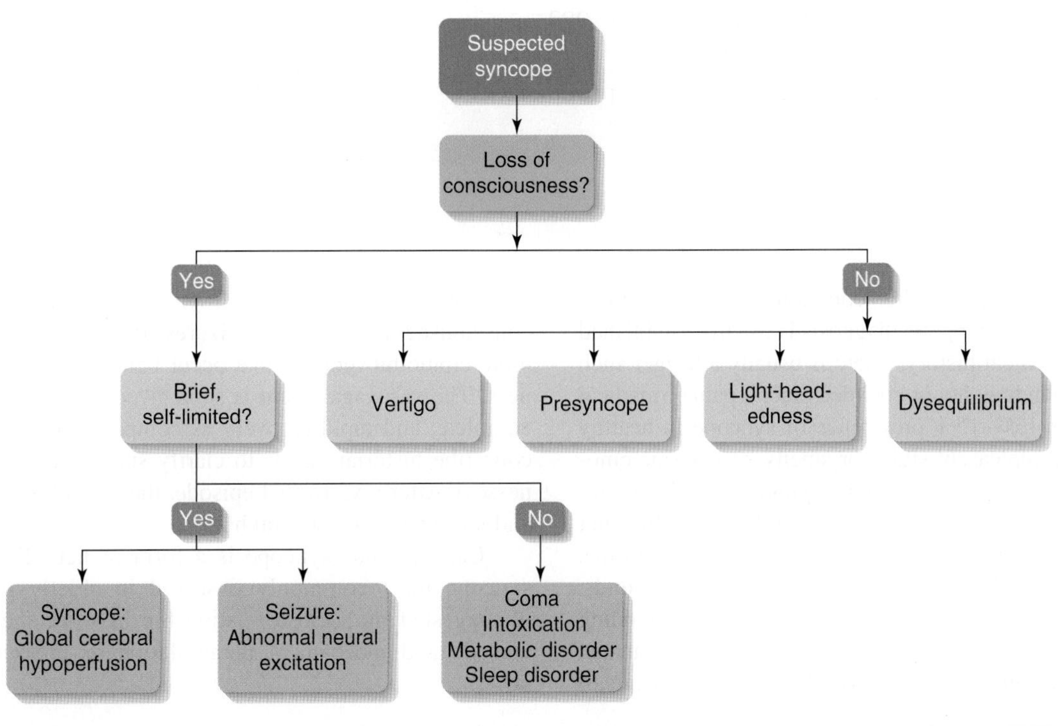

FIGURE 29–1 Initial diagnostic approach: Suspected syncope. Presyncope may require an evaluation similar to syncope.

Distinguishing Seizures From Syncope[12,13]

Questions	Probable Diagnosis	LR+
Do you wake up with a cut tongue after your episodes?	Seizure	16.5
Do you have a sense of déjà vu or jamais vu before your episodes?	Seizure	3.4
Is emotional stress associated with losing consciousness?	Seizure	3.8
Has anyone ever noted your head turning during an episode?	Seizure	13.5
Has anyone ever noted that you:		
• Are unresponsive or have unusual posturing or jerking limbs during an episode?	Seizure	3.0 (unresponsiveness), 12.9 (unusual posturing), 5.6 (jerking limbs)
• Have no memory of your episodes afterward?	Seizure	4.0 (no memory of episode)
Has anyone ever noticed that you are confused after an episode?	Seizure	3.0
Did bystanders notice you were blue during the episode?	Seizure	5.8
Did you experience muscle pain after the episode?	Seizure	3.4
Have you ever had light-headed spells?	Syncope	0.27 (for seizure)
At times do you sweat before your spells?	Syncope	0.17 (for seizure)
Do you experience shortness of breath before your spells?	Syncope	0.08 (for seizure)
Is prolonged sitting or standing associated with your spells?	Syncope	0.05 (for seizure)

Vasovagal syncope, or the "common faint," is the most common form of syncope. Its diagnosis is usually established by a detailed medical history. There is usually a trigger such as prolonged standing, hot or crowded places, pain or medical instrumentation (5%–15% prevalence of syncope in healthy blood donors), unpleasant sights or smells, or extreme emotion such as fear. Typical prodromal symptoms include nausea, vomiting, sweating, feeling cold or hot, and blurring vision. However, elderly patients may report no prodrome. The onset is relatively rapid, usually within 10 to 20 seconds. The patient loses voluntary muscle control, falling if standing or slumping over if sitting. Pallor suggests vasovagal syncope, whereas cyanosis implies seizure. Brief jerking movements of the arms and legs may occur in syncope, typically after loss of consciousness. Grand mal seizures produce more prolonged tonic-clonic movements that occur before loss of consciousness. The vasovagal event is short-lived with a spontaneous, complete, and rapid recovery as compared with pseudosyncope (the historian needs to clarify such features from witnesses). After a vasovagal episode, the patient may feel tired and lack energy for several hours.

Carotid sinus syncope is a form of neurally mediated syncope most commonly observed in elderly patients. It is suggested by a close relationship between the syncopal episode and mechanical manipulation or pressure on the neck.

Use focused questions to determine: the circumstances just prior to the episode, the onset of the episode, what bystanders observed during the episode (eg, duration, rapidity of recovery, arm or leg movement, duration and onset, presence of incontinence), and background information on past medical and family history. Answers to these questions will help narrow the differential diagnosis.

QUESTIONS	THINK ABOUT ...
Do you have heart disease or heart failure?	Cardiac syncope
Do you have a family history of sudden death?	Arrhythmias Long QT syndrome Brugada syndrome
Do you have chest or neck pain with your episodes?	Coronary artery disease Glossopharyngeal neuralgia
Does exercise bring on your symptoms?	Valvular (aortic) stenosis Pulmonary hypertension Subclavian steal Severe coronary artery disease
Do you pass out with changes in position?	Atrial myxoma or thrombus
Do you lose consciousness in the supine position?	Arrhythmia
Do you notice palpitations or a fast heart rate before your episodes?	Arrhythmia
Are you taking any medication?	Medication-induced (see box titled, "Drugs Associated With Syncope or Presyncope"). Hypoglycemic agents typically produce more prolonged symptoms incompatible with syncope.
Do you have a history of seizures?	Epilepsy
Do you have a history of stroke or transient ischemic attack?	Cerebrovascular disease (vertebrobasilar transient ischemic attack)
Do you have the sensation that the room is spinning (vertigo)? Do you have double vision, difficulty speaking, or weakness or numbness on one side of the body?	Cerebrovascular disease (vertebrobasilar transient ischemic attack)
Do you have a history of diabetes with neuropathy?	Autonomic neuropathy
Do you have a history of Parkinson's disease or other autonomic neuropathy?	Parkinsonism Subacute combined systems atrophy
Do your episodes occur after coughing, urinating, defecating, or swallowing?	Situational syncope
Do your episodes occur during a migraine attack?	Basilar artery migraine
Do you have severe throat or facial pain with your episodes?	Glossopharyngeal neuralgia

—Continued next page

Continued—

Do your episodes occur in hot crowded environments? *With prolonged standing? After experiencing intense pain, fear, or emotion? After unexpected sights, sounds, or smells?*	Vasovagal syncope
Do either of your parents have problems with fainting due to vasovagal syncope?	Vasovagal syncope
Do you notice nausea, vomiting, or feeling cold or fatigued before the episodes?	Vasovagal syncope
Are you pale during or after the episodes?	Vasovagal syncope
Do you injure yourself during the episodes?	Seizure Arrhythmia
Do you have black tarry stools, bloody stools, or hematemesis?	Orthostatic hypotension from gastrointestinal bleeding (see Chapter 36)
Do you have severe diarrhea, frequent urination, or prolonged vomiting?	Volume depletion
Do your episodes occur within 1 hour of eating meals?	Postprandial hypotension
Do you have diabetes, alcoholism, or chronic kidney disease?	Autonomic insufficiency
Do your symptoms occur with abrupt neck movements, especially looking upward, or with pressure on the neck?	Carotid sinus syncope

Drugs Associated With Syncope or Presyncope[16]

Cardiovascular

β-Blockers

Vasodilators (α-blockers, calcium channel blockers, nitrates, hydralazine, angiotensin-converting enzyme inhibitors)

Antiarrhythmics

Diuretics

Centrally acting antihypertensives (clonidine, methyldopa)

Central nervous system

Antidepressants (tricyclics, monoamine oxidase inhibitors)

Antipsychotics (phenothiazines)

Sedatives (barbiturates, ethanol)

Antiparkinsonian agents

Anticonvulsants

Narcotic analgesics
Anxiolytic agents (benzodiazepines)
Drugs that prolong the QT interval[a]
Cardiovascular (disopyramide, dofetilide, ibutilide, procainamide, quinidine, sotalol, bepridil, amiodarone)
Cisapride
Calcium channel blockers (lidoflazine, not marketed in the United States)
Anti-infective agents (clarithromycin, erythromycin, halofantrine, pentamidine, sparfloxacin)
Antiemetic agents (domperidone, droperidol)
Antipsychotic agents (chlorpromazine, haloperidol, mesoridazine, thioridazine, pimozide)
Antihistamines (terfenadine and astemizole, no longer marketed in United States)
Methadone
Arsenic trioxide

[a]*Further details can be found at www.torsades.org; syncope is reported with newly introduced medications every year. Always check to make sure a medication the patient is taking is not associated with syncope.*

DIAGNOSTIC APPROACH (INCLUDING ALGORITHMS)[17–24]

There are 3 key questions in the evaluation of every patient with syncope:

1. Does the patient really have syncope?
2. Does the patient have underlying heart disease?
3. Are there historical features that suggest a specific diagnosis?

The answers to these questions come from a detailed medical history obtained from the patient and any eyewitnesses. Based on history and physical examination alone, the etiology of syncope can be established in at least 45% of cases.[17,18] Adding electrocardiography to the initial evaluation increases diagnostic yield to greater than 50% and may add prognostic information. See Figures 29–1 and 29–2 for the diagnostic approach algorithms for suspected syncope and syncope, respectively.

CAVEATS

- Establish that the patient has suffered true loss of consciousness (not one of the other causes of dizziness).
- Seizures, metabolic disorders (eg, hypoglycemia), and alcohol or other intoxications are suggested by a much longer episode.
- When interviewing eyewitnesses, try to distinguish isolated involuntary (myoclonic) jerk movements, which can occur with syncope, from the tonic-clonic movements characteristic of a seizure.
- Older patients are more likely to have a serious (cardiac) cause but may be less likely to recall details of the episode (eg, premonitory features).[8,22]
- The elderly often have multifactorial syncope. Do not stop taking the history after finding a single plausible explanation for the patient's symptoms.
- The cause of syncope can be diagnosed by history alone in 45% to 55% of cases.

PROGNOSIS

Prognosis of syncope is related to the underlying cause. Reflex-mediated syncope has an excellent prognosis unless the provocative event is a serious cause (eg, myocardial infarction). Vasovagal syncope requires only reassurance and patient education (eg, sit or lie down or perform the leg-crossing maneuver at the first warning of prodromal symptoms). Cardiovascular causes are associated with increased mortality and require appropriate treatment for the specific condition. Primary autonomic insufficiency is treated supportively. Secondary autonomic insufficiency from diabetes mellitus is difficult to treat. The prognosis of other secondary causes of autonomic insufficiency (eg, chronic kidney disease, amyloidosis, paraneoplastic, Chagas disease) depends on the underlying disease. Lastly, most patients with a simple faint (vasovagal syncope) never seek medical attention and have an excellent prognosis.

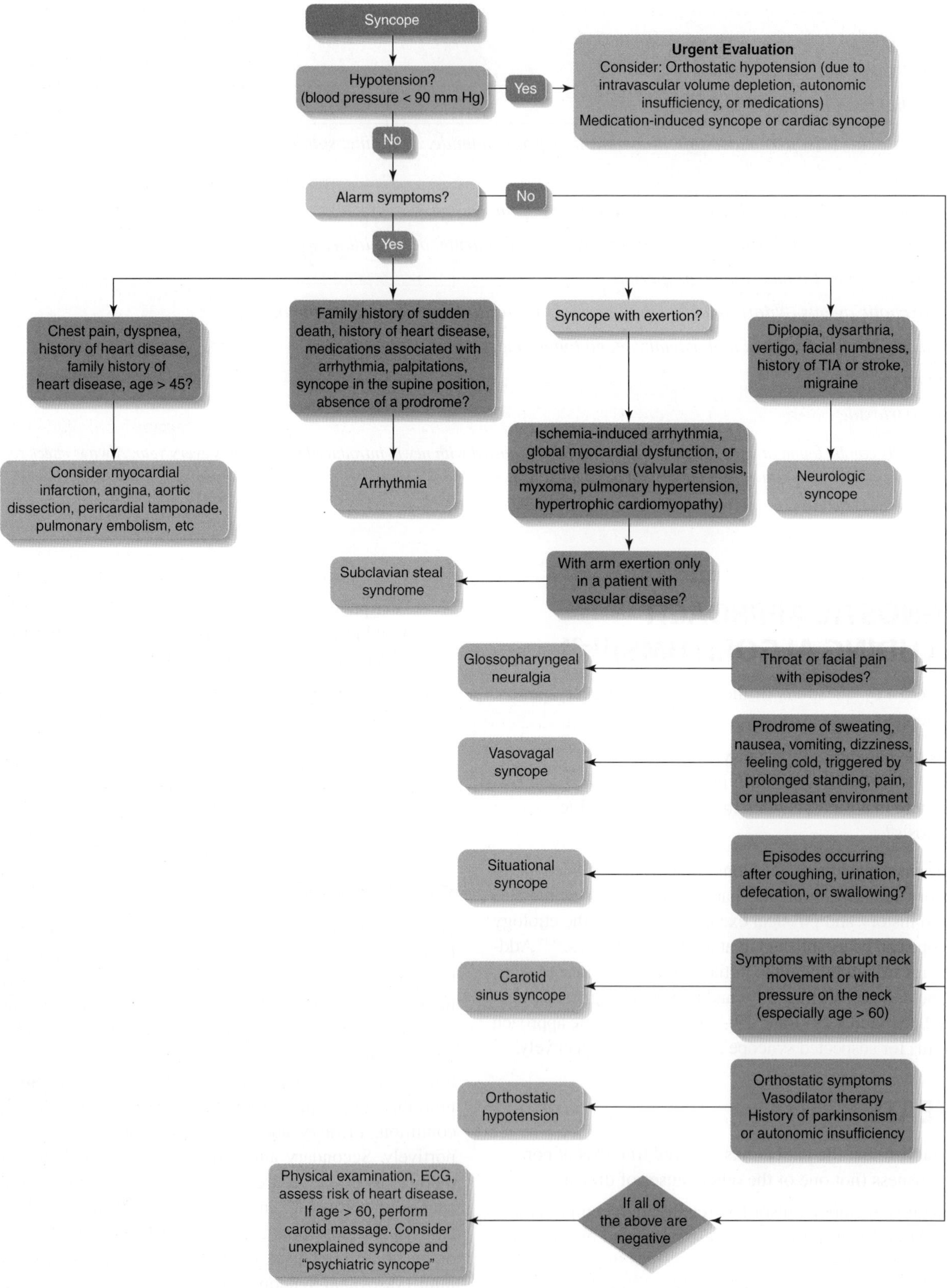

FIGURE 29–2 Diagnostic approach: Syncope. ECG, electrocardiogram; TIA, transient ischemic attack. (Modified from Brignole M, Alboni P, Benditt D, et al. Task Force on Syncope, European Society of Cardiology. Guidelines on management (diagnosis and treatment) of syncope. *Eur Heart J.* 2001;22:1256–1306.)

CASE SCENARIO | Resolution

A 20-year-old college wrestler comes to your office with his mother because she is concerned that he has "passed out" in church. While attending Sunday services during the summer, he has twice become dizzy while standing and slumped to the floor. He was briefly "out of it" but revived quickly when taken outside. On each occasion, he insisted on completing the religious service.

ADDITIONAL HISTORY

On both occasions, the church was crowded and hot, and the congregation had been standing for a prolonged period. He initially felt a graying out of his vision, then his hearing began to fade, and finally, he felt suddenly very hot and sweaty. The next thing he remembers was being surrounded by people fanning him as he came to consciousness. His mother reported that he slumped down to the floor very suddenly and looked "pale and clammy." He spontaneously recovered and was only momentarily confused. The other episode occurred the previous summer under similar circumstances. He is taking no medications, has no history of cardiac disease, and denies palpitations. There is no history of seizures. He keeps himself fit and exercises regularly to keep in shape for the wrestling season. There is no family history of sudden death, although a paternal grandfather died in his seventies of "heart attack." His mother and father are healthy.

Question: What is the most likely diagnosis?

A. Sinus node dysfunction
B. Long QT syndrome
C. Seizure
D. Vasovagal syncope
E. Orthostatic hypotension

Test Your Knowledge

1. You evaluate a 52-year-old nurse who lost consciousness while reading in bed. Her husband witnessed the episode and phoned 911.

   Which historical feature is most concerning for a serious cause of syncope?

   A. Loss of consciousness
   B. Spontaneous, prompt, and complete recovery
   C. Sweating and nausea
   D. Occurrence in the supine position

2. Which of the following is *not* a cause of syncope?

   A. Carotid distribution transient ischemic attack
   B. Severe aortic stenosis
   C. Pulmonary embolism
   D. Paroxysmal supraventricular tachycardia
   E. Left atrial myxoma

3. A 25-year-old medical student agrees to have 75 mL of blood drawn for a scientific study. While the phlebotomist is attempting to draw the blood, she encounters difficulty and begins manipulating the needle and probing. The medical student becomes pale, cold, and clammy. A few seconds later, he slumps over in the chair and has several brief jerking movements of the arms and legs. He is helped down to the floor and promptly regains consciousness. After a few brief moments of confusion, he appears normal and is quite embarrassed.

   What is the most likely diagnosis?

   A. Seizure
   B. Orthostatic hypotension
   C. Carotid sinus syncope
   D. Vasovagal syncope

4. A 66-year-old man with history of 2 prior myocardial infarctions, coronary artery bypass grafting, hypertension, and congestive heart failure suddenly turns pale and slumps over in his chair and onto the floor while eating breakfast with his wife. He appears cold, sweaty, clammy, and unconscious. She phones 911. By the time the emergency medical technicians arrive 15 minutes later, he is groggy but awake. His pulse and blood pressure are normal, and he refuses to go with them to the hospital because he feels fine.

   Which of the following most suggests that he has a serious condition?

   A. History of heart disease
   B. Loss of consciousness
   C. Sweating
   D. Pallor

References

1. Day SC, Cook EF, Funkenstein H, Goldman L. Evaluation and outcome of emergency room patients with transient loss of consciousness. *Am J Med.* 1982;73:15–23.
2. Sarasin FP, Louis-Simonet M, Carballo D. Prospective evaluation of patients with syncope: a population based study. *Am J Med.* 2001;111:177–184.
3. Silverstein MD, Singer DE, Mulley A. Patients with syncope admitted to medical intensive care units. *JAMA.* 1982;248:1185–1189.
4. Eagle KA, Black HR. The impact of diagnostic tests in diagnosing syncope. *Yale J Biol Med.* 1983;56:1–8.
5. Ben-Chetrit E, Flugelman M, Eliakim M. Syncope: a retrospective study of 101 hospitalized patients. *Isr J Med Sci.* 1985;21:950–953.
6. Martin GJ, Adams SL, Martin HG, et al. Prospective evaluation of syncope. *Ann Emerg Med.* 1984;13:499–504.
7. Chen LY, Gersh BJ, Hodge DO, et al. Prevalence and clinical outcomes of patients with multiple potential causes of syncope. *Mayo Clin Proc.* 2003;78:414–420.
8. Lipsitz LA, Pluchino FC, Wei YC, Rowe JW. Syncope in institutionalized elderly: the impact of multiple pathologic conditions and situational stress. *J Chronic Dis.* 1986;39:619–630.
9. Bizios AS, Sheldon RS. Vasovagal syncope: state or trait? *Curr Opin Cardiol.* 2008;24:68–73.
10. Alboni P, Brignole M, Menozzi C, et al. Diagnostic value of history in patients with syncope with or without heart disease. *J Am Coll Cardiol.* 2001;37:1921–1928.
11. Quinn JV, Stiehl IG, McDermott DA, et al. Derivation of the San Francisco Syncope Rule to predict patients with short-term serious outcomes. *Ann Emerg Med.* 2004;43:224–232.
12. Sheldon R, Rose S, Ritchie D, et al. Historical criteria that distinguish syncope from seizures. *J Am Coll Cardiol.* 2002;40:142–148.
13. McKeon A, Vaughan C, Delanty N. Seizure versus syncope. *Lancet Neurol.* 2006;5:171–180.
14. Calkins H, Shyr Y, Frumin H, Schork A, Morady F. The value of the clinical history in the differentiation of syncope due to ventricular tachycardia, atrioventricular block, and neurocardiogenic syncope. *Am J Med.* 1995;98:365–373.
15. Oh JH, Hanusa BH, Kapoor WN. Do symptoms predict cardiac arrhythmias and mortality in patients with syncope? *Arch Intern Med.* 1999;159:375–380.
16. Roden DM. Drug-induced prolongation of the QT interval. *N Engl J Med.* 2004;350:1013–1022.
17. Linzer M, Yang EH, Estes NA 3rd, et al. Diagnosing syncope. Part 1: value of history, physical examination, and electrocardiography: Clinical Efficacy Assessment Project of the American College of Physicians. *Ann Intern Med.* 1997;126:989–996.
18. Linzer M, Yang EH, Estes NA 3rd, et al. Diagnosing syncope. Part 2: unexplained syncope: Clinical Efficacy Assessment Project of the American College of Physicians. *Ann Intern Med.* 1997;126:76–86.
19. Brignole M, Alboni P, Benditt D, et al. Task Force on Syncope, European Society of Cardiology. Guidelines on management (diagnosis and treatment) of syncope. *Eur Heart J.* 2001;22:1256–1306.
20. Goldschlager N, Epstein AE, Grubb BP, et al. Etiologic considerations in the patient with syncope and an apparently normal heart. Practice Guidelines Subcommittee, North American Society of Pacing and Electrophysiology. *Arch Intern Med.* 2003;163:151–162.
21. Medow MN, Stewart JM, Sanyal S, et al. Pathophysiology, diagnosis, and treatment of orthostatic hypotension and vasovagal syncope. *Cardiol Rev.* 2008;16:4–20.
22. Tan MP, Parry SW. Vasovagal syncope in the older patient. *J Am Coll Cardiol.* 2008;51:599-606.
23. Benditt DG, Nguyen JT. Syncope. *J Am Coll Cardiol.* 2009;53:1741–1751.
24. Jhanjee R, Can I, Benditt DG. Syncope. *Dis Mon.* 2009;55:532–585.

Suggested Reading

Benditt DG, Blanc J-J, Brignole M, Sutton R. *The Evaluation and Treatment of Syncope. A Handbook for Clinical Practice.* 2nd ed. Malden, MA: Blackwell Futura Publishing, 2006.

Garcia-Civera R, Baron-Esquivas G, Blanc J-J, et al. *Syncope Cases.* Malden, MA: Blackwell Futura Publishing, 2006.

Grubb BP, Olshansky B, eds. *Syncope: Mechanisms and Management.* 2nd ed. Malden, MA: Blackwell Futura Publishing, 2005.

Chapter 30

Edema

Jeff Wiese, MD, and Michelle Guidry, MD

CASE SCENARIO

A 54-year-old man comes to your office because of worsening "leg swelling." The swelling began 3 months ago and has steadily increased since that time. He also notes polyuria and generalized fatigue.

- **What additional questions would you ask to characterize the edema?**
- **What are the 5 pathophysiologic categories that induce peripheral edema?**
- **Can a definitive cause of the edema be determined by historical information alone?**
- **What historical questions will be useful in determining the appropriate evaluation of the edema?**

INTRODUCTION

Edema is the accumulation of fluid in the interstitial space between cells. It is categorized into 5 subtypes based on the Starling law of fluid flow across a membrane:

$$\text{Edema} = K[(P_{in} - P_{out}) - (Onc_{in} - Onc_{out})]$$

where K = vessel permeability
P_{in} = intravascular hydrostatic pressure
P_{out} = interstitial hydrostatic pressure
Onc_{in} = intravascular oncotic pressure
Onc_{out} = interstitial oncotic pressure

Fluid is kept in the intravascular space by the capillary walls that selectively allow small amounts of fluid to leave the vascular space to deliver water, oxygen, and nutrients to the body cells. Under normal circumstances, only a small amount of fluid leaves the vascular space and is returned to the vascular space via lymphatic drainage. The permeability constant of the capillary membrane regulates how much fluid leaks out (K). The high protein concentration in the blood also prevents excessive fluid from leaving the intravascular space by osmotically retaining water in the vessels (Onc_{in}).

Edema typically results when the pressure in the vessels (P_{in}) overrides the semipermeable capillary membrane, pushing more volume into the extravascular space.

Edema can also arise when the lymphatic drainage of the tissues is obstructed, the capillary membrane permeability is increased (K), or the blood protein concentration is decreased (Onc_{in}). Increased protein concentration in the interstitium (Onc_{out}) is rarely a cause of edema, although excess fat in the interstitium may draw and hold water into the interstitial space causing edema (lipedema).

The most efficient method of diagnosing the etiology of edema is to sequentially consider each of these 4 forces that augment fluid leaving the intravascular space and entering the interstitial space.

KEY TERMS

Anasarca	Edema involving all aspects of the body: upper and lower extremities and the face.
Ascites	Collection of fluid in the peritoneal cavity.
Lipedema	Edema caused by fluid retained in the interstitial space by lipids in the dermis.
Lymphedema	Edema caused by obstruction of lymphatic drainage of the tissues.
Myxedema	Edema resulting from hypothyroidism (see below).
Pretibial myxedema	Not technically edema, the swelling on the anterior shins is due to coalescing of subcutaneous plaques due to Graves disease antibodies infiltrating dermal tissue.

ETIOLOGY

Patients with edema but no additional symptoms are most likely to have venous stasis or medications as the cause. Patients with additional complaints are more likely to have systemic diseases such as congestive heart failure, renal disease, or cirrhosis. Determining the onset of the edema, the presence or absence of additional symptoms (ie, dyspnea, increased abdominal girth, polyuria), or comorbid disease (ie, diabetes, heart failure, ischemic coronary disease, liver disease) can quickly narrow the differential diagnosis.

Differential Diagnosis

	Prevalence
Varicose veins or venous stasis	30%
Congestive heart failure	30%
Lipedema	10%
Cirrhosis	10%
Nephrotic syndrome	5%
Hypothyroidism	5%
Venous thrombosis/ obstruction	3%
Medications	3%
Anaphylaxis	1%
Lymphatic obstruction	1%
Protein-losing enteropathy	1%
Malnutrition	1%

GETTING STARTED WITH THE HISTORY

- Review medication list prior to seeing the patient and validate during the interview.
- Avoid leading questions. It may be necessary to follow-up with a few closed-ended questions directed at the most likely disorder.
- Determine the time course and progression of the edema.

Questions	Remember
When did the swelling begin? How has the swelling progressed since that time?	Let patients use their own words. Avoid interrupting.
Do you have a history of heart, kidney, liver, or thyroid disease?	Listen to the patient's description for diagnostic clues.
Tell me about your diet.	Try to assemble the patient's description into a chronologic story as you obtain the history.

INTERVIEW FRAMEWORK

- Assess for alarm symptoms.
- Ask about symptoms of heart failure.
- Ask about alcohol use and other risk factors for liver disease.
- Ask about risk factors for venous stasis and vascular injury.
- Take a dietary history.
- Determine the temporal pattern and duration of symptoms, accompanying symptoms, and precipitating factors.

IDENTIFYING ALARM SYMPTOMS

With the exception of anaphylaxis, edema is rarely life threatening. Congestive heart failure can be life threatening, but the risk is due to pulmonary congestion from the heart failure and not the edema itself. A deep venous thrombosis is considered life threatening because it can lead to pulmonary embolism.

Serious Diagnoses

- Congestive heart failure
- Anaphylaxis
- Liver failure
- Deep venous thrombosis leading to pulmonary embolism

Alarm Symptoms	Consider
New medication Exposure to latex or chemicals	Anaphylaxis
Chest discomfort, shortness of breath, orthopnea, or paroxysmal nocturnal dyspnea	Valve stenosis or insufficiency Cardiac ischemia
Loss of consciousness (syncope) Feeling like going to pass out, especially when walking (presyncope)	Outflow tract obstruction (eg, aortic stenosis, hypertrophic cardiomyopathy, primary pulmonary hypertension, or atrial myxoma) Pulmonary embolus
Alcohol abuse Unprotected sex (hepatitis B and C) Use of injection drugs (hepatitis C) Use of illicit drugs (eg, mushrooms or Ecstasy)	Liver failure
Abdominal swelling (ascites)	Above conditions plus constrictive pericarditis
Sedentary position for a prolonged time (eg, bedridden, long travel)? Smoking History of blood clots Use of oral contraceptives, especially in smokers	Pulmonary embolism

FOCUSED QUESTIONS

Considering each pathophysiologic category separately is the best method for determining the cause of edema.

Increased Permeability

Increased permeability affects all tissue beds equally; edema of the upper and lower extremities (and face) suggests increased permeability as the etiology.

QUESTIONS	THINK ABOUT...
What medications are you taking, and how long have you taken each? *Do you take over-the-counter medications?*	**Anaphylaxis:** Most medications can cause edema by way of anaphylaxis. Histamine is released in response to the allergen, increasing vessel permeability and causing edema. Anaphylaxis may develop at any time after starting a medication.
Are you taking an angiotensin-converting enzyme (ACE) inhibitor or calcium channel blocker?	**ACE inhibitor– or calcium channel blocker–induced edema:** ACE degrades circulating bradykinin, which is released naturally from tissue injury to promote extravasation of fluid (and white blood cells) at sites of injury. High circulating bradykinin levels can cause unwarranted edema. Calcium channel blockers cause edema by an unknown mechanism.

—Continued next page

Continued—

Do you feel tired or have dry skin, coarse hair, or intolerance to cold?	**Hypothyroidism:** Hypothyroidism causes increased vessel permeability and increased circulating volume due to excess antidiuretic hormone production.
Does the edema come and go suddenly? *Do you note hives or trouble breathing when you experience the edema?*	**Hereditary angioedema:** Hereditary angioedema is due to a deficiency in C1 esterase. Without this enzyme, C1 accumulates, stimulating the complement cascade that eventually results in excess histamine release and angioedema. Hereditary angioedema almost always involves the lips and face and occasionally the airway and gastrointestinal tract.

Increased Intravascular Pressure

Increased intravascular pressure is due to either volume overload or obstruction of venous blood return to the heart. Because pressure is greatest in the lower extremities (due to gravity), edema due to increased intravascular pressure always begins in the lower extremities and ascends superiorly to the site of the obstruction. Venous pressure is higher in the left leg because the left iliac vein must cross under the aorta to join the vena cava. Therefore, edema due to increased intravascular pressure typically begins in the left leg, eventually becoming bilateral.

A. Volume Overload

QUESTIONS	THINK ABOUT...
Have you noticed a decrease in your urinary output?	Renal, cardiac, and hepatic disease
What types of food do you eat?	Excessive sodium is contained in the following foods: potato chips, salted peanuts, fast food, canned foods, and Chinese food. Be certain to ask how much salt the patient adds to food.
Is the patient receiving intravenous medications?	Some medications are formulated as the anion portion of a salt and must be combined with a cation such as sodium for solubility. The sodium concentration can be considerable, especially for every 4-hour dosing of a medication (eg, ticarcillin).
What intravenous fluids is the patient receiving?	The recommended sodium intake per day is less than 3 g. One liter of normal saline is 0.9% sodium, or 9 g.
Do you work outdoors or in hot climates?	**Steroid-induced edema:** In hot climates, many people will have minor lower extremity edema by the end of the day due to elevated aldosterone levels (stimulated by the loss of volume due to sweating). The edema resolves as the patient is prone overnight.
Are you taking steroids?	Most steroids stimulate the aldosterone receptor, resulting in sodium and water retention.
Do you have marked weakness or stretch marks on the abdomen?	**Cushing's syndrome:** Excess cortisol stimulates the aldosterone receptor, causing sodium and water retention.

B. Venous or Lymphatic Obstruction

The best method is to start at the aortic root and work backward, remembering that any valvular obstruction or incompetence will result in increased pressure in the venous system proximal to the obstruction. All abnormalities from the aortic root to the left atrium may cause shortness of breath, as blood is "backed up" into the lungs.

QUESTIONS	THINK ABOUT...
Have you had chest pain or loss of consciousness or felt short of breath?	**Aortic stenosis:** Stenosis of the aortic valve impairs forward blood flow, resulting in pooling of the blood in the lungs causing dyspnea. The elevated left ventricular pressure increases myocardial work and impairs subendocardial blood flow, resulting in cardiac ischemia and chest pain. The lack of blood flow to the brain results in syncope.
Are you short of breath? *Do you use injection drugs?*	**Aortic insufficiency:** The incompetent valve increases left ventricular pressure and thus pulmonary vein pressure, causing dyspnea. The most common cause of acute aortic insufficiency is infection of the aortic valve (endocarditis).
Do you have a history of heart attack? *Have you recently given birth?* *Have you received cancer chemotherapy in the past?* *Are you short of breath?*	**Cardiomyopathy:** Cardiomyopathy is a decrease in left ventricular function due to myocyte damage from hypertension, ischemic heart disease, diabetes, and rarely chemotherapeutic agents, viral infections, or the postpartum state. The decreased left ventricular function elevates venous pressure in the lungs (dyspnea) and the systemic veins (edema).
Do you have a history of ischemic heart disease? *Do you use injection drugs?* *Did you have rheumatic fever as a child?*	**Mitral regurgitation or stenosis:** The most common cause of mitral stenosis is rheumatic heart disease. The most common causes of mitral insufficiency are dilation of the left ventricle due to heart failure (the dilating ventricle pulls the valve leaflets apart), myocardial infarction involving the papillary muscles (connecting the mitral valve to the left ventricle), or infection of the valve.
Did you have rheumatic fever as a child? *Have you taken the dietary supplement fenfluramine?*	**Pulmonic stenosis or insufficiency**
Do you use injection drugs? *Did you have rheumatic fever as a child?*	**Tricuspid stenosis or insufficiency:** The most common causes of tricuspid stenosis or insufficiency are endocarditis and rheumatic heart disease; tricuspid regurgitation is also caused by any cardiomyopathy.
Have you had tuberculosis? *Have you been diagnosed with lung or breast cancer?*	**Constrictive pericarditis:** Constrictive pericarditis impairs the right ventricle from expanding to accommodate venous blood return to the heart. The most common causes include tuberculosis, lung or breast cancer, and previous pericarditis of any cause.
Do you smoke?	**Cardiac tamponade:** Tamponade is collection of fluid between the pericardium and the heart that impairs the heart from accommodating systemic and pulmonary venous volume.
Do you have a history of tuberculosis or lung cancer? *Are your face and arms swollen more than your legs?*	**Superior vena cava syndrome:** Superior vena cava syndrome results from a mass (infectious or malignant) that encases the superior vena cava preventing venous blood from returning to the heart. The edema is localized to the arms and face.

—Continued next page

Continued—

Have you noticed abdominal swelling?	**Abdominal mass or pregnancy:** An abdominal mass that obstructs the inferior cava will prevent venous volume from returning to the right heart.
Do you have a history of blood clots? *Do you smoke?* *Have you been in a prolonged state of immobility (airplane ride, bedridden)?* *Do you take oral contraceptives?* *Do you have a past diagnosis of cancer?*	**Deep venous thrombosis:** The Virchow triad of risk factors for intravascular thrombosis includes stasis, hypercoagulability, and vessel injury. The most common causes of hypercoagulability include smoking, estrogen use, and genetic predisposition (factor V Leiden, prothrombin mutation 20210, antithrombin III deficiency).
Is the edema localized to the left leg?	**May-Thurner syndrome:** May-Thurner syndrome is compression of the left iliac vein as it crosses under the aorta to get to the inferior vena cava. Definitive diagnosis is made by venogram.
Have you noticed prominent veins on your legs?	Varicose veins
Do you have a history of cancer? *Do you have yellow nails?* *Have you traveled to tropical areas?*	**Lymphatic obstruction:** The most common cause of lymphatic insufficiency is a malignancy obstructing lymph flow. The yellow nail syndrome is a genetic syndrome composed of yellow nails and lymphatic insufficiency. Parasitic infection may also obstruct the lymphatic chain (elephantiasis due to filariasis).

Decreased Oncotic Pressure

Decreased oncotic pressure results from a deficiency in albumin, either due to inadequate production or accelerated loss.

QUESTIONS	THINK ABOUT...
Have you had diarrhea?	**Protein-losing enteropathy:** This is due to impairment of the bowel's ability to absorb protein. The increased oncotic pressure in the bowel lumen causes diarrhea.
How much alcohol do you drink? *Have you had viral hepatitis?* *Have you had liver disease?*	**Cirrhosis:** Damage to the liver tissue impairs its ability to convert absorbed protein to albumin. See Chapter 37 for questions that may reveal the cause of liver disease and other symptoms associated with liver failure.
Have you noticed foamy urine? *Do you have a history of kidney disease?* *Do you have diabetes or hypertension?*	**Nephrotic syndrome:** Nephrotic syndrome is loss of the protein in the urine. The most common causes in adults are diabetes, hypertension, minimal change disease, and focal segmental glomerulosclerosis. Excessive protein in the urine causes it to be foamy.

DIAGNOSTIC APPROACH (INCLUDING ALGORITHM)

The diagnostic algorithm for edema is shown in Figure 30–1.

CAVEATS

- Peripheral edema is graded on a 1 to 4 scale based on the pit recovery time (PRT). To assess the PRT, apply pressure with one finger over the area of edema for 5 seconds. Release the pressure and assess the time required for the pit to return to normal. Each 1 point on the scale corresponds to 30 seconds of PRT (1+ edema = < 30 seconds PRT; 2+ edema = 30–60 seconds PRT, etc.). The higher the PRT, the greater the likelihood that the edema is due to increased hydrostatic pressure (ie, congestive heart failure).

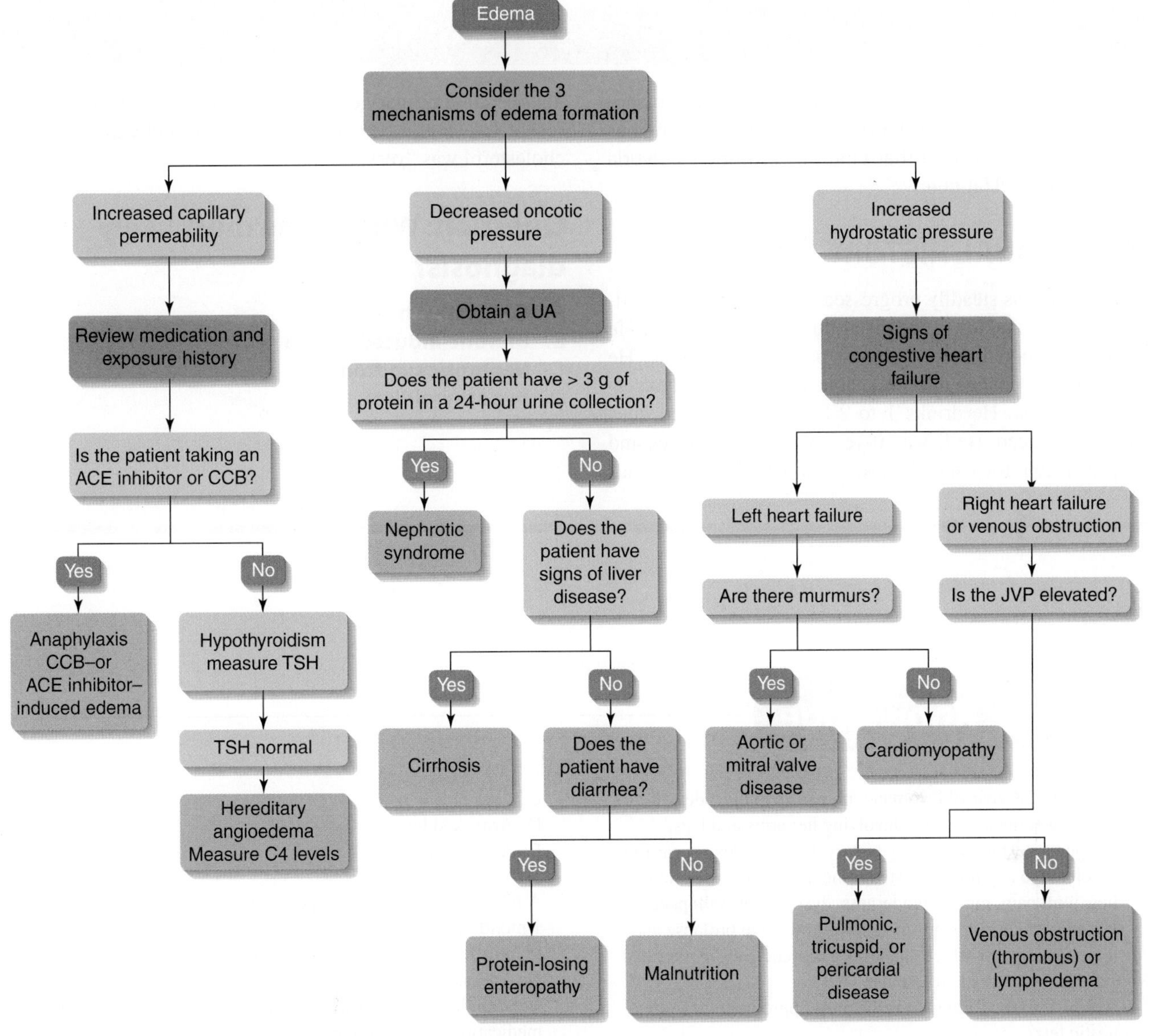

FIGURE 30–1 Diagnostic approach: Edema. ACE, angiotensin-converting enzyme; CCB, calcium channel blocker; JVP, jugular venous pressure; TSH, thyroid-stimulating hormone; UA, urinalysis.

- Mild to moderate heart failure results in edema involving the legs, feet, and toes. Severe heart failure leads to edema involving the legs and feet but sparing the toes. The inadequate cardiac output causes peripheral vascular constriction to maintain core mean arterial pressure, which decreases blood flow to the toes, thus diminishing edema in the toes.
- Edema involving the legs but sparing the feet is lipedema, or fluid retained by fat in the interstitial space. Because there is no fat on the top of the feet, they are spared. Decreasing intravascular volume with diuretics will not mobilize the fluid of lipedema.

PROGNOSIS

The prognosis for edema depends on the underlying etiology.

CASE SCENARIO | Resolution

A 54-year-old man comes to your office because of worsening "leg swelling." The swelling began 3 months ago and has steadily increased since that time. He also notes polyuria and generalized fatigue.

ADDITIONAL HISTORY

The edema has steadily progressed over 3 months, extending from his ankles to his distal thighs on both sides. He denies exertional dyspnea, chest pain, or palpations. He has noted no change in bowel habits but does report excessive urination. He drinks 1 to 2 beers per day and does not use tobacco. He has a 10-year history of diabetes and hypertension, for which he takes oral medications. He has not been to a primary care provider for some time but was recently seen at a community health fair and was told his cholesterol was "very high."

Question: What is the most likely diagnosis?

A. Congestive heart failure
B. Diuretic-induced edema
C. Nephrotic syndrome
D. Hypothyroidism

Test Your Knowledge

1. You see a 28-year-old woman with recurrent episodes of facial swelling and edema involving her arms and legs. Despite an extensive dietary history, the episodes appear to be unrelated to any food ingestion. She denies skin abnormalities, joint pain, muscle tenderness, dyspnea, or orthopnea. Her past medical history includes mitral valve prolapse and hypertension, for which she takes a diuretic. Her mother had similar symptoms as a teenager.
   Which of the following is the most appropriate next diagnostic test?
   A. C4 (complement) levels
   B. Antinuclear antibody (ANA) level
   C. Echocardiogram
   D. Thyroid function tests

2. A 20-year-old woman presents with recurrent, unilateral leg swelling. She has had multiple ultrasound examinations, all of which have been negative for deep vein thrombosis.
   Which of the following distributions of edema would be most consistent with a diagnosis of May-Thurner syndrome?
   A. Left leg
   B. Right leg
   C. Legs only
   D. Arms and legs
   E. Arms only

3. A 62-year-old man with hypertension presents with edema for 1 month in both lower extremities, extending from the ankles to mid-shins. He denies dyspnea, abdominal swelling, fatigue, weakness, or changes in exercise tolerance. He reports constipation but no diarrhea and no urinary symptoms. His only medication is amlodipine.
   Which of the following is the most appropriate diagnostic step?
   A. Liver enzymes and coagulation studies
   B. Echocardiogram
   C. Thyroid function tests
   D. Discontinue amlodipine

Suggested Reading

Adler O, Kalidindi S, Butt A, Hussain KM. Chordae tendineae rupture resulting in pulmonary edema in a patient with discrete subvalvular aortic stenosis—a case report and literature review. *Angiology.* 2003;54:613–617.

Blankfield RP, Finkelhor RS, Alexander JJ, et al. Etiology and diagnosis of bilateral leg edema in primary care. *Am J Med.* 1998;105:192–197.

Cho S, Atwood JE. Peripheral edema. *Am J Med.* 2002;113:580–586.

Elwell RJ, Spencer AP, Eisele G. Combined furosemide and human albumin treatment for diuretic-resistant edema. *Ann Pharmacother.* 2003;37:695–700.

Fishel RS, Are C, Barbul A. Vessel injury and capillary leak. *Crit Care Med.* 2003;31(8 Suppl):S502–S511.

Macdonald JM, Sims N, Mayrovitz HN. Lymphedema, lipedema, and the open wound: the role of compression therapy. *Surg Clin North Am.* 2003;83:639–658.

Sica DA. Calcium channel blocker-related peripheral edema: can it be resolved? *J Clin Hypertens.* 2003;5:291–294, 297.

Sica DA. Metolazone and its role in edema management. *Congest Heart Fail.* 2003;9:100–105.

Szuba A, Shin WS, Strauss HW, Rockson S. The third circulation: radionuclide lymphoscintigraphy in the evaluation of lymphedema. *J Nucl Med.* 2003;44:43–57.

Yoshida S, Sakuma K, Ueda O. Acute mitral regurgitation due to total rupture in the anterior papillary muscle after acute myocardial infarction successfully treated by emergency surgery. *Jpn J Thorac Cardiovasc Surg.* 2003;51:208–210.

SECTION

VII GASTROINTESTINAL SYSTEM

Chapter 31

Abdominal Pain

Thomas E. Baudendistel, MD, and Amarpreet Sandhu, DO

CASE SCENARIO

A 62-year-old man with a history of hyperlipidemia, hypertension, and coronary artery disease presents to your primary care practice with abdominal pain for 6 months. His pain gets worse after eating meals.

- **What are the other important questions to ask this patient?**
- **What is the differential diagnosis of acute and chronic abdominal pain?**
- **Can you make a definite diagnosis through an open-ended history followed by focused questions?**

INTRODUCTION

Abdominal pain is a commonly encountered clinical problem, accounting for nearly 10% of all visits to emergency departments. Nearly 25% of all patients evaluated for abdominal pain in such settings require hospitalization. What is the reason for such a high rate of hospitalization? The etiology of abdominal pain is often, at least initially, uncertain. Approximately 25% of the patients leave the emergency setting without a definite diagnosis. The frequency of this clinical problem and the associated diagnostic uncertainty mandate a further discussion of abdominal pain. A better understanding of the historical features associated with different causes of abdominal pain will expedite appropriate diagnosis and treatment.

KEY TERMS

Acute abdomen	An abdominal condition that requires immediate surgical intervention.[1,2] Patients with an acute abdomen represent only a fraction of those with acute abdominal pain.
Acute abdominal pain	Acute abdominal pain has an onset over minutes but can persist for days.[3] Sometimes, very severe abdominal pain is described as acute, which is appropriate only if the pain is a new problem. An acute exacerbation of chronic abdominal pain should not be described as acute abdominal pain.
Biliary colic	Pain caused by acute transient obstruction of the cystic duct, usually due to the passage of a gallstone. Patients commonly describe the pain as occurring "in waves." This may be due to peristaltic contractions against a fixed obstruction.
Chronic abdominal pain	Abdominal pain that is present for at least 6 months without a diagnosis despite an appropriate evaluation.
Nonspecific abdominal pain	Pain poorly localized to a specific area of the abdomen. It is often inadequately explained by any specific diagnosis.
Peritoneum	The membrane derived from embryonic mesoderm that covers the viscera and lines the walls of the abdominal and pelvic cavities. The part of the peritoneum that lines the viscera is called the visceral peritoneum. The parietal peritoneum lines the abdominal and pelvic cavities. Autonomic nerves innervate the visceral peritoneum, whereas spinal somatic nerves innervate the parietal peritoneum.[1]

—Continued next page

Continued—

Referred pain	Referred pain is experienced distant from the site of origin.[4] The referral of visceral pain to distant sites is not well understood but may involve both somatic and visceral input to the dorsal horn of the spinal cord.
Somatic pain	Somatic pain emanates from the parietal peritoneum. The somatic nerves innervating the parietal peritoneum contain A-delta neurons.[1] These nerves are fast transmitters and typically produce very sharp, localized pain.
Visceral pain	Pain emanating from the visceral peritoneum. The visceral peritoneum contains C fibers, which transmit slowly, resulting in poorly localized, dull, achy pain.[1] The innervation of the visceral peritoneum is bilateral, resulting in pain that often refers to the midline. Visceral pain often results from distention of an organ (eg, inflamed gallbladder, impacted kidney stones, or small bowel obstruction).

ETIOLOGY (INCLUDING PREVALENCE OF VARIOUS CAUSES)

The prevalence of the various causes of acute abdominal pain depends on the age of the patient. The epidemiology of chronic abdominal pain has not been well studied.

Differential Diagnosis

	Prevalence[a]		
	Total (%)	*> 60 years old (%)*	*< 60 years old (%)*
Abdominal pain, nonspecific	34.9	9.6–22.5	43
Aortic aneurysm, ruptured	1.3	3	0.1
Appendicitis, acute	12–26	3.5–6.7	25
Biliary			
• Cholangitis			
• Cholecystitis		26–40.8	
• Cholelithiasis	5.1	8.9	2.6
Colon, other diseases		3.5–3.7	
• Colitis			
Diverticulitis	3.9	3.4–8.5	0.8
Gastroenteritis	0.3	0	0.6
Gynecologic	1.1	0.2	1.7
Hernia, incarcerated		4.8–9.6	
Inflammatory bowel disease	0.8	1.1	0.7
Ileus		7.3–10.7	
Intestinal obstruction	14.8	28	6.1
Malignancy, abdominal	3	5.5–13.2	1.4
Pancreatitis	2.4	1.9–5.1	1.5

Peptic ulcer disease	3.3	3.3–8.4	2.5
Pelvic inflammatory disease			
Sickle cell crisis			
Testicular • Epididymitis • Testicular torsion			
Trauma, abdominal	3.1	0.4	4.9
Urologic • Bladder distention • Cystitis • Nephrolithiasis • Pyelonephritis	5.9	3.2	7.6
Vascular occlusion, mesenteric	0.6	1.5	0

[a] In patients presenting to the emergency department with acute abdominal pain[5,6]; prevalence is unknown when not indicated.

GETTING STARTED WITH THE HISTORY

- Allow patients to describe their symptoms in their own words.
- Avoid leading questions. Initiate the discussion with open-ended questions.
- Complete the history taking with closed-ended questions directed at the most likely disorder.
- Review the list of medicines the patient is taking prior to seeing the patient and validate during the interview. Remember to ask about over-the-counter and herbal medicines.
- Inquire about alcohol and illicit drug use.

Questions	Remember
I'm sorry to hear that you're having abdominal pain. Can you tell me more about it?	Allow the patient to describe his or her story without interruption.
When did your abdominal pain begin?	Listen carefully for details that may help formulate a differential diagnosis.
I can tell that this abdominal pain is very uncomfortable for you; I'd like to ask you some questions so I can understand what is causing your pain.	Reassurance will put the patient at ease and facilitate the interview.

INTERVIEW FRAMEWORK

- Determine whether the pain is acute or chronic abdominal pain (or an acute exacerbation of chronic abdominal pain). The differential diagnosis differs depending on the acuity of the pain.
- Assess for alarm symptoms.
- Identify the primary location of the pain (if possible), and determine whether the pain has moved to another location[4]:
  - Right upper quadrant (RUQ) pain
  - Epigastric pain
  - Left upper quadrant (LUQ) pain
  - Right flank pain
  - Periumbilical pain
  - Left flank pain
  - Right lower quadrant (RLQ) pain
  - Hypogastric pain (midline below the umbilicus)
  - Left lower quadrant (LLQ) pain
  - Diffuse abdominal pain
- Inquire about abdominal pain characteristics using the cardinal symptom features (PQRST):

Provocation	What makes the pain worse or better?
Quality	What is the character of the pain?
Radiation	Does the pain radiate?
Severity	Rate the pain on a scale from 0 to 10 (with 0 being no pain and 10 being the worst pain possible).
Timing/Treatment	How long have you had the pain? Has the pain been persistent or intermittent over this period of time? What has been done to treat the pain?

IDENTIFYING ALARM SYMPTOMS

There are many potentially serious causes of abdominal pain. Identification of these diagnoses requires detailed questioning aimed at identifying the characteristic features of the disease.

After asking open-ended questions, ask specifically about the presence of alarm symptoms. The patient's response will help guide further diagnostic evaluation.

Serious Diagnoses

	Comment
Abdominal aortic aneurysm (AAA)	• Most AAAs are asymptomatic until rupture. • Abdominal or back pain suggests expansion of the AAA. • The first symptom of an AAA may be thrombosis or embolization to a distal site. • Only 50% of patients survive a ruptured AAA.
Adnexal torsion	Presents as sudden onset of pain in the lower abdomen on the affected side. Urinary urgency, nausea, and vomiting may accompany the pain.
Adrenal insufficiency, acute	Hypotension is the most concerning feature; often accompanied by abdominal pain, fever, confusion, fatigue, nausea, and vomiting.
Aortic dissection, thoracic	• Acute abdominal pain occurs in 22% of dissections of the ascending aorta (Stanford Classification type A) and in 43% of those involving the aorta distal to the origin of the left subclavian artery (Stanford Classification type B). • 40%–50% of untreated patients with dissection of the proximal aorta die within 48 hours. For those who survive beyond 48 hours, 1-year mortality is 90%.[7] • Patients present with sharp, "tearing" pain in the chest, back, or abdomen. The pain is maximal at its onset, as opposed to the crescendo nature of acute myocardial infarction. The pain may move inferiorly over time, which likely corresponds to extension of the aortic dissection.
Appendicitis	• Lifetime risk in general population is 7%.[3] • Patients often initially develop constant, nonspecific periumbilical or diffuse abdominal discomfort. Over a matter of hours, the pain localizes to the RLQ and is associated with anorexia, nausea, and vomiting. Localized tenderness may not develop in patients with a retrocecal appendix because the appendix is not in contact with the parietal peritoneum. Patients often report constipation, although some will have diarrhea.

Biliary process	
• Cholangitis	Charcot's triad (fever, RUQ abdominal pain, and jaundice) occurs in 50%–75% of patients with cholangitis.
• Cholecystitis	• 75% of patients have nausea and vomiting.[3] • Most commonly, persistent and severe RUQ and epigastric pain may occur. It can radiate to the right shoulder or back. • Acute cholecystitis is usually due to gallstones. Risk factors for gallstone disease include female gender, age > 40, and obesity. • Acalculous cholecystitis in the absence of gallstones can occur in critically ill patients.
Bowel obstruction	• 50% of patients have had prior abdominal surgery.[3] • Patients typically have crampy, periumbilical pain, which occurs in paroxysmal waves every few minutes. • Untreated strangulated obstruction is associated with 100% mortality.
Celiac sprue	The most common symptoms include diarrhea, flatulence, weight loss, abdominal discomfort, and bloating.
Diabetic ketoacidosis	• Mortality has decreased from 8% 20 years ago to 0.67% currently. • Nearly 50% of patients have abdominal pain.
Diverticulitis	• Symptoms include LLQ pain (70%), nausea and vomiting (20%–62%), constipation (50%), diarrhea (25%–35%), and urinary symptoms (10%–15%). • Right-sided colonic diverticulitis is less common in Western countries but accounts for up to 75% of diverticulitis in Asians.
Endometriosis	• Approximately 50% of teenage women who undergo laparoscopy for evaluation of pelvic pain or dysmenorrhea have endometriosis. • Symptoms include pelvic pain, rectal pain, dysmenorrhea, and dyspareunia. Aching pain tends to begin several days before menses and worsens until menses abates. Some patients are asymptomatic. The presence or extent of endometriosis does not correlate with symptoms.
Familial Mediterranean fever	• Symptoms include recurrent attacks of abdominal pain (due to serositis) and fever lasting several days. • 65% of first attacks begin before age 10 and 90% before age 20.
Hernia, incarcerated	• The lifetime risk of developing a groin hernia is 25% in men and < 5% in women. • 90% of groin hernias are inguinal, and 10% are femoral. • Inguinal hernias are more common in men than women (9:1) and occur more frequently on the right side. • Femoral hernias are more common in women than men (4:1); 40% of femoral hernias present with incarceration or strangulation. • The most common symptom is a sensation of "heaviness" with activities that increase intra-abdominal pressure (ie, straining or lifting). Pain should raise concern for incarceration. Peritoneal signs often accompany bowel strangulation. *—Continued next page*

Continued—	
Hypercalcemia	• Up to 20% incidence of peptic ulcer disease (PUD) and nephrolithiasis among patients with primary hyperparathyroidism. Both conditions can cause acute abdominal pain. • Hypercalcemia causes different kinds of abdominal pain, depending on the complication (ie, constipation, nephrolithiasis, or pancreatitis).
Inflammatory bowel disease	
• Crohn's disease	• The symptoms of Crohn's disease are much more variable than ulcerative colitis; 80% of patients have small bowel involvement, usually in the distal ileum. • Common symptoms include abdominal pain, fever, weight loss, and diarrhea with or without bleeding. Up to 10% of patients do not have diarrhea.
• Ulcerative colitis	• Symptoms are due to inflammation of the mucosal surface of the colon, which almost always involves the rectum. The disease may extend proximally and continuously to involve other parts of the colon. Bloody diarrhea is the principal symptom. Defecation may relieve the lower abdominal cramps.
Intestinal ischemia, acute	• Patients complain of sudden onset of crampy abdominal pain. • Acute intestinal ischemia may be due to occlusive disease in either the arterial or venous system. • Arterial mesenteric ischemia accounts for 60%–70% of acute intestinal ischemia with mortality rate of 60%. Risk factors include atherosclerosis, low cardiac output states, recent myocardial infarction, and cardiac valvular disease. • Symptoms of colitis may occur if the inferior mesenteric artery is compromised. • Left unrecognized, ischemia may lead to bowel infarction, analogous to myocardial infarction.
Intestinal ischemia, chronic	• Typical patient is a smoker with atherosclerotic vascular disease. • Nearly 50% of patients have either peripheral vascular disease or coronary artery disease. • Patients typically complain of dull, crampy periumbilical pain within 1 hour of eating a meal. Symptoms usually subside over the ensuing hours until the next meal. • About 80% will have weight loss at presentation because patients often avoid eating in order to prevent pain.
Irritable bowel syndrome	• Common idiopathic disorder characterized by chronic abdominal pain and bloating typically relieved by a bowel movement, passage of mucus, change in the number of bowel movements or stool consistency (harder or softer), and episodic diarrhea alternating with constipation (see Chapter 32). • Symptoms usually worsened by stress and eating.
Malignancy, occult	• 33% of patients with renal cell carcinoma present with flank pain or abdominal mass. • 85% of patients with pancreatic cancer have abdominal pain.

Myocardial infarction or ischemia	• Myocardial infarction can cause dull epigastric discomfort and is sometimes confused with PUD.
Pyelonephritis, acute	• Patients present with fever, nausea, vomiting, and flank pain. Pain can be abdominal or pelvic, and patients may have symptoms of urinary tract infection.
Nephrolithiasis	• Nephrolithiasis may be asymptomatic. Renal stones most commonly cause pain when they pass from the pelvis into the ureter. The pain is typically paroxysmal, related to stone movement and subsequent ureteral contractions. The pain migrates as the stone moves through the ureter (see Chapter 42).
Pancreatitis, acute	• Abdominal pain occurs in nearly 100% of patients. The pain typically starts in the epigastrium and radiates to the back. The pain resolves after the acute attack. • Common causes include gallstones (40%) and alcohol (35%, more common in men). • Nausea and vomiting occur in 90% of patients.
Pancreatitis, chronic	• Abdominal pain may initially be episodic but often becomes continuous with intermittent exacerbations. • Presenting signs include exocrine and endocrine dysfunction, including steatorrhea and glucose intolerance.
Pelvic inflammatory disease	• The abdominal pain usually occurs bilaterally in the lower abdominal quadrants. The pain often begins during or shortly after the beginning of menses. In 33% of patients, the onset of pain is accompanied by abnormal uterine bleeding. Coitus and sudden movements may worsen the pain. Up to 10% of patients have perihepatitis, which presents with RUQ pain (Fitz-Hugh–Curtis syndrome). Only about 50% of patients are febrile. Many women have minimal symptoms.
PUD	• Patients may have a wide range of symptoms, none of which are sensitive or specific. These include "burning" epigastric pain and fullness, postprandial belching, bloating, anorexia, nausea, and vomiting. Pain due to a duodenal ulcer classically occurs several hours after a meal when the stomach is empty, whereas gastric ulcer usually causes severe pain soon after a meal. Pain caused by a duodenal ulcer is typically more responsive to antacid therapy or food than is pain caused by a gastric ulcer.
Porphyria, acute intermittent (AIP)	• AIP is the most common and most severe of the porphyrias due to enzymatic deficiencies in the heme biosynthetic pathway. • Abdominal pain is the most common symptom and often the first sign of an acute attack. • Occurs most commonly in young postpubertal women.
Pregnancy, ectopic	• Symptoms include lower quadrant abdominal pain (99%), amenorrhea (74%), and vaginal bleeding (56%).[3] • 50% of patients are asymptomatic before rupture.
Pulmonary infarct	• Abdominal pain, when present, is pleuritic and typically occurs in the upper quadrants.
Sickle cell crisis	• Acute hepatic crisis occurs in 10% of patients, resulting in RUQ pain. *—Continued next page*

Continued—	
Testicular torsion	• Predominantly occurs in neonates and postpubertal boys, but nearly 40% occur in patients older than 21 years. • Sudden scrotal pain is the most common symptom.
Vasculitis	• Vasculitis may occur in the setting of inflammatory bowel disease, especially Crohn's disease. • Antiphospholipid antibody syndrome may present with abdominal pain due to intestinal ischemia. • 25% of patients with polyarteritis nodosa have abdominal pain. • Churg-Strauss syndrome presents with a classic triad of symptoms: allergic rhinitis, asthma, and peripheral eosinophilia. A vasculitis of the small and medium-sized vessels often occurs. • Abdominal pain occurs in nearly 50% of people with Henoch-Schönlein purpura, a small vessel vasculitis that more commonly affects children than adults. The classic tetrad includes rash, abdominal pain, arthralgia, and renal disease. • Behçet disease is more common among men in the Middle East and women in Asia. Symptoms include recurrent oral and genital ulcers, uveitis, skin lesions, and arthritis. A multisystem vasculitis may occur. • Takayasu arteritis, most common in young Asian women, primarily affects the aorta and its branches but can present with intestinal ischemia.

Alarm Symptoms	Serious Causes	Positive Likelihood Ratio (LR+)[a]	Negative Likelihood Ratio (LR–)[a]	Benign Causes
Cardiovascular symptoms				
Nausea and vomiting	Myocardial infarction	1.9[8]		Gastroenteritis
Constitutional symptoms				
Fever	Appendicitis	1.94[9]	0.58[9]	Viral syndrome
	Cholangitis			
	Cholecystitis	1.5[10]	0.9[10]	
	Diverticulitis			
Gastrointestinal symptoms				
Acholic stools Tea-colored urine	Biliary obstruction			Dehydration causes concentrated urine; not to be confused with bilirubinuria

Black-colored stools	Gastrointestinal bleeding			Iron supplements may cause dark stools
Bloody stools				
Hematemesis				
Constipation	Bowel obstruction			Dehydration
	Hypercalcemia			
Nausea or vomiting	Appendicitis	0.69–1.2[9]	0.7–1.12[9]	Gastroenteritis
	Bowel obstruction	1.0–1.5[10]	0.6–1.0[10]	
	Cholecystitis			
	Hernia, incarcerated or strangulated			
	Pancreatitis			
Pain before vomiting	Appendicitis	2.76[9]		
Migration of periumbilical pain to the RLQ	Appendicitis	3.18[9]	0.5[9]	
RLQ pain	Appendicitis	7.31–8.46[9]	0.28[9]	Mesenteric adenitis
RUQ pain	Cholecystitis	1.5–1.6[10]	0.4–0.7[10]	
Miscellaneous				
Jaundice	Biliary obstruction			
	Cholangitis			
Neurologic deficit, focal	Aortic dissection	6.6–33[7]	0.71–0.87[7]	
Pain, abrupt onset	Aortic dissection	1.6[7]	0.3[7]	
Pain, abrupt and tearing in nature	Aortic dissection	2.6[7]		
Pain, migratory	Aortic dissection	1.1–7.6[7]	0.6–0.97[7]	
Pain, tearing quality	Aortic dissection	1.2–10.8[7]	0.4–0.99[7]	

[a]Each LR applies to the adjacent serious cause.

FOCUSED QUESTIONS

After listening to the patient describe his or her abdominal pain with consideration to possible alarm symptoms, the following questions will help narrow the differential diagnosis.

QUESTIONS (REMEMBER "PQRST")	THINK ABOUT...
Provoke	
Does eating worsen the pain?	Pancreatitis, gastric ulcer, mesenteric ischemia
Does eating alleviate the pain?	Duodenal ulcer, gastroesophageal reflux disease
Quality or associated symptoms	
Is the pain associated with nausea and vomiting?	Pancreatitis, bowel obstruction, biliary colic
Is the pain "tearing"?	Aortic dissection
Is the pain "crampy"?	Distention of a hollow tube (ie, bowel, bile duct, or ureter)
Is the pain associated with emesis of undigested food?	Esophageal obstruction
Is the pain associated with emesis of undigested food with acidic, digestive juices from the stomach but no bile?	Gastroparesis or gastric outlet obstruction
Is the emesis bloody?	Gastroesophageal reflux disease, esophageal or gastric varices, PUD, gastric cancer, aortoenteric fistula
Radiation	
Does the pain radiate to the back?	Pancreatitis, duodenal ulcer, gastric ulcer, aortic dissection
Does the pain radiate to the right shoulder?	Biliary colic, cholecystitis
Does the pain radiate to the left shoulder?	Splenomegaly or splenic infarction
Does the pain radiate to the left arm or neck?	Myocardial ischemia
Severity	
Did the pain in your right lower abdomen suddenly improve from an 8 or 9 to a 2 or 3? (on a scale of 0 to 10)	Perforated appendix
Did the pain hurt the most at its onset?	Aortic dissection
Timing/treatment	
Is the pain continuous with intermittent waves of worsening pain?	Biliary colic, renal colic, small bowel obstruction
Are there multiple waves of pain that increase in intensity, then stop abruptly for short periods of time?	Small bowel obstruction
Did you recently take antibiotics?	Colitis due to *Clostridium difficile*
Does the pain occur once monthly around 2 weeks after the beginning of your menses, occasionally associated with vaginal spotting?	Mittelschmerz

DIAGNOSTIC APPROACH (INCLUDING ALGORITHM)

The first goal in the evaluation of abdominal pain is to consider diagnoses that might require urgent management with surgery or endoscopy. Urgent intervention will be required in a minority of patients presenting with abdominal pain. For all other patients with abdominal pain, the differential diagnosis is best narrowed based on localization of the pain. See Figure 31–1 for the diagnostic approach algorithm for abdominal pain.

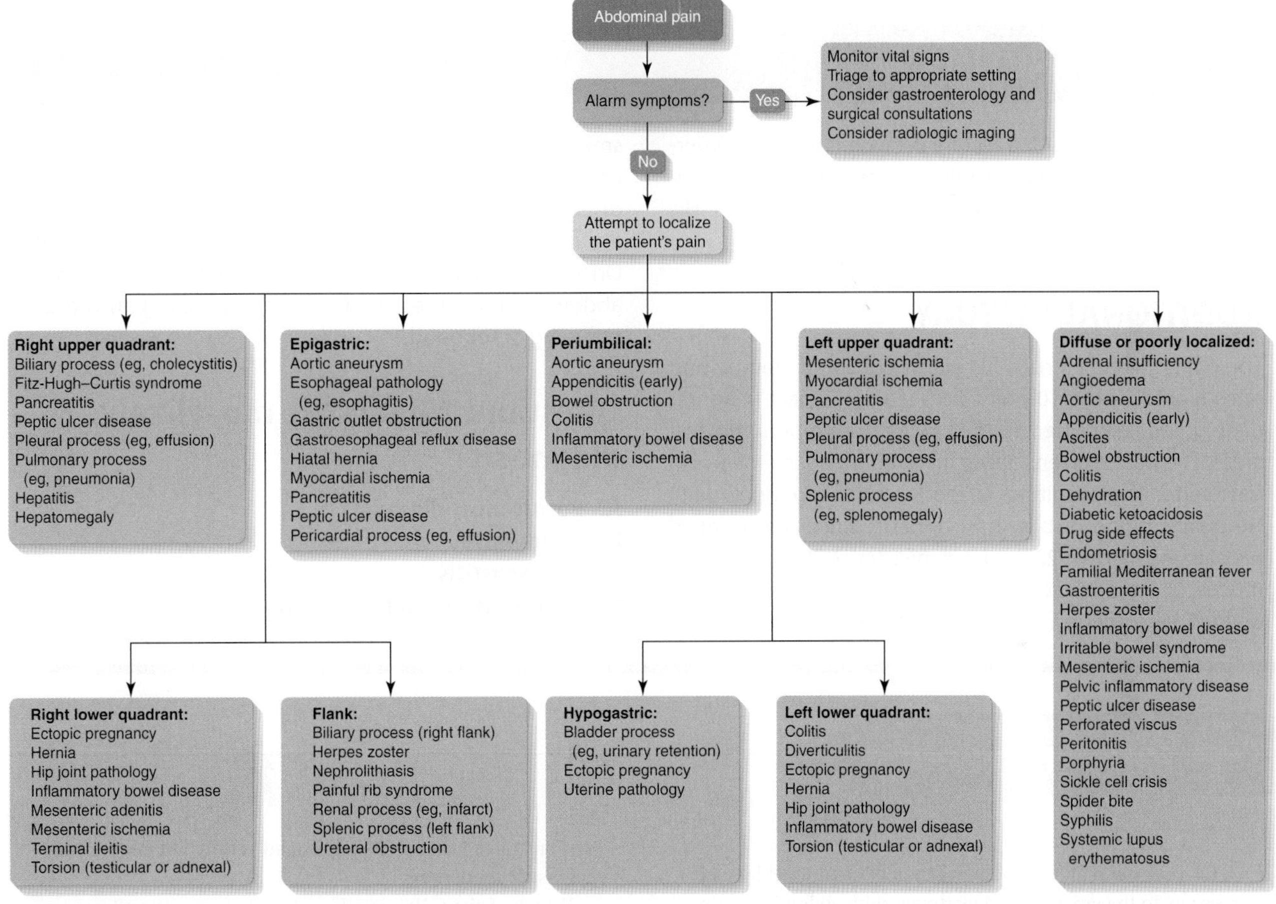

FIGURE 31–1 Diagnostic approach: Abdominal pain.

CAVEATS

- Although nonspecific abdominal pain accounts for up to 33% of patients with acute abdominal pain, it remains a diagnosis of exclusion. Consider a broad differential diagnosis before arriving at such a conclusion.
- The signs and symptoms of acute abdominal pain can change markedly over a period of minutes to hours. Serial abdominal examinations can increase the diagnostic yield.
- The severity of abdominal pain may be underestimated in the elderly, the very young, patients with diabetes mellitus, and immunocompromised patients (ie, patients receiving long-term corticosteroid therapy).
- Many patients cannot provide a history that readily fits into a specific diagnostic category. Barriers, including a different native language, emotional distress, or psychiatric illness, may delay a rapid and accurate diagnosis. Under such circumstances, it is important to recognize that the history may be incomplete. The use of laboratory and imaging studies should supplement the appropriate diagnostic evaluation.

PROGNOSIS

While most hospitals and clinics have sophisticated imaging and laboratory technologies, it is expensive and inefficient to order an abdominal computed tomography scan on every patient with acute abdominal pain. Paradoxically, imaging may also delay a thorough history and physical examination, which might otherwise have led to the appropriate diagnosis. Triage based on history and physical examination is important because abdominal pain may result from a wide range of disorders with markedly different prognoses.

The prognosis of appropriately treated gastroesophageal reflux disease is very good. The prognosis for appendicitis depends on age. The overall mortality rate for patients who receive appropriate therapy is less than 1%, but is 5 to 15 times higher in the elderly.[9] A delay in diagnosis may underlie this mortality difference, which highlights the importance of rapid and thoughtful diagnostic evaluation of patients with acute abdominal pain.

CASE SCENARIO | Resolution

A 62-year-old man with a history of hyperlipidemia, hypertension, and coronary artery disease presents to your primary care practice with abdominal pain for 6 months. His pain gets worse after eating meals.

ADDITIONAL HISTORY

The patient characterizes his pain as dull and crampy and rates it as a 5 on a 10-point pain scale. His pain is nonradiating and is localized to the epigastric and periumbilical areas. The pain worsens about an hour after each meal and gets better after vomiting. All foods tend to trigger his pain. He denies blood or bile in his emesis. Since the onset of his pain, he has lost 20 lbs. He denies fever, chills, or blood, mucus, or fat in his stool. He denies heartburn or previous abdominal surgeries. He is a school teacher who stopped smoking 10 years ago and drinks alcohol socially. He does not use illicit drugs, and he has no family history of heart disease, diabetes, or malignancy. His medications include aspirin, simvastatin, hydrochlorothiazide, and metoprolol. On physical examination, he is well appearing with mild abdominal tenderness in the periumbilical region without guarding or rebound.

Question: What is the most likely diagnosis?

A. Peptic ulcer disease
B. Pancreatitis
C. Cholecystitis
D. Chronic mesenteric ischemia

Test Your Knowledge

1. A 24-year-old man with no past medical or surgical history presents to the emergency department with abdominal pain and fever of 101°F. Six hours ago, he felt nauseated and began to notice a vague periumbilical pain that is now severe (10/10), constant, and sharp, and has migrated to the right lower quadrant. On physical examination, he is febrile and restless, and he is tender in the right lower quadrant.

   What is the most likely diagnosis?

   A. Testicular torsion
   B. Appendicitis
   C. Ischemic colitis
   D. Pancreatitis
   E. Small bowel obstruction

2. A 48-year-old healthy obese woman comes to your clinic with a 1-day history of nonradiating epigastric burning pain that started 2 hours after eating lunch, which she rates as a 4 on 10-point pain scale. She describes similar pains in the past few months but never as severe. The pain is worse when lying flat in bed at night and has been relieved in the past by antacids. She denies fevers, weight loss, changes in her bowel movements, or radiation to her back. Physical examination demonstrates normal vital signs and is only notable for mild epigastric tenderness.

   Which of the following disorders do you suspect?

   A. Cholecystitis
   B. Pancreatitis
   C. Peptic ulcer disease
   D. Aortic dissection
   E. Celiac sprue

3. A 30-year-old alcoholic man with no past medical or surgical history is brought in by ambulance to the ED with severe (7/10) epigastric abdominal pain. The pain started 5 hours after the ingestion of a large meal. It radiates to the back and is associated with nausea and nonbloody, nonbilious emesis. He denies any problems or pain with urinating. On physical examination, he is afebrile, tachycardic, and tender without rebound in the epigastrium and left upper quadrant.

   What is the most likely diagnosis?

   A. Peptic ulcer disease
   B. Cholecystitis
   C. Appendicitis
   D. Nephrolithiasis
   E. Pancreatitis

ACKNOWLEDGEMENT

The authors wish to acknowledge Joseph Ming Wah Li, MD, for his major contributions to a previous version of this chapter.

References

1. Martin RF, Rossi RL. The acute abdomen: an overview and algorithms. *Surg Clin North Am.* 1997;77:1227–1243.
2. Jung PA, Merrell RC. Acute abdomen. *Gastroenterol Clin North Am.* 1988;17:227–244.
3. Stone R. Acute abdominal pain. *Lippincotts Prim Care Pract.* 1998;2:341–357.
4. Kelso LA, Kugelmas M. Nontraumatic abdominal pain. *AACN Clin Issues.* 1997;8:437–448.
5. Irvin T. Abdominal pain: a surgical audit of 1190 emergency admissions. *Br J Surg.* 1989;76:1121–1125.
6. Fenyo G. Acute abdominal disease in the elderly: experience from two series in Stockholm. *Am J Surg.* 1982;143:751–754.
7. Klompas M. Does this patient have an acute thoracic aortic dissection? *JAMA.* 2002;287:2262–2272.
8. Panju A, Hemmelgarn B, Guyatt G, Simel D. Is this patient having a myocardial infarction? *JAMA.* 1998;280:1256–1263.
9. Wagner JM, McKinney WP, Carpenter JL. Does this patient have appendicitis? *JAMA.* 1996;276:1589–1594.
10. Trowbridge RL, Rutkowski NK, Shojania KG. Does this patient have cholecystitis? *JAMA.* 2003;289:80–86.

Suggested Reading

Cartwright SL, Knudson MP. Evaluation of acute abdominal pain in adults. *Am Fam Physician.* 2008;77:971–978.

Flasar MH, Goldberg E. Acute abdominal pain. *Med Clin North Am.* 2006;90:481–503.

Langell JT, Mulvihill SJ. Gastrointestinal perforation and the acute abdomen. *Med Clin North Am.* 2008;92:599–625.

Lin SF, Lin JD, Huang YY. Diabetic ketoacidosis: comparison of patient characteristics, clinical presentations and outcomes today and 20 years ago. *Chang Gung Med J.* 2005;28:24–30.

Lyon C, Clark DC. Diagnosis of acute abdominal pain in older patients. *Am Fam Physician.* 2006;74:1537–1544.

McKinsey JF, Gewertz BL. Acute mesenteric ischemia. *Surg Clin North Am.* 1997;77:307–318.

Ranji SR, Goldman LE, Simel DL, Shojania KG. Do opiates affect the clinical evaluation of patients with acute abdominal pain? *JAMA.* 2006;296:1764–1774.

Silen W. *Cope's Early Diagnosis of the Acute Abdomen.* 19th ed. New York, NY: Oxford University Press, 1996.

Chapter 32

Constipation

Auguste H. Fortin VI, MD, MPH

CASE SCENARIO

A 37-year-old woman comes to your clinic for "constipation," which she has had since childhood. She states that a work-up by her pediatrician turned up nothing. She reports intermittent, crampy abdominal pain that reaches 8 out of 10 in severity and is relieved "mostly" by a bowel movement. She has a bowel movement nearly every day, but her stools are usually hard. When the pain occurs, her stools are "really hard." She was recently laid off from her job and has noted an increase in her abdominal pain and hard stools.

- **Does she really have constipation?**
- **What additional questions would you ask to learn more about her symptoms?**
- **Do her symptoms suggest a serious disease?**
- **How helpful is the history in diagnosing the etiology of constipation?**

INTRODUCTION

Constipation is a common digestive symptom, with a prevalence of 2% to 28%, depending on the definition used.[1–3] The classic definition—fewer than 3 bowel movements per week—has been expanded to acknowledge patients' broader use of the term. In a survey of healthy young adults, 52% defined constipation as straining to pass fecal material, 44% thought it was the process of passing hard stools, and 34% believed it was the inability to have a bowel movement at will. Only 32% believed that constipation was the infrequent passage of stool (definitions were not mutually exclusive).[4]

Some patients describe themselves as constipated, even though they have one or more bowel movements a day, whereas others with fewer than 3 per week do not. Constipation leads to 2.5 million physician visits per year[5] and more than $800 million in expenditures on laxatives.[6] There is an increased prevalence among the elderly and female population. Other risk factors include limited physical activity, low socioeconomic status, and low caloric intake. In a national Canadian survey, 34% of persons with constipation had seen a physician for their symptoms.[7]

Constipation may reflect serious disease, but most people with this symptom have a benign, functional disorder. Effective history taking can help guide further evaluation. Knowing the alarm features that suggest serious causes of constipation and using a sensitive interviewing style will help you appropriately evaluate this often embarrassing symptom.

KEY TERMS

Organic illness	Associated with detectable structural changes in an organ.
Functional illness	This term is being redefined but currently means there is no simple single organic explanation for a patient's symptoms.
Acute constipation	Symptoms for < 3 months.
Chronic constipation	Symptoms persisting > 3 months, often for many years.

—Continued next page

Continued—

Irritable bowel syndrome (IBS)	A functional gastrointestinal syndrome without a single organic cause, characterized by chronic abdominal pain and bloating relieved by a bowel movement, feelings of incomplete evacuation and/or passage of mucus, change in the number of bowel movements or change in stool consistency (harder or softer), episodic diarrhea alternating with constipation, and periods of normal bowel function. Symptoms are usually exacerbated by stress.
Constipation-predominant IBS	A form of IBS wherein constipation alternates with periods of normal bowel function.
Defecatory disorders	Conditions in which the puborectalis and external anal sphincter muscles either fail to relax or contract more vigorously in response to increased rectal pressure during defecation, leading to constipation (eg, pelvic floor dyssynergia, anismus, outlet obstruction, rectal prolapse).
Chronic functional constipation	Chronic constipation in the absence of any known organic cause. Also known as idiopathic chronic constipation.
Normal transit constipation	Also known as functional constipation. Normal stool transit through the colon and normal stool frequency, but a perception of constipation.
Slow transit constipation	Delayed passage of feces through the colon. May be due to colonic hypomotility or hypermotile, disorganized peristalsis causing retropulsion of stool.
Somatization	The expression of psychological distress through physical symptoms such as constipation.

ETIOLOGY AND DIFFERENTIAL DIAGNOSIS

Many illnesses and medications can cause constipation. Acute-onset constipation is more likely to be organic or medication-induced, whereas most patients with chronic constipation have a functional condition affecting the colon or anorectum. The pathophysiology of idiopathic chronic constipation, particularly the brain's influence on gut function, is poorly understood. Idiopathic chronic constipation (like other functional gastrointestinal disorders) is associated with depression, anxiety, somatization, and a history of sexual abuse.[8,9] In gastroenterology practice, approximately 40% of patients with chronic functional constipation report a history of sexual abuse. This number is twice both the prevalence in patients with organic intestinal disorders and the estimated national prevalence.[8,9]

Functional chronic constipation may be associated with slow or disordered colonic motility (slow transit constipation), abnormal functioning of the pelvic floor muscles during defecation (defecatory disorder), or constipation-predominant irritable bowel syndrome (IBS).

Constipation is more common with age and in women. There are few data on the epidemiology of constipation in patients presenting to primary care providers. One study classified people with chronic constipation according to their responses in a structured telephone interview.[3] Although the group surveyed was not a nationwide sample, overall prevalence of constipation was 14.7%. Approximately 33% had "functional" (normal transit) constipation, and another 33% had a defecatory disorder. Approximately 15% were classified as having IBS. Approximately 25% had a combination of IBS and an "outlet" defecatory disorder. Nearly half of respondents had been symptomatic with constipation for 5 or more years. Of those with "functional" constipation, 8.3% had a medical condition (eg, diabetes mellitus, Parkinson's disease, multiple sclerosis) or took a medication (eg, opiate analgesics) associated with constipation.

Constipation in infants and children has a different differential diagnosis[6]; this chapter focuses on constipation in adolescents and adults.

Differential Diagnosis

Anorectal obstruction
Anal fissure
Colon or rectal cancer
Colonic polyps
Fecal impaction
Ileus
Megarectum (a feces-filled rectum with nerve or muscle abnormalities that prevent function of the external anal sphincter and puborectalis muscle; most common in the elderly)

Strictures (diverticular, inflammatory bowel disease, postradiation, or postischemic)
Thrombosed hemorrhoids
Defecatory disorders
Pregnancy
Metabolic and endocrine conditions
Diabetes mellitus
Hypercalcemia
Hyperparathyroidism
Hypokalemia
Hypomagnesemia
Hypothyroidism
Lead poisoning
Pregnancy
Uremia
Neurogenic disorders
Autonomic neuropathy
Chagas disease
Hirschsprung disease
Neurofibromatosis
Central nervous system disorders
Multiple sclerosis
Parkinsonism
Spinal cord tumor or injury
Cerebrovascular accident
Muscular and connective tissue disorders
Amyloidosis
Systemic sclerosis
Myotonic dystrophy
Medication side effect
Antacids (aluminum- and calcium-containing)
Anticholinergics
Antidiarrheals
Antidepressants
Antipsychotics
Antispasmodics
Calcium supplements
Cholestyramine
Clonidine
Iron supplements
Levodopa
Nonsteroidal anti-inflammatory drugs (NSAIDs)
Opiate analgesics
Sympathomimetics
Verapamil
Colorectal motility dysfunction
Slow transit constipation
Constipation-predominant IBS
Defecatory disorders
Idiopathic chronic constipation
Psychosocial
Depression
Low-fiber diet
Sedentary lifestyle
Somatization

INTERVIEW FRAMEWORK

- Begin with patient-centered inquiry (see next section, "Getting Started with the History").
- Determine whether the patient actually has constipation. Range of normal is from 3 bowel movements per week to several per day. Patients preoccupied with their bowels may have unreasonable expectation of "regularity."
- Determine whether constipation is acute or chronic. Long-standing constipation is less likely to be due to serious disease and more likely to be functional.
- Assess for alarm features (see below).
- If constipation is chronic, determine patient's idea of "normal" bowel function.
- Assess for the presence of chronic functional constipation.
- Assess for symptoms of other medical conditions causing constipation (eg, hypothyroidism, IBS).
- Obtain a complete medication list, including over-the-counter medications and alternative therapies.
- Obtain a dietary history to estimate fiber and fluid intake.
- Use the Bristol Stool Scale (Figure 32–1) to estimate stool transit time.

Bristol Stool Chart

Type 1	Separate hard lumps, like nuts (hard to pass)
Type 2	Sausage-shaped but lumpy
Type 3	Like a sausage but with cracks on the surface
Type 4	Like a sausage or snake, smooth and soft
Type 5	Soft blobs with clear-cut edges
Type 6	Fluffy pieces with ragged edges, a mushy stool
Type 7	Watery, no solid pieces. **Entirely Liquid**

FIGURE 32.1 Bristol Stool Chart.

GETTING STARTED WITH THE HISTORY

- Allow the patient to fully describe his or her constipation before asking any clinician-centered questions. Use open-ended questions to draw out the symptom story (see Chapter 3). This will give you diagnostically important data and let the patient feel heard.
- Listen for how the constipation affects the patient's life and ask what he/she thinks might be causing it (the personal story; see Chapter 3).
- Seek out emotion and address it (see Chapter 3). Patients may be afraid that constipation signals cancer or other serious disease. Responding empathically to emotion helps build a strong clinician–patient relationship and can also allow sensitive or embarrassing psychosocial issues to be broached.

IDENTIFYING ALARM SYMPTOMS

Acute-onset constipation with fever, abdominal pain, weight loss, or rectal bleeding suggests serious organic illness such as colon cancer or stricture, as does a family history of inflammatory bowel disease or cancer. Constipation with an age of onset over 50 is also a red flag because of the increased incidence of colon cancer, diverticulitis, hypothyroidism, and Parkinson's disease.

Serious Diagnoses

- Colon cancer
- Strictures
- Spinal cord tumors/trauma
- Bowel obstruction or ileus

FOCUSED QUESTIONS

After using patient-centered interviewing skills to draw out the patient's symptom story of constipation, personal story, and emotional story (see Chapter 3), assess for alarm symptoms (see above) and narrow the differential diagnosis with the following questions.

First, determine if the patient actually has constipation. A consensus conference definition of chronic constipation is as follows[10]:

At least 3 months, which need not be consecutive, in the preceding 6 months of 2 or more of the following:

1. Straining during at least 25% of defecations
2. Lumpy or hard stools in at least 25% of defecations
3. Sensation of incomplete evacuation in at least 25% of defecations
4. Sensation of anorectal obstruction/blockage in at least 25% of defecations

Questions	Remember
Tell me about your constipation.	Avoid interrupting.
What do you mean when you say that you are constipated?	Listen for clues of organic illness or psychosocial distress.
What do you think might be causing your symptoms?	Hearing the patient's explanatory model can help allay fears, uncover cultural issues, etc.
How has this been for you?	Seek out emotion and use empathy.

Alarm Symptoms	If Present, Consider Serious Causes...	However, Benign Causes for This Feature Include...
Unintentional weight loss	Colon cancer Depression	
Recent onset	Colon cancer Metabolic or endocrine disorder	Medication side effect Psychosocial stressor Immobility
Hematochezia, melena	(Serious conditions tend to have blood mixed in with stool.) Colon cancer Diverticulosis Stricture Anal fissure or ulcer (blood on outside of stool)	Hemorrhoids (blood on the outside of stool and/or drops of blood in toilet water)
Significant abdominal pain	Cancer Diverticulitis	IBS Side effect of medications such as metformin, antidepressants, or NSAIDs Hemorrhoids
Change in stool caliber ("Have your stools gotten narrow, like a pencil, or flattened, like a ribbon?")	Colon cancer Stricture Anal fissure	IBS
Nausea, vomiting	Bowel obstruction (eg, from tumor or stricture)	IBS
Fever	Diverticulitis Cancer	
Back pain, saddle anesthesia, leg weakness/numbness, difficulty urinating	Spinal cord process (eg, cauda equina syndrome)	

5. Manual maneuvers to facilitate at least 25% of defecations (eg, digital evacuation, support of the pelvic floor) and/or
6. Fewer than 3 defecations per week

Having the patient keep a bowel diary for 2 weeks can also be helpful.

QUESTIONS	THINK ABOUT...
Acute onset of severe constipation	
Are you able to pass gas?	Failure to pass gas suggests complete intestinal obstruction

—Continued next page

Continued—	
Do you have abdominal pain or cramps?	Intestinal obstruction (eg, cancer, diverticulitis, IBS, ileus)
Do you have nausea or vomiting?	Intestinal obstruction
Are you having fecal incontinence?	Fecal impaction
Have you recently started any new medicines? (also ask about illicit drug use)	Medication side effect
Tell me what you've eaten in the last 24 hours, starting with just before coming to this visit and working backward. Does this represent a change in your diet?	Decrease in fiber or liquids can cause constipation
Has your level of activity recently changed?	Bed rest or sedentary state often leads to constipation
What were your bowel habits like before this episode?	Prior abnormal bowel habits: chronic condition progressing to complete intestinal obstruction
	Bouts of constipation alternating with diarrhea: colon cancer, IBS, diabetic autonomic neuropathy, fecal impaction
Have you had abdominal surgery or radiation?	Strictures Adhesions
Have you suffered a back injury?	Spinal cord trauma
Do you have new weakness in your legs? Numbness around your rectum or genitals? Difficulty passing urine?	Spinal cord damage from tumor or trauma
Chronic constipation	
How often do you have bowel movements? For you, what would normal bowel function be?	Patients with fewer than 2 stools per week are more likely to have slow transit constipation
What is the most distressing symptom for you?	May provide clue to etiology (see next 5 questions for defecatory disorders)
Do you have difficulty passing even soft stools or enema liquid?	Defecatory disorder
Do you ever need to press around your vagina/rectum with your fingers in order to move your bowels?	Defecatory disorder
Do you ever need to evacuate your bowels with your finger?	Defecatory disorder
Do you feel like your bowels are blocked?	Defecatory disorder
Do you have difficulty letting go or relaxing your muscles to have a bowel movement?	Defecatory disorder
Do you have the sensation of incomplete evacuation?	IBS
Do you have abdominal pain and bloating that is associated with bowel movements?	IBS Intestinal obstruction
How often do you experience an urge to move your bowels? Do you always heed it?	Chronic failure to heed may lead to chronic rectal distention, lax muscle tone, slow transit time, and chronic constipation

What medicines do you take, including over-the-counter and alternative remedies?	Medication side effect
What laxatives, enemas, or suppositories do you use? *What dosage? How often?*	Laxative abuse can lead to chronic constipation. After purging with a laxative or enema, it can take several days for enough stool to accumulate for another bowel movement.
Are you ever able to have a bowel movement without using a laxative?	"No" suggests slow transit constipation
Does increasing your fiber intake improve your constipation?	Normal transit constipation
Tell me what you've eaten and drunk in the last 24 hours, starting with just before coming to this visit and working backward.	A diet low in fiber or liquids can lead to constipation
Have you had any pregnancies? Deliveries?	Multiparity is associated with defecatory disorder
Has your level of activity recently changed?	Bed rest or sedentary lifestyle can cause constipation
How is your sleep? Appetite? Mood? Concentration? Interest in things? (see Chapter 64)	Depression can lead to constipation
Have you had any weight gain, decreased energy levels, or swelling in your legs?	Hypothyroidism
Have you had increased urinary frequency or increased thirst, or been told that you have diabetes?	Diabetes and autonomic neuropathy
In your life, have you been hit, slapped, kicked, or otherwise physically hurt by someone? *In your life, has anyone ever displayed their genitals to you against your will, inappropriately touched your genitals, or forced you to have sexual contact against your will?*	Idiopathic chronic constipation and defecatory disorders are often associated with a history of physical or sexual abuse, often unknown to the physician.[8,9] The odds ratio (OR) for functional gastrointestinal disorder in patients with sexual abuse is 2.8.[8] Although you may choose not to ask in an initial visit, it is important to consider in patients with refractory constipation.
Quality	
Are your stools thin like a pencil or ribbon?	Narrowing of the distal colon, sigmoid, or rectum from colon cancer or stricture
Do you pass mucus?	IBS
Are your stools watery?	In debilitated or elderly persons, consider fecal impaction (liquid stool passing around the obstructing fecal mass)
Do you have constipation alternating with diarrhea?	IBS
	Colorectal cancer
Are your stools mixed with blood?	Colon cancer
Are the outside of your stools streaked with blood?	Anal disorder (hemorrhoids, fissures, ulcers)
Are your stools black?	Bismuth subsalicylate, iron supplements, upper gastrointestinal bleeding (see Chapter 36)

—*Continued next page*

Continued—

Time course	
When did your constipation begin?	Postoperative: adhesions, ileus
	Recent: colon cancer, fecal impaction, medication side effect, psychological stress
	Long-standing: IBS, chronic idiopathic constipation
	Lifelong: Hirschsprung disease
Associated symptoms	
Have you had abdominal pain or discomfort for 3 or more days per month in the last 3 months that is improved by a bowel movement? Is the discomfort associated with a change in the number of bowel movements? Is the discomfort associated with a change in the consistency of your stools?	IBS, if 2 or more of these associated symptoms present for more than 6 months[11]
Modifying symptoms	
Do you notice any change in your symptoms with stress?	Increase in symptoms with psychosocial stress suggests IBS
Family history	
Has a parent or sibling ever been diagnosed with colorectal cancer or had a colon polyp?	Colon cancer; the risk of colon cancer is increased approximately 2-fold if a first-degree relative had colorectal cancer or adenoma[12]

DIAGNOSTIC APPROACH (INCLUDING ALGORITHM)

After determining that the patient has constipation, follow the diagnostic algorithm shown in Figure 32–2. Pain as a predominant symptom, without alarm features, makes constipation-predominant IBS, intestinal obstruction, or medication side effect likely.

Next, assess the time course. Chronic functional constipation may be due to a defecatory disorder or to slow colonic transit. The Bristol Stool Scale[13] (see Figure 32–1) can help estimate colonic transit time; lower values, particularly Type 1 or Type 2, indicate slow colonic transit time.

See Figure 32–2 for the diagnostic approach algorithm for constipation.

CAVEATS

- Many patients with chronic constipation have chronic functional constipation, a condition associated with somatization and occasionally a history of sexual abuse.[8,9]
- New-onset constipation, especially in the elderly, should be taken seriously and evaluated further.
- Constipation associated with abdominal pain or bloating is more likely to be due to mechanical obstruction (eg, colon cancer, strictures, fecal impaction), but these symptoms also commonly occur in IBS, a benign, functional condition. Acute onset of symptoms supports the former; pain relieved with bowel movement suggests the latter.
- After purging with a laxative or enema, it can take several days for enough stool to accumulate for another bowel movement. This delay does not indicate constipation. Patients may need to be educated about this phenomenon.
- Patients who complain of chronic constipation may do so because of difficulty passing stool rather than because of infrequent bowel movements.
- It is not always possible to distinguish organic and functional disorders by history alone; further diagnostic evaluation (eg, endoscopy, radio-opaque marker transit time) is often required.
- Data are conflicting about whether it is possible to distinguish slow transit constipation from defecatory disorders by history alone.[3,14–16]

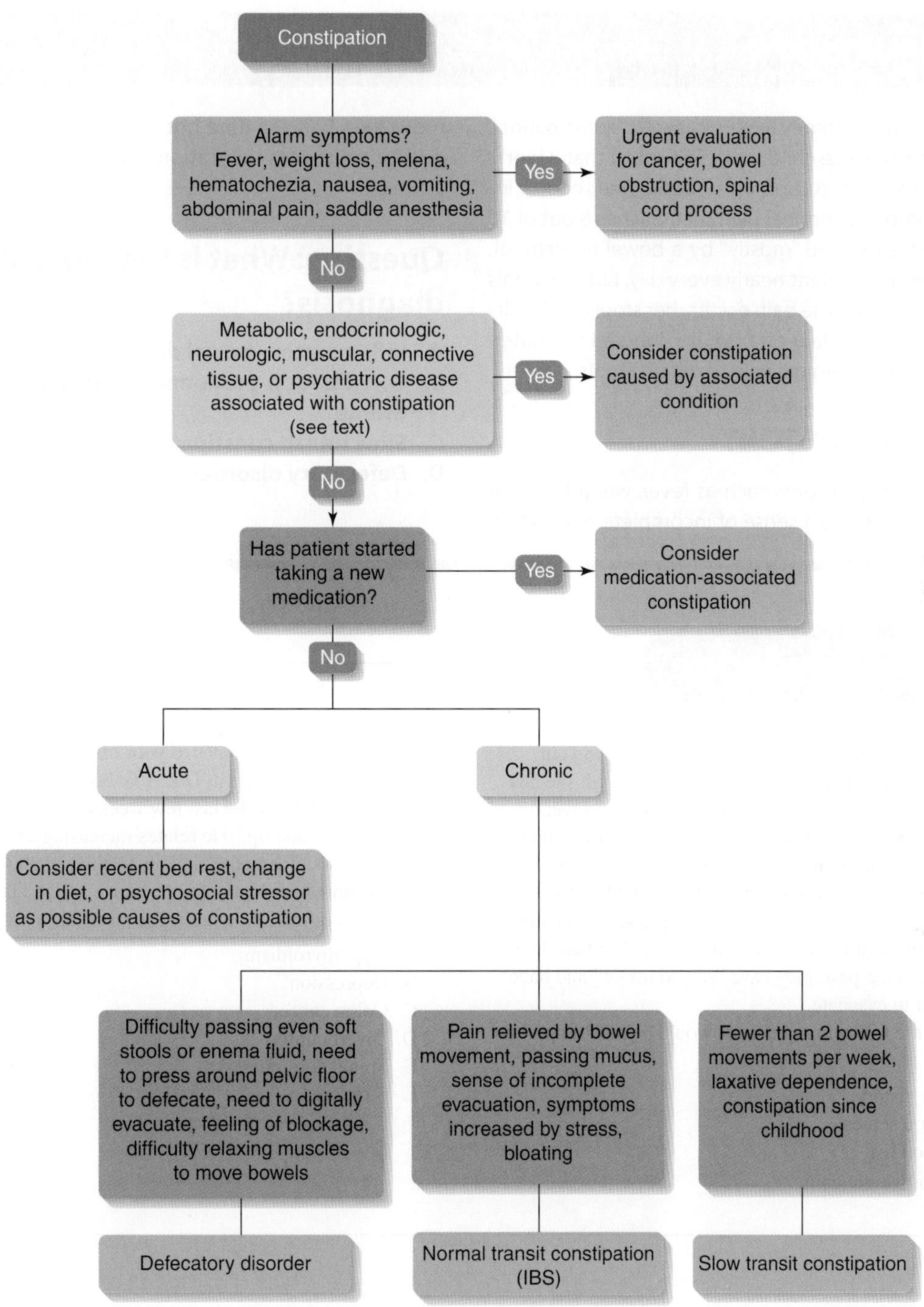

FIGURE 32.2 Diagnostic algorithm: Constipation. IBS, irritable bowel syndrome.

PROGNOSIS

The survival of patients with colon cancer depends on the stage at which the cancer is diagnosed. Advanced disease is more likely when colon cancer presents as acute-onset constipation from obstruction. Strictures usually require surgical intervention. Constipation caused by other conditions (eg, hypothyroidism, medication side effect) usually responds to treatment of the underlying disorder. Chronic functional constipation is difficult to treat, but quality of life can be improved, particularly if a history of sexual or physical abuse is uncovered and addressed.

CASE SCENARIO | Resolution

A 37-year-old woman comes to your clinic for "constipation," which she has had since childhood. She states that a work-up by her pediatrician turned up nothing. She reports intermittent, crampy abdominal pain that reaches 8 out of 10 in severity and is relieved "mostly" by a bowel movement. She has a bowel movement nearly every day, but her stools are usually hard. When the pain occurs, her stools are "really hard." She was recently laid off from her job and has noted an increase in her abdominal pain and hard stools.

ADDITIONAL HISTORY

She has no alarm symptoms such as fever, weight loss, or rectal bleeding. She has a sense of incomplete evacuation more than half the time but does not have to use her fingers to assist with defecation. She denies history of sexual abuse.

Question: What is the most likely diagnosis?

A. Inflammatory bowel disease
B. Constipation-predominant irritable bowel syndrome
C. Slow transit constipation
D. Defecatory disorder

Test Your Knowledge

1. An otherwise healthy 36-year-old woman comes to your office because of constipation for 2 years. Although she has a bowel movement every day, she has to strain for several minutes to pass stool. She admits with embarrassment that she occasionally has to insert her fingers in her vagina and push posteriorly in order to evacuate the stool. Her stools, when finally passed, are sometimes soft. She says over-the-counter laxatives "just don't seem to do much." When she has tried enemas in the past, they have "stayed inside" and have been difficult to evacuate.

   Which of the following questions would be most important to ask?

   A. Obstetric history
   B. Depression screen
   C. Medication list
   D. History of weight gain

2. A 67-year-old man comes to your office for constipation. He says, "I just don't get it, Doc. I've been as regular as a clock all my life, but for the last few weeks, I've been getting more and more bound up." He relates increasing abdominal pain, nausea, loss of appetite, and an 11-lbs weight loss. He has noted some blood on the toilet tissue and in his stools.

   Which of the following is the most likely diagnosis?

   A. Hypothyroidism
   B. Depression
   C. Colon cancer
   D. Diverticulitis
   E. Spinal cord process
   F. Stricture

References

1. Drossman DA, Li Z, Andruzzi E, et al. U.S. householder survey of functional gastrointestinal disorders. Prevalence, sociodemography, and health impact. *Dig Dis Sci.* 1993;38:1569–1580.
2. Locke GR 3rd. The epidemiology of functional gastrointestinal disorders in North America. *Gastroenterol Clin North Am.* 1996;25:1–19.
3. Stewart WF, Liberman JN, Sandler RS, et al. Epidemiology of Constipation (EPOC) study in the United States: relation of clinical subtypes to sociodemographic features. *Am J Gastroenterol.* 1999;94:3530–3540.
4. Sandler RS, Drossman DA. Bowel habits in young adults not seeking health care. *Dig Dis Sci.* 1987;32:841–845.
5. Sonnenberg A, Koch TR. Physician visits in the United States for constipation: 1958 to 1986. *Dig Dis Sci.* 1989;34:606–611.
6. Arce DA, Ermocilla CA, Costa H. Evaluation of constipation. *Am Fam Physician.* 2002;65:2283–2290.
7. Pare P, Ferrazzi S, Thompson WG, et al. An epidemiological survey of constipation in Canada: definitions, rates, demographics, and predictors of health care seeking. *Am J Gastroenterol.* 2001;96:3130–3137.
8. Drossman DA, Talley NJ, Leserman J, et al. Sexual and physical abuse and gastrointestinal illness. Review and recommendations. *Ann Intern Med.* 1995;123:782–794.

9. Leroi AM, Bernier C, Watier A, et al. Prevalence of sexual abuse among patients with functional disorders of the lower gastrointestinal tract. *Int J Colorectal Dis*. 1995;10:200–206.
10. Locke GR 3rd, Pemberton JH, Phillips SF. AGA technical review on constipation. American Gastroenterological Association. *Gastroenterology*. 2000;119:1766–1778.
11. Longstreth GF, Thompson WG, Chey WD, et al. Functional bowel disorders. *Gastroenterology*. 2006;130:1480–1491.
12. Johns LE, Houlston RS. A systematic review and meta-analysis of familial colorectal cancer risk. *Am J Gastroenterol*. 2001;96:2992–3003.
13. Heaton KW, O'Donnell LJD. An office guide to whole-gut transit time: patients' recollection of their stool form. *J Clin Gastroenterol*. 1994;19:28–30.
14. Cash BD, Chang L, Sabesin SM, Vitat P. Update on the management of adults with chronic idiopathic constipation. *J Fam Pract*. 2007;56(6 Suppl):S13–S19.
15. Glia A, Lindberg G, Nilsson LH, et al. Clinical value of symptom assessment in patients with constipation. *Dis Colon Rectum*. 1999;42:1401–1408.
16. Rao SS. Constipation: evaluation and treatment. *Gastroenterol Clin North Am*. 2003;32:659–683.

Suggested Reading

Lembo A, Camilleri M. Chronic constipation. *N Engl J Med*. 2003;349:1360–1368.

Longstreth GF, Thompson WG, Chey WD, et al. Functional bowel disorders. *Gastroenterology*. 2006;130:1480–1491.

Rao SS. Constipation: evaluation and treatment of colonic and anorectal motility disorders. *Gastroenterol Clin North Am*. 2007:36;687–711.

Chapter 33

Diarrhea

Alexander R. Carbo, MD, and Gerald W. Smetana, MD

CASE SCENARIO

A 42-year-old woman visits her primary care physician, reporting 6 weeks of abdominal pain accompanied by bloody diarrhea. This occasionally wakes her from sleep.

- **What additional questions would you ask to learn more about her diarrhea?**
- **How is diarrhea classified?**
- **Can you make a diagnosis through an open-ended history followed by focused questions?**
- **How can you use the patient history to distinguish between benign causes of diarrhea and serious ones?**

INTRODUCTION

Diarrhea accounts for up to 28 million office visits and 1.8 million hospital admissions in the United States each year, with up to 200 million total cases per year.[1] The yearly incidence in adult patients has been reported to be 3% to 63% per year, depending on the referral source. In the United States, several billion dollars are spent annually on medical care and lost productivity due to diarrhea.[1] Although a strict definition of diarrhea includes stool frequency and stool weight, many patients use the term when they experience increased stool liquidity. This chapter aims to clarify some key components of the history when interviewing a patient with diarrhea.

KEY TERMS

Acute diarrhea	Diarrhea lasting < 2 weeks.
Chronic diarrhea	Diarrhea lasting at least 4 weeks.
Diarrhea	Increased frequency of stools (> 3 per day) with increased stool weight (> 200 g/d). However, patients may use the term "diarrhea" to describe increased liquidity. In one series of patients referred to a gastrointestinal (GI) clinic for diarrhea, only 40% of patients actually had output > 200 g/d.[2]
Dysentery	The passage of bloody stools.
Irritable bowel syndrome (IBS)	A functional disorder characterized by the Rome III criteria, which include "Recurrent abdominal pain or discomfort at least three days per month in the last three months with symptom onset at least six months prior to the diagnosis, associated with two or more of the following: improvement with defecation, onset associated with a change in frequency of stool, and/or onset associated with a change in form (appearance) of stool."[3]
Organic versus functional diarrhea	Diarrhea with a known structural or biochemical explanation (ie, infection, inflammation, neoplasm) versus that without a known underlying cause.[3]
Persistent diarrhea	Diarrhea lasting 2–4 weeks. This time frame includes more prolonged and atypical presentations of acute diarrhea. Clinicians should not consider diarrhea to be chronic (and sufficient to evaluate for chronic diarrhea) unless it persists for at least 4 weeks.
Pseudodiarrhea, hyperdefecation	Increased frequency of defecation, but no increase in stool weight or change in stool consistency.
Tenesmus	Spasm of the anal sphincter associated with cramping and ineffective straining at stool.

ETIOLOGY

Because most episodes of diarrhea are self-limited, many patients never seek medical attention. For this reason, prevalence data must be viewed in the proper context: Patients referred to specialists are more likely to have chronic diarrhea, and conditions with alarm symptoms may be overrepresented. The prevalence of common etiologies of diarrhea in a primary care setting is unknown.

Differential Diagnosis

	Prevalence[a]	Prevalence[b]
Functional diarrhea	45%	21%
Infectious diarrhea	11%	
Inflammatory bowel disease (IBD)	7%	3%
Malabsorption	5%	11%
Laxative use	4%	2%
Medication-related (includes caffeine and alcohol)	4%	
Postoperative diarrhea	2.5%	20%
Malignancies	1%	
Collagenous colitis		15%
Idiopathic		20%
Hyperthyroidism		
Ischemic colitis		

[a]Among patients referred to a GI clinic with a complaint of diarrhea[2]; prevalence is unknown when not indicated.

[b]Among patients referred to a tertiary medical center with "undiagnosed or difficult to manage chronic diarrhea"[4]; prevalence is unknown when not indicated.

GETTING STARTED WITH THE HISTORY

- Let patients give the history in their own words by saying, for example, "Tell me about the diarrhea."
- Avoid interrupting.
- Assess for related symptoms, beginning with open-ended questions, such as "Are you having any other symptoms?"

INTERVIEW FRAMEWORK

- The most important first step in taking the history is to determine duration. The goal is to differentiate between acute and chronic diarrhea, because the respective differential diagnoses differ substantially. Keep in mind that chronic diarrhea will initially present as acute diarrhea that does not resolve over time.
- In acute diarrhea, the initial focus is to determine whether the patient is volume depleted.
- Identify alarm features for both acute and chronic diarrhea.
- Consider comorbidities, accompanying symptoms, and precipitating factors.

IDENTIFYING ALARM SYMPTOMS

Most episodes of acute diarrhea will be self-limited. The astute clinician should look for signs of volume depletion such as thirst, fatigue, or dizziness that may warrant intravenous fluid resuscitation and/or hospitalization. Also look for alarm features in order to identify serious diagnoses.

In assessing chronic diarrhea, ask about alarm features and symptoms of organic illness that would prompt further evaluation.

Serious Diagnoses

The main goal is to distinguish functional (ie, IBS) and self-limited (ie, gastroenteritis) causes of diarrhea from those due to organic etiologies. Alarm symptoms and features can help differentiate between the two groups. Serious diagnoses include neoplasm, IBD (Crohn's disease and ulcerative colitis), infection, intermittent bowel obstruction, systemic disease, and malabsorption.

FOCUSED QUESTIONS

After making a distinction between acute and chronic diarrhea and assessing for alarm features, focused questions will narrow

Alarm Features	Serious Causes	Benign Causes
Weight loss (> 5 lbs)	• With normal appetite: hyperthyroidism, malabsorption • Weight loss precedes diarrhea: neoplasm, diabetes mellitus, tuberculosis, malabsorption[5]	
Fever	• Invasive pathogens *(Salmonella, Shigella, Campylobacter)* • Cytotoxic organisms with mucosal inflammation *(Clostridium difficile)*[6] • IBD	Enteric viruses
Bloody stools (dysentery)	• IBD (ulcerative colitis) • Malignancy • Ischemic colitis • Infection with *Salmonella, Shigella, Campylobacter*, enterohemorrhagic *Escherichia coli* (O157:H7), *Entamoeba histolytica*	• Hemorrhoids • Beet ingestion (may cause red, but not bloody, stool)
Awakening from sleep	Generally associated with organic (not functional) causes (eg, IBD, diabetes mellitus)	Self-limited viral syndrome
Family history of colon cancer, IBD, multiple endocrine neoplasia, or celiac sprue	Only useful if positive, because these conditions can develop in patients without a family history	
Age > 50 with change in symptoms	Organic etiology	
Immunocompromised host	Infection	

the differential diagnosis. By asking about the quality and time course of the diarrhea, along with associated symptoms, clinicians can begin to differentiate functional diarrhea (ie, IBS) from other causes. Although the history is the first step toward making a diagnosis, further evaluation such as physical examination, stool studies, and imaging techniques may be necessary.

QUESTIONS	THINK ABOUT...
Quality	
Have you had more bowel movements than usual?	Frequent watery voluminous stools usually signify a small bowel etiology. Smaller volumes with lower abdominal pain point toward a large bowel etiology.
Do you have abdominal pain? If so, where is the pain? Can you point to one spot that is bothering you?	
• *Periumbilical*	Small bowel pathology
• *Lower abdominal*	Large bowel pathology: Ulcerative colitis, bacterial dysentery, herpes simplex virus, gonorrhea, *Chlamydia*, *E histolytica*[7]

—Continued next page

Continued—

• *Generalized*	IBS
	Ischemic bowel
	Celiac sprue
Do you have a sense of incomplete emptying of your rectum or the need to move your bowels but only mucus passes (tenesmus)?	Anorectal inflammation such as ulcerative colitis or infectious dysentery
Is this pain relieved after a bowel movement?	IBS
Has there been passage of mucus?	IBS
	Ulcerative colitis
Is the stool greasy or oily and difficult to flush?	Steatorrhea due to malabsorption
Time course	
Did this begin abruptly?	Viral or bacterial infection; idiopathic secretory diarrhea[4]
Did it come on gradually over time?	IBS
	IBD
Associated symptoms	
Do you have abdominal bloating?	IBS
	Lactose intolerance
	Viral enteritis
	Antibiotic administration
	Nonulcer dyspepsia
	Celiac sprue[8]
Have you noticed an increased amount of flatus?	IBS
	Carbohydrate malabsorption
	Viral enteritis
Do you have a feeling of straining, urgency, or incomplete evacuation?	Ulcerative colitis
	IBS
	Proctitis
Do you have nausea or vomiting?	Viral gastroenteritis
	Bowel obstruction
Do you have symptoms outside of your abdomen (extraintestinal symptoms)?	
• *Arthritis (joint pain, swelling, redness)*	Reactive arthritis after infection, IBD
• *Arthritis, urethritis, or conjunctivitis*	Reiter syndrome (usually after infection with *Salmonella enteritidis* or *Shigella, Yersinia, Campylobacter*)[9]

Modifying symptoms and relevant additional history

Do milk or dairy products worsen your symptoms?	Lactose intolerance
Have you noticed symptoms after eating rye, wheat, or barley?	Celiac sprue
Do you chew sugarless gum?	Sorbitol ingestion
Do your symptoms persist if you stop eating?	Secretory diarrhea
Have you traveled recently?	
• *South or Central America, Mexico, Southeast Asia*	Various infectious etiologies: enterotoxigenic *E coli* (most common), *Shigella,* rotavirus, *Salmonella, Campylobacter, Giardia, E histolytica*[6]
• *Russia*	*Cryptosporidium*
	Giardia[6]
• *Mountainous areas in United States*	*Giardia*[6]
Did you drink any stream water?	*Giardia*
Have you recently taken any antibiotics?	*C difficile,* antibiotic-associated diarrhea
Have you recently begun taking any new medications?	Hydroxymethylglutaryl-coenzyme A (HMG-CoA) reductase inhibitors (statins), proton pump inhibitors, and selective serotonin reuptake inhibitors may cause diarrhea
Have you been hospitalized recently or been to an extended care facility?	*C difficile*, medication-related
Have you ever had surgery such as vagotomy, intestinal resection, or cholecystectomy?	Diarrhea occurs due to lack of absorptive surface, decreased transit time, and malabsorption of bile acids[8]
Has anyone else that you shared a meal with developed these symptoms?	Food-borne outbreaks[6,7]:
What did you eat?	• < 6 hours after ingestion: *Staphylococcus aureus* (after mayonnaise, potato/egg salad, custards, poultry), *Bacillus cereus* (classically after fried rice)
When did you eat it?	
Did you develop other symptoms?	• 8–14 hours after ingestion: *Clostridium perfringens* (after poorly reheated meats or poultry) • 8–72 hours after eating seafood: *Vibrio* species • > 14 hours with vomiting: Viral agents • With dysentery: Enterohemorrhagic *E coli* • With fever or dysentery: *Salmonella, Shigella, Campylobacter*

Modifying symptoms and relevant additional history

Do you work in a daycare center?	Rotavirus (sudden, with vomiting)
	Shigella
	Giardia
	Cryptosporidium[6]

—Continued next page

Continued—

Do you have any pets, such as iguanas or turtles?	*Salmonella*[7]
Do you engage in anal intercourse?	Herpes simplex virus, gonorrhea, *Chlamydia* (direct inoculation causing proctitis), *Shigella, Salmonella, Campylobacter, Giardia, E histolytica, Cryptosporidium* (fecal–oral transmission)[6]
Do you have human immunodeficiency virus (HIV) infection?	*Cryptosporidium*
	Microsporidium
	Isospora
	Cytomegalovirus
	Mycobacterium avium complex
Do any diseases run in your family?	IBD
	Multiple endocrine neoplasia
Do you use laxatives?	Laxative abuse
Are you happy with your body image?	Laxative abuse
Have you had associated body flushing?	Carcinoid syndrome

As previously noted, many patients with diarrhea never seek medical attention; therefore, the denominator in prevalence studies is often uncertain. Fortunately, a recent systematic review evaluated the presence of particular symptoms in patients with IBS.[10] Taken individually, each clinical feature was insufficient to diagnose IBS; this syndrome is diagnosed with a constellation of symptoms.

Symptom	Sensitivity	Specificity	LR+ for IBS	LR– for IBS
Lower abdominal pain	0.90	0.32	1.3	0.29
Mucus per rectum	0.45	0.65	1.2	0.88
Incomplete evacuation	0.74	0.45	1.3	0.62
Looser stool at onset of pain	0.58	0.73	2.1	0.59
More frequent stools at onset of pain	0.53	0.72	1.9	0.67
Pain relieved by defecation	0.60	0.66	1.8	0.62
Abdominal distension	0.39	0.77	1.7	0.79

LR, likelihood ratio.

DIAGNOSTIC APPROACH (INCLUDING ALGORITHM)

See Figure 33–1 for the diagnostic approach algorithm for diarrhea.

CAVEATS

- This review focuses only on adult patients. A different spectrum of disease may apply to infants and children.
- Many patients with diarrhea do not seek medical care. Conditions with alarm symptoms may be overrepresented in the published literature series.
- Some patients have greater than 300 g of stool per day due to a high-fiber diet but do not complain of diarrhea because their stool consistency is normal.[11]
- Remember to differentiate acute from chronic diarrhea, because failure to do so will lead to consideration of an incorrect differential diagnosis.

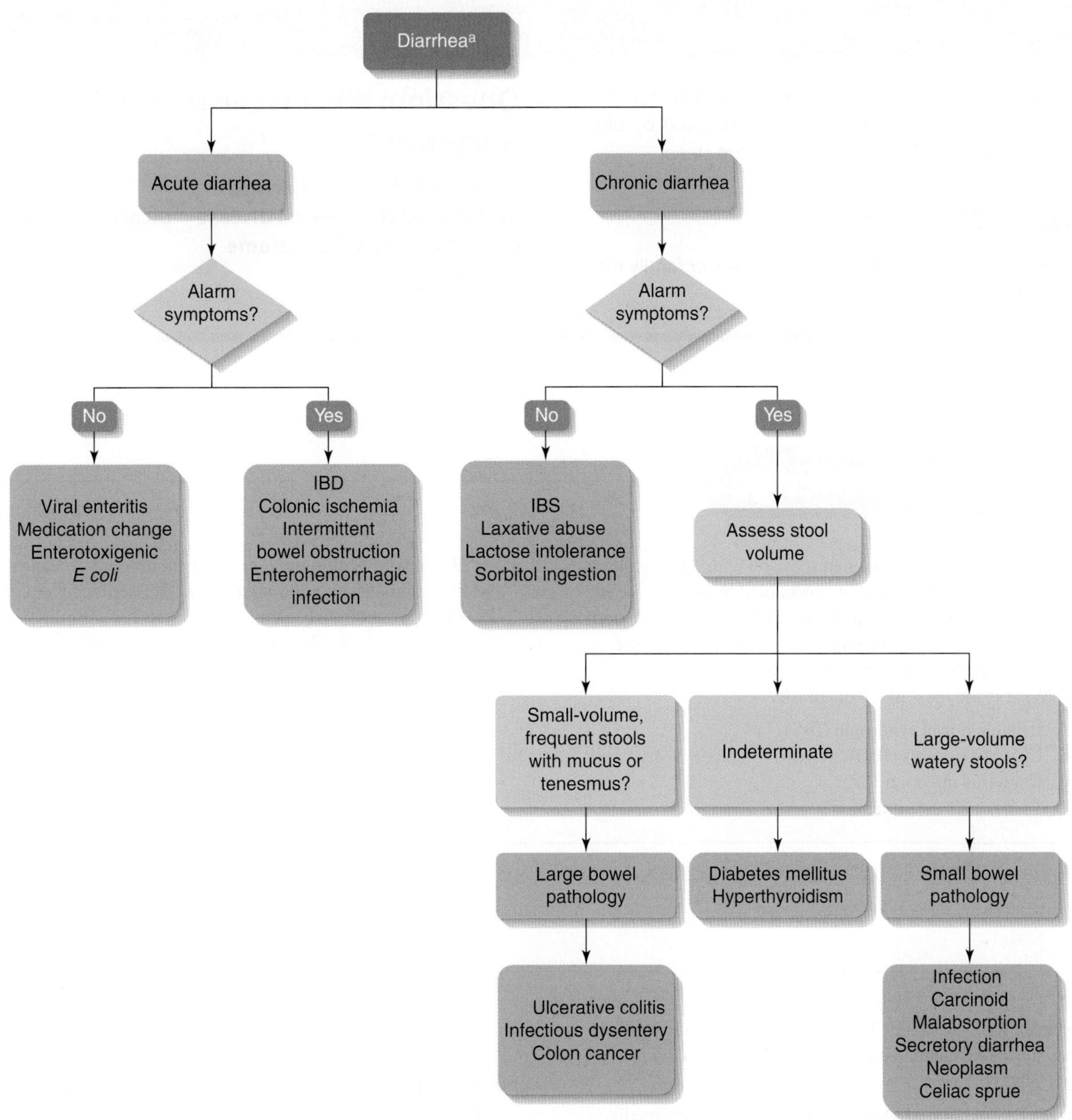

FIGURE 33–1 Diagnostic approach: Diarrhea. IBD, inflammatory bowel disease; IBS, irritable bowel syndrome.
[a]If hypovolemic, give fluid resuscitation. If patient is immunocompromised, consider broader infectious work-up.

- Be sure to review a patient's medications, including over-the-counter medications, because these agents can cause diarrhea.
- Ask about fecal incontinence, the involuntary release of rectal contents, because many patients may confuse this with diarrhea. Although diarrhea may lead to incontinence, there are many nondiarrheal causes.
- Laxative abuse is a frequently overlooked cause of chronic diarrhea. Four percent of patients visiting GI clinics and up to 20% of those referred to tertiary centers have laxative abuse as the cause for chronic diarrhea. Despite seeking medical attention for diarrhea, many of these patients will deny laxative use.[8]

PROGNOSIS

Most diarrheal episodes are self-limited. However, patients with alarm symptoms and signs of volume depletion at the extremes of age are particularly at risk for mortality. Of the average 3000 annual deaths attributed to diarrhea in the United States, 51% were in those older than 74 years, 78% were in those older than 55 years, and 11% were in those younger than 5 years.[1]

CASE SCENARIO | Resolution

A 42-year-old woman presents to her primary care physician with 6 weeks of abdominal pain accompanied by bloody diarrhea. This occasionally wakes her from sleep.

ADDITIONAL HISTORY

She denies any sick contacts, recent travel, or family history of neoplasm.

Question: What is the most likely diagnosis?

A. Acute infectious diarrhea
B. Inflammatory bowel disease—ulcerative colitis
C. Irritable bowel syndrome
D. Celiac sprue

Test Your Knowledge

1. A 41-year-old healthy woman sees you with a 10-month history of abdominal pain, accompanied by an increase in stool frequency and a more watery consistency of her stool. She reports that her pain improves with defecation. She denies fever, bleeding, or weight loss.
   What is the most likely diagnosis?
   A. Irritable bowel syndrome (IBS)
   B. Ulcerative colitis (IBD)
   C. Rotavirus infection
   D. *Escherichia coli* infection

2. A 23-year-old healthy man develops nonbloody diarrhea several hours after attending a picnic. He denies fever, bleeding, or abdominal pain.
   What is the most likely cause of his symptoms?
   A. *Escherichia coli* O157:H7
   B. *Salmonella*
   C. *Staphylococcus aureus*
   D. Celiac sprue

References

1. Guerrant RL, Van Gilder T, Steiner TS, et al. Practice guidelines for the management of infectious diarrhea. *Clin Infect Dis.* 2001;32:331–351.
2. Bytzer P, Stokholm M, Andersen I, et al. Aetiology, medical history, and faecal weight in adult patients referred for diarrhoea. A prospective study. *Scand J Gastroenterol.* 1990;25:572–578.
3. Longstreth GF, Thompson WG, Chey WD, et al. Functional bowel disorders. *Gastroenterology.* 2006;130:1480–1491.
4. Fine, KD, Schiller LR. AGA technical review on the evaluation and management of chronic diarrhea. *Gastroenterology.* 1999;116:1464–1486.
5. Krosner JA, Mertz DC. Evaluation of the adult patient with diarrhea. *Prim Care Clin Office Pract.* 1996;23:629–647.
6. DuPont HL. Guidelines on acute infectious diarrhea in adults. The Practice Parameters Committee of the American College of Gastroenterology. *Am J Gastroenterol.* 1997;92:1962–1975.
7. Hogan DE. The emergency department approach to diarrhea. *Emerg Med Clin North Am.* 1996;14:673–694.
8. Donowitz M, Kokke FT, Saidi R. Evaluation of patients with chronic diarrhea. *N Engl J Med.* 1995;332:725–729.
9. Dworkin MS, Shoemaker PC, Goldoft MJ, et al. Reactive arthritis and Reiter's syndrome following an outbreak of gastroenteritis caused by *Salmonella enteritidis. Clin Infect Dis.* 2001;22:1010–1014.
10. Ford AC, Talley NJ, Veldhuyzen van Zanten SJ, et al. Will the history and physical examination help establish that irritable bowel syndrome is causing this patient's lower gastrointestinal tract symptoms? *JAMA.* 2008;300:1793–1805.
11. Schiller LR. Diarrhea. *Med Clin North Am.* 2000;84:1259–1274.

Suggested Reading

DuPont HL. Bacterial diarrhea. *N Engl J Med*. 2009;361:1560–1569.

Hammer J, Eslick GD, Howell SC, et al. Diagnostic yield of alarm features in irritable bowel syndrome and functional dyspepsia. *Gut*. 2004;53:666–672.

Somers SC, Lembo A. Irritable bowel syndrome: evaluation and treatment. *Gastroenterol Clin.* 2003;32:507–529.

Talley NJ, Weaver AL, Zinsmeister AR, et al. Self-reported diarrhea: what does it mean? *Am J Gastroenterol.* 1994;89:1160–1164.

Chapter 34

Dyspepsia

Sara B. Fazio, MD, FACP

CASE SCENARIO

A 40-year-old woman presents with 3 months of vague abdominal discomfort. It is predominantly epigastric in location but is often accompanied by a sense of "fullness" that makes it difficult for her to eat. Over the past few weeks, she has also noted a burning sensation in her upper abdomen and reports increased abdominal bloating, as well as postprandial nausea.

- **What additional questions would be important to ask to clarify the cause of her dyspepsia?**
- **How do you classify dyspepsia?**
- **What historical features or symptoms would prompt concern for a serious diagnosis?**
- **How can the history help you distinguish between the various types of dyspepsia?**

INTRODUCTION

Dyspepsia is a general term that refers to symptoms originating from the upper gastrointestinal tract. As such, it may encompass a variety of symptoms. Typically, patients will describe epigastric pain but may also complain of heartburn, nausea, vomiting, abdominal distention, heartburn, early satiety, and anorexia. The condition occurs in approximately 25% to 40% of the population, with a range of 13% to 40%, although the majority of patients do not seek medical care.[1,2] Dyspepsia is responsible for 2% to 5% of visits to a primary care physician[3] and accounts for 40% to 70% of gastrointestinal complaints in general practice.[4] An organic cause is found in 40% to 50% of cases, most often gastric ulcer, gastroesophageal reflux disease, and gastric cancer, but in approximately 50% of cases, no cause is found, and the patient is deemed to have functional or "nonulcer" dyspepsia.[3] The approach to a dyspeptic patient should be 2-fold: attempting to elicit a symptom complex that may be helpful in diagnosing a specific condition and excluding worrisome or "alarm" symptoms.

KEY TERMS

Dysphagia	Difficulty swallowing; food getting stuck.
Flatulence	Passing of gas.
Functional dyspepsia	Symptom without an anatomic correlate for pain; also known as "nonulcer" dyspepsia.
Gastroparesis	Hypoactive bowel activity; often associated with autonomic neuropathy of diabetes. Characterized by abdominal distention, bloating, nausea, and flatulence.
GERD	Gastroesophageal reflux disease.
Irritable bowel syndrome (IBS)	Abdominal pain or discomfort associated with change in stool frequency or consistency and often relieved by defecation.
Negative predictive value	The probability of not having the suspected disease when a particular symptom is absent.

—Continued next page

Continued—

NSAID	Nonsteroidal anti-inflammatory drug.
Organic dyspepsia	Dyspepsia associated with a specific diagnosis.
Positive likelihood ratio	The increase in odds for a particular diagnosis if a symptom or factor is present.
Positive predictive value	The probability of the suspected disease in a patient with a particular symptom.
Regurgitation	Reflux of gastrointestinal contents into the esophagus or mouth, or both.

ETIOLOGY

The cause of dyspepsia proves to be benign in most patients. The most common diagnoses among patients who have undergone endoscopy include functional dyspepsia (prevalence approximating 50%), peptic ulcer disease (10%), esophagitis (20%), endoscopy-negative reflux disease (20%), and gastric or esophageal cancer (1%).[5] The prevalence of a particular condition varies depending on the population being studied. For example, in one series, gastric ulcer constituted 30% of dyspepsia diagnoses in persons under the age of 30 but 60% in persons over the age of 60.[6] Similarly, gastric malignancy is much more common in patients over the age of 45 to 55 and in persons of East Asian descent. In addition, it is often difficult to extrapolate data from studies performed in tertiary care centers (ie, gastroenterology clinics) to the general primary care setting because the incidence of any pathologic finding is likely to be higher in the former.

Differential Diagnosis

Benign Causes	Prevalence[a]
Functional dyspepsia	50%[5]
Peptic ulcer disease (gastric or duodenal ulcer)	10%[5]
GERD	20%[5]
Esophagitis	20%[5]
Gastritis and duodenitis	
Biliary tract disease	
Gastroparesis	
IBS	
Pancreatitis	
Medications (NSAIDs, antibiotics, potassium, iron, alcohol, theophylline, acarbose, alendronate, metformin, corticosteroids, narcotics)	
Celiac disease	
Lactose intolerance	
Metabolic disturbances (hyperthyroidism, hypothyroidism, diabetes, hyperparathyroidism, adrenal insufficiency)	

[a]Among general population with dyspepsia; prevalence is unknown when not indicated.

GETTING STARTED WITH THE HISTORY

Although obtaining a complete history from a patient with dyspepsia is important, the presence of symptoms alone has not been found to be very helpful in establishing a specific diagnosis.[1] Clinicians correctly diagnose only 45% to 50% of adults on initial presentation.[7] However, certain clusters of symptoms have been found to have a high negative predictive value for organic causes of dyspepsia.[8] In other words, the presence of these features makes a serious cause unlikely. For example, in one study, the diagnosis of functional dyspepsia was much more likely if the patient had upper abdominal pain that was not severe and if there was an absence of nocturnal pain, nausea, vomiting, or weight loss.[7]

It is important to ask open-ended questions at the beginning of the interview to allow the patient to provide as much of the history as possible without specific prompting. Because clinicians use the term "dyspepsia" to describe a variety of symptoms, it is important to allow the patient to describe the symptoms in detail to avoid coming to a diagnosis prematurely.

Questions	Remember
Tell me more about the symptoms you are having.	Allow the patient to tell the story in his or her own words.
Describe the discomfort that you are feeling.	Begin to create a differential diagnosis in your mind as you are listening to the patient's story.
Go over the last episode you had from beginning to end, describing everything that you felt.	

INTERVIEW FRAMEWORK

After asking open-ended questions, directed questions should help classify a dyspeptic patient into 1 of 3 categories of benign disease:

1. *Ulcer-like dyspepsia.* Discomfort is typically well localized and often relieved by food or antacids. Patients often complain of nighttime symptoms.
2. *Dysmotility-like dyspepsia.* Discomfort is aggravated by meals and associated with bloating or fullness. Nausea, vomiting, and early satiety are frequent complaints.
3. *Reflux-like dyspepsia.* This type is characterized by a burning sensation that radiates into the chest or throat and is associated with a sour taste in the mouth. The symptoms are worse when lying down or after intake of spicy foods, fatty foods, alcohol, chocolate, peppermint, or caffeinated beverages. Patients may report regurgitation or the effortless passage of stomach contents into the mouth. Dysphagia may progressively worsen over time, particularly for solids, which often indicates the presence of an esophageal stricture.

Assessment of alarm symptoms, which are suggestive of a more serious disease, is equally important. A paradigm to organize specific questions includes asking about the following:

- Onset
- Duration
- Frequency
- Location
- Character of pain or discomfort
- Radiation
- Associated symptoms
- Exacerbating factors
- Relieving factors

IDENTIFYING ALARM SYMPTOMS

Most serious causes for dyspepsia are rare, with the exception of duodenal or peptic ulcer disease. Duodenal and peptic ulcer diseases have been included here because they can cause a gastrointestinal hemorrhage or perforation if left untreated. Gastric or esophageal malignancy, the most feared diagnosis, has a prevalence of 1% among patients with dyspepsia. Patients with malignancy tend to be older and to seek medical attention earlier (due to severity of symptoms) than persons with a benign disease.[1]

Differential Diagnosis

Serious Causes	Prevalence[a]
Gastric or esophageal cancer	1%[2]
Duodenal or gastric ulcer	10%[2]
Infiltrative diseases of the stomach (Crohn's disease, sarcoidosis)	
Ischemic colitis	
Hepatoma	
Pancreatic cancer	
Ischemic heart disease	

[a]Among the general population with dyspepsia; prevalence is unknown when not indicated.

One of the most important functions of the history for a patient with dyspepsia is the identification of alarm symptoms or features. Definitions of alarm features vary but generally include any of the following:

- Weight loss
- Bleeding
- Anemia
- Dysphagia
- Severe pain
- Protracted vomiting

Age over 45 is often listed as an alarm feature because the incidence of gastric malignancy is higher in this age group. However, it is important to remember that even among this age group, the likelihood of malignancy in a patient with dyspepsia is still less than 3%.[4] Many patients with a diagnosis of malignancy have one or more alarm features. However, these features are not specific for malignancy, as illustrated by a study of 20,000 patients who underwent endoscopy for evaluation of dyspepsia. Only 3% of patients with any of 4 major predictors (age > 45, male sex, anemia, or bleeding) proved to have a malignancy (positive predictive value). However, the negative predictive value was 99% (99% of patients with no significant major predictors had no malignancy).[9] Thus, the absence of any alarm features is perhaps the most helpful diagnostic tool.[10]

Alarm Features	If Present, Consider Serious Causes...	Positive Likelihood Ratio (LR+)[a]	However, Benign Causes Include...
Weight loss	Gastric or esophageal malignancy		Peptic ulcer disease
	Intra-abdominal malignancy		Malabsorption
	Colon cancer		Metabolic disturbance
	Ischemic colitis		
Bleeding	Gastric or esophageal malignancy	2.90[9]	
	Colon cancer		
	Peptic or duodenal ulcer		
	Ischemic colitis		
Anemia	Gastric or esophageal malignancy	2.28[9]	Peptic ulcer disease
	Intra-abdominal malignancy		
Dysphagia	Gastric or esophageal malignancy		Esophageal stricture
			Esophagitis
Age > 45	Gastric or esophageal malignancy	1.72[9]	Any etiology
	Intra-abdominal malignancy		
	Colon cancer		
Male sex	Gastric or esophageal malignancy	1.40[9]	Any etiology

[a]Each LR applies to the adjacent serious cause.

FOCUSED QUESTIONS

After asking open-ended questions and considering alarm symptoms, ask the following questions in order to narrow the differential diagnosis.

QUESTIONS	THINK ABOUT...
Have you ever had a gastric or duodenal ulcer?	Peptic ulcer disease is much more common in a person with a prior history.
Do you have a family history of ulcer disease?	Peptic ulcer disease
Do you smoke?	Peptic ulcer disease
	Reflux esophagitis
	Gastric cancer
Do you have a history of heavy alcohol use?	Gastritis
	Reflux esophagitis
	Peptic ulcer disease
	Pancreatitis
	Esophageal cancer
How often do you take NSAIDs?	NSAID use increases the likelihood of gastrointestinal bleeding in a patient with dyspepsia by a factor of 7 (odds ratio, 7.1).[11]
Are you over the age of 45?	Age > 45 (and particularly > 55) increases the likelihood of a gastric or esophageal malignancy.
How long have you had this discomfort?	More serious diagnoses tend to have a shorter interval until presentation; thus, a patient who has had dyspepsia for years with no associated symptoms is more likely to have a benign diagnosis.
Quality	
Is the pain:	
• *Burning?*	Gastritis
	Duodenal ulcer
	Gastric ulcer
• *Stabbing?*	Pancreatitis
	Duodenal ulcer
	Gastric ulcer
• *Severe/unbearable?*	Acute pancreatitis
	Perforated viscus
• *Crampy/colicky?*	Biliary colic
	IBS
	Intestinal obstruction

—Continued next page

Continued—

Where is the pain localized?	
• *Epigastric*	Gastritis
	Esophagitis
	Duodenal ulcer
	Peptic ulcer
	Pancreatitis
	Gastric or esophageal malignancy
	Pancreatic cancer
	Colon cancer (in transverse colon)
	Functional dyspepsia
• *Substernal*	Ischemic heart disease
	Esophagitis
• *Right upper quadrant*	Biliary colic
	IBS
	Hepatoma
• *Periumbilical*	Small bowel disease
	Small bowel obstruction
• *Left upper quadrant*	IBS
	Lesion in tail of pancreas
Does the pain:	
• *Remain in the same place?*	Gastric ulcer
• *Radiate from the epigastrium to the back?*	Pancreatitis
	Posterior penetration of peptic ulcer
• *Radiate from the epigastrium to the chest or neck?*	GERD
	Ischemic heart disease
	Esophageal spasm
Is the pain:	
• *Constant?*	Gastric malignancy
• *Intermittent?*	Gastritis
	Peptic ulcer disease
	Biliary colic
	IBS
	Medication-related dyspepsia

Time course	
Tell me about the onset of the discomfort.	
• *Abrupt onset*	Acute pancreatitis
	Perforated viscus
	Vascular thrombosis
• *Gradual increase in intensity*	Peptic ulcer disease
	Biliary colic
How long does it last?	
• *Steady for 30 minutes to 2 hours before gradually subsiding*	Peptic ulcer disease
• *Reaches peak intensity in 15–45 minutes and subsides over several hours*	Biliary colic
Does the pain wake you from sleep?	Peptic ulcer disease
Associated symptoms	
Do you have nausea, or are you vomiting?	Peptic ulcer disease
	Gastric cancer
	Biliary colic
Do you have melena?	Peptic ulcer disease
	Gastric cancer
	Colon cancer
Do you have chronic cough or hoarseness?	GERD
Is your urine dark? Have you noticed a yellow tone in your skin?	Biliary disease
Are you belching?	Biliary disease
	IBS
	GERD
Does your abdomen feel full?	IBS
Do you have heartburn, a bitter taste in your mouth, or regurgitation of food contents?	GERD
Are you passing gas?	IBS
	Malabsorption
	Biliary disease

—Continued next page

Continued—

Have you lost weight?	Gastric or esophageal cancer
	Peptic ulcer disease
	Colon cancer
	Intra-abdominal malignancy
	Malabsorption
Is swallowing difficult?	GERD
	Esophagitis
	Esophageal stricture
	Esophageal cancer
Are you bloated?	IBS
Have you had a change in stool frequency or consistency?	IBS, often associated with "alternating constipation and diarrhea" as well as pencil-thin stools
Are you constipated?	Colon cancer
	IBS
Is there mucus with passage of stool?	IBS
	Inflammatory bowel disease
Is bright red blood present with passage of stool?	Colon cancer
	Diverticulosis
	Briskly bleeding peptic ulcer
	Hemorrhoids
	Inflammatory bowel disease
Modifying symptoms	
Are symptoms:	
• *Worse after eating?*	Gastric ulcer
	GERD
• *Worse before eating and relieved by food?*	Duodenal ulcer
• *Worse after:*	
◦ *Drinking milk?*	Lactose intolerance
◦ *Eating fatty or fried foods?*	Biliary colic
	IBS
◦ *Eating gluten-containing foods (ie, wheat, barley, rye)?*	Celiac disease
◦ *Consuming citrus fruits?*	Gastritis
	GERD
◦ *Drinking alcohol?*	Gastritis
	GERD
	Peptic ulcer disease
	Pancreatitis

• *Worse when lying down?*	GERD
	Pancreatitis
• *Relieved by defecation?*	IBS
• *Precipitated by stress?*	IBS
	Gastritis
• *Related to menstrual cycle?*	Nongastrointestinal etiology; consider endometriosis, dysfunctional uterine bleeding, ovarian cyst

DIAGNOSTIC APPROACH (INCLUDING ALGORITHM)

The first step is to determine whether any alarm features are present. If absent, the likelihood of a benign etiology is much higher. If present, immediate evaluation with endoscopy should take place. Among the benign etiologies of dyspepsia, consider 3 subclassifications: ulcer-like dyspepsia, reflux-like dyspepsia, and dysmotility-like dyspepsia. The recently revised Rome III criteria recommend classifying functional dyspepsia as either postprandial distress syndrome or epigastric pain syndrome.[12] Although distinct from dyspepsia, biliary colic symptoms can often overlap and should also be considered. Certain symptom groupings, if present, will help clarify the diagnosis. See Figure 34–1 for diagnostic approach algorithm for dyspepsia.

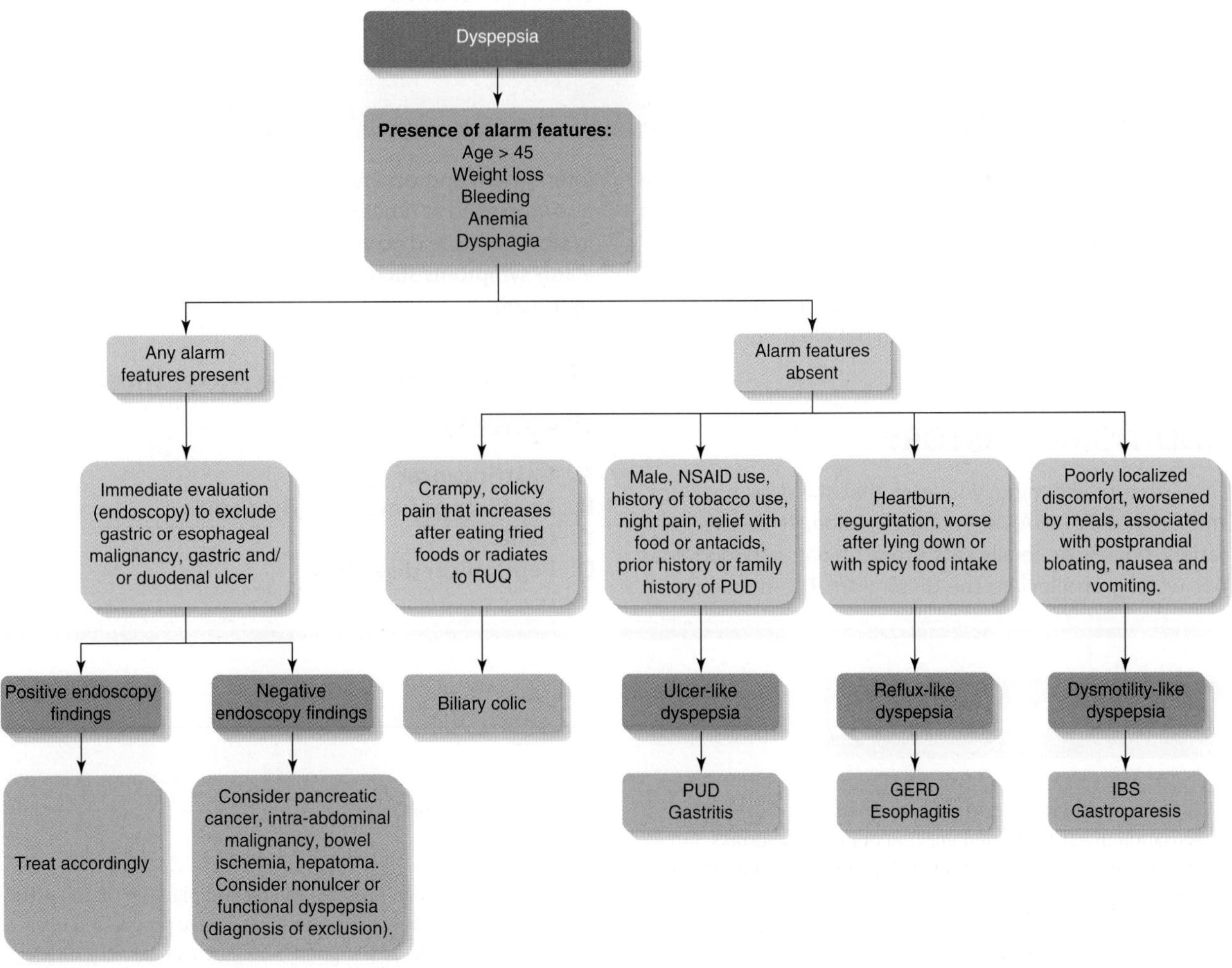

FIGURE 34–1 Diagnostic approach: Dyspepsia. GERD, gastroesophageal reflux disease; IBS, irritable bowel syndrome; NSAID, nonsteroidal anti-inflammatory drug; PUD, peptic ulcer disease; RUQ, right upper quadrant.

CAVEATS

- Dyspepsia refers to a constellation of symptoms arising from the upper gastrointestinal tract and, as such, has a very broad differential diagnosis.
- Most causes of dyspepsia are benign; the presence of alarm features may help distinguish a patient with a more serious condition. Such patients must be referred for endoscopic evaluation.
- Extensive symptom overlap occurs between different groups of patients with dyspepsia.[1] The value of the medical history is unfortunately limited as a tool to discriminate between different etiologies. Thus, although history is important, physical examination and diagnostic studies are also important parts of the evaluation.
- Avoid narrowing the differential diagnosis too early. A patient who complains of generalized epigastric discomfort may have a primary cardiac and not gastrointestinal etiology.
- Taking a complete medication history is of paramount importance. Many herbal products and over-the-counter medications can cause dyspepsia, and the patient is unlikely to bring them up unless you ask the patient directly.
- Gastric malignancies are rare but are more common in patients older than age 45 years; in patients with a family history of gastric cancer, gastric surgery, or infection with *Helicobacter pylori*; and in patients who have immigrated from an endemic area (eg, Japan, Costa Rica, China, Brazil).[4]

PROGNOSIS

Most patients with dyspepsia have an excellent prognosis because the most common etiologies are nonulcer dyspepsia, GERD, and peptic ulcer disease. However, dyspepsia can have a significant impact on quality of life, with large societal and individual costs, including multiple physician visits, diagnostic tests, the cost of medications for treatment, and loss of productivity. The symptoms can be quite disabling and distressing. If untreated, peptic ulcer disease can be associated with significant morbidity. Gastric cancer is uncommon, but approximately 95% of symptomatic lesions are discovered at an advanced stage, when the 5-year survival is 10%.[4]

CASE SCENARIO | Resolution

A 40-year-old woman presents with 3 months of vague abdominal discomfort. It is predominantly epigastric in location but is often accompanied by a sense of "fullness" that makes it difficult for her to eat. Over the past few weeks, she has also noted a burning sensation in her upper abdomen and reports increased abdominal bloating, as well as postprandial nausea.

ADDITIONAL HISTORY

On further questioning, you learn that she does not drink, smoke, or take NSAIDs. Eating occasionally causes early satiety, but she generally eats 3 meals a day, and food does not worsen or alleviate the discomfort. The discomfort is intermittent and occurs on some days but not others. It is also worsened at times of stress. There has been no change in stool habits and no vomiting or hematemesis. She has no alarm symptoms such as weight loss, bleeding, anemia, or dysphagia.

Question: What is the most likely diagnosis?

A. Gastric cancer
B. Nonulcer or functional dyspepsia
C. GERD
D. Peptic ulcer disease

Test Your Knowledge

1. A 25-year-old graduate student complains of a burning sensation in her throat and upper abdomen. She drinks 3 to 4 cups of coffee per day and often skips meals. Symptoms are often worse at bedtime.

   Which of the following symptoms would be most consistent with a diagnosis of gastroesophageal reflux?

   A. Weight loss
   B. Flatulence
   C. Chronic cough
   D. Vomiting

2. A 55-year-old man presents to you complaining of epigastric pain and early satiety. His symptoms have progressed over the past 6 months to the point where he can eat very little and has lost 10 lbs. He complains of severe constipation and occasional black stool.

Which of the following features is *not* an alarm symptom that should prompt immediate endoscopy?

A. Age over 45
B. Weight loss
C. Constipation
D. Black stool

3. Your next patient is a 30-year-old man with a chief complaint of abdominal pain. The pain intensifies in the absence of food and generally is relieved once he eats. He reports vomiting several times a week.

Which of the following features, if present, would suggest a diagnosis of peptic ulcer disease?

A. Pain worsening upon lying down
B. Pain colicky in nature
C. Difficulty with swallowing
D. History of prolonged NSAID use

References

1. Bazaldua OV, Schneider FD. Evaluation and management of dyspepsia. *Am Fam Physician.* 1999;60:1773–1784.
2. Zagari RM, Fuccio L, Bazzoli F. Investigating dyspepsia. *BMJ.* 2008;337:a1400.
3. Fisher RS, Parkman HP. Management of nonulcer dyspepsia. *N Engl J Med.* 1998;339:1376–1381.
4. McQuaid K. Dyspepsia. In: Feldman M, Friedman LS, Sleisenger MH, Scharshmidt BF, eds. *Sleisenger and Fordtran's Gastrointestinal and Liver Disease*. 7th ed. New York, NY: WB Saunders and Company, 2002:102.
5. Moayyedi P, Talley NJ, Fennerty MB, Vakil N. Can the clinical history distinguish between organic and functional dyspepsia? *JAMA*. 2006;295:1566–1576.
6. Richter JE. Dyspepsia: organic causes and differential characteristics from functional dyspepsia. *Scand J Gastroenterol Suppl.* 1991;182:11–16.
7. Muris JW, Starmans R, Pop P, et al. Discriminant value of symptoms in patients with dyspepsia. *J Fam Pract.* 1994;38:139–143.
8. Zell SC, Budhraja M. An approach to dyspepsia in the ambulatory care setting: evaluation based on risk stratification. *J Gen Intern Med.* 1989;4:144–150.
9. Wallace MB, Durkalski VL, Vaughan J, et al. Age and alarm symptoms do not predict endoscopic findings among patients with dyspepsia: a multicentre database study. *Gut.* 2001;49: 29–34.
10. Stephens MR, Lewis WG, White S, et al. Prognostic significance of alarm symptoms in patients with gastric cancer. *Br J Surg*. 2005;92:840–846.
11. Kurata JH, Nogawa AN, Noritake D. NSAIDs increase risk of gastrointestinal bleeding in primary care patients with dyspepsia. *J Fam Pract.* 1997;45:227–235.
12. Lacy BE, Cash BD. A 32-year-old woman with chronic abdominal pain. *JAMA*. 2008;299:555–565.

Suggested Reading

Bytzer P, Talley NJ. Dyspepsia. *Ann Intern Med.* 2001;134:815–822.

Longstreth GF. Functional dyspepsia—managing the conundrum. *N Engl J Med*. 2006;354:791–793.

McNamara DA, Buckley M, O'Morain CA. Nonulcer dyspepsia. Current concepts and management. *Gastroenterol Clin North Am.* 2000;29:807–818.

Talley NJ, Vakil NB, Moayyedi P. American Gastroenterological Association technical review: on the evaluation of dyspepsia. *Gastroenterology.* 2005;129:1756–1780.

Chapter 35

Dysphagia

Anthony Lembo, MD, and Filippo Cremonini, MD

CASE SCENARIO

A 52-year-old gentleman comes to your office with a history of intermittent difficulty swallowing solid food. His symptoms have been present for the past 5 years. He points to his supraclavicular notch when describing where the food feels stuck, although he is able to chew his food and transfer it into his posterior pharynx without difficulty. He does not choke or cough while eating. Drinking water will usually relieve his symptoms, although on several occasions he has self-induced vomiting. His symptoms are slightly worse now than they were several years ago, which prompted today's visit.

- **Would you classify his dysphagia as esophageal or oropharyngeal?**
- **What symptoms help determine whether his dysphagia is due to a mechanical or motor (ie, motility) abnormality?**
- **How can you use the patient's history to distinguish between a benign and malignant cause of his dysphagia?**

INTRODUCTION

The word dysphagia derives from the Greek words *dys* (with difficulty) and *phagein* (to eat) and is defined as difficulty in swallowing. It is the sensation of hesitation or delay in passage of food during swallowing. Therefore, dysphagia differs from odynophagia, which refers to pain with swallowing. It also differs from globus, which is the sensation of a lump or tightness in the throat unrelated to swallowing. The complaint of dysphagia, especially when it is a new symptom, should always be taken seriously because it is the most common presenting symptom of neoplasm of the esophagus.

Dysphagia can be classified as either oropharyngeal or esophageal.[1] These are distinct processes that require different evaluation and management. Oropharyngeal (or transfer) dysphagia occurs from disorders that affect the oropharyngeal area, typically from neurologic or myogenic abnormalities as well as oropharyngeal tumors. Esophageal dysphagia occurs from disorders of the esophagus and is most commonly due to mechanical obstruction or altered motility of the esophagus. A detailed history can distinguish between the 2 types of dysphagia and with further evaluation can establish the diagnosis in 80% to 85% of cases.[2]

KEY TERMS

Esophageal dysphagia	Difficulty in passage of a bolus from the upper esophagus to the stomach.
Globus	Sensation of lump or tightness in the throat unrelated to swallowing.
Mechanical disorder	Obstruction of the esophageal lumen.
Motor disorder of the esophagus	Dyscoordination of the esophageal contractions.
Odynophagia	Pain with swallowing.
Oropharyngeal dysphagia	Difficulty initiating the swallowing process (ie, passage of a bolus from the mouth to the proximal esophagus).

ETIOLOGY

The exact prevalence of dysphagia is unknown. Current studies estimate the prevalence of dysphagia to be between 16% and 22% among individuals over 50 years of age.[3] The estimated prevalence of dysphagia in younger people is lower. For example, in a population survey of persons age 30 to 64 years living in the Midwest, the prevalence of dysphagia was 6% to 9%.[4] Up to 25% of hospitalized patients and 33% of nursing home residents experience dysphagia.[5] Most nursing home residents with dysphagia have oropharyngeal dysphagia.[6] Oropharyngeal dysphagia complicates up to 67% of strokes and places these patients at increased risk for aspiration pneumonia. The 12-month mortality rate in these persons is as high as 45%.[7]

A study at the Mayo Clinic showed that of 499 patients with esophageal dysphagia, 47% had an obstructive lesion in the esophagus (eg, ring, web, stricture, cancer), 32% had dysphagia related to disturbed esophageal motility (eg, spasm, scleroderma, achalasia), and 21% had no demonstrable structural or motor abnormalities in the esophagus or oropharynx. Older age, male sex, the presence of weight loss, heartburn, and a history of prior esophageal dilation significantly predicted mechanical causes of dysphagia.[8]

Eosinophilic esophagitis (EE) is increasing recognized as a cause of dysphagia in the pediatric as well as the adult population. EE can result in narrowing and stricturing of the esophagus and is a common cause for food impaction, especially in young adults. EE is diagnosed by the presence of 15 eosinophils per high-power field on light microscopy. Recent data suggest that dilatation of the esophagus in patients with EE is associated with increased rate of esophageal perforation. The treatment is avoidance of dietary allergens, topical steroids, and anti–interleukin-5 antibody if necessary.

Differential Diagnosis

Oropharyngeal dysphagia	*Examples*
Neuromuscular causes	Stroke Cerebral palsy Multiple sclerosis Myasthenia gravis Amyotrophic lateral sclerosis Parkinson's disease Myopathies Polymyositis/dermatomyositis
Structural causes	Zenker diverticulum Head and neck tumors Cervical spondylosis Vertebral osteophytes Pharyngeal webs (Plummer-Vinson syndrome)
Iatrogenic causes	Radiation therapy Corrosive pill injury Anticholinergic medications (dries mucous membranes)
Esophageal dysphagia	***Examples***
Motor disorders	Achalasia Diffuse esophageal spasm Nutcracker esophagus

	Scleroderma
	Sjögren syndrome
	Chagas disease
Mechanical, intrinsic	Tumors (esophageal carcinoma, lymphoma)
	Strictures
	Lower esophageal rings (Schatzki ring)
	Esophageal webs and rings
	Eosinophilic (allergic) esophagitis (EE)
	Foreign bodies
Mechanical, extrinsic	Right-sided aorta
	Left atrial enlargement
	Aberrant vessels
	Mediastinal lymphadenopathy
	Substernal thyroid
Iatrogenic	Pill esophagitis (doxycycline, nonsteroidal anti-inflammatory drugs [NSAIDs], alendronate, potassium chloride tablets)
Infectious	Candidal esophagitis
	Herpes esophagitis
	Cytomegalovirus (CMV) esophagitis

GETTING STARTED WITH THE HISTORY

- Ask the patient to describe what happens when he or she swallows.
- Ask open-ended questions.
- Distinguish between oropharyngeal and esophageal dysphagia, remembering that in up to 80% of cases of dysphagia, it is possible to establish the cause based on history alone.
- Determine which types of food result in dysphagia (solids, liquids, or both). Dysphagia to both solids and liquids is suggestive of a motor disorder, whereas dysphagia to solids alone is more likely due to a mechanical obstruction.
- Determine the time course. The new onset of symptoms that progressively worsen over weeks to months requires prompt evaluation because of the concern for malignancy.

Questions	**Remember**
Tell me what happens when you swallow.	Avoid interrupting.
When did you first notice that you were having difficulty swallowing? Are your symptoms getting worse?	Do not ask focused questions until the patient is done describing his or her symptoms in detail.
Describe what happens when you try to eat solid foods.	Ask the patient to describe these events in detail.
Describe what happens when you drink liquids.	

INTERVIEW FRAMEWORK

- Evaluate the patient's medication list before the interview and consider the potential contribution of the medications in dysphagia.
- Determine whether the patient has symptoms with ingestion of solids only or both liquids and solids to distinguish between mechanical obstruction and neuromuscular disorders.
- Determine whether symptoms are progressive or intermittent.
- Determine whether the patient has any associated symptoms or comorbid conditions, such as history of stroke, neurologic disorders, tobacco use, or history of reflux disease.
- Assess for additional alarm symptoms (ie, weight loss, bleeding, fevers, hematemesis, advanced age).
- Establish characteristic features of the dysphagia such as onset, duration, frequency, location, and precipitating or alleviating factors. If a patient has not offered this information with your open-ended questioning, be sure to ask directed questions.

IDENTIFYING ALARM SYMPTOMS

- Older patients presenting with progressive dysphagia, particularly those with a past history of alcohol abuse, smoking, obesity, or gastroesophageal reflux, should raise concern about an underlying oropharyngeal or esophageal malignancy.

Serious Diagnoses

Diagnosis	Remarks	Prevalence
Oropharyngeal or laryngeal carcinoma	Associated with tobacco and chronic alcohol use.	82% of all patients with oropharyngeal or laryngeal carcinoma experience dysphagia.[9]
Stroke	Most common cause of oropharyngeal dysphagia. Onset is often abrupt.	45% of all stroke patients experience dysphagia at 3 months.
Head injury		
Parkinson's disease	Common cause of oropharyngeal dysphagia.	81% of patients with Parkinson's disease have mild dysphagia.
Multiple sclerosis		24%–34% of patients with multiple sclerosis have permanent dysphagia.[10]
Amyotrophic lateral sclerosis	Characterized by progressive dysphagia.	
Huntington's chorea		
Myasthenia gravis	Dysphagia becomes progressively worse with repetitive swallows.	67% of patients have dysphagia at the time of diagnosis.
Esophageal carcinoma	Progressive dysphagia to solids, and then to both solids and liquids, is the most common presentation. Squamous cancer of the esophagus is associated with smoking and alcohol use. Adenocarcinoma of the esophagus is associated with gastroesophageal reflux, smoking, and obesity.	6%–17% of patients presenting with dysphagia in the primary care setting prove to have carcinoma.
Mediastinal tumors		
Vascular structures (dysphagia lusoria)		
Muscular dystrophies	Can present with dysphagia and ptosis later in life.	

Alarm Symptoms	If Present, Consider Serious Causes...	However, Benign Causes for This Feature Include...
Weight loss	Malignancy	Peptic stricture
Progressive symptoms	Malignancy	
	Neurodegenerative disorders	
Symptoms are worse with solids than with liquids	Malignancy	Peptic stricture Esophageal web or ring Foreign bodies
Blood in stools	Malignancy	
Otalgia (ear pain) with dysphagia	Hypopharyngeal lesion (eg, squamous cell cancer or thyroid cancer)	
Hoarseness (dysphonia) or pain with speaking and dysphagia	Muscular dystrophies	
Dysarthria	Stroke	

FOCUSED QUESTIONS

After hearing the story in the patient's own words and considering possible alarm symptoms, ask the following questions to narrow the differential diagnosis.

QUESTIONS	THINK ABOUT...
Do you cough, choke, or sense food coming back through your nose after swallowing?	Oropharyngeal dysphagia
Does it feel as if food is getting stuck within the first few seconds of swallowing?	Oropharyngeal dysphagia
Do you have difficulty swallowing liquids, solids, or both?	Liquids and solids = motor disorder Solids progressing to include liquids = mechanical obstruction
Are your symptoms getting worse?	Rapidly progressive symptoms are worrisome for malignancy
Do you always have trouble swallowing, or are your symptoms intermittent?	Intermittent, nonprogressive symptoms suggest a distal esophageal web or ring
Have you received radiation therapy in the past?	Radiation esophagitis
Do you take your medications with fluids?	Pill esophagitis. Most commonly associated with ingestion of iron supplements, aspirin, potassium, doxycycline, and alendronate.
Do you take your medications immediately before going to bed?	
Do you have a medical condition that suppresses your immune system (eg, human immunodeficiency virus [HIV], chronic steroid use, chemotherapy)?	Candidal, herpes simplex virus (HSV), or CMV esophagitis

—Continued next page

Continued—

Quality	
Is food sticking or getting stuck after you swallow?	Esophageal dysphagia
Have you experienced nasal regurgitation?	Oropharyngeal dysphagia
Do you have difficulty initiating a swallow?	Oropharyngeal dysphagia
Do you choke or cough when you try to swallow?	Oropharyngeal dysphagia
Have your symptoms remained the same over a long period of time, or are they getting worse?	Nonprogressive symptoms indicate benign structural lesions such as Schatzki ring or web
Location	
Where exactly does the food stick or hang up?	Oropharyngeal dysphagia: Patients frequently point to their cervical region
	Esophageal dysphagia: The lesion is at or below the region to which they point
Time course and frequency	
Are your symptoms episodic?	Episodic dysphagia to solids over a long period of time suggests a benign disease such as a lower esophageal ring
How long have you had these symptoms?	Dysphagia of short duration suggests an inflammatory process
Associated symptoms	
Do you hear a gurgling noise when you swallow?	Zenker diverticulum
Do you feel like you have bad breath?	Halitosis is associated with Zenker diverticulum
Do you regurgitate old foods?	Distal esophageal obstruction
	Zenker diverticulum
	Achalasia
Is it painful to swallow?	Esophageal mucosal inflammation (ie, esophagitis)
Do you experience chest pain?	Motor disorders of the esophagus (ie, diffuse esophageal spasm, achalasia, and scleroderma)
Do you ever have to bear down or raise your arms over your head to help a food bolus pass?	Motor disorders
Are your symptoms worse with very hot or cold liquids?	Motor disorders
Do you have a long-standing history of heartburn?	Peptic stricture
Are your symptoms relieved by repeated swallows?	Motor disorders
Have you ever experienced the sudden onset of dysphagia after swallowing pieces of meat?	Esophageal ring
	"Steak house syndrome" (Recurrent episodes of obstruction in distal esophagus often after eating a piece of steak or bread. The obstruction is the result of a lower esophageal ring and is usually relieved by drinking large amounts of water.)

Are your symptoms worse when you swallow cold foods?	Motor disorders
Do you suffer from food allergies or have other allergic diseases (eg, asthma)?	EE

DIAGNOSTIC APPROACH (INCLUDING ALGORITHM)

The diagnostic approach algorithm for dysphagia is shown in Figure 35–1.

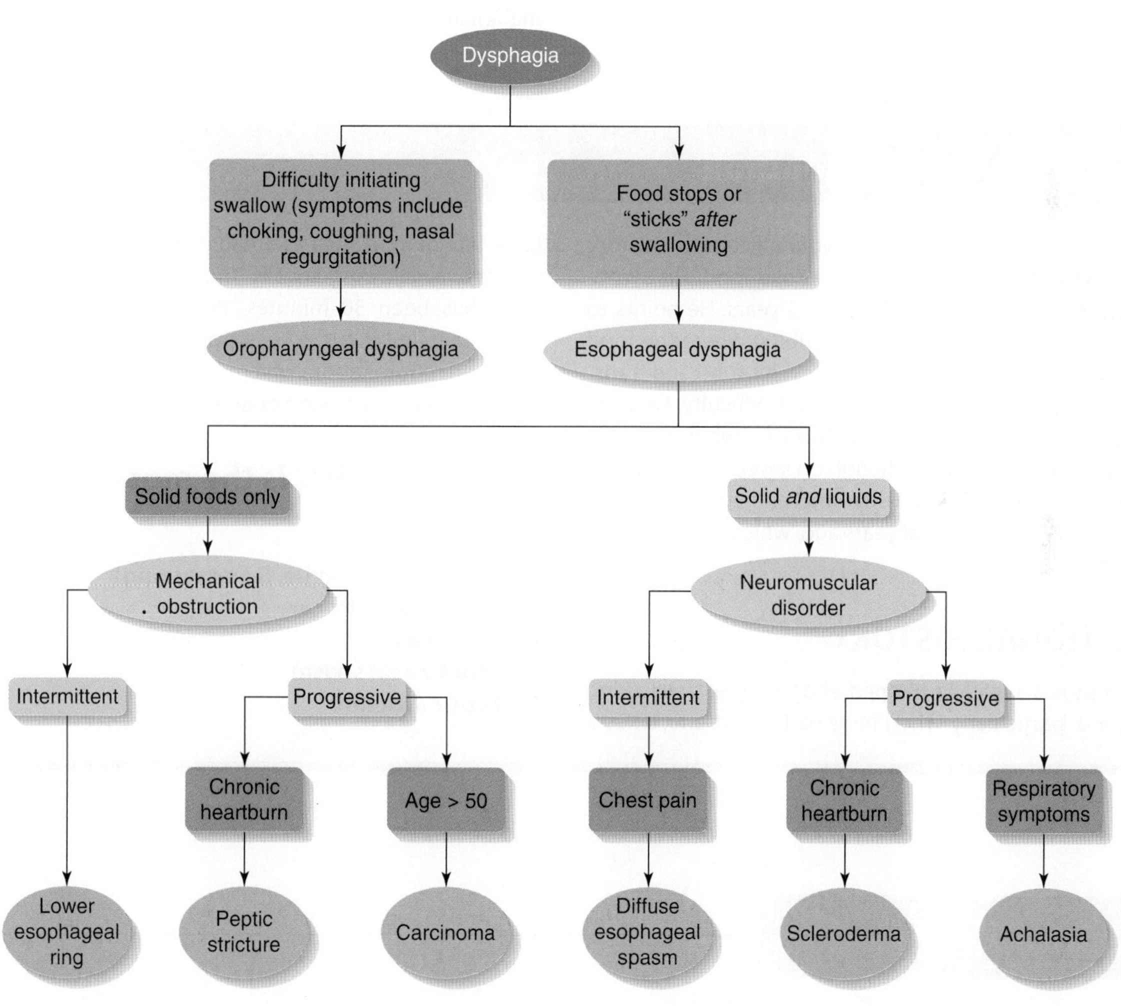

FIGURE 35–1 Diagnostic approach: Dysphagia.

CAVEATS

- Dysphagia should always be taken seriously and should prompt further evaluation. Dysphagia is never functional and always mandates a careful evaluation.
- The duration and frequency of a patient's dysphagia provide useful clues and can help make the diagnosis.
- Distinguish between oropharyngeal and esophageal dysphagia at the beginning of the interview.
- Patients with dysphagia due to esophageal disease, such as a peptic stricture, often perceive the obstruction to be in the suprasternal notch even though the obstruction is distal.
- Dysphagia in young persons (men > women) may be secondary to EE, especially in patients with disorders such as asthma and atopic dermatitis.

- Dysphagia to solid food is most often due to a mechanical obstruction, whereas dysphagia to solid and liquid food is often due to a motor (motility) disorder.
- Dysphagia can occur from impingement of the esophagus by a vascular anomaly (dysphagia lusoria) such as an aberrant right subclavian artery.
- A history of dry mouth or eyes may indicate inadequate salivary production. In such cases, it is particularly important to obtain a detailed review of medications. Anticholinergics, antihistamines, and certain antihypertensives can reduce salivary flow. Consider Sjögren syndrome when these sicca symptoms are present.
- If a food gets stuck and only regurgitation will relieve the symptom, the patient probably has a mechanical obstruction. However, if certain physical maneuvers assist the passage of food, then the patient likely has a motility disorder.

PROGNOSIS

The prognosis in patients with dysphagia varies from excellent to poor depending on its cause and severity. In patients with benign mechanical causes for esophageal dysphagia, the prognosis is generally excellent. In contrast, the prognosis of malignant causes for dysphagia is generally poor.

CASE SCENARIO | Resolution

A 52-year-old gentleman comes to your office with a history of intermittent difficulty swallowing solid food. His symptoms have been present for the past 5 years. He points to his supraclavicular notch when describing where the food feels stuck, although he is able to chew his food and transfer it into his posterior pharynx without difficulty. He does not choke or cough while eating. Drinking water will usually relieve his symptoms, although on several occasions he has self-induced vomiting. His symptoms are slightly worse now than they were several years ago, which prompted today's visit.

ADDITIONAL HISTORY

His symptoms typically happen shortly after swallowing solid food, particularly when he is eating fast and takes a large bite of food such as bread or meat. He does not have difficulty swallowing liquids. The longest he has had food stuck has been 30 minutes, during which time he had severe pain in his chest. He reports rare episodes of heartburn and regurgitation, which have been relieved with antacids. He denies smoking or excessive alcohol use.

Question: What is the most likely diagnosis?

A. Esophageal ring (ie, Schatzki ring)
B. Esophageal cancer
C. Achalasia
D. Esophageal spasm
E. Peptic stricture

Test Your Knowledge

1. You see a 22-year-old man with recent onset of solid food dysphagia. His symptoms have gradually worsened, and he has experienced several bouts of food impaction. He has a history of asthma and allergic rhinitis and believes that he has multiple food allergies as well.
   What is the most likely cause of his dysphagia?

   A. Achalasia
   B. Eosinophilic esophagitis
   C. Schatzki ring
   D. Esophageal spasm

2. Your patient, a 42-year-old woman, has a history of progressive dysphagia to solids and liquids for approximately 10 years. Recently, she has begun to lose weight and now sleeps sitting up to avoid regurgitating liquid. She notes chest fullness with some pain.
   What is the most likely diagnosis?

   A. Achalasia
   B. Peptic stricture
   C. Esophageal cancer
   D. Oropharyngeal dysphagia

References

1. Cohen S, Parkman H. Diseases of the esophagus. In: Goldman L, ed. *Cecil's Textbook of Medicine.* New York, NY: WB Saunders & Company, 2000.
2. Spieker M. Evaluating dysphagia. *Am Fam Physician.* 2000;61:3639–3648.
3. Lind C. Dysphagia: evaluation and treatment. *Gastroenterol Clin.* 2003;32:553–575.
4. Talley N, Weaver A, Zinmeister A, Melton L. Onset and disappearance of gastrointestinal symptoms and functional gastrointestinal disorders. *Am J Epidemiol.* 1992;136:65–77.
5. Layne KA, Losinski DS, Zenner PM, Ament JA. Using the Fleming index of dysphagia to establish prevalence. *Dysphagia.* 1989;4:39–42.
6. Lynn R. Dysphagia. In: Edmundowicz S, ed. *20 Common Problems in Gastroenterology.* New York, NY: McGraw-Hill, 2002.
7. Croghan JM, Burke EM, Caplan S, Denman S. Pilot study of 12-month outcomes of nursing home patients with aspiration on videofluoroscopy. *Dysphagia.* 1994;9:141–146.
8. Kim C, Weaver A, Hsu J, et al. Discriminate value of esophageal symptoms: a study of the initial clinical findings in 499 patients with dysphagia of various causes. *Mayo Clin Proc.* 1993;68:948–954.
9. Chua KS, Reddy SK, Lee MC, Patt RB. Pain and loss of function in head and neck cancer survivors. *J Pain Symptom Manage.* 1999;18:193–202.
10. De Pauw A, Dejaeger E, D'hooghe B, Carton H. Dysphagia in multiple sclerosis. *Clin Neurol Neurosurg.* 2003;104:345–351.

Suggested Reading

Fauci AS, Braunwald E, Kasper DL, et al., eds. Dysphagia. In: *Harrison's Principles of Internal Medicine.* 19th ed. New York, NY: McGraw-Hill Medical, 2008.

Goyal & Shaker GI Motility Online. Available at: http://www.nature.com/gimo.

Richter J. Dysphagia, odynophagia, heartburn and other esophageal symptoms. In: *Sleisenger's and Fordtram's Gastrointestinal and Liver Disease.* New York, NY: Elsevier, 2002.

Chapter 36

Acute Gastrointestinal Bleeding

Amandeep Shergill, MD, and Kenneth R. McQuaid, MD

CASE SCENARIO

A 72-year-old man presents to the emergency department for evaluation of dizziness, weakness, and black, tarry stools. He has a history of diabetes, coronary artery disease, and myocardial infarction 1 year ago that was treated with a drug-eluting stent. He takes both aspirin and clopidogrel.

- **What additional questions would you ask to learn more about his symptoms?**
- **How do you approach gastrointestinal bleeding?**
- **Can you make a diagnosis with a good history?**

INTRODUCTION

Gastrointestinal (GI) bleeding is a common medical condition. Most patients with acute GI bleeding present to the emergency department or develop bleeding while hospitalized for another reason. The respective annual incidence of acute upper and lower GI bleeding is 100 to 200 and 20 to 27 cases per 100,000 population.[1–7] Distinguishing between upper and lower GI bleeding is critical because the differential diagnosis and management vary. The prognosis ranges from trivial to life threatening.

Patients with acute GI bleeding require rapid evaluation and treatment. The initial history and physical examination provide information about the severity, duration, location, and possible etiology of GI bleeding. This initial assessment guides initial fluid resuscitation, triage within the hospital, timing of diagnostic procedures, and therapy.

KEY TERMS

Hematemesis	Vomiting of bright red (fresh) blood or old "coffee-ground" material.
Hematochezia	Bright red blood, maroon blood, or clots per rectum.
Melena	Black, tarry, foul-smelling stools.
Upper gastrointestinal bleeding (UGIB)	Bleeding that originates proximal to the ligament of Treitz (ie, esophagus, stomach, or duodenum). Manifests in 3 ways: (1) hematemesis, (2) melena, or (3) hematochezia.
Lower gastrointestinal bleeding (LGIB)	Bleeding that originates distal to the ligament of Treitz (ie, small intestine [5%] or colon [95%]). Manifested by hematochezia.
Hemodynamic instability	Systolic blood pressure < 100 mm Hg and/or pulse > 100 beats per minute. Indicates significant intravascular volume loss.
Positive nasogastric aspirate	The presence of bright red blood, clots, or coffee-ground material aspirated from nasogastric tube; confirms UGIB. Red blood suggests active bleeding.

ETIOLOGY

UGIB originates from sources above the ligament of Treitz. Lack of hematemesis does not exclude UGIB because bleeding may be intermittent or arise from the distal duodenum. LGIB originates from sources beyond the ligament of Treitz. Melena usually indicates UGIB; however, bleeding from the small intestine or proximal colon with slow transit time may also cause melena. Hematochezia usually indicates LGIB, although 10% of episodes result from brisk UGIB.

Historically, approximately 50% of UGIB was attributed to peptic ulcer disease (PUD).[8] However, in a recent analysis of the Clinical Outcomes Research Initiative (CORI) national database that includes community, academic, and Veterans Affairs endoscopy practices, the most common abnormality on an esophagogastroduodenoscopy for UGIB was "mucosal abnormality" (40%).[9] PUD was the second most common diagnosis (21%), followed by esophageal inflammation (~15%), varices (11%), arteriovenous malformations (~5%), Mallory-Weiss tear (~3%), and tumors (~1%).[9]

Clinical characteristics help classify patients with UGIB into high-risk and low-risk categories. The Glasgow-Blatchford bleeding score (GBS) was validated in a large, prospective study.[10] It is based on clinical variables (sex, initial systolic blood pressure, heart rate, and presentation with melena or syncope), laboratory variables (hemoglobin and blood urea nitrogen), and past medical history of significant hepatic or cardiac comorbidities. A GBS of 0 indicates a low risk of death or need of intervention and identifies patients who may be managed on an outpatient basis.[10]

The nasogastric aspirate also is helpful in distinguishing high-risk from low-risk bleeding lesions. Bloody nasogastric aspirates have a sensitivity of 48%, specificity of 75%, and positive predictive value (PPV) of 45% for high-risk lesions. Clear nasogastric aspirates have a specificity of 94% and PPV of 85% for predicting low-risk lesions at endoscopy.[11] It may be helpful to perform a nasogastric aspirate in a patient whose clinical characteristics, as defined above, suggest a low risk of bleeding. A bloody nasogastric aspirate in such a patient would increase the pretest probability for a high-risk lesion, warranting hospital admission and urgent evaluation.

UGIB related to PUD can be further risk stratified by endoscopic characteristics. The highest risk lesions are ulcers with active bleeding seen on endoscopy, which account for 18% of bleeding ulcers. Nonbleeding visible vessels (17%) and adherent clots (17%) are also considered to be high-risk stigmata. Flat spots (20%) and clean-based ulcers (42%) are considered low-risk lesions.[8]

LGIB is most commonly caused by diverticular bleeding (17%–40%), followed by colonic vascular ectasias (2%–30%), colitis (9%–21%), colonic neoplasia or postpolypectomy bleeding (11%–14%), and anorectal lesions (4%–10%).[6]

Patients presenting with a presumed LGIB also can be clinically classified as low, moderate, or high risk for severe bleeding. Severe bleeding is defined as continued bleeding (> 2-unit transfusion requirement and/or 6%–8% decrease in hematocrit or recurrent rectal bleeding after 24 hours of stability).[12] A validated clinical prediction rule uses 7 factors: heart rate ≥ 100/min, systolic blood pressure ≤ 115 mm Hg, syncope, nontender abdominal examination, rectal bleeding during the first 4 hours of evaluation, aspirin use, and multiple comorbid illnesses. Patients with no risk factors are at low risk for severe bleeding (< 10%), and those with 3 or more risk factors are at high risk for severe bleeding (80%).[12]

Differential Diagnosis

Cause	Description	Frequency
Common causes of UGIB[9]		
Mucosal abnormality	Small mucosal breaks (< 3 mm) commonly caused by nonsteroidal anti-inflammatory drugs (NSAIDs) or severe physiologic stress ("stress gastritis")	40%
Peptic ulcers	Ulcerations > 3 mm in size caused by *Helicobacter pylori* or NSAIDs	20%
Esophageal inflammation	Esophageal injury, commonly called "esophagitis," which can be secondary to reflux, medications, or infection	15%
Gastroesophageal varices	Dilated veins in the esophagus or stomach caused by portal hypertension, usually secondary to cirrhosis	11%
Angiodysplasia or vascular ectasias	Congenital or acquired abnormal dilation of submucosal veins and capillaries	5%
Mallory-Weiss tear	Mucosal laceration at the gastroesophageal junction, commonly occurring after retching	3%

Uncommon causes of UGIB		
Gastric antral vascular ectasia	Diffuse vascular ectasias of antrum ("watermelon stomach")	2%–5%
Portal hypertensive gastropathy	Dilated submucosal veins caused by portal hypertension	< 5%
Tumors	Adenocarcinoma, lymphoma, or stromal tumors	1%–5%
Dieulafoy lesion	Rupture of a large, tortuous artery in the proximal stomach	1%–5%
Aortoenteric fistula	Fistula between aorta and duodenum, most commonly in patients with prior abdominal aortic aneurysm surgery	< 1%
Hemobilia	Bleeding from liver lesion into bile duct	< 1%
Hemosuccus pancreaticus	Bleeding from pancreatic lesion into pancreatic duct	< 1%
Colonic sources of LGIB[6]		*Account for > 95% of LGIB*
Diverticulosis	Herniations of the mucosa through intestinal wall at sites of penetrating arteries. Bleeding occurs in < 5% of patients and stops spontaneously in 75% of episodes.	17%–40%
Angiodysplasia or vascular ectasia	Most commonly found in the cecum or ascending colon	2%–30%
Colorectal malignancy/ postpolypectomy hemorrhage	Colorectal cancer usually presents with occult bleeding or blood mixed with stool, uncommonly with severe bleeding. Postpolypectomy bleeding occurs in 1 of 300 patients after colonoscopic removal of polyps. More than 70% stop spontaneously.	11%–14%
Colitis	In ischemic colitis, impaired colonic blood supply caused by reduced cardiac output or occlusion of mesenteric arteries. Bleeding usually is self-limited. Infectious colitis is often manifested by dysentery (ie, blood mixed with stool and pus), caused by *Shigella, Campylobacter, Salmonella, or Escherichia coli* O157:H7 infection. Inflammatory bowel disease includes ulcerative colitis and Crohn's disease; bloody diarrhea is common with ulcerative colitis, but major bleeding is uncommon.	9%–21%
Anorectal causes	Includes hemorrhoids, rectal varices, and anal fissures, which commonly present with minor hematochezia. Usually characterized by blood streaking stool and dripping into toilet during defecation. Uncommonly cause serious LGIB.	4%–10%
Stercoral ulcers	Rectal ulcerations caused by chronic constipation	1%–2%
Radiation proctitis	Occurs months to years after pelvic radiation	1%–2%

—Continued next page

Continued—		
Small intestine sources		***Account for < 5% of LGIB***
Angiodysplasias or vascular ectasias	Commonly cause chronic, occult bleeding leading to anemia; but may cause acute, severe bleeding.	3%–5%
Meckel's diverticulum	Vitelline duct remnant located in terminal ileum. Most common cause of small bowel bleeding in patients younger than 25 years.	
Crohn's disease	Most common in terminal ileum or proximal colon	< 1%
NSAID-induced ulcers	Erosions, ulcers, or webs can occur throughout the small intestine, but clinically significant bleeding is uncommon.	1%–2%
Tumors	Adenocarcinoma, lymphoma, carcinoid, stromal tumors	< 1%

GETTING STARTED WITH THE HISTORY

The first step in evaluating patients with acute GI bleeding is to assess the severity of the bleeding to determine whether hemodynamic resuscitation is necessary. The provider should initially perform a focused history, obtain the patient's vital signs (pulse and blood pressure), and insert intravenous catheters for fluid replacement. This preliminary assessment should:

- Determine whether the patient has lost substantial volumes of blood.
- Seek clues as to whether the bleeding is ongoing or may have stopped.
- Determine whether the bleeding is likely originating from the upper or lower GI tract.

Questions	**Remember**
Describe what you saw in the toilet bowl.	Melena suggests UGIB or slow LGIB. Hematochezia suggests either LGIB or massive UGIB. Blood mixed with or coating stool suggests a hemodynamically insignificant bleed from an anorectal source.
Have you had vomiting? If so, describe what it looks like.	Hematemesis indicates an UGIB. Coffee-ground emesis suggests that the bleeding has slowed or stopped. Bright red emesis indicates recent or ongoing bleeding.
When did you first notice the bleeding?	Bleeding that began more than 4–6 hours earlier may have resulted in significant blood loss.
How many times have you had hematochezia or vomiting?	Repeated episodes suggest significant blood loss.
Have you been passing or vomiting cups of blood or only streaks or small clots?	Although patient estimations of blood loss are of questionable value, bloody streaks or small clots mixed with emesis or stool suggest minor blood loss.
When was the last time you passed a black or bloody stool?	Blood in the GI tract is a potent cathartic. If no melena or hematochezia has occurred in the last 4–6 hours, bleeding may have slowed or stopped.
Do you have any dizziness?	Dizziness suggests significant intravascular volume loss.
Obtain the patient's vital signs (blood pressure and pulse) while supine. If normal, obtain vital signs after patient assumes a sitting or standing position.	See below.

INTERVIEW FRAMEWORK

After the initial assessment and appropriate fluid resuscitation, a more complete history and physical examination should be obtained. Most causes of bleeding can be ascertained from the patient's presenting symptoms and past medical history. Details of the current bleeding episode, prior bleeding episodes, recent GI symptoms, past medical history, medications, and social history will provide clues to the most likely source and help determine whether the patient should be admitted to an intensive care unit or regular hospital unit.

- A past history of GI bleeding or other GI disorders may suggest potential causes of the current bleeding.
- Aspirin, NSAIDs, and other antiplatelet agents may cause or potentiate UGIB or LGIB due to their ulcerogenic and antiplatelet effects. Anticoagulants (heparin, warfarin) may exacerbate but do not cause GI bleeding.

IDENTIFYING ALARM SIGNS AND SYMPTOMS

The sight of GI bleeding is frightening to patients and providers alike. Certain symptoms and signs suggest massive GI bleeding or raise concern that the patient is at increased risk for morbidity and mortality. Such patients usually warrant admission to the intensive care unit.

- Reassure and calm the patient, who may be anxious and frightened.
- Vital signs: Supine systolic blood pressure less than 100 mm Hg or pulse greater than 100 beats per minute indicates significant (> 20%) intravascular volume loss and the need for immediate fluid resuscitation. Orthostatic hypotension or tachycardia indicates intravascular volume loss of 10% to 20%.
- Hematochezia with hematemesis or a positive nasogastric lavage indicates active, life-threatening UGIB and should prompt urgent evaluation and therapy.
- Elderly patients may have concomitant cardiovascular disease, placing them at increased risk for adverse events from bleeding, hypotension, or anemia.
- Dizziness and light-headedness suggest significant intravascular volume depletion.
- Patients with chronic liver disease may have severe bleeding due to portal hypertension and coagulopathy and are at increased risk for complications.
- GI bleeding in hospitalized patients carries increased risk of morbidity and mortality compared with bleeding that begins in outpatients, irrespective of the cause.

Alarm Symptoms	Serious Causes	Benign Causes
Ongoing hematemesis, bright red blood per nasogastric tube with hematochezia, or unstable vital signs	Massive UGIB due to esophageal or gastric varices Peptic ulcer disease (PUD) Aortoenteric fistula	
Ongoing hematemesis or bright red blood from nasogastric tube with melena	Esophageal or gastric varices Peptic ulcer with arterial bleed Dieulafoy lesion Aortoenteric fistula	Mallory-Weiss tear Erosive esophagitis Erosive gastritis Portal hypertensive gastropathy
Ongoing, brisk hematochezia with no blood from nasogastric lavage	LGIB due to diverticulosis, vascular ectasia, or NSAID ulcers	Radiation proctitis Stercoral ulcers Inflammatory bowel disease

—Continued next page

Continued—		
	If vital signs unstable, also consider UGIB from duodenal ulcer or aortoenteric fistula (without blood refluxing into stomach)	Hemorrhoids
Weight loss	Neoplasm	Peptic ulcer with gastric outlet obstruction
Acute onset of lower abdominal or midabdominal pain followed by bleeding	Mesenteric or colonic ischemia	Ulcerative colitis Crohn's disease Cramps from cathartic effects of blood
Prior aortic repair	Aortoenteric fistula	
Shortness of breath, chest pain, light-headedness	Cardiac ischemia secondary to significant blood loss	Anxiety
UGIB that begins in hospitalized, critically ill patient	Stress-related erosions or ulcers of stomach or duodenum	Esophagitis NSAID-induced gastric erosions

FOCUSED QUESTIONS

After taking the initial history, obtaining vital signs, and assessing for alarm symptoms, perform a more complete history focusing on associated GI symptoms, past medical history, medications, and social history.

QUESTIONS	THINK ABOUT...
Associated symptoms	
Have you had:	
• *Vomiting, retching?*	Mallory-Weiss tear (< 50% have a history of vomiting or retching)
• *Heartburn?*	Erosive esophagitis
• *Odynophagia (pain on swallowing)?*	Pill-induced esophageal ulceration Infections (cytomegalovirus [CMV], *Candida*, herpesvirus)
• *Dysphagia?*	Esophageal neoplasm
	Gastroesophageal reflux with esophageal stricture
• *Dyspepsia (epigastric discomfort or pain)?*	PUD or erosive gastritis; however, patients with bleeding from PUD may be asymptomatic
• *Evidence of chronic liver disease (jaundice, scleral icterus, ascites, spider telangiectasias, palmar erythema, gynecomastia, hepatosplenomegaly)?*	Esophageal or gastric varices Portal hypertensive gastropathy

• *Bloody diarrhea (dysentery)?*	Infectious diarrhea or inflammatory bowel disease (ulcerative colitis, less likely Crohn's disease); symptoms for > 2 weeks suggest inflammatory bowel disease
• *Straining with defecation, constipation?*	Distal colonic or rectal neoplasm
	Hemorrhoids
	Stercoral ulcer
Past medical history	
Do you have:	
• *History of peptic ulcer?*	Ulcer recurrence
• *History of gastric surgery or gastric bypass?*	Ulcer at anastomosis between intestine and stomach
• *History of immunodeficiency (human immunodeficiency virus [HIV] with low CD4 count, immunosuppression, chemotherapy)?*	CMV ulcers
	Fungal infections
	Kaposi sarcoma
• *History of esophageal, gastric, or colonic neoplasm?*	Recurrence of neoplasm
• *History of diverticulosis?*	Diverticulosis is the major cause of clinically significant LGIB
• *History of inflammatory bowel disease?*	Ulcerative colitis is a more common cause of bleeding, usually manifested by bloody diarrhea. Crohn's disease uncommonly presents with acute bleeding from ulceration.
• *History of radiation therapy?*	Postradiation esophagitis or proctitis
• *History of coronary artery disease or peripheral artery disease?*	Increased risk of ischemic bowel disease. Also, likely use of antiplatelet agents and/or anticoagulants.
• *Chronic kidney disease?*	Increased risk of angiodysplasias. Potential for worsened bleeding from any cause due to uremic platelet dysfunction.
• *Osteoarthritis?*	Likely use of NSAIDs
• *History of hepatitis or known chronic liver disease?*	Increased risk of bleeding from varices or portal hypertensive gastropathy
Have you had an endoscopy or colonoscopy with biopsy, sphincterotomy, or polypectomy within prior 2 weeks?	Bleeding from biopsy or polypectomy site
Medications	
What medications are you taking?	
• *Aspirin, NSAIDs*	Erosions or peptic ulcer in stomach, duodenum, small bowel, or proximal colon. Due to antiplatelet effects, may potentiate bleeding from upper or lower GI tract source.
• *Anticoagulants (eg, warfarin, heparin, enoxaparin, clopidogrel)*	Do not directly cause GI bleeding, but potentiate bleeding from pre-existing lesions within GI tract

—Continued next page

Continued—	
• *Immunosuppressants (chemotherapy, prednisone, antirejection drugs)*	Opportunistic infections (CMV, herpes simplex virus, *Candida*)
• *Recent use of antibiotics?*	*Clostridium difficile* colitis
• *Bisphosphonates (alendronate), potassium, quinidine, iron, antibiotics*	Pill-induced esophageal ulcer (usually does not cause significant bleeding)
Social history	
Is the patient:	
• *An immigrant from a developing country (Mexico, Central America, Africa, Asia)?*	In a patient with UGIB, peptic ulcer may be due to chronic infection with *H pylori.*
	If patient > 40 years of age, also consider *H pylori*–associated gastric cancer or lymphoma.
• *A US resident from lower socioeconomic background (especially blacks and Hispanics)?*	In a patient with UGIB, peptic ulcer may be due to chronic infection with *H pylori.*
	If patient > 40 years of age, also consider *H pylori*–associated gastric cancer or lymphoma.
Do you drink alcohol? How much? Do you have a history of drinking alcohol?	Gastroesophageal varices or portal hypertensive gastropathy secondary to alcoholic cirrhosis
Have you traveled recently? If so, where?	Infectious diarrhea
Do you engage in sexual activity with increased risk of anal–oral contamination?	Infectious diarrhea

DIAGNOSTIC APPROACH (INCLUDING ALGORITHM)

The first step is to assess the severity of bleeding, whether the bleeding is likely from an upper or lower source, and whether it is ongoing. All patients with hemodynamic instability, evidence of ongoing bleeding, or significant comorbidities should be admitted to the intensive care unit for resuscitation and stabilization prior to endoscopic evaluation. Patients with suspected UGIB should undergo endoscopy. Patients with suspected LGIB should undergo evaluation with colonoscopy after a rapid purge. See Figures 36–1 and 36–2 for diagnostic approach algorithms for UGIB and LGIB, respectively.

CAVEATS

- UGIB and LGIB cause overlapping symptoms and share broad differential diagnoses.
- Nasopharyngeal and pulmonary disorders also cause epistaxis or hemoptysis, which may be misinterpreted as hematemesis.
- Lesions in the duodenum do not always cause hematemesis or a positive nasogastric lavage, because the bleeding may not reflux into the stomach.

PROGNOSIS

The overall mortality rates from UGIB and LGIB are < 10% and < 5%, respectively. Approximately 80% of GI bleeding stops spontaneously. Persistent or recurrent bleeding markedly increases the risk of morbidity and mortality. The 2 most important prognostic factors are the cause of bleeding and the presence of comorbid illnesses.[13–15] Bleeding originating from gastroesophageal varices, ulcers with visible blood vessels, or advanced malignancies have an increased risk of adverse outcome. Patients with serious comorbid illnesses, especially coronary ischemia or heart failure, advanced liver disease, renal failure, or disseminated malignancy have increased rates of rebleeding and mortality. Other independent risk factors for mortality from GI bleeding include age and the presence of shock (systolic blood pressure < 100 mm Hg) on admission.[13,14] For both upper and lower GI bleeding, endoscopy may help localize the source of bleeding, determine the risk of rebleeding, and provide therapy if indicated. If adequate visualization cannot be achieved due to vigorous bleeding or if there is hemodynamic instability, angiography with attempted embolization of the bleeding lesion should be considered. Surgery may be required for treatment of persistent or recurrent bleeding that cannot be treated with endoscopy or embolization.

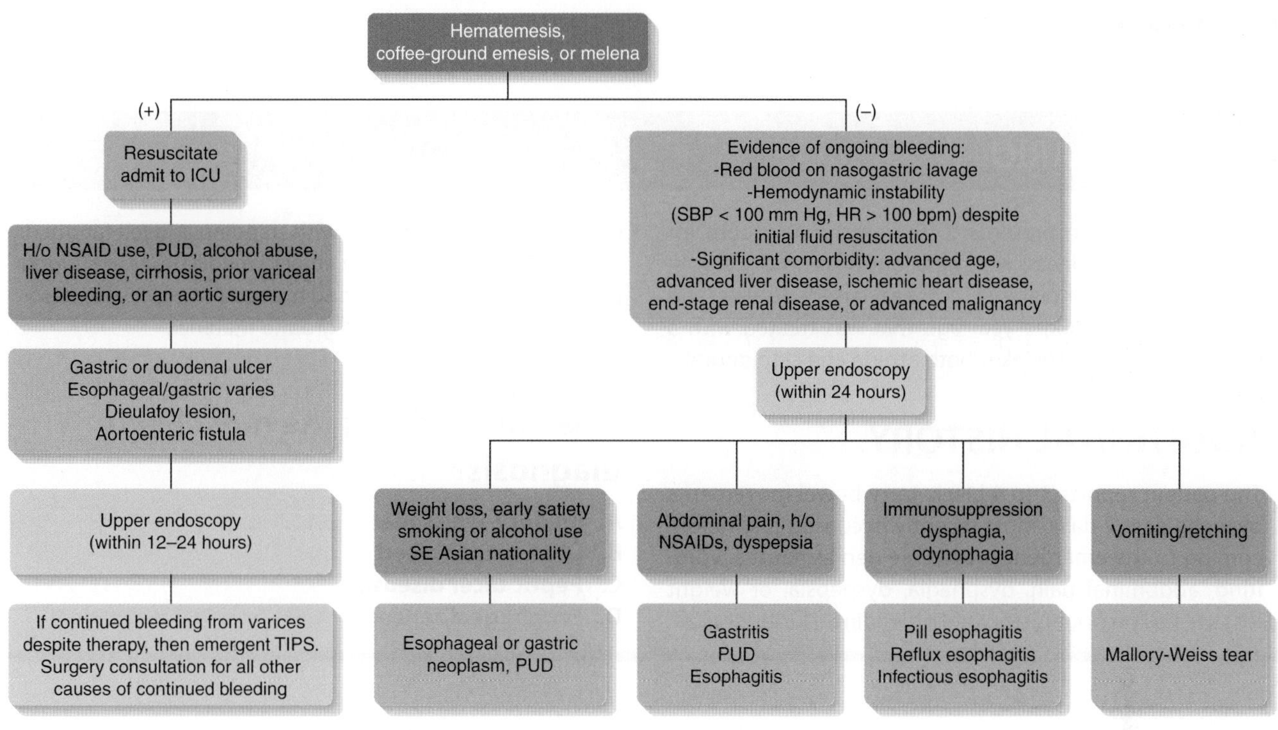

FIGURE 36–1 Diagnostic approach: Upper gastrointestinal bleeding. h/o, history of; HR, heart rate; ICU, intensive care unit; NSAID, nonsteroidal anti-inflammatory drug; PUD, peptic ulcer disease; SBP, systolic blood pressure; SE, southeast; TIPS, transvenous intrahepatic portosystemic shunt.

Hematochezia,
maroon-colored stools

Presence of alarm features: Ongoing bleeding, age > 60, hemodynamic instability, dyspnea, or chest pain

(+)

Resuscitate
admit to ICU

Nasogastric lavage

(+)

Go to UGIB algorithm

(–)

H/o diverticular bleed, vascular surgery, renal insufficiency, NSAID use

Diverticular bleed, aortoenteric fistula, colonic or small bowel ulcer, angiodysplasias

Rapid purge followed by colonoscopy. If brisk, active bleed: Radionuclide study or angiography. Consider surgical consultation, especially if > 6 U PRBCs.

(–)

H/o diverticular bleed, vascular disease, renal insufficiency, NSAID use, hypotension

Diverticular bleed, colonic or small bowel ulcer, angio-dysplasia, colonic ischemia, neoplasm

If ischemia supected: Flexible sigmoidoscopy Otherwise: Rapid purge for colonoscopy

Blood mixed in stool, constipation, straining with defecation, H/o pelvic radiation

Hemorrhoids anal fissure, neoplasm, radiation proctitis, stercoral ulcer

Outpatient colonoscopy

Bloody diarrhea

Infectious diarrhea, inflammatory bowel disease

Send stool cultures. If continued bleeding or no evidence of infection, then colonoscopy

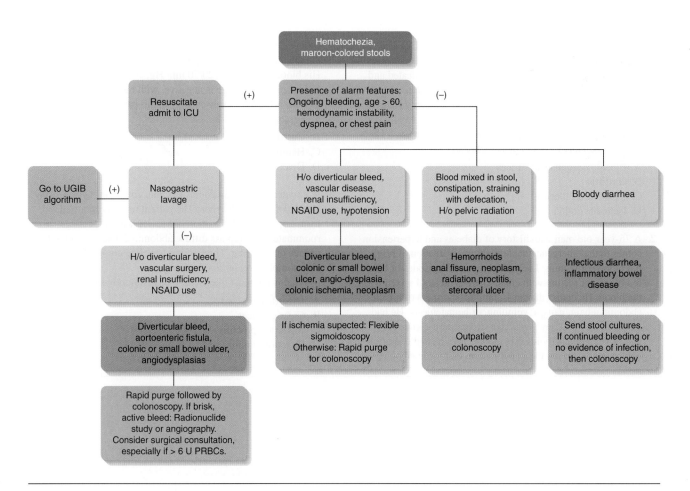

FIGURE 36–2 Diagnostic approach: Lower gastrointestinal bleeding. h/o, history of; ICU, intensive care unit; NSAID, nonsteroidal anti-inflammatory drug; PRBCs, packed red blood cells; U, units; UGIB, upper gastrointestinal bleeding.

CASE SCENARIO | Resolution

A 72-year-old man presents to the emergency room for evaluation of dizziness, weakness, and black, tarry stools. He has a history of diabetes, coronary artery disease, and myocardial infarction 1 year ago that was treated with a drug-eluting stent. He takes both aspirin and clopidogrel.

ADDITIONAL HISTORY

The patient reports 3 to 4 black, tarry bowel movements over the past 2 days, most recently occurring just before coming to the emergency room. He denies nausea, vomiting, abdominal pain, dysphagia, dyspepsia, or weight loss. He has no prior history of GI bleeding. During the last episode, he noted dizziness with standing and felt fatigued. He has not been taking any antacid medications. His blood pressure is 105/80 mm Hg, and his heart rate is 95. His nasogastric lavage shows coffee-ground material.

Question: What is the most likely diagnosis?

A. Mallory-Weiss tear
B. Diverticular bleed
C. Peptic ulcer disease
D. Esophageal cancer

Test Your Knowledge

1. A 56-year-old man with a history of significant alcohol abuse and alcoholic cirrhosis comes to the emergency department complaining of maroon stool. The patient is intoxicated and uncooperative during the history. He has a heart rate of 118 and a blood pressure of 95/60 mm Hg. He suddenly starts to vomit red blood.

   Which of the following is the most likely diagnosis for the patient's hematemesis and hematochezia?

   A. Bleeding esophageal varices
   B. Gastritis
   C. Diverticular bleed
   D. Ischemic colitis

2. A 76-year-old man with history of diabetes and hypertension comes to the emergency department for evaluation of bright red blood per rectum. The patient reports 3 episodes of bright red blood per rectum with clots. There is no stool mixed with the blood. He denies dizziness, fatigue, shortness of breath, abdominal pain, nausea, vomiting, or hematemesis. He had a normal colonoscopy 1 year ago except for diverticulosis and internal hemorrhoids. Six months ago, he had one prior episode of bright red blood per rectum that resolved on its own and for which he did not seek medical care. On physical examination, he is well appearing and in no acute distress. His blood pressure is 120/70 mm Hg, and his heart rate is 80. His nasogastric lavage is negative, with bilious fluid.

   What is the most likely etiology of this patient's hematochezia?

   A. Esophagitis
   B. Gastric cancer
   C. Hemorrhoids
   D. Diverticulosis

3. A 22-year-old woman comes to clinic complaining of a 4-day history of bloody diarrhea. The patient recently returned from a spring break vacation in Mexico with her college roommates. She reports diffuse abdominal discomfort but no nausea or vomiting. Three of her traveling companions were also complaining of bloody diarrhea.

   What is the most likely cause of her bloody stools?

   A. Diverticular bleed
   B. Gastric cancer
   C. Radiation proctitis
   D. Infectious colitis

References

1. Blatchford O, Davidson LA, Murray WR, Blatchford M, Pell J. Acute upper gastrointestinal haemorrhage in west of Scotland: case ascertainment study. *BMJ*. 1997;315:510–514.
2. Esrailian E, Gralnek IM. Nonvariceal upper gastrointestinal bleeding: epidemiology and diagnosis. *Gastroenterol Clin North Am*. 2005;34:589–605.
3. Longstreth GF. Epidemiology of hospitalization for acute upper gastrointestinal hemorrhage: a population-based study. *Am J Gastroenterol*. 1995;90:206–210.
4. Longstreth GF. Epidemiology and outcome of patients hospitalized with acute lower gastrointestinal hemorrhage: a population-based study. *Am J Gastroenterol*. 1997;92:419–424.
5. Rockall TA, Logan RF, Devlin HB, Northfield TC. Incidence of and mortality from acute upper gastrointestinal haemorrhage in the United Kingdom. Steering Committee and Members of the National Audit of Acute Upper Gastrointestinal Haemorrhage. *BMJ*. 1995;311:222–226.
6. Zuccaro G. Epidemiology of lower gastrointestinal bleeding. *Best Pract Res Clin Gastroenterol*. 2008;22:225–232.
7. Zuckerman GR, Prakash C. Acute lower intestinal bleeding. Part II: etiology, therapy, and outcomes. *Gastrointest Endosc*. 1999;49:228–238.
8. Laine L, Peterson WL. Bleeding peptic ulcer. *N Engl J Med*. 1994;331:717–727.
9. Boonpongmanee S, Fleischer DE, Pezzullo JC, et al. The frequency of peptic ulcer as a cause of upper-GI bleeding is exaggerated. *Gastrointest Endosc*. 2004;59:788–794.
10. Stanley AJ, Ashley D, Dalton HR, et al. Outpatient management of patients with low-risk upper-gastrointestinal haemorrhage: multicentre validation and prospective evaluation. *Lancet*. 2009;373:42–47.
11. Aljebreen AM, Fallone CA, Barkun AN. Nasogastric aspirate predicts high-risk endoscopic lesions in patients with acute upper-GI bleeding. *Gastrointest Endosc*. 2004;59:172–178.
12. Strate LL, Saltzman JR, Ookubo R, Mutinga ML, Syngal S. Validation of a clinical prediction rule for severe acute lower intestinal bleeding. *Am J Gastroenterol*. 2005;100:1821–1827.
13. Barkun AN, Bardou M, Kuipers EJ, Sung J, Hunt RH, Martel M, Sinclair P. International consensus recommendations on the management of patients with nonvariceal upper gastrointestinal bleeding. *Ann Intern Med*. 2010;152:101–113.
14. Rockall TA, Logan RF, Devlin HB, Northfield TC. Risk assessment after acute upper gastrointestinal haemorrhage. *Gut*. 1996;38:316–321.
15. Chiu PW, Ng EK. Predicting poor outcome from acute upper gastrointestinal hemorrhage. *Gastroenterol Clin North Am*. 2009;38:215–230.

Suggested Reading

Garcia-Tsao G, Bosch J. Management of varices and variceal hemorrhage in cirrhosis. *N Engl J Med*. 2010;362:823–832.

Gralnek IM, Barkun AN, Bardou M. Management of acute bleeding from a peptic ulcer. *N Engl J Med*. 2008;359:928–937.

Laine L, McQuaid KR. Endoscopic therapy for bleeding ulcers: an evidence-based approach based on meta-analyses of randomized controlled trials. *Clin Gastroenterol Hepatol*. 2009;7:33–47.

Strate LL, Naumann CR. The role of colonoscopy and radiological procedures in the management of acute lower intestinal bleeding. *Clin Gastroenterol Hepatol*. 2010;8:333–343.

Chapter 37

Jaundice

Thomas E. Baudendistel, MD, and Dayana Carcamo-Molina, MD

CASE SCENARIO

A 67-year-old man with type 2 diabetes presents to your primary care practice following 3 weeks of intermittent nausea and vomiting. His wife insisted he see a doctor because his skin and eyes are yellow. He has noticed that his pants are looser, but he has no other complaints.

- **What are other important questions to ask this patient?**
- **What is the differential diagnosis of jaundice? Of painless jaundice?**

INTRODUCTION

Jaundice is a yellow discoloration of body tissues due to an excess of bilirubin, a pigment produced during the metabolism of heme. Normally, serum bilirubin should never exceed 1 to 1.5 mg/dL. Levels above 2 mg/dL result in detectable jaundice, first in the sclerae, next under the tongue and along the tympanic membranes, and finally in the skin. Thus, cutaneous jaundice implies higher levels of bilirubin than isolated scleral icterus.

A thorough dietary and medication history can exclude the yellow skin discoloration of carotenemia, isotretinoin, or rifampin overdose, all of which spare the sclerae. Once these mimickers are excluded, jaundice must be recognized as a manifestation of advanced hepatocellular or cholestatic liver disease or, less commonly, hemolysis or abnormal bilirubin metabolism. The history should proceed in 2 parallel routes: (1) arrive rapidly at a likely diagnosis and (2) identify alarm features that may necessitate urgent intervention.

KEY TERMS

Budd-Chiari syndrome	Hepatic vein obstruction, often due to an underlying hypercoagulable state (eg, oral contraceptives, polycythemia vera, paroxysmal nocturnal hemoglobinuria, antiphospholipid antibody syndrome); the acute form classically presents with tender hepatomegaly, jaundice, and ascites.
Cholestasis	Retention of bile in the liver, due to intra- or extrahepatic obstruction or biliary stasis.
Conjugated bilirubin	Formed in the liver when unconjugated bilirubin is metabolized, then released into bile; may be filtered by the glomerulus and appear in the urine.
Fulminant hepatic failure	Onset of hepatic encephalopathy within 8 weeks of liver injury, often accompanied by coagulopathy. Common causes include acute viral hepatitis, ingestions (eg, acetaminophen or *Amanita* mushrooms), and hepatic ischemia. Less common causes include Wilson's disease, autoimmune hepatitis, acute Budd-Chiari syndrome, other infections, and malignancy.
Hepatocellular jaundice	Accumulation of conjugated bilirubin in the serum due to hepatocyte dysfunction.
Hyperbilirubinemia	Elevated serum levels of bilirubin (> 1.2 mg/dL).
Icterus	Synonymous with jaundice.
Infiltrative liver disease	Subset of liver disease marked by cholestasis due to diffuse involvement within the liver including granulomatous disease (sarcoidosis, Wegener's granulomatosis, fungal and mycobacterial infections), amyloidosis, Wilson's disease, hemochromatosis, lymphoma, and metastatic cancer.

—*Continued next page*

Continued—	
Jaundice	Yellow pigmentation of the skin and sclerae.
Nonalcoholic fatty liver disease (NAFLD)	Parenchymal liver disease common in patients with the metabolic syndrome (phenotype is obese diabetic with hyperlipidemia but can also occur in obese patients without other comorbidities).
Obstructive jaundice	Excess conjugated bilirubin in the serum due to impaired bile flow in the intrahepatic or extrahepatic bile ducts.
Unconjugated bilirubin	The main circulating form of bilirubin, produced upon heme breakdown and delivered to the liver for further metabolism.

ETIOLOGY

The numerous causes of jaundice can be divided into 4 broad categories (Figure 37–1):

1. Impaired bilirubin metabolism
   a. Excess bilirubin production
   b. Impaired bilirubin uptake
   c. Impaired conjugation of bilirubin
2. Impaired secretion of bile into bile canaliculi
3. Liver disease
4. Obstruction of the bile ducts

Most disorders in the first category cause unconjugated hyperbilirubinemia and, with the exceptions of sepsis and acute hemolytic reactions, are milder. Predominantly conjugated hyperbilirubinemia is more common and generally implies a more serious condition. In adults, most jaundice results from gallstone disease, cancer (pancreatic and hepatobiliary), sepsis, and cirrhosis (due to alcohol abuse, chronic viral hepatitis, or NAFLD).

Differential Diagnosis

Disorder	Prevalence Among Patients Hospitalized With Jaundice[1,2,a]
Pancreatic or biliary carcinoma	20%–35%
Sepsis or shock	22%
Alcoholic cirrhosis	10%–21%
Gallstone disease	13%
NAFLD	
Drug or toxin-mediated hepatitis (most commonly acetaminophen)	5.8%
Acute viral hepatitis	1.7%
Autoimmune hepatitis	1.7%
Other Amyloidosis Congenital disorder (Gilbert, Crigler-Najjar, Dubin-Johnson, Rotor syndromes) Hemochromatosis Hemolysis Primary biliary cirrhosis Primary sclerosing cholangitis Sarcoidosis Wilson's disease	< 1%

[a]Blanks indicate that the prevalence is unknown.

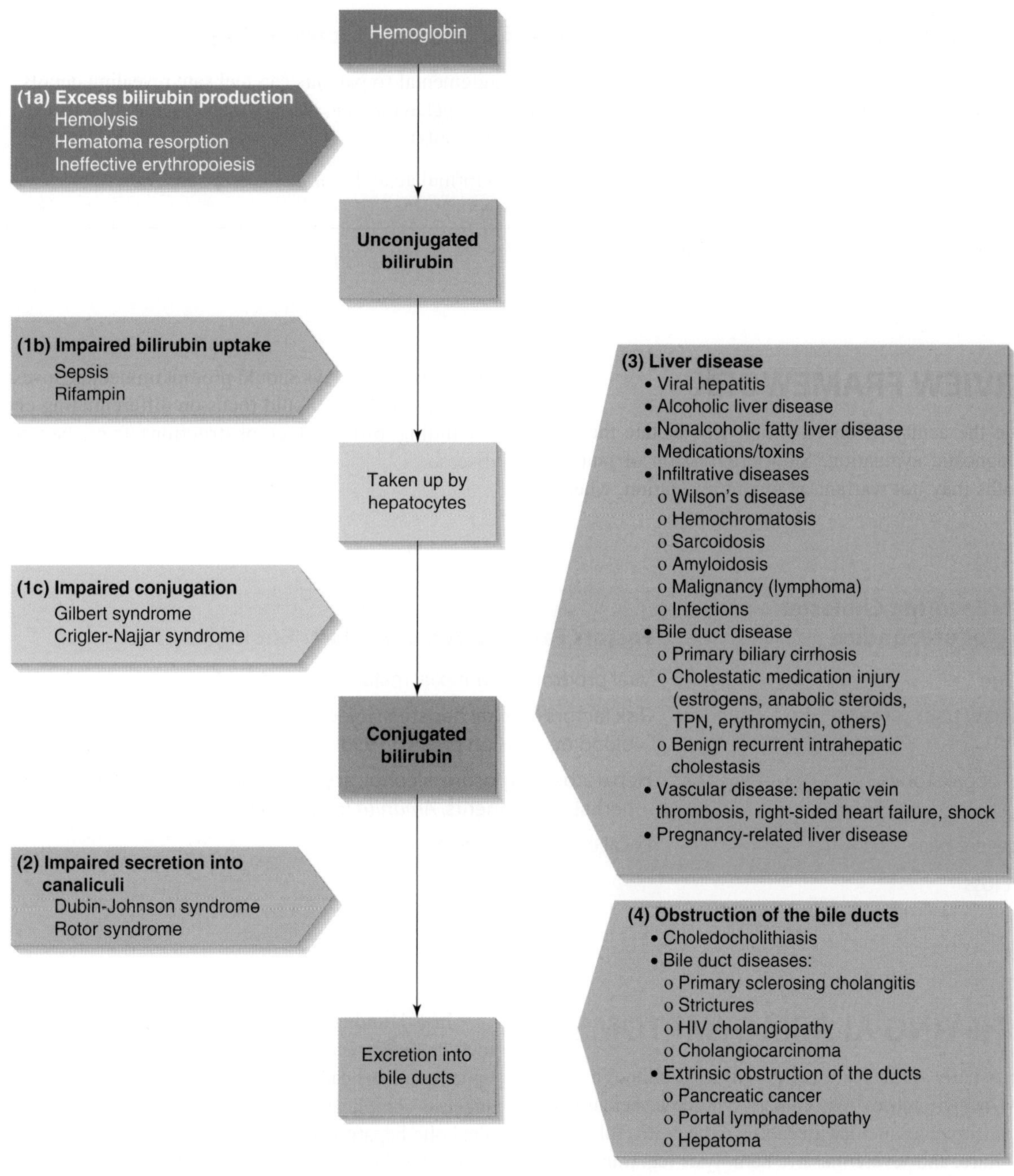

FIGURE 37–1 Causes of jaundice based on mechanism of bilirubin accumulation. HIV, human immunodeficiency virus; TPN, total parental nutrition. Note: Darker shading reflects predominantly unconjugated hyperbilirubinemia; lighter shading indicates conjugated hyperbilirubinemia.

GETTING STARTED WITH THE HISTORY

Jaundice seldom occurs as an isolated event and is often a late manifestation of a chronic illness. However, the patient may not immediately relate jaundice, which is a skin or eye complaint, to other symptoms. Therefore, allow the patient time to disclose other key etiologic information.

Open-Ended Questions	Tips for Effective Interviewing
Tell me how you were feeling when you first noticed the color change.	Be nonjudgmental so patients can feel safe revealing details of high-risk behaviors (eg, alcohol intake, illicit drug use, suicide attempts).
What other symptoms have accompanied this color change?	Begin to formulate and rank items on your differential diagnosis.
When did you last feel your health was normal?	

INTERVIEW FRAMEWORK

Determine the acuity of onset, which will dictate the pace of the diagnostic evaluation. Slow progression of jaundice over months may not warrant an urgent evaluation, whereas rapid onset over days should prompt immediate investigation. Early questioning should focus on differentiating cholestatic (including biliary duct obstruction) from hepatocellular disease.

Factors Favoring Cholestatic Etiologies of Jaundice	Factors Favoring Hepatocellular Etiologies of Jaundice
Older age	Viral prodrome (anorexia, malaise, fatigue)
Prior biliary tract surgery	Risk factors for viral hepatitis: injection drug use, sexual promiscuity, blood transfusion prior to 1990
History of gallstones	Hepatotoxin exposure: alcohol, acetaminophen, new medications or herbal supplements, *Amanita* mushrooms
More severe pain	Local outbreak of hepatitis
Weight loss	

IDENTIFYING ALARM SYMPTOMS

Jaundice usually indicates a serious illness, although there are a few benign causes (eg, Gilbert syndrome, hematoma). Medical emergencies include ascending cholangitis, fulminant hepatic failure, and severe/massive hemolysis (eg, transfusion reaction, disseminated intravascular coagulation, thrombotic thrombocytopenic purpura, *Clostridium perfringens* sepsis, or falciparum malaria).

In a jaundiced patient, clues to a potential emergency include fever, confusion, evidence of coagulopathy, and right upper quadrant pain. The presence of fever or abdominal pain suggests complications from gallstones, sepsis, or acute viral or alcoholic hepatitis. Encephalopathy and coagulopathy suggest impending hepatic failure; the latter concern should prompt immediate consideration of liver transplantation. Painless jaundice classically suggests pancreatic or hepatobiliary cancer.

Alarm Feature	If Present in a Jaundiced Patient, Consider Serious Causes…	However, Benign Causes for This Include…
Fever[a]	Cholangitis Gallstone disease Acute hepatitis (viral, toxin/alcohol, medication-induced) Sepsis	Hematoma

Right upper quadrant pain[a]	Cholangitis Gallstone disease Acute hepatitis Budd-Chiari syndrome Right-sided heart failure	Varicella zoster Right lower lobe pneumonia Right-sided pleural effusion Peptic ulcer disease Atypical renal colic Musculoskeletal pain
Confusion or altered mentation[a]	Cholangitis Hepatic encephalopathy Sepsis Intracranial bleed due to coagulopathy Hypoglycemia Seizure	Delirium of any cause
Mucosal or cutaneous bleeding	Thrombocytopenia due to fulminant hepatic failure or hypersplenism Disseminated intravascular coagulation Falciparum malaria	Minor trauma to the affected sites
Back pain	Acute severe hemolysis	Musculoskeletal pain
Pregnancy	Hyperemesis gravidarum Acute fatty liver of pregnancy Eclampsia HELLP syndrome Intrahepatic cholestasis of pregnancy	
Dark urine	Hemoglobinuria from acute hemolysis Bilirubinuria (due to any cause of conjugated hyperbilirubinemia) Gross hematuria from coagulopathy	Dehydration, medications (rifampin: orange urine; beets: red urine) Myoglobinuria due to rhabdomyolysis
Involuntary weight loss	Pancreatic or hepatobiliary cancer	

HELLP, hemolysis, elevated liver enzymes, and low platelet count.

[a]**Charcot's triad** refers to jaundice, fever, and right upper quadrant pain, classically associated with cholangitis and present in 22%–75% of cases of cholangitis. The addition of altered mentation and hypotension compose **Reynolds' pentad**, a surgical or endoscopic emergency.[3,4]

FOCUSED QUESTIONS

QUESTIONS	THINK ABOUT...
If answered in the affirmative	
Have you had previous biliary surgery?	Retained stones after cholecystectomy Biliary stricture Obstruction from recurrent malignancy
Have you recently ingested any acetaminophen, new medications, herbal supplements, or wild mushrooms?	Fulminant hepatic failure from numerous medications (eg, acetaminophen, isoniazid, anticonvulsants) or *Amanita* mushrooms

—Continued next page

Continued—

Do you drink alcohol?	Acute alcoholic hepatitis, chronic alcoholic cirrhosis, and "therapeutic misadventure"—liver injury at therapeutic doses of acetaminophen in an alcoholic
Have you ever used injection drugs?	Hepatitis C: 65% prevalence among injection drug users[5]
Are you younger than age 20?	Familial disorders of bilirubin metabolism (Gilbert, Crigler-Najjar, Dubin-Johnson, and Rotor syndromes)
Are you between the ages of 15 and 40?	Wilson's disease Autoimmune hepatitis (especially in women) Primary sclerosing cholangitis (especially in men)
Are you older than 40?	Increased risk of primary biliary cirrhosis (especially in women) Hemochromatosis Cancer of the pancreas or bile ducts
Have you been recently exposed to anyone with hepatitis?	Hepatitis A is a common cause of food-borne outbreaks of hepatitis. Hepatitis B can be transmitted through sexual activity (hepatitis C to a much lesser extent).
Have you received any blood transfusions?	Acute transfusion reaction may rarely cause massive hemolysis. Past blood transfusions may increase the risk for hepatitis B and C; this risk is low today, but transfusions prior to 1990 were not routinely tested for hepatitis C.
Does anyone in your family have hepatitis or a history of jaundice?	Hepatitis B transmitted vertically from mother to child at the time of birth may remain asymptomatic for years; familial causes include hemochromatosis, Wilson's disease, and Gilbert, Crigler-Najjar, Dubin-Johnson, and Rotor syndromes.
Have you become jaundiced with prior illnesses?	Gilbert syndrome, present in 10% of whites, often coincides with a viral illness.
Are you diabetic?	Diabetes and obesity are risk factors for NAFLD; diabetes may also be a manifestation of hemochromatosis.
Do you have sickle cell disease?	Sickle cell patients have 2 reasons for jaundice: chronic hemolysis due to sickled hemoglobin and predisposition to pigment gallstone formation (resulting in biliary colic).
Do you have a history of ulcerative colitis?	Primary sclerosing cholangitis develops in 1%–4% of patients with ulcerative colitis, whereas 67% of patients with primary sclerosing cholangitis have ulcerative colitis.
Do you have a history of heart failure?	Decompensated heart failure Constrictive pericarditis
Have you or has anyone in your family ever had blood clots?	Hypercoagulable states may result in Budd-Chiari syndrome.

Time course	
Was onset abrupt?	Choledocholithiasis Cholangitis Acute hepatitis Acute Budd-Chiari syndrome Hemolysis Sepsis
Was onset over weeks to months?	Pancreatic and hepatobiliary cancers Any cause of chronic cirrhosis Infiltrative liver disease Heart failure
Are episodes recurrent and self-limited?	Biliary colic and familial disorders of bilirubin metabolism (eg, Gilbert syndrome)
Associated symptoms	
Do you have:	
• *Epigastric pain?*	Pancreatitis Pancreatic cancer
• *Nausea or vomiting?*	Choledocholithiasis Cholangitis Acute hepatitis (viral, toxin/alcohol, medication-induced) Budd-Chiari syndrome Sepsis
• *Prodrome of malaise, fatigue, and anorexia?*	Viral hepatitis Pancreatic or hepatobiliary cancer
• *Clay-colored stools?*	Biliary duct obstruction
• *Silver stool?*	Cancer at the head of the pancreas causing melena without bile (tumor obstructs bile duct and may bleed into intestinal lumen)
• *Hematuria or flank pain?*	Renal cell carcinoma with associated paraneoplastic reversible hepatic dysfunction (Stauffer syndrome)
• *Increased abdominal girth?*	Suggests either ascites (due to decompensated chronic liver disease or Budd-Chiari syndrome) or abdominal mass (hepatoma, pancreatic cancer, lymphoma)
• *Pruritus?*	Subacute or chronic cholestatic process such as primary biliary cirrhosis, medication injury (estrogens, oral contraceptives, anabolic steroids, erythromycin, parenteral nutrition), benign recurrent intrahepatic cholestasis, intrahepatic cholestasis of pregnancy
• *Increased or easy bruisability?*	Coagulopathy due to impaired clotting factor synthesis from cirrhosis
• *Missed menses?*	Pregnancy
• *Arthralgias?*	Prodrome of viral hepatitis; also seen in hemochromatosis

DIAGNOSTIC APPROACH (INCLUDING ALGORITHM)

Figure 37–2 shows the diagnostic approach algorithm for jaundice.

CAVEATS

- Most patients will not complain of "jaundice" per se, but rather of discolored eyes or skin or of the accompanying symptoms that may be more concerning to the patient.

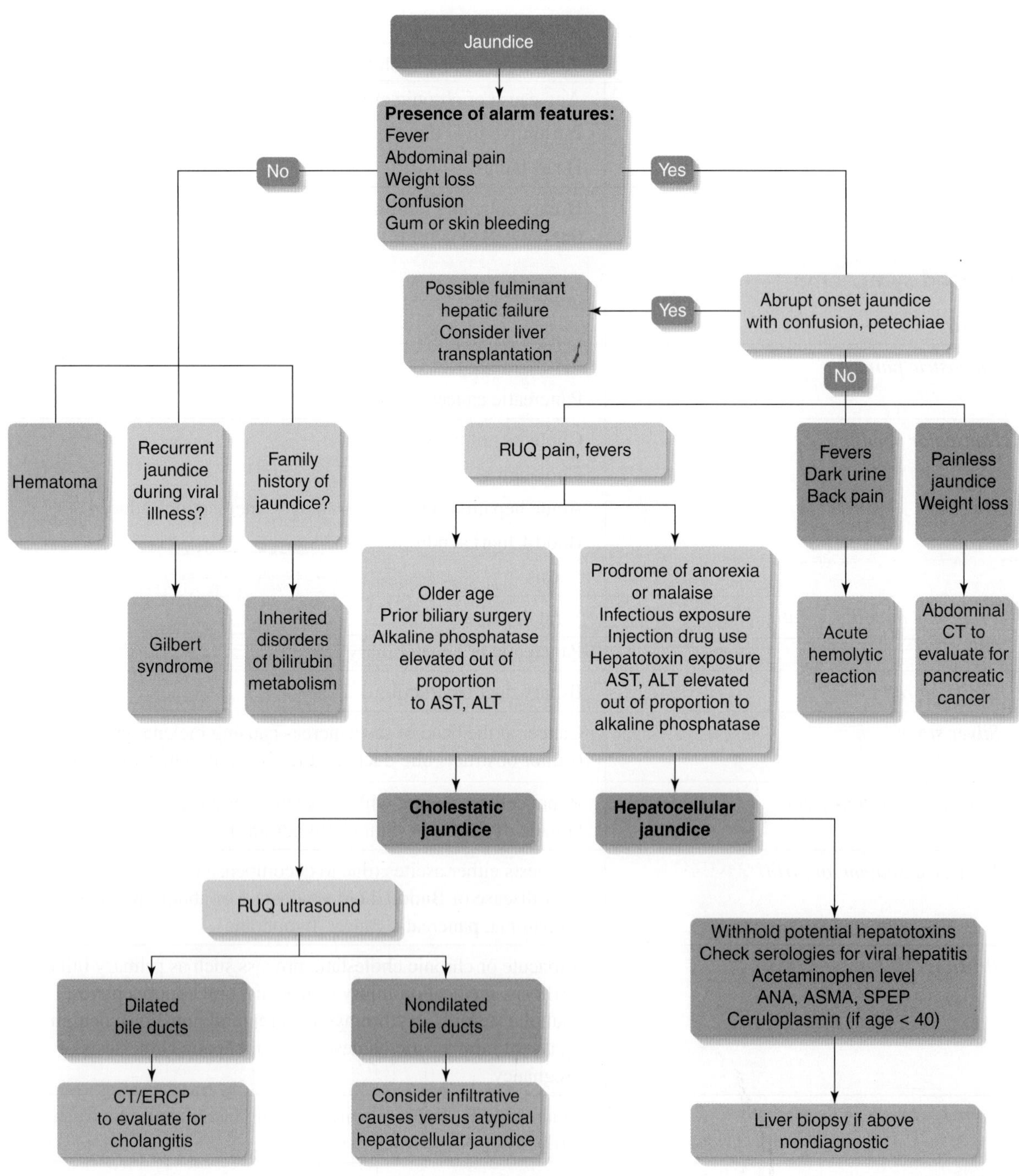

FIGURE 37–2 Diagnostic approach: Jaundice. ALT, alanine aminotransferase; ANA, antinuclear antibody; ASMA, anti-smooth muscle antibody; AST, aspartate aminotransferase; CT, computed tomography; ERCP, endoscopic retrograde cholangiopancreatography; RUQ, right upper quadrant; SPEP, serum protein electrophoresis.

- Prevalence data must be interpreted with caution: The main outpatient causes of jaundice in the United States are biliary obstruction and decompensated alcoholic liver disease. Sepsis and hepatic ischemia emerge as common causes in the inpatient setting.[5]
- Life-threatening causes of jaundice fall under 1 of 2 broad categories: liver injury or biliary tract obstruction. Unfortunately, the history alone is limited in its ability to reliably discriminate between the 2, and combined history and physical are only 80% accurate.[6] Physical examination, laboratory evaluation, and often abdominal imaging are needed to arrive at an accurate diagnosis.
- A complete ingestion history is vital, including acetaminophen and other medications, toxins (eg, alcohol), foods (eg, *Amanita* mushrooms), and herbal remedies. Even medications taken at therapeutic doses can result in fulminant hepatic failure. Combinations of medications or hepatotoxins can provoke a toxic reaction at lower doses, such as seen with concomitant alcoholic liver disease and acetaminophen use.

PROGNOSIS

The mortality rate among hospitalized patients with jaundice was 32% in one study[2] but varied by underlying cause. Highest mortality rates were seen with sepsis or hypotensive liver injury, followed closely by malignancy and cirrhosis; whereas gallstone disease had a more favorable prognosis. Fulminant hepatic failure of any cause warrants immediate evaluation for liver transplantation.

Pancreatic cancer has a dismal overall prognosis, with 5-year survival rates between 2% and 5%. Select patients with smaller tumors involving the pancreas head may reach survival rates of 20% to 40%.

Among patients infected with hepatitis C virus, chronic disease will develop in 80%, and 20% will progress to cirrhosis over 20 years. For an immunocompetent adult infected with hepatitis B, chronic infection will develop in less than 5%. Only the small subset of chronically infected hepatitis B patients with actively replicating virus is at risk for progressing to cirrhosis. Once hepatitis B or C results in cirrhosis, the annual risk of developing hepatocellular carcinoma is 3% to 5%, and screening for hepatocellular carcinoma is warranted.[1]

CASE SCENARIO | Resolution

A 67-year-old man with type 2 diabetes presents to your primary care practice following 3 weeks of intermittent nausea and vomiting. His wife insisted he see a doctor because his skin and eyes are yellow. He has noticed that his pants are looser, but he has no other complaints.

ADDITIONAL HISTORY

On further questioning, he denies fevers, chills, and abdominal pain. He reports moderate anorexia and states that his urine is dark and his stools are becoming lighter in color. There have been no outbreaks of food-borne illnesses where he lives, and he has not traveled outside of the United States recently. He has a history of heavy alcohol use in the past but quit 15 years ago. His only medication is metformin, which he has been taking for several years. He does not take herbal supplements, has never received a blood transfusion, and has never used intravenous or illicit drugs. There is no family or personal history of hepatitis, liver disease, inflammatory bowel disease, or cancer. He has smoked one pack of cigarette daily for over 30 years. On physical examination, he is not cachectic, but the sclerae are icteric and his skin is visibly jaundiced. No palpable masses or tenderness are present on abdominal examination.

Question: What is the most likely diagnosis?

A. Primary sclerosing cholangitis
B. Adenocarcinoma of the pancreas
C. Chronic viral hepatitis C infection
D. Ascending cholangitis

Test Your Knowledge

1. A 45-year-old obese man was brought to your primary care clinic by a coworker who found the patient confused in the office earlier that day. The patient acknowledged feeling unwell for the past several days, with low-grade fevers and chills, nausea, and right upper quadrant abdominal pain. He also reports a "yellow tinge" to his skin. He has no other past medical history, takes no medications or herbal supplements, is not sexually active, and denies alcohol or illicit drug use. On examination, he is found to have a blood pressure of 90/50 mm Hg and a temperature of 101.7°F and is tender to palpation in the right upper quadrant of his abdomen.
   What is this patient's presentation most consistent with?
   A. Ascending cholangitis
   B. Acute viral hepatitis C
   C. Nonalcoholic fatty liver disease
   D. Hepatic congestion from right-sided heart failure
   E. Chronic viral hepatitis B

2. A 55-year-old obese woman with diabetes mellitus and hypertriglyceridemia visits you for routine follow-up. On examination, the patient is afebrile and has normal vital signs but has scleral icterus. Her skin is normal, and the abdomen is obese with mild hepatomegaly but no tenderness.
   Which of the following disorders do you suspect?
   A. Acute cholecystitis
   B. Carotenemia
   C. Nonalcoholic fatty liver disease
   D. HELLP syndrome
   E. Acute viral hepatitis

3. A 20-year-old college student presents to student health clinic with 3 days of fevers, runny nose, sore throat, and malaise. She has no abdominal pain, nausea, or vomiting, and she denies taking any medications, alcohol, supplements, or illicit drugs. On examination, she has a temperature of 100.3°F. She has pharyngeal erythema without exudates, and there is mild bilateral anterior cervical lymphadenopathy. Her sclerae are icteric and her abdomen is nontender without hepatosplenomegaly. On further questioning, she recalls having similar episodes of her eyes turning yellow when she was sick ever since she was a child; in those instances, her eye color always returned to normal once her illness resolved.
   What is the most likely diagnosis?
   A. Biliary colic
   B. Acute intermittent porphyria
   C. Gilbert syndrome
   D. Cirrhosis
   E. Hemochromatosis

ACKNOWLEDGEMENT

The authors wish to acknowledge Estella M. Geraghty, MD, for her major contributions to a previous version of this chapter.

References

1. Reisman Y, Gips CH, Lavelle SM, Wilson JH. Clinical presentation of (subclinical) jaundice—the Euricterus Project in The Netherlands. United Dutch Hospitals and Euricterus Project Management Group. *Hepatogastroenterology*. 1996;43:1190–1195.
2. Whitehead MW, Kingham JGC. The causes of obvious jaundice in South West Wales: perceptions versus reality. *Gut*. 2001;48:409–413.
3. Csendes A, Diaz JC, Burdiles P, et al. Risk factors and classification of acute suppurative cholangitis. *Br J Surg*. 1992;79:655–658.
4. Saik RP, Greenburg AG, Farris JM, Peskin GW. Spectrum of cholangitis. *Am J Surg*. 1975;130:143–150.
5. Garfein RS, Vlahov D, Galai N, et al. Viral infections in short-term injection drug users: the prevalence of the hepatitis C, hepatitis B, human immunodeficiency, and human T-lymphotropic viruses. *Am J Public Health*. 1996;86:655–661.
6. Reisman Y, van Dam GM, Gips CH, et al. Physicians' working diagnosis compared to the Euricterus Real Life Date Diagnostic Tool in three jaundice databases: Euricterus Dutch, independent prospective, and independent retrospective. *Hepatogastroenterology*. 1997;44:1367–1375.

Suggested Reading

Almeda-Valdes P, Cuevas-Ramos D, Aguilar-Salinas A. Metabolic syndrome and non-alcoholic fatty liver disease. *Ann Hepatol.* 2009;8:18–24.

Edwards CQ, Kushner JP. Screening for hemochromatosis. *N Engl J Med.* 1993;328:1616–1620.

Elwood DR. Cholecystitis. *Surg Clin North Am.* 2008;88:1241–1252.

Kim WR, Lindor KD, Locke GR, et al. Epidemiology and natural history of primary biliary cirrhosis in a U.S. community. *Gastroenterology.* 2000;119:1631–1636.

O'Grady JG, Alexander GJM, Hayllar KM, Williams R. Early indicators of prognosis in fulminant hepatic failure. *Gastroenterology.* 1989;97:439–445.

Pasanen PA, Partanen KP, Pikkarainen PH, et al. A comparison of ultrasound, computed tomography and endoscopic retrograde cholangiopancreatography in the differential diagnosis of benign and malignant jaundice and cholestasis. *Eur J Surg.* 1993;159:23–29.

Chapter 38

Nausea and Vomiting

Randall E. Lee, MD

CASE SCENARIO

A 24-year-old woman presents to your urgent care clinic complaining of nausea and vomiting for the past 4 weeks.

- **What additional questions should you ask to determine the severity of her condition?**
- **Can you narrow the differential diagnosis of her "nausea and vomiting" through your use of open-ended questions followed by more focused queries?**

INTRODUCTION

Nausea and vomiting are common symptoms experienced across all age groups. Although they are often manifestations of minor self-limited illnesses, these symptoms may also be harbingers of life-threatening disease. Nausea and vomiting cause significant worldwide reductions in worker productivity and increases in healthcare costs, particularly among pregnant women, patients receiving cancer chemotherapy, and patients recovering from surgery. Nausea is frequently, but not always, associated with vomiting.[1]

KEY TERMS[1]

Chronic nausea and vomiting	The persistence of the symptoms for > 1 month.
Early satiety	The sensation of feeling full after eating an unusually small amount of food.
Nausea	The unpleasant sensation of the imminent need to vomit that may or may not ultimately lead to actual vomiting.
Postchemotherapy nausea and vomiting (PCNV)	3 types: acute, within 24 hours; delayed, after 24 hours later; and anticipatory, just before the next chemotherapy dose.
Recurrent vomiting	3 or more episodes.
Regurgitation	The passive retrograde flow of esophageal contents into the mouth without the muscular activity associated with vomiting and without antecedent nausea.
Retching	The "dry heaves." Spasmodic respiratory movements against a closed glottis with contractions of the abdominal musculature without expulsion of any gastric contents. Retching often immediately precedes vomiting.
Rumination	Chewing and swallowing of regurgitated food that has come back into the mouth through a voluntary increase in intra-abdominal pressure within minutes of eating or during eating.
Vomiting	The forceful oral expulsion of gastric contents associated with contraction of the abdominal and chest wall musculature.

ETIOLOGY

The initial differential diagnosis of nausea and vomiting is broad but may be narrowed significantly by the clinical context.

The evaluation of an infant or young child who has acute vomiting merits special consideration. For instance, the possibility of a toxic ingestion is much more likely in a child than an adult. Despite a declining incidence, Reye's syndrome remains a consideration in an acutely vomiting child who has had a recent viral infection (and has been given aspirin products).

Similarly, the differential diagnosis for a recurrently vomiting infant or young child should be expanded to include congenital abnormalities (eg, malrotation, pyloric stenosis, esophageal atresia). Remember, vomiting in infants may simply be regurgitation due to physiologic gastroesophageal reflux.

A positive family history along with associated neurologic symptoms should raise suspicion for inherited metabolic disorders (eg, urea cycle enzyme deficiencies, Wilson's disease) or neurogastrointestinal disorders (eg, cyclic vomiting syndrome).

Differential Diagnosis

	Percentage of Patients With Specific Diagnosis Who Have Nausea and Vomiting[a]
Acute nausea and vomiting	
Gastrointestinal infections and toxins (gastroenteritis, hepatitis, food poisoning)	
Medications (chemotherapeutics, antibiotics, analgesics, etc)	Cancer patients receiving narcotics for pain control: 40%–70%[1] Patients receiving cisplatin chemotherapy: 90%[1] Post general anesthesia: 37% nausea, 23% vomiting[1]
Visceral pain (pancreatitis, appendicitis, biliary colic, acute small bowel obstruction, renal colic, intestinal ischemia, myocardial infarction)	
Conditions affecting central nervous system (CNS) (eg, labyrinthitis, motion/space sickness, head trauma, stroke, Reye syndrome, meningitis, increased intracranial pressure)	Skull fracture: 28% adults, 33% children[2]
Metabolic (pregnancy, ketoacidosis, uremia)	First trimester of pregnancy: 70%[1]
Radiation	Radiation therapy to abdomen: 80%[1]
Chronic nausea and vomiting	
Gastric (mechanical obstruction or functional dysmotility; ie, gastroparesis, dyspepsia) Small intestinal dysmotility (pseudo-obstruction, scleroderma) Metabolic (pregnancy, hyperthyroidism, adrenal insufficiency) CNS (increased intracranial pressure due to tumor, pseudotumor cerebri, cerebral edema, or encephalopathy) Psychogenic (eating disorder) Cyclic vomiting syndrome	

[a]Prevalence is unknown when not indicated.

GETTING STARTED WITH THE HISTORY

- The approach to a patient with nausea and vomiting begins by clearly defining the symptoms and characterizing their duration, severity, and associated factors.
- Assess the patient for alarm symptoms that require immediate intervention.
- Distinguish between acute and chronic symptoms to narrow the broad differential diagnosis.
- Finally, ask focused questions to further refine the differential diagnosis.

Open-Ended Questions	Tips for Effective Interviewing
Tell me about your nausea and vomiting. *Tell me about the first time this happened.*	Allow the patient to tell the story without interruption.
What do you think is the cause of your nausea and vomiting? Have you been able to establish a pattern? *Think about your most recent episode of nausea and vomiting. What did you do that day, starting from when you woke up in the morning?*	When the patient pauses, prompt for more information by asking "What else?"

INTERVIEW FRAMEWORK

- Define the patient's symptoms based on the above definitions or key terms. For instance, is the patient truly experiencing vomiting, or is it regurgitation?
- Assess the patient for alarm symptoms.
- Determine the following symptom characteristics:
  - Duration of nausea and vomiting (acute or chronic?)
  - Frequency of the symptoms
  - Severity of the nausea and vomiting
  - Relationship of the vomiting to meals and medications
  - Quality and quantity of vomitus
- Determine associated symptoms.
- Determine modifying symptoms.

IDENTIFYING ALARM SYMPTOMS

Serious Diagnoses

	Prevalence[a]
Hyperemesis gravidarum	0.3%–2.0%[3]
Acute fatty liver of pregnancy (AFLP)	0.008%[3]
HELLP syndrome (hemolytic anemia, elevated liver enzymes, low platelet count)	0.6% in pregnant women (5%–10% of women with preeclampsia)[3]
Intra-abdominal emergency (obstruction, perforation, peritonitis)	
Acute myocardial infarction	
CNS disorder (skull fracture, infection, increased intracranial pressure, bleed)	
Toxic ingestion	
Upper gastrointestinal bleeding	

[a]Prevalence is unknown when not indicated.

Alarm Symptoms	If Present, Consider Serious Causes	Positive Likelihood Ratio (LR+)	Possible Benign Causes
Large-volume hematemesis (grossly bloody or black, like coffee grounds)	Major upper gastrointestinal bleeding from peptic ulcer, varices, or Mallory-Weiss tear		
History of head trauma	Skull fracture	Adult, LR+ 4.17 Child, LR+ 2.82[2]	

—Continued next page

Continued—			
Headache	Intracranial bleed, mass, or infection	Jolt accentuation of headache, LR+ 2.4 for meningitis[4]	Migraine
Neck stiffness	Meningitis		
Altered mental status	Intracranial bleed, mass, infection, or encephalopathy		
Right lower quadrant pain	Acute appendicitis	LR+ 8.0[5]	
Migration of periumbilical pain to right lower quadrant	Acute appendicitis	LR+ 3.1[5]	
Abdominal pain before vomiting	Acute appendicitis	LR+ 2.76[5]	
Abdominal pain that worsens with jolting movements, such as going down stairs (peritoneal pain)	Peritonitis		
Upper abdominal pain: steady pain lasting > 30 minutes (biliary colic)	Acute cholecystitis		
Acute chest pain	Acute myocardial infarction	Pain radiation to left arm, LR+ 2.3 Pain radiation to both left and right arms, LR+ 7.1[6]	Gastroesophageal reflux disease
Postural symptoms, lethargy, unable to retain oral liquids for > 8 hours in a child (12 hours in an adult)	Hypovolemia and/or electrolyte imbalances requiring urgent treatment		
Paresthesias, blurred vision, dysphagia, muscle weakness	Food-borne toxins (botulinum, ciguatera, paralytic shellfish toxin)		

FOCUSED QUESTIONS

QUESTIONS	THINK ABOUT...
Do you also have diarrhea? Do others in your community (family, day care, cruise ship, summer camp) also have vomiting and diarrhea?	Viral gastroenteritis Food-borne illness
Do you have any symptoms of pregnancy, such as late menstrual period or breast swelling, tingling, or tenderness?	Early pregnancy (LR+ 2.70)[7]

Are you pregnant (first trimester)?	Hyperemesis gravidarum
Are you pregnant (second or third trimester)?	AFLP or HELLP syndrome
Does the room feel like it is moving? (vertigo)	Labyrinthitis (see Chapter 6)
Have you been receiving chemotherapy for cancer?	Post chemotherapy nausea and vomiting
Has your weight gone up and down (30–40 lb) this past year? Do you always vomit into the toilet and never on the floor or in public? Do you make yourself vomit?	Eating disorder (see Chapter 15)
Do you vomit without retching? Do you rechew and/or reswallow your vomitus?	Rumination syndrome; not true vomiting
Do you have a history of kidney disease or failure?	Uremia
Do you have a history of peptic ulcer? Have you been taking nonsteroidal anti-inflammatory drugs (NSAIDs) or aspirin?	Peptic ulcer or gastric outlet obstruction
Do you feel full after eating just a small amount of food (early satiety)?	Gastric malignancy, gastric outlet obstruction
Do you chew on your hair?	Bezoar
Do you have a history of heart disease?	Acute myocardial infarction, digoxin toxicity
Have you had previous abdominal surgery?	Intestinal obstruction due to adhesions
Is anyone else who ate or drank the same thing also having nausea and vomiting?	Food poisoning
Did the symptoms occur within a few hours after eating or drinking something?	Food poisoning due to *Staphylococcus aureus* or *Bacillus cereus* toxins
Did you eat raw shellfish?	Food poisoning due to *Vibrio vulnificus*
Did you eat shellfish, and do you have numbness and tingling around your mouth?	Paralytic shellfish poisoning (saxitoxin)
Did you eat home canned or preserved food? Do you have trouble swallowing? Is your mouth dry? Is your vision blurry?	Botulism[8]
Did you eat raw fish?	Anisakiasis
Did you drink liquids that were stored in a metal container? Do you also have a metallic taste?	Heavy metal ingestion (zinc, copper, tin, iron, cadmium)
Did the bumps in the car ride make your abdominal pain worse?	Peritonitis
Do you have diabetes?	Diabetic ketoacidosis or gastroparesis
Does the child's ear hurt? Is the child rubbing or pulling on the ear?	Acute otitis media LR+ 3 to 7.3[9] (see Chapter 17)
Did the child recently have the flu or a cold? Did the child receive aspirin?	Reye's syndrome
Is there a family history of early childhood death?	Inherited metabolic disorders (urea cycle disorders, Wilson's disease)

—Continued next page

Continued—

Quality	
Is the vomitus grossly bloody?	Peptic ulcer Esophageal varices Mallory-Weiss tear
Does the vomitus contain partially digested food?	Gastroparesis Gastric outlet obstruction
Is the vomitus bilious (containing green bile)?	Small bowel obstruction
Is it feculent?	Bowel obstruction
Does it contain undigested food regurgitated (not truly vomited)?	Achalasia Zenker diverticulum Esophageal stenosis
Do you have nausea without vomiting?	Pregnancy
Is vomiting projectile?	Pyloric stenosis Increased intracranial pressure
Time course	
Do you vomit:	
• *In the morning before breakfast?*	Pregnancy Increased intracranial pressure
• *≥ 1 hour after eating?*	Gastroparesis Gastric outlet obstruction
• *During or soon after a meal?*	Gastric ulcer Eating disorder
• *Soon after taking medications?*	Medication side effect
• *In a recurrent but intermittent pattern?*	Cyclic vomiting syndrome
Associated symptoms	
Do you have:	
• *Diarrhea, headache, myalgia, or fever?*	Viral gastroenteritis
• *Headache, neck stiffness, altered mentation, or photophobia?*	Meningitis
• *Low weight or weight loss?*	Eating disorder Gastrointestinal malignancy
• *Lack of concern regarding weight loss or vomiting?*	Eating disorder
• *Jaundice, dark urine, or light stools?*	Hepatitis Choledocholithiasis
• *Chest pain or cold sweats (diaphoresis)?*	Myocardial infarction
• *Crampy, colicky abdominal pain?*	Bowel obstruction
• *Upper abdominal pain (biliary colic)?*	Cholecystitis or cholelithiasis

• *Epigastric abdominal pain radiating to the back?*	Pancreatitis
• *Abdominal pain that worsens with jolting movements?*	Bowel perforation Peritonitis
• *Migraine headaches?*	Cyclic vomiting syndrome
• *Vertigo?*	Labyrinthitis
Modifying symptoms	
Do you get sick:	
• *Only as a passenger in a vehicle?*	Motion sickness/sea sickness/space sickness
• *Only during periods of stress?*	Psychogenic

DIAGNOSTIC APPROACH (INCLUDING ALGORITHM)

The diagnostic approach to the patient with nausea and vomiting has 2 basic goals: (1) determine the need for immediate intervention, and (2) identify the specific cause of the symptoms. The comprehensive history and subsequent physical examination narrow the differential diagnosis by determining whether the symptoms are acute or chronic, and then directs the selection of diagnostic tests such as blood tests, esophagogastroduodenoscopy, computed tomography, abdominal ultrasonography, and barium radiographs. Figure 38–1 shows the diagnostic approach algorithm for nausea and vomiting.

CAVEATS

- By itself, a history of nausea and vomiting has poor predictive value (LR+ of 1.3 and LR– of 0.64) for the diagnosis of acute meningitis in adults.[4]
- No single clinical finding has sufficient diagnostic power to establish or exclude a diagnosis of acute cholecystitis in a patient with upper abdominal pain without further testing, such as abdominal ultrasonography.[10]
- The gold standard for diagnosing early pregnancy is a urine or serum human chorionic gonadotropin pregnancy test.

PROGNOSIS

The prognosis depends on the underlying cause of the nausea and vomiting. A careful history and physical examination alone generally yield the etiology and subsequent therapy of acute nausea and vomiting. In contrast, determining the cause of chronic nausea and vomiting may be more elusive and require more diagnostic testing. The management of chronic symptoms generally is more challenging and may require comanagement with mental health professionals. Eating disorders in general and anorexia nervosa in particular tend to have relapsing courses.

CASE SCENARIO | Resolution

A 24-year-old woman presents to your urgent care clinic complaining of nausea and vomiting for the past 4 weeks.

ADDITIONAL HISTORY

She had no prior gastrointestinal problems until the onset of symptoms 4 weeks ago. She generally develops nausea about 1/2 hour after eating and then vomits nonbloody material about an hour later. Solid food causes more symptoms than liquids, and the amount of food needed to cause symptoms has been decreasing. Otherwise, she cannot establish any aggravating or alleviating factors. Her weight involuntarily dropped about 3 kg since the onset of symptoms. She has no associated postural symptoms, fevers, diaphoresis, headache, neck stiffness, vertigo, chest pain, abdominal pain, or altered mental state. No close contacts have the same symptoms. She has not had any abdominal surgery. Her last menstrual period was 2 weeks ago and on schedule. Two years ago, she was honorably discharged from the US Army after injuring her knees while on duty in Afghanistan. Currently she is a sophomore majoring in mechanical engineering at the state university, funded by the GI Bill. Other than over-the-counter NSAIDs for chronic knee pain and oral contraceptives, she uses no regular medications and has no allergies.

Question: What is the most likely diagnosis?

A. Eating disorder
B. Peptic ulcer with partial gastric outlet obstruction
C. Early pregnancy
D. Gastroesophageal reflux disease

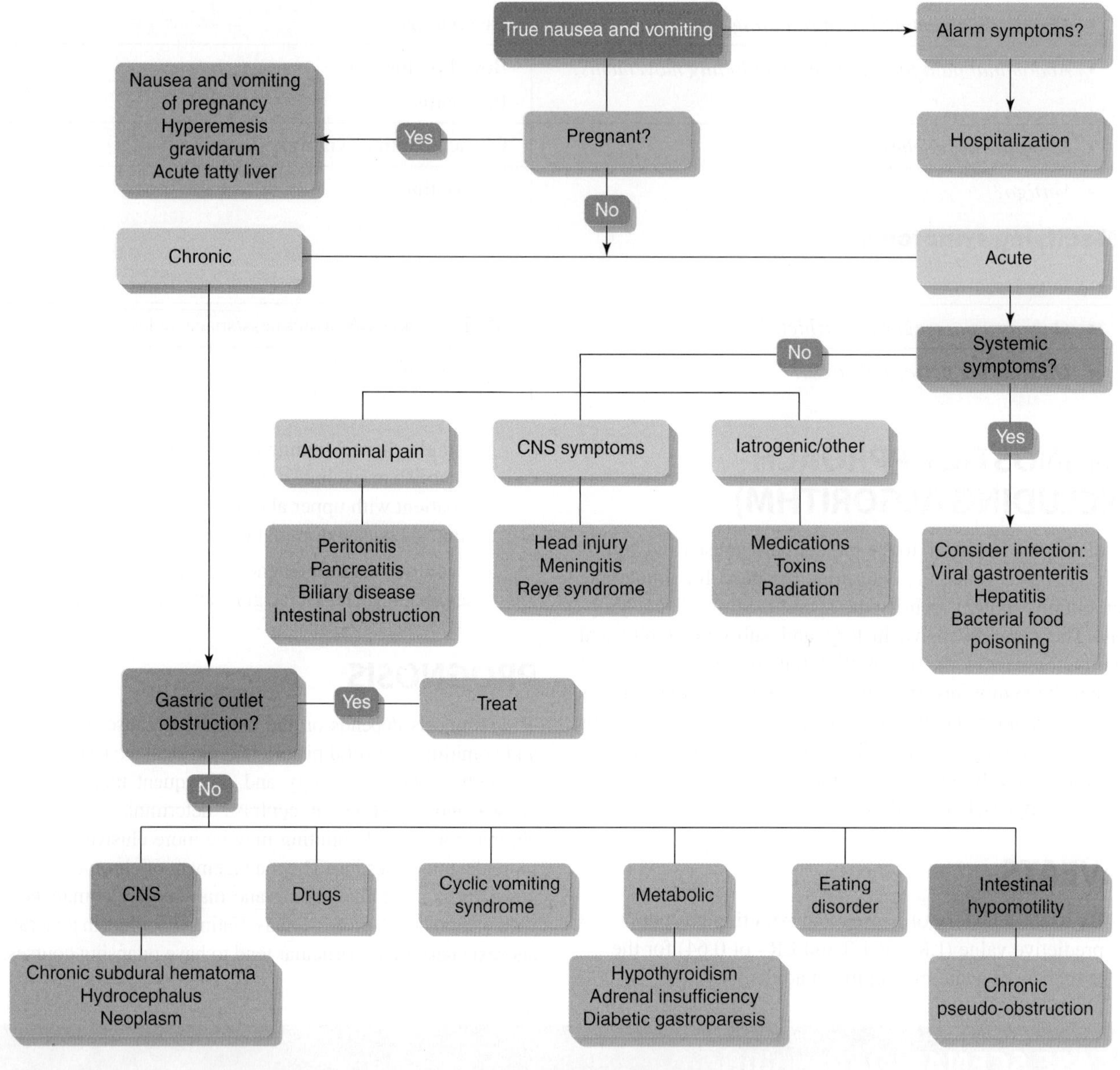

FIGURE 38–1 Diagnostic approach: Nausea and vomiting. CNS, central nervous system.

Test Your Knowledge

1. A previously healthy 45-year-old man went home from work after lunch with fatigue and nausea. Shortly thereafter, he developed severe vomiting.

   Which of the following is *not* an alarm symptom that merits possible hospitalization?

   A. Diarrhea
   B. Lip numbness
   C. Abdominal pain accentuated by jolting movements
   D. Large-volume hematemesis
   E. Confusion

2. A 55-year-old overweight woman presents to clinic with nausea, vomiting, and abdominal pain. She had no prior gastrointestinal symptoms until about 16 hours ago when she developed increasingly severe upper abdominal discomfort, followed by nausea and nonbloody emesis and subjective fever and chills, but no jaundice.

   Which of the following can best establish or exclude a diagnosis of acute cholecystitis?

   A. Physical examination showing right upper quadrant tenderness with inspiratory arrest (Murphy sign)

B. Liver chemistry panel (aspartate aminotransferase [AST], alanine aminotransferase [ALT], alkaline phosphatase, total and direct bilirubin, albumin)
C. Complete blood count
D. Right upper abdominal ultrasonography
E. No further testing needed

3. A 33-year-old overweight woman presents with recurrent nausea and vomiting. For about 20 years, she has had a near continuous sense of nausea with episodes of nonbloody vomiting. She has no abdominal pain and cannot establish a pattern to the vomiting. Treatment with antiemetics and proton pump inhibitors is not helpful. She brings a large stack of outside medical records documenting repeatedly normal endoscopic, pathologic, and radiologic evaluations.

   Which of the following is most likely to yield a diagnostic and therapeutic benefit to this patient?

   A. Referral for esophagogastroduodenoscopy
   B. *Helicobacter pylori* antibody testing
   C. Computed tomography scan of the abdomen and pelvis
   D. Detailed psychosocial history with attention to possible trauma 20 years ago
   E. Upper gastrointestinal radiographic series

References

1. American Gastroenterological Association Clinical Practice and Practice Economics Committee. AGA technical review on nausea and vomiting. *Gastroenterology.* 2001;120:263–286.
2. Nee PA, Hadfield JM, Yates DW, Faragher EB. Significance of vomiting after head injury. *J Neurol Neurosurg Psychiatry.* 1999;66:470–473.
3. Joshi D, James A, Quaglia A, Westbrook R, Heneghan M. Liver disease in pregnancy. *Lancet.* 2010;375:594–605.
4. Hatala R, Attai J, Bent S. Make the diagnosis: meningitis, adult. In: Simel D, Rennie D, eds. *The Rational Clinical Examination: Evidence-Based Clinical Diagnosis*. New York, NY: McGraw-Hill, 2009.
5. Wagner J, Shojania K. Make the diagnosis: appendicitis, adult. In: Simel D, Rennie D, eds. *The Rational Clinical Examination: Evidence-Based Clinical Diagnosis*. New York, NY: McGraw-Hill, 2009.
6. Simel D, Goodacre S, Newby L. Update: myocardial infarction. In: Simel D, Rennie D, eds. *The Rational Clinical Examination: Evidence-Based Clinical Diagnosis*. New York, NY: McGraw-Hill, 2009.
7. Bastian L, Piscitelli J. Make the diagnosis: early pregnancy. In: Simel D, Rennie D, eds. *The Rational Clinical Examination: Evidence-Based Clinical Diagnosis*. New York, NY: McGraw-Hill, 2009.
8. Lawrence D, Dobmeier S, Bechtel L, Holstege C. Food poisoning. *Emerg Med Clin North Am.* 2007;25:357–373.
9. Simel D, Rothman R, Keitz S. Make the diagnosis: otitis media, child. In: Simel D, Rennie D, eds. *The Rational Clinical Examination: Evidence-Based Clinical Diagnosis*. New York, NY: McGraw-Hill, 2009.
10. Trowbridge R, Shojania K, Rosenthanl A. Update: acute cholecystitis. In: Simel D, Rennie D, eds. *The Rational Clinical Examination: Evidence-Based Clinical Diagnosis*. New York, NY: McGraw-Hill, 2009.

Suggested Reading

American Gastroenterological Association Clinical Practice and Practice Economics Committee. American Gastroenterological Association Medical Position Statement: nausea and vomiting. *Gastroenterology.* 2001;120:261–262.

Li B, Lefevre F, Chelimsky GG, et al. North American Society for Pediatric Gastroenterology, Hepatology, and Nutrition consensus statement on the diagnosis and management of cyclic vomiting syndrome. *J Pediatr Gastroenterol Nutr.* 2008;47:379–393.

Malagelada J, Malagelada C. Nausea and vomiting. In: Feldman M, Friedman L, Brandt L, eds. *Sleisenger & Fordtran's Gastrointestinal and Liver Disease: Pathophysiology, Diagnosis, Management.* 9th ed. New York, NY: Saunders, 2010:197–206.

Miller C, Golden N. An introduction to eating disorders: clinical presentation, epidemiology, and prognosis. *Nutr Clin Pract.* 2010;25:110–115.

Pigott D. Foodborne illness. *Emerg Med Clin North Am.* 2008;26:475–497.

Chapter 39

Anorectal Pain

Matthew C. Baker, David S. Fefferman, MD, & Ciarán P. Kelly, MD

CASE SCENARIO

A 60-year-old gentleman presents to you with a 3-day history of constant perianal pain and bright red blood seen in the toilet bowl. This morning, he noticed a small swollen mass at his anus when washing in the shower. He experienced a similar episode of pain and bleeding several months ago, which he attributed to hemorrhoids, but his symptoms today are far more severe.

- **What else in this patient's history might help to establish the diagnosis?**
- **What characteristics of the pain and bleeding are important to know?**
- **If the patient is correct about having hemorrhoids, are they likely internal or external?**
- **Does this history cause concern for anal cancer?**
- **Can you make the diagnosis based on this history alone?**

INTRODUCTION

Symptoms of anorectal disease are common. However, due to the reluctance of both patients and clinicians to discuss these symptoms in detail, problems may be attributed hastily to internal hemorrhoids and not investigated adequately. In many cases, a thorough history will point to a specific diagnosis, or at least help target the physical examination and indicate the appropriate special tests. No matter how clear the history seems to be, a perianal inspection and digital anorectal examination are mandatory unless the anal canal is too tender or too stenotic to allow this examination. Anoscopy is an important adjunct to the physical examination in patients with anorectal symptoms. After a detailed history, physical examination, and anoscopy, further or more invasive diagnostic testing may be unnecessary.

KEY TERMS

Anal fissure	A cut or tear of the anal mucosa.
Coccydynia	Referred pain from injured, inflamed, or hypersensitive coccyx.
Defecatory dysfunction or anismus	Dysfunction, weakness, or faulty coordination of the muscles that affect defecation.
Fecal impaction	Obstruction of the anal outlet with stool.
Fistula	Abnormal tunnel of infection or inflammation into the perianal skin, usually originating from an anal gland.
Foreign body	An item placed within the rectum for therapeutic or recreational purposes can cause rectal irritation, obstruction (if retained), or trauma including tearing of the anal mucosa and a painful anal fissure.

—Continued next page

Continued—

Hemorrhoid	Dilation of the superior or inferior hemorrhoidal venous plexus (cushions) resulting in internal or external hemorrhoids, respectively.
Levator ani syndrome	Idiopathic dull ache possibly resulting from dysmotility of the muscles supporting the rectum and anus.
Perianal abscess	Collection of infection within or adjacent to the perianal space.
Proctalgia fugax	Idiopathic recurrent sharp pain in the anus or rectum lasting several seconds and that is usually unrelated to bowel movements.
Proctitis	Inflammation, infection, or ischemia of the rectum.
Prostatitis	Infection or inflammation of the prostate gland.
Pruritus ani	This is not an etiology of anorectal pain but rather a symptom of itching in the skin of the anal canal or perianal region. It has a variety of causes including many of those listed above in addition to local irritation of the perianal skin from fecal soilage, infection (bacterial, fungal, viral, parasitic), inflammation, and dermatologic abnormalities. It may also be idiopathic.
Sacral nerve compression	Referred pain from compression or inflammation of sacral nerve.

ETIOLOGY

The pathophysiology of pain from the anorectum varies greatly depending on the disorder. However, useful groupings include: local causes, referred causes, and functional disorders (for which no known pathophysiologic mechanism has been demonstrated). Because of the varied mechanisms, it is difficult to differentiate between them by history alone, without performing a physical examination. Basic knowledge of the different innervations of the anal mucosa and rectal mucosa, which are separated anatomically by the dentate line, may help localize the lesion. The anal mucosa is innervated by pain sensory nerve fibers, which, when irritated or inflamed, produce sharp, well-localized symptoms. Conversely, lesions of the rectum, which contain only stretch fibers, result in poorly localized pressure sensations.

Differential Diagnosis

There have been no published studies summarizing the prevalence of disease or predictive value of symptoms in patients presenting with anorectal pain. Population surveys have found that 80% of people with anorectal symptoms do not seek medical attention.[1] Because many symptoms are falsely attributed to hemorrhoids, the relative prevalence of other anorectal disorders may be underestimated. The relative prevalence of the different etiologies for anorectal pain in the general population is provided below. Although anal or rectal carcinoma is an uncommon cause of rectal pain, this serious diagnosis should be considered in every patient.

Local Causes	Frequency
Anal fissure	Very common
Thrombosed external hemorrhoid	Very common
Perianal abscess	Common
Thrombosed/prolapsed internal hemorrhoid	Common
Defecatory dysfunction or anismus	Common
Fistula	Infrequent
Proctitis	Infrequent
Fecal impaction	Infrequent
Anal or rectal neoplasm (benign or malignant tumors of the anal canal or rectum)	Rare

Referred Pain	**Frequency**
Coccydynia	Rare
Sacral nerve compression	Rare
Prostatitis	Rare
Uterine disease	Rare
• Referred pain from inflamed or enlarged uterus	
• Direct compression or invasion of rectum	
Pelvic inflammatory disease	Rare
• Referred pain from inflamed reproductive organs	
Functional Syndromes	**Frequency**
Proctalgia fugax	Common
Levator ani syndrome	Rare

GETTING STARTED WITH THE HISTORY

Ask open-ended questions initially. Determine the onset of symptoms, frequency, and association with bowel movements. Obtain a detailed history of bowel movements including frequency, consistency, urgency, episodes of fecal incontinence, the presence of blood in the stool, bleeding after defecation, or the presence of a palpable swelling in the anal area during or after defecation.

Next, ask targeted follow-up questions to obtain a complete and detailed history. Obtaining a past medical history, including complete surgical and gynecologic histories, is imperative. Assess the family history specifically for gastrointestinal malignancies and inflammatory bowel disease (IBD). Inquire about medication use including the use of enemas or suppositories. Ask specifically about anal instrumentation or trauma (including the insertion of digits or participation in receptive anal intercourse) that is temporally related to the onset or alteration of anorectal symptoms.

Questions	**Remember**
Tell me about the symptoms you are experiencing.	Let patients use their own words.
What were the events surrounding the first time you experienced the symptoms? *Under what circumstances do your symptoms typically occur?* *What do you think may be causing your symptoms?*	Refrain from using the word pain; the patient may be experiencing other sensations, such as a dull ache, a poorly defined sense of discomfort, or even pruritus.

INTERVIEW FRAMEWORK

Characterize the type, onset, duration, frequency, and severity of pain or discomfort.

Assess for the following:

- The temporal association of symptoms with bowel movements.
- The presence of blood with, after, or separate from bowel movements.
- The presence or absence of a palpable mass, lump, or bulge.
- If a palpable mass, lump, or bulge is present, determine whether it develops only when straining during defecation and resolves spontaneously or following manual reduction.
- The presence of alarm symptoms.

IDENTIFYING ALARM SYMPTOMS

Although a rare cause of anorectal pain, neoplasia should be considered in every patient. Even though a change in bowel habits, blood in the stool, or constitutional symptoms (weight loss, fatigue, fever) may be due to benign conditions, these features increase suspicion for a more serious process that may warrant colonoscopic and/or radiologic evaluation. Similarly, acute onset of pain with fever or abdominal pain and tenderness, especially with a history of IBD, should raise concern for serious inflammatory or infectious conditions including intra-abdominal or perirectal abscess.

Serious Diagnoses

- Anorectal cancer
- Perirectal or pelvic abscess
- Intraperitoneal infection
- IBD

Alarm Symptoms	Serious Causes	Benign Causes
Weight loss	Cancer Infection IBD	
Chronic anemia	Cancer IBD Infection	
Blood in the stool	Cancer IBD Infection	Hemorrhoidal bleeding Anal fissure Polyp
Dark blood or blood mixed with the stool	Suggests a bleeding source more proximal than the anorectum	
Fevers	Infection IBD Cancer	
Abdominal pain	Abscess Infection IBD	Fecal impaction and obstruction Levator ani syndrome Coccydynia Uterine disease
Gradual increase in pain over days	Abscess	Fecal impaction and obstruction
Loss of sensation or muscle weakness	Neoplasm or infection affecting the spinal cord, nerve roots, or peripheral nerves	
Change in bowel habits in patients older than 50 years	Colon cancer	

FOCUSED QUESTIONS

QUESTIONS	POSSIBLE ETIOLOGY
Pain related to bowel movements	
Did your pain begin when you were moving your bowels?	Anal fissure Thrombosed or prolapsed internal hemorrhoid
Did you develop sharp pain while passing a large hard bowel movement?	Anal fissure

Do you experience pain that feels like being cut by glass when you pass a stool?	Anal fissure
Do you notice small amounts of red blood on the toilet paper after you pass a bowel movement?	Anal fissure, bleeding internal hemorrhoid
Did you experience a dull pain or sensation of rectal fullness start after prolonged straining?	Thrombosed or prolapsed internal hemorrhoid Rectal prolapse
Did you develop a sudden onset of severe sharp pain associated with the development of a tender perianal swelling?	Thrombosed external hemorrhoid
Do you feel a sensation of rectal pressure with a recurrent urge to defecate and passage of small amounts of feces or mucus?	Proctitis
Pain not related to bowel movements	
Do you feel pain regardless of bowel movements with a full, tender area just beside the anus or on the buttock?	Perianal abscess or fistula
Do you feel pain regardless of bowel movements with a small amount of bloody or pus-like discharge from an area just beside the anus?	Perianal fistula
Do you have pain associated with vesicles, blisters, or ulcers in the area near the anus?	Perianal infection (herpes simplex virus [HSV], chancroid) or inflammation
Are your symptoms related in time to the onset of your menses?	Endometriosis
Do you experience pain deep in the pelvis during sexual intercourse?	Endometriosis Pelvic inflammatory disease Uterine pathology
Does your pain come on suddenly, lasting only seconds to minutes?	Proctalgia fugax
Does your pain come on episodically including at night?	Proctalgia fugax
Did your pain start after a fall or other trauma to the tailbone?	Coccydynia
Is there tenderness of your sacrum or coccyx?	Coccydynia
Is your pain made worse by movement of your legs or back?	Sacral nerve lesion
Pain characteristics	
Is your pain sharp?	Anal fissure
Is your pain centered on your anal canal and on the skin around the anal opening?	Thrombosed external hemorrhoid Perirectal abscess or fistula Anal fissure
Is your pain dull?	Proctitis
Is your pain hard to localize precisely but in the general area inside the rectum?	Fecal impaction Defecatory dysfunction Thrombosed/prolapsed internal hemorrhoid Prostatitis Uterine disease Rectal cancer Referred pain

—Continued next page

Continued—

Was your pain mild initially but then gradually got more severe over several days?	Perianal infection or abscess Obstruction
Associated symptoms and history	
Do you pass drips of blood into the toilet after a bowel movement without feeling pain?	Bleeding from internal hemorrhoid
Do you notice rectal bleeding around the beginning of your period?	Colonic endometriosis
Do you notice pus-like material draining from an area beside the anus?	Perianal fistula
Do you have a lump, bulge, or a mass in the area of the anus?	Thrombosed external hemorrhoid Prolapsed internal hemorrhoid Rectal prolapse Infection IBD Cancer
Did you develop a new tender lump close to the anus associated with the sudden onset of pain?	Thrombosed external hemorrhoid
Do you notice a soft painless lump at the anus that develops while you strain at stool and can be pushed back inside?	Prolapsed internal hemorrhoid Rectal prolapse
Do you notice a soft painless lump at the anus that develops while you strain at stool, that can be pushed back inside and at times drips bright red blood?	Prolapsed, bleeding internal hemorrhoid
Do you sometimes or always have constipation or difficulty passing a bowel movement?	Anal fissure Internal hemorrhoid Fecal impaction Trauma during attempted digital disimpaction or administration of an enema
Did anything enter your anus or rectum during sex or to help you to pass a bowel movement?	Anorectal trauma Infection Retained foreign body
Do you or does a relative of yours have a history of cancer of the colon, rectum, bowel, or intestine (most relevant if cancer developed at age younger than 50 years)?	Colonic neoplasia
Do you or does a relative of yours have a history of inflammatory bowel disease, Crohn's disease, colitis, or ulcerative colitis?	Ulcerative colitis Ulcerative proctitis Crohn's proctocolitis or perianal Crohn's disease
Have you noticed small bumps, blisters, or ulcers in or around the anal opening?	Perianal infection (HSV, chancroid) or inflammation

DIAGNOSTIC APPROACH (INCLUDING ALGORITHMS)

The first step is to identify whether or not the anorectal pain is associated with defecation. If it is, the nature of the pain will help determine the cause. A sharp, well-localized pain is likely due to an anal fissure or thrombosed external hemorrhoid, whereas a dull rectal ache is more concerning for rectal prolapse, a thrombosed internal hemorrhoid, or fecal impaction. Figure 39–1 shows the diagnostic approach algorithm for anorectal pain with defecation.

If the pain occurs without defecation, it is important to determine whether the pain is episodic or constant. Episodic pain that only lasts a few seconds with no identifiable trigger is suggestive of proctalgia fugax or levator ani syndrome. Depending on the trigger, other conditions to consider are endometriosis, coccydynia, and sacral nerve irritation. If the pain is constant, neoplasm must be considered. Anorectal cancer can present with or without constitutional symptoms. If constitutional symptoms are present, other conditions such as perianal fistula and perirectal abscess should also be considered. Figure 39–2 shows the diagnostic approach algorithm for anorectal pain without defecation.

CAVEATS

- Anorectal pain is common and often caused by anal fissures, thrombosed external hemorrhoids, and perirectal abscesses. Despite a clear history suggesting a benign cause and the rarity of anorectal cancers presenting with pain, cancer must be considered in every patient, especially the elderly.
- Due to the reluctance of both patients and clinicians to discuss anorectal symptoms and function in detail, problems may be hastily attributed to hemorrhoids and not investigated adequately.
- Evaluate every patient with a thorough history, review of symptoms, and physical examination including perianal and digital rectal examinations. When applicable, perform anoscopy. In a young patient without alarm symptoms and no risk factors for infectious or neoplastic disease, an initial management plan can be instituted without further testing. However, further investigations such as stool testing, colonoscopy, or abdominal imaging are indicated in patients of advanced age and in those with alarm symptoms or evident risk factors for infection or neoplasia.

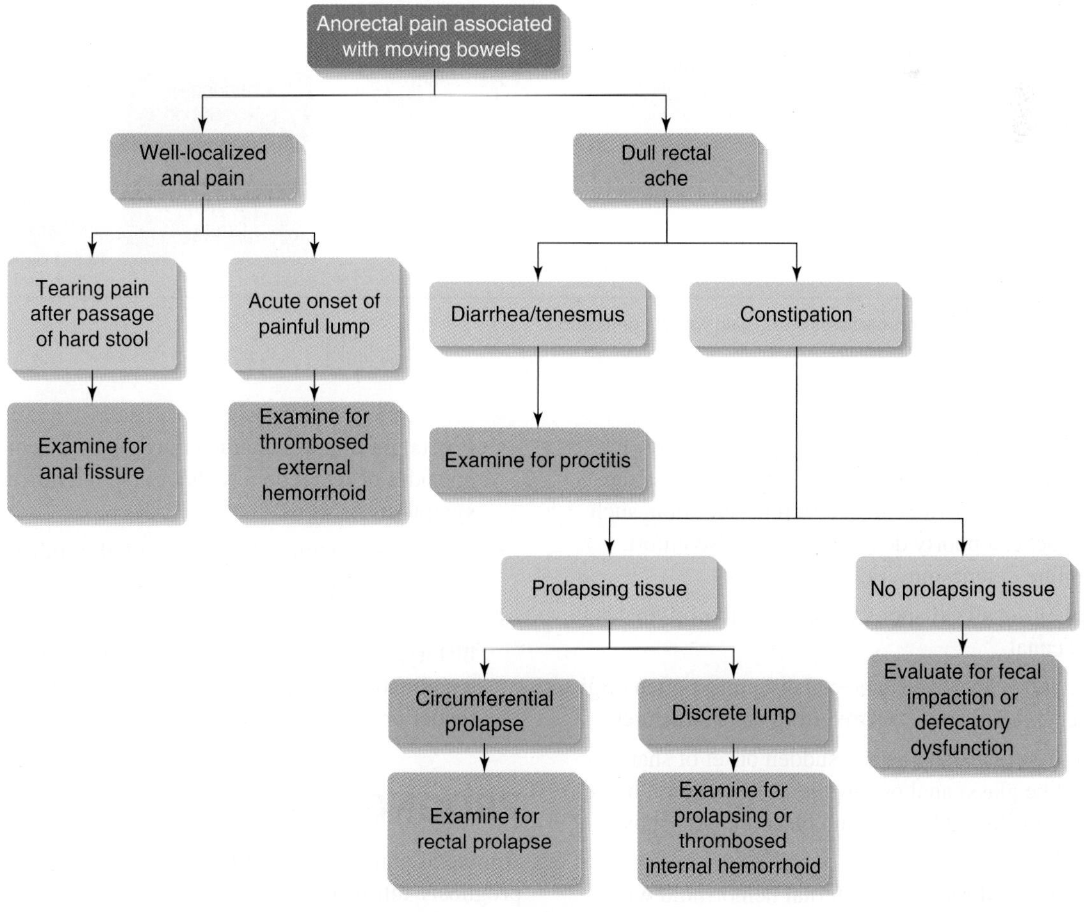

FIGURE 39–1 Diagnostic approach: Anorectal pain with defecation.

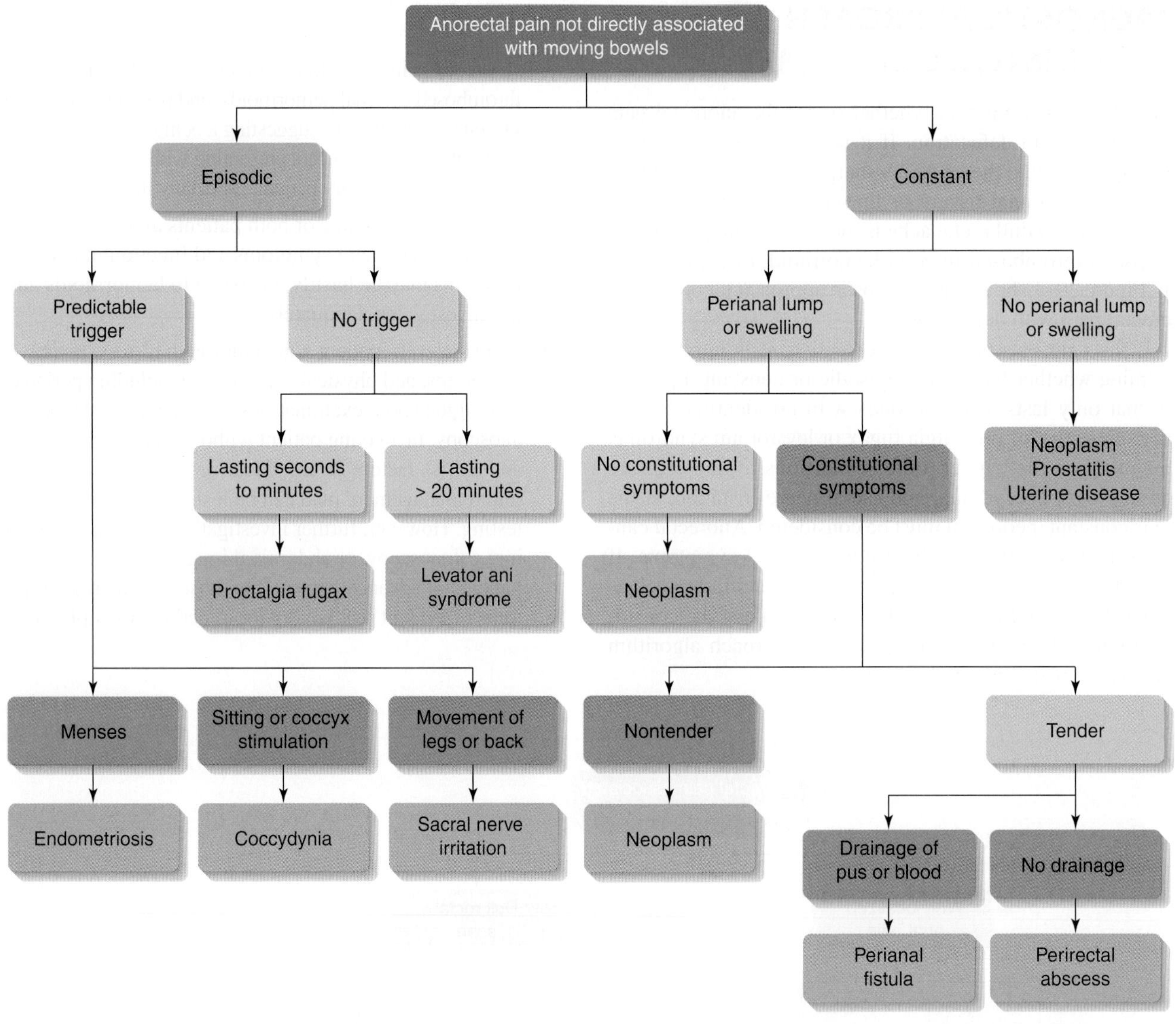

FIGURE 39–2 Diagnostic approach: Anorectal pain without defecation.

- When obtaining a history, ask the patient exactly what he or she means by pain in the rectal area because the patient may be experiencing a different sensation, such as a dull ache, a poorly defined sense of discomfort, rectal fullness, tenesmus, or even pruritus.
- Sharp, well-localized anorectal pain usually originates in the anal canal.
- Diffuse, poorly localized anorectal discomfort often originates in the rectum or is referred from other structures.
- An anal fissure usually causes sudden onset of sharp (cutting like glass) anal pain while passing a hard bowel movement followed by pain and bleeding with subsequent bowel movements.
- Patients with a thrombosed external hemorrhoid will describe the sudden onset of severe perianal pain and a tender perianal swelling.
- Proctalgia fugax is characterized by recurrent brief episodes of rectal pain without other significant symptoms or signs.
- Coccydynia frequently follows a fall or other trauma and is associated with tenderness of the coccyx.
- No matter how clear the diagnosis seems to be by history, a perianal inspection and digital anorectal examination is mandatory unless the anal canal is too tender or too stenotic.

PROGNOSIS

Anorectal pain can be due to a wide array of conditions; the prognosis ultimately depends on the diagnosis. For benign causes such as hemorrhoids and anal fissures, the prognosis is very good, and these disorders typically respond well to medical management. Most cases improve with lifestyle modification, stool softeners, and pain relief with ice packs and local anesthetics. Pain caused by proctitis due to an underlying sexually transmitted infection typically resolves after treatment of the infection. Conditions such as complete rectal prolapse require surgery, which typically involves some degree of resection and fixation to nearby structures. Patients with functional anorectal disorders, such as proctalgia fugax and levator ani syndrome, often have protracted courses because there is a lack of effective therapies. Rectal cancer, depending on the staging, is treated with a combination of surgery, radiation, and chemotherapy, and the prognosis is based on the stage of disease at the time of diagnosis.

CASE SCENARIO | Resolution

A 60-year-old gentleman presents to you with a 3-day history of constant perianal pain and bright red blood seen in the toilet bowl. This morning, he noticed a small swollen mass at his anus when washing in the shower. He experienced a similar episode of pain and bleeding several months ago, which he attributed to hemorrhoids, but his symptoms today are far more severe.

ADDITIONAL HISTORY

The patient is otherwise healthy and has no history of a serious medical condition such as Crohn's disease or cancer. He has been in a monogamous relationship with his wife for almost 40 years and has never had a sexually transmitted infection. He describes his current pain as excruciating and constant throughout the day. He estimates the amount of blood in the toilet bowl to be about 1 tablespoon. He has not had any other drainage from the area and denies any recent fevers or chills. Upon further questioning, he endorses chronic constipation that seems to have worsened over the last few months, resulting in increased straining with defecation.

Question: What is the most likely diagnosis?

A. Perianal abscess
B. Thrombosed external hemorrhoid
C. Anal fissure
D. Anal cancer
E. Rectal prolapse

Test Your Knowledge

1. Your patient, a 77-year-old gentleman with a smoking history of 100 pack-years, presents with several months of dull rectal pain and tenesmus. This has been associated with blood in the stool and recently with significant constipation.
   Which of the following additional symptoms is most concerning for rectal cancer?
   A. Sharp, stabbing pain with defecation
   B. Vesicles in the perianal region
   C. Weight loss
   D. Recurrent respiratory infections

2. Mrs. Jones, a 23-year-old G1P0 woman, sees you at 30 weeks of gestation because of severe pain with defecation. Pain occurs with bowel movements, and she has noted blood on the toilet paper.
   Which of the following is the most helpful when distinguishing between an anal fissure and a thrombosed external hemorrhoid?
   A. The color of the blood
   B. A tender lump
   C. Pain that wakes the patient up at night
   D. Constitutional symptoms

3. A 48-year-old man who has been your patient for 14 years and is in good general health reports continued episodes of rectal pain that last a few seconds and then disappear completely. The pain seems to be worse with sitting than with standing or lying down.
   Which of the following symptoms suggests a diagnosis of proctalgia fugax?
   A. Anorectal pain associated with dysuria and urinary urgency
   B. Sudden, brief paroxysms of pain
   C. Bright red blood per rectum
   D. Intermittent anal discharge

Reference

1. Nelson RL, Abcarian H, Davis FG, Persky V. Prevalence of benign anorectal disease in a randomly selected population. *Dis Colon Rectum.* 1995;38:341–344.

Suggested Reading

Bharucha A, Wald A, Enck P, Rao S. Functional anorectal disorders. *Gastroenterology*. 2006;130:1510–1518.

Billingham RP, Isler JT, Kimmins MH, et al. The diagnosis and management of common anorectal disorders. *Curr Probl Surg*. 2004;41:586–645.

Felt-Bersma R, Bartelsman J. Haemorrhoids, rectal prolapse, anal fissure, peri-anal fistulae and sexually transmitted diseases. *Best Pract Res Clin Gastroenterol*. 2009;23:575–592.

Gopal DV. Diseases of the rectum and anus: a clinical approach to common disorders. *Clin Cornerstone*. 2002;4:34–48.

Halverson A. Hemorrhoids. *Clin Colon Rectal Surg*. 2007;20:77–85.

Hull T. Examination and diseases of the anorectum. In: Feldman M, Friedman LS, Sleisenger MH, eds. *Sleisenger & Fordtran's Gastrointestinal and Liver Disease*. 7th ed. New York, NY: WB Saunders Co, 2002:2277–2293.

Pfenninger JL, Zainea GG. Common anorectal conditions. Part I. Symptoms and complaints. *Am Fam Physician*. 2001;63: 2391–2398.

Pfenninger JL, Zainea GG. Common anorectal conditions. Part II. Lesions. *Am Fam Physician*. 2001;64:77–88.

SECTION

VIII

GENITOURINARY SYSTEM

Chapter 40

Dysuria

Sara L. Swenson, MD

CASE SCENARIO

You receive a telephone call from a 32-year-old woman who complains of burning with urination over the past 12 hours. She also feels an intense need to urinate but reports difficulty voiding more than a small amount. She has experienced similar symptoms in the past and requests that you call in a prescription for antibiotics to her pharmacy.

- **What additional questions will you ask her?**
- **What aspects of the patient history will enable you most efficiently to differentiate between benign and serious diagnoses?**
- **Which questions, if any, can help you determine whether it is safe to treat her over the telephone?**

INTRODUCTION

Dysuria is defined as pain, burning, or discomfort experienced during or immediately after urination. Although it has a broad differential diagnosis, dysuria usually results from infection or inflammation of the bladder and/or urethra.[1] The patient's age, sex, and sexual history can help the clinician quickly delineate the most likely causes of dysuria. When infection seems less likely, the characteristics and duration of the pain, associated symptoms, and the patient's medical comorbidities can effectively narrow the differential diagnosis.

KEY TERMS

Acute dysuria	Dysuria of less than 1 week in duration.
Internal dysuria	Dysuria that is localized to the internal genital structures (urethra, bladder, suprapubic area).
External dysuria	Dysuria that is localized to external genital structures (labia minora and majora) and occurs as urine exits the body.
Urgency	A sudden, compelling need to urinate that is often accompanied by bladder discomfort and the inability to void more than a minimal quantity of urine.
Frequency	Urinating more frequently than usual without an increase in total urine volume due to the bladder's decreased capacity to hold urine.
Nocturia	Waking up to urinate 2 or more times during the night.
Voiding symptoms	Symptoms that occur at the time of urination. These include a slow or intermittent urine stream, difficulty initiating urination (hesitancy), prolonged termination of urination (dribbling), and dysuria.
Storage symptoms	Symptoms that occur during bladder storage and filling. These include urinary urgency or frequency, nocturia, and incontinence.
Urinary tract infection (UTI)	An infection of the urethra, bladder, prostate, or kidney. Lower UTI implies infection of the urethra and/or bladder (ie, urethrocystitis or cystitis). Upper UTI usually indicates infection of the kidney (ie, pyelonephritis).

—Continued next page

Continued—	
Complicated UTI	UTI in individuals with functional or structural abnormalities of the urinary tract. Such individuals are at higher risk of treatment failure.
Positive likelihood ratio	The increase in the odds of a diagnosis if a given clinical factor is present.
Negative likelihood ratio	The decrease in the odds of a diagnosis if a given clinical factor is absent.

ETIOLOGY

Dysuria usually reflects irritation or inflammation of the external genitalia (urethral meatus, labia majora/minora) or the lower (urethra, bladder) or upper (ureters, kidneys) genitourinary tract. Less commonly, referred pain from other pelvic or abdominal organs can lead to dysuria. Infection of the urinary tract (including the urethra, bladder, or prostate) is by far the most common cause of dysuria. Little data exist regarding the prevalence of other causes of dysuria.

Dysuria in Women

Dysuria affects women, particularly younger, sexually active women, much more commonly than men. Nearly 25% of adult women experience an acute episode of dysuria each year.[2] In adult women with dysuria and vaginal discharge, vulvovaginitis is much more common than UTI. In women with dysuria but no vaginal symptoms, UTI is more common.[3] Among sexually active adolescent women, urethritis caused by sexually transmitted infections may be more common than bacterial UTI; thus, the presence or absence of vaginal symptoms may not accurately distinguish between UTIs and sexually transmitted infections (STIs) in this population.[4] Dysuria in older women also arises from noninfectious causes, such as atrophic vaginitis.

Dysuria in Men

UTIs in men younger than 50 are uncommon; in this population, dysuria usually results from urethritis (due to STIs) or prostatitis. In older men, urinary symptoms are quite common and increase with increasing age. Over half of men over age 55 and 70% of men over age 80 report lower urinary tract symptoms. However, they report dysuria much less often than frequency, urgency, and incomplete voiding.[5] About 60% of men with dysuria will have infections of the urinary tract, prostate, or epididymus,[6] and the incidence of UTI increases with increasing age.[1] Benign prostatic hyperplasia is also a common cause of dysuria in older men.

	Prevalence	
Infection	**Women**	**Men**
Bacterial urethrocystitis[a]	26%–50%[4,7]	
Urethritis due to Chlamydia trachomatis[a]	5%–22%[4,8]	4%[9]
Urethritis due to Neisseria gonorrhoeae[a]	Up to 10%[4,8]	0.1%[10]
Pyelonephritis[b]	0.3%[13]	
Prostatitis (acute and chronic)		4%–10%[11,12]
Epididymitis		
Inflammation		
Atrophic vaginitis	3%–47%	
Irritant or allergic reactions		
Lichen sclerosis		
Lichen planus		
Vulvovestibulitis (vulvodynia)		

Reactive arthritis	
Behçet's syndrome	< 1%
Urethral or vesicular calculi	
Painful bladder syndrome/interstitial cystitis	
Radiation	< 1%
Drug side effects (chemotherapy, dopamine)	
Mechanical	
Cystocele	
Urethral stricture	
Bladder neck obstruction (benign prostatic hyperplasia)	< 1%
Urinary catheter insertion	
Neoplasm	
Cancers of the penis, prostate, vagina, or bladder	
Metastatic cancers	Rare
Referred	
Shingles/postherpetic neuralgia	
Sacral nerve compression or injury (osteoarthritis, degenerative disk disease, spinal stenosis)	
Pudendal nerve injury (childbirth or pelvic surgery)	
Neurologic	
Multiple sclerosis	
Neurofibromatosis	
Parkinson's disease/multiple system atrophy	
Hormonally mediated	
Atrophic vaginitis	
Endometriosis	

[a]In women, prevalence among those with urinary symptoms. In men, annual population incidence.

[b]Annual population incidence.

GETTING STARTED WITH THE HISTORY

- Efficiency is important when evaluating dysuria. Because most patients have an infectious etiology, start with questions to help confirm the presence of a UTI.
- Elicit a sexual history. Many causes of dysuria are provoked by or transmitted through sexual intercourse. Use open-ended questions and a nonjudgmental attitude to minimize patient discomfort and enhance the accuracy of the history.
- Briefly explore the patient's agenda. Most patients with recurrent UTI simply want expedient treatment, but some may have concerns about a new STI or even cancer.
- An effective history can determine whether a woman with dysuria can be safely treated over the telephone or requires a more in-depth evaluation, including physical examination and laboratory testing.

Open-Ended Questions	Tips for Effective Interviewing
Tell me about your symptoms.	Begin with an open-ended question to avoid premature closure.
I will need to ask some questions about your sexual practices to help me find out what's causing your symptoms. Are you currently sexually active (or having sex)?	Normalize asking about sexual practices. If the patient seems uncomfortable, you can say, "These are questions I ask all my patients."
How many sexual partners have you had in the past year?	Avoid assumptions about sexual orientation or marital status. Focus on assessing behavior.
Do you have sex with men, women, or both?	

INTERVIEW FRAMEWORK

- Focus on symptom location, onset, and duration as well as associated urinary, genital, pelvic, and systemic symptoms.
- Ask about symptoms that support the diagnosis of a UTI, such as recent-onset dysuria, urinary urgency, frequency, nocturia, suprapubic pain, and cloudy urine.
- UTIs tend to recur, especially in young, sexually active women. Streamline the interview by comparing a patient's current symptoms with past experiences. When symptoms recur in a woman who has previously had cystitis, her pretest probability of UTI is 90%.[3]
- In sexually active men and young women, especially those who report urethral or vaginal discharge, consider sexually transmitted infections.
- In the past medical history, also ask about prior STIs and pelvic, urologic, or back surgeries. In women, include a gynecologic history.
- In older individuals, explore factors that may increase the risk of UTI (eg, atrophic vaginitis, benign prostatic hyperplasia, chronic prostatitis, urinary tract instrumentation).

Questions	Remember
When urinating, do you experience a burning sensation, as if the urine were hot?	Dysuria is usually caused by inflammation of the lower urinary tract.
Are you urinating more frequently than usual during the day?	Assess for associated symptoms that support a diagnosis of UTI.
Do you feel a strong sensation that you need to urinate immediately?	Infection or inflammation of the bladder also decreases its capacity, resulting in urinary frequency, nocturia, incontinence, and discomfort with holding even small amounts of urine, leading to urinary urgency.
Have you been treated for a urinary tract infection in the past?	If a woman's symptoms match those of a prior infection, it is very likely that she has a recurrent UTI.
Did your symptoms improve after treatment with antibiotics?	If the patient's current symptoms differ from those of previous infections, further investigation will be necessary.
How do your current symptoms compare to those you had at that time?	

IDENTIFYING ALARM SYMPTOMS

Most causes of dysuria are benign and easily treated. Nonetheless, clinicians should ask about symptoms that portend a more serious diagnosis. Dysuria with an insidious onset raises the possibility of rare neoplastic etiologies. Dysuria in the presence of systemic symptoms (eg, fever or chills, abdominal or flank pain, nausea and vomiting) should prompt the consideration of other acute bacterial causes of dysuria such as pyelonephritis, acute prostatitis, epididymitis, or pelvic inflammatory disease. In women, the likelihood of pyelonephritis increases with recent spermicide use, new incontinence in the past month, UTI in the past year, diabetes, a history of UTI in the patient's mother, and sexual intercourse more than once in the past week.[13]

Alarm Symptoms	Serious Causes	More Common Causes
Fever or chills	Urosepsis	Pyelonephritis, epididymitis, acute prostatitis
Flank pain		Pyelonephritis
Flank pain with hematuria	Renal cancer	Nephrolithiasis
Hematuria	Bladder cancer	Hemorrhagic cystitis
Penile discharge, mass or ulcer, pain at tip of penis	Penile cancer	Urethritis (chlamydia, gonorrhea, herpes simplex virus)
Scrotal pain/swelling		Epididymitis
Pelvic pain, dyspareunia	Endometriosis Pelvic inflammatory disease	
Vaginal bleeding	Vaginal cancer Pelvic inflammatory disease	Menstruation
Painful oral ulcers, arthritis, eye findings	Behçet's syndrome Reactive arthritis	
Painful genital ulcers	Behçet's syndrome	Herpes simplex virus
Suprapubic pain, incontinence, obstructive urinary symptoms (weak stream, hesitancy)	Neurologic disease (multiple sclerosis, Parkinson's disease)	Bladder outlet obstruction due to benign prostatic hyperplasia or urethral stricture

FOCUSED QUESTIONS

After confirming the presence of dysuria, assess the likelihood of the various diagnoses by asking questions regarding the quality of the dysuria, its time course, associated symptoms, and pertinent sexual and past medical history.

QUESTIONS	THINK ABOUT...
Time course	
How long have you had pain with urination?	
• *1–2 days?*	Bacterial cystitis Acute bacterial prostatitis Bacterial epididymitis
• *2–7 days?*	Urethritis/epididymitis (gonorrhea, chlamydia, herpes simplex virus)
• *More than 14 days?*	Chlamydia infection (in women)
• *Weeks to months?*	Interstitial cystitis Chronic bacterial prostatitis Chronic prostatitis/pelvic pain syndrome (men) Vulvodynia (women)

—Continued next page

Continued—

Is the pain associated with your menstrual cycle?	
• *Cyclic pain several days before onset*	Endometriosis
• *During or immediately after onset*	Pelvic inflammatory disease
Did your symptoms start after having sex?	Recurrent UTI. Women whose symptoms begin after sexual intercourse have 12 times the odds of recurrent UTI than those whose symptoms do not.[14]
At what point during urination does your pain occur?	
• *At the beginning of urination?*	Urethritis
• *At the end of urination?*	Cystitis or prostatitis
Does your pain get worse after you consume certain foods or drinks?	Interstitial cystitis or painful bladder syndrome[15]
Does your pain increase when your bladder is full and improve after urination?	Interstitial cystitis or painful bladder syndrome[15]
Urine symptoms	
Do you urinate more frequently than usual during the day?	Urinary *frequency* suggests increased urine production (polyuria), decreased bladder capacity (bladder inflammation or infection), or incomplete bladder emptying (benign prostatic hyperplasia, neurologic disease). Polyuria is not usually associated with dysuria.
Do you have an intense sensation of needing to urinate immediately?	Urinary *urgency* results from irritability of the inflamed bladder and decreased bladder compliance. It is common in cystitis, bladder cancer, radiation damage, and neurogenic bladder dysfunction.
Is the urge to urinate so immediate that you sometimes urinate before you can get to the bathroom?	Urinary *incontinence* may occur with bladder inflammation (acute cystitis), upper motor neuron lesions, detrusor muscle instability, and obstruction or irritation by bladder tumors. Neurologic disorders (multiple sclerosis, Parkinson's disease, prior stroke) can uncommonly present with voiding symptoms. Chronic incontinence is a risk factor for UTI in postmenopausal women.[16]
Is the amount of urine with each episode less than usual?	Bladder inflammation from infection, irritants, systemic disease, or interstitial cystitis Incomplete bladder emptying
Has the appearance of your urine changed?	Cloudy urine has a positive likelihood ratio of approximately 2.0 for UTI.
Does your urine smell of ammonia?	UTI with urea splitting (eg, *Proteus* species)
(For men) Do you have pain with urination without frequency or urgency?	Urethritis
(For men) Is your urinary stream weaker than usual? *Does it take longer than usual to begin urination?* *Do you experience dribbling or slow urine flow at the end of urination?*	Voiding symptoms (weak or intermittent stream, hesitancy, dribbling, and dysuria) commonly occur with bladder outlet obstruction from benign prostatic hyperplasia or urethral stricture.

Associated symptoms	
With fever...	
Do you have flank pain or nausea and vomiting?	Pyelonephritis
Are your testicles painful or swollen?	Bacterial epididymitis or prostatitis can cause unilateral testicular symptoms.
Do you have rectal discomfort, pain, or discharge?	Prostatitis (pain only) or proctitis due to gonorrhea, chlamydia, or herpes simplex virus (HSV)
Have you noticed any swollen lymph nodes in your groin area or new headaches?	Primary genital HSV
With hematuria...	
Have you noticed any blood in your urine?	Hemorrhagic cystitis (acute onset) Bladder cell cancer, benign prostatic hyperplasia (intermittent or chronic)
Are you having pain in your mid-back (flank pain)?	Nephrolithiasis (usually acute onset) Renal cell cancer (chronic)
With vaginal or urethral discharge...	
What color is the discharge?	Purulent or mucopurulent discharge characterizes urethritis or cervicitis due to gonorrhea or chlamydia. Importantly, most women with these infections will be asymptomatic.
(For women) Do you have burning or pain in your external genital area?	External genital discomfort (with or without urination) suggests candidal vulvovaginitis.
(For women) Do you have lower abdominal pain or vaginal bleeding?	Pelvic inflammatory disease
(For men) Is the discharge bloody?	Bloody urethral discharge can occur with urethral cancer (rare).
Other associated symptoms	
Have you felt more tired than usual? *Have you been losing weight without trying?*	Renal cell cancer Bladder cancer
Have you had joint aches, mouth ulcers, or eye symptoms?	Behçet's syndrome Reactive arthritis (Reiter syndrome)
Have you had painful genital ulcers?	HSV (common) Behçet's syndrome (rare)
(For women) Have you felt vaginal dryness?	Atrophic vaginitis
(For women) Do you feel discomfort or the sensation of something in your vagina when you urinate?	Cystocele. Weakness of the anterior vaginal wall causes the bladder to protrude into the vagina during urination.

—Continued next page

Continued—

Sexual history	
Are you sexually active?	Sexually transmitted infections (chlamydia, gonorrhea, trichomoniasis). Sexually active adolescent women and young men are at highest risk of STIs.
Do you have a new sexual partner?	Chlamydia or gonorrhea
How many times have you had sexual intercourse in the past week?	More than one episode per week increases the risk of pyelonephritis.[13]
(For women) Is sexual intercourse painful?	Dyspareunia during initial penetration suggests vulvovaginitis, atrophic vaginitis, or urethritis. Dyspareunia with deep penetration occurs with endometriosis.
(For women) What do you use to prevent pregnancy?	Irritant or allergic reactions to condoms or spermicide. Spermicide use is also associated with an increased risk of UTI.
(For men) Do you have sex with men?	Insertive anal intercourse is a risk factor for cystitis in men.[2,16]
Surgical history	
Tell me about any surgeries you have had.	
Any vaginal or pelvic surgery? *Any severe tearing with childbirth?*	Pudendal nerve or pelvic muscle injury can uncommonly present with dysuria.
Have you recently had any bladder procedures or had a urinary catheter placed?	Bladder (eg, Foley) catheterization or instrumentation increases the risk of UTI. Ureteral stents can cause dysuria.
Social history	
Did you ever smoke cigarettes? *What jobs have you held?*	Bladder cancer. Cigarette smoking and chemical exposures, especially in the paint, metal-working, and rubber-processing industries, are known risk factors.
Have you ever lived or traveled in the Middle East, North or sub-Saharan Africa, or India?	Urinary schistosomiasis

DIAGNOSTIC APPROACH (INCLUDING ALGORITHM)

In adult women with acute dysuria, the pretest probability of UTI is relatively high (approximately 50%), and the clinician should begin by considering a lower UTI. If UTI is suspected, the clinician should ask about upper UTI symptoms and ascertain whether the UTI is complicated. Women with certain symptom combinations, such as the presence of at least 2 urinary symptoms and absence of vaginal discharge or irritation, have a pretest probability of UTI of at least 90% and can safely be treated empirically.[7] UTI is also the most likely diagnosis in women who self-diagnose their current symptoms as a UTI.[7] Women at high risk for STI or who report vaginal discharge are at lower risk of UTI and should be evaluated for other causes of dysuria.[4,18] Men and those with alarm symptoms or chronic dysuria require a more in-depth history and investigation. See Figure 40–1 for the diagnostic approach algorithm for a female patient with dysuria.[7,17]

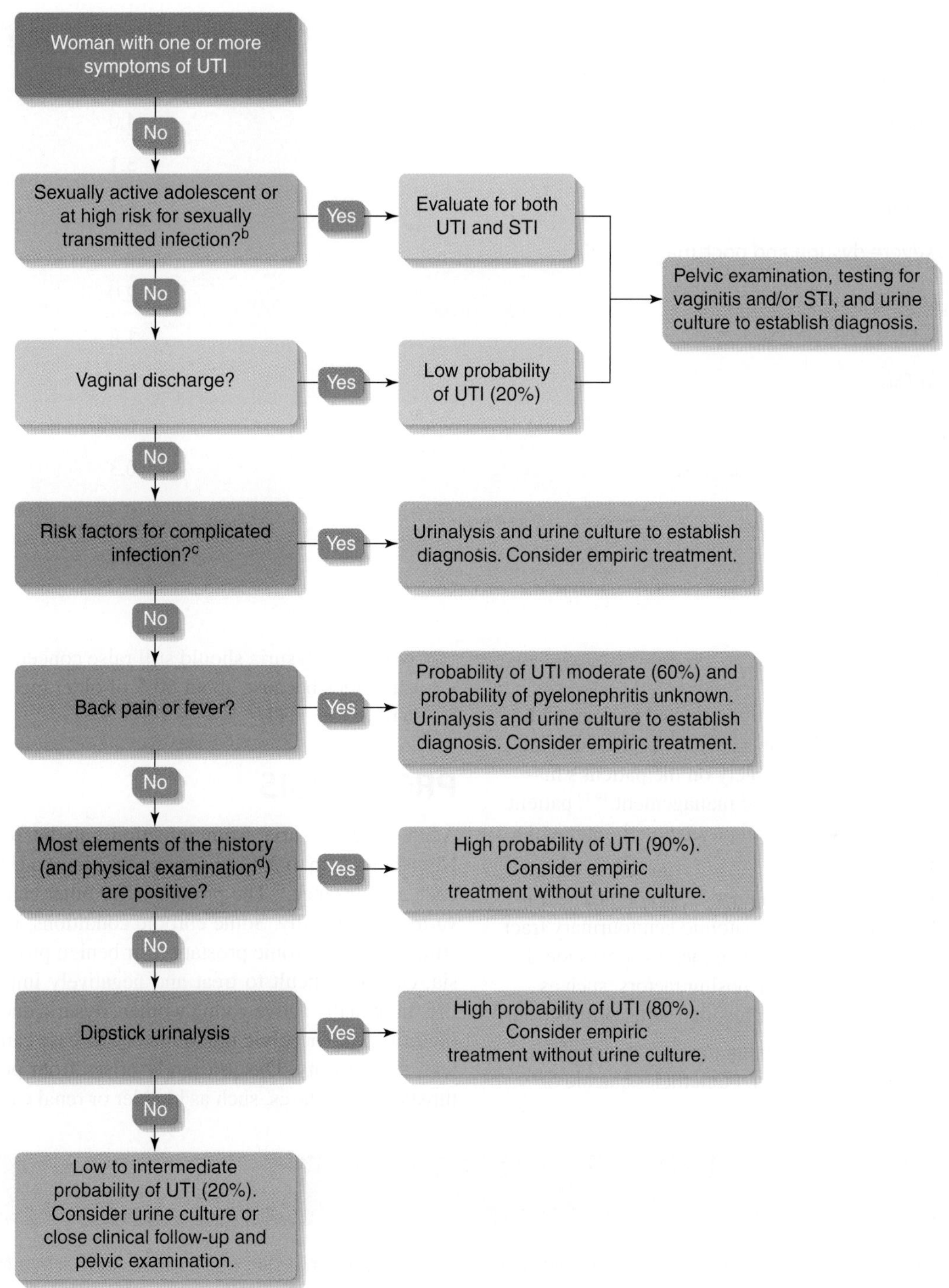

FIGURE 40–1 Diagnostic approach: Evaluation of the female patient with dysuria. STI, sexually transmitted infection; UTI, urinary tract infection.

[a]Adapted from Bent S, et al. *JAMA*. 2002; 287:2701–2710.

[b]In sexually active adolescents with urinary symptoms, the risk of STI may exceed that of UTI, and women can have both simultaneously. Women should undergo chlamydia testing if they are sexually active and younger than 25 or have a history of STIs, a new sexual partner, more than one male sexual partner, inconsistent condom use, or a history of exchanging sex for money or drugs.

[c]pregnancy, diabetes, immunosuppression, pyelonephritis in the past year, neurogenic bladder, indwelling bladder catheter, recent urinary tract instrumentation, or a history of nephrolithiasis.

[d]Important physical examination findings include costovertebral angle tenderness,7 cloudy-appearing urine, and urine with a strong odor.[17]

Symptom	Likelihood Ratio for UTI[4,7,18]
Dysuria, frequency, and no vaginal discharge/irritation	24.6
Positive self-diagnosis	4.0
No vaginal discharge	3.1
No vaginal irritation	2.7
Moderate to severe dysuria and nocturia	2.1
Hematuria	2.0
Frequency	1.8
Genital discomfort	0.67
Dyspareunia	0.59
Vaginal discharge/irritation and no dysuria	0.3
Vaginal discharge	0.3
Vaginal irritation	0.2

CAVEATS

- There is increasing evidence that selected women with acute uncomplicated UTI can safely be treated via management strategies that rely solely on the patient's history, including telephone-based management,[19,20] patient self-treatment,[16] or use of a patient-operated, interactive computer algorithm.[21]
- UTIs are uncommon in men under 35 but do not necessarily warrant evaluation for anatomic genitourinary tract abnormalities. In contrast, UTIs in men over 50 should prompt consideration of predisposing factors, such as chronic bacterial prostatitis or bladder outlet obstruction.
- Voiding symptoms due to benign prostatic hyperplasia commonly occur in older men. Nonetheless, acute or worsened dysuria should still raise concern for other etiologies because about 60% of older men with dysuria will have a UTI.[6]

PROGNOSIS

Acute-onset dysuria from infection can be readily treated. Nonetheless, up to 25% of women who have a UTI will experience a recurrence.[22] The prognosis for other causes of dysuria varies substantially. Some chronic conditions, including interstitial cystitis, chronic prostatitis, or benign prostatic hyperplasia, can be difficult to treat and negatively impact quality of life. In sexually active young women, dysuria due to chlamydia urethritis and/or pelvic inflammatory disease can, if untreated, lead to infertility. Dysuria rarely arises from potentially life-threatening diseases, such as bladder or renal cancer.

CASE SCENARIO | Resolution

You receive a telephone call from a 32-year-old woman who complains of burning with urination over the past 12 hours. She also feels an intense need to urinate but reports difficulty voiding more than a small amount. She has experienced similar symptoms in the past and requests that you call in a prescription for antibiotics to her pharmacy.

ADDITIONAL HISTORY

Your patient states that she had similar symptoms 6 months ago, which were diagnosed as a urinary tract infection. Her symptoms at that time resolved completely with antibiotic treatment. She denies any current vaginal irritation or discharge. She has had one male sexual partner for the past 2 years, does not use condoms, and has not had any sexually transmitted diseases. She denies fever, chills, nausea, vomiting, and back, pelvic, or abdominal pain. She does not have diabetes and is not pregnant.

Question: What is the most likely diagnosis?

A. Pyelonephritis
B. Urethrocystitis due to herpes simplex virus
C. Lower urinary tract infection
D. Vaginal candidiasis

Test Your Knowledge

1. You are seeing a 67-year-old man who reports mild dysuria for the past 3 months.
   Which of the following symptoms would be *least* concerning for bladder cancer?
   A. One episode of bloody urine last week
   B. An 18 pack-year smoking history
   C. Associated symptoms of difficulty initiating urination and a weak urinary stream
   D. Associated symptoms of urinary frequency and urgency

2. You have just diagnosed bacterial urinary tract infection (UTI) in a 56-year-old woman. She reports 3 UTIs in the past year and is concerned about why they keep recurring. She has multiple sclerosis and was diagnosed with type 2 diabetes 1 year ago. She has chronic, intermittent urinary incontinence, which is large volume and occurs without warning in both the daytime and at night. She denies vaginal dryness, dyspareunia, hematuria, or unilateral back pain but had a kidney stone 10 years earlier.
   What is the most likely explanation for her recurrent urinary tract infections?
   A. Retained kidney stone
   B. Diabetes
   C. Atrophic vaginitis
   D. Chronic incontinence

3. Each of the following women presents with dysuria and has not had a medical evaluation for over a year.
   Which patient does *not* need testing for chlamydia?
   A. 19-year-old sexually active woman who consistently uses condoms
   B. 32-year-old woman with a new male sexual partner
   C. 26-year-old woman who has not been sexually active for the past year
   D. 27-year-old married woman who had chlamydia at age 26

4. You are seeing an 80-year-old man with a 2-day history of dysuria and increased urinary frequency. These symptoms have worsened over the last day, and this morning, he was unable to urinate. He also developed fever, shaking chills, and lower abdominal pain. He underwent bladder catheterization during a hospitalization 1 week ago. He denies back pain, hematuria, and scrotal swelling or pain.
   What is the most likely diagnosis?
   A. Prostate cancer
   B. Bacterial epididymitis
   C. Bladder outlet obstruction from benign prostatic hyperplasia
   D. Acute bacterial prostatitis

References

1. Bremnor JD, Sadovsky R. Evaluation of dysuria in adults. *Am Fam Physician.* 2002;65:1589–1596.
2. Hooton TM, Stamm WE. Diagnosis and treatment of uncomplicated urinary tract infection. *Infect Dis Clin North Am.* 1997;11:551–581.
3. Fihn SD. Acute uncomplicated urinary tract infection in women. *N Engl J Med.* 2003;349:259–266.
4. Huppert JS, Biro F, Lan D, et al. Urinary symptoms in adolescent females: STI or UTI? *J Adolesc Health.* 2007;40: 418–424.
5. Kellogg-Parsons J, Bergstrom J, Silberstein J, Barrett-Conner E. Prevalence and characteristics of lower urinary tract symptoms in men aged 80 years and older. *Urology.* 2008;72:318–321.
6. Roberts RG, Hartlaub PP. Evaluation of dysuria in men. *Am Fam Physician.* 1999;60:865–872.
7. Bent S, Nallamothu BK, Simel D, Fihn SD, Saint S. Does this woman have an acute uncomplicated urinary tract infection? *JAMA.* 2002;287:2701–2710.
8. Komaroff AL, O'Leary MP, Eamranond P. Dysuria in adult women. UpToDate. Available at: www.uptodate.com. Updated September 21, 2009.
9. Brodine SK, Shafer MA, Shaffer RA, et al. Asymptomatic sexually transmitted disease prevalence in four military populations: application of DNA amplification assays for chlamydia and gonorrhea screening. *J Infect Dis.* 1998;178: 1202–1204.
10. Centers for Disease Control and Prevention. Gonorrhea. Available at: http://www.cdc.gov/std/stats08/gonorrhea.htm. Accessed October 22, 2011.
11. Clemens JQ, Meenan RT, Rosetti MCO, et al. Prevalence of and risk factors for prostatitis: population based assessment using physician assigned diagnosis. *J Urol.* 2007;178:1333–1337.
12. Nickel JC, Downey J, Hunter D, Clark J. Prevalence of prostatitis-like symptoms in a population based study using the National Institutes of Health chronic prostatitis symptom index. *J Urol.* 2001;165:842–845.
13. Scholes D, Hooton TM, Roberts PL, et al. Risk factors associated with acute pyelonephritis in healthy women. *Ann Intern Med.* 2005;142:20–27.
14. Gopal M, Northington G, Arya L. Clinical symptoms predictive of recurring urinary tract infections. *Am J Obstet Gynecol.* 2007;197:74.e1–e4.
15. Warren JW, Brown J, Tracy JK. Evidence-based criteria for pain of interstitial cystitis/painful bladder syndrome in women. *Urology.* 2008;71:444–448.
16. Nicolle LE. Uncomplicated urinary tract infection in adults including uncomplicated pyelonephritis. *Urol Clin North Am.* 2008;35:1–12.

17. Little P, Turner S, Rumbsy K, et al. Developing clinical rules to predict urinary tract infection in primary care settings: sensitivity and specificity of near patient tests (dipsticks) and clinical scores. *Br J Gen Pract*. 2006;56:606–612.
18. Medina-Bombardo D, Segui-Diaz M, Roca-Fusalba C, et al. What is the predictive value of urinary symptoms in diagnosing urinary tract infection in women? *Fam Pract.* 2003;20: 103–107.
19. Saint S, Scholes D, Fihn SD, Farrell RG, Stamm WE. The effectiveness of a clinical practice guideline for the management of presumed uncomplicated urinary tract infection in women. *Am J Med.* 1999;106:636–641.
20. Barry HC, Hickner J, Ebell MH, Ettenhofer T. A randomized controlled trial of telephone management of suspected urinary tract infections in women. *J Fam Pract.* 2001;50:589–594.
21. Aagaard EM, Nadler P, Adler J, Maselli J, Gonzales R. An interactive computer kiosk module for the treatment of recurrent uncomplicated cystitis in women. *J Gen Intern Med.* 2006; 21:1156–1159.
22. Car J. Urinary tract infections in women: diagnosis and management in primary care. *BMJ*. 2006;332:94–97.

Suggested Reading

Bent S, Nallamothu BK, Simel D, Fihn SD, Saint S. Does this woman have an acute uncomplicated urinary tract infection? *JAMA*. 2002;287:2701–2710.

Gupta K, Hooton TM, Roberts PL, Stamm WE. Patient-initiated treatment of uncomplicated recurrent urinary tract infections in young women. *Ann Intern Med.* 2001;135:9–16.

Chapter 41

Hematuria

Virginia U. Collier, MD, FACP

CASE SCENARIO

A previously healthy 18-year-old woman is seen in your office complaining of a 3-day episode of "red urine," which has now resolved. She is frightened because this has never happened to her before.

- **What additional symptoms should the historian ask about in a patient with this complaint?**
- **Can you make a diagnosis based on history alone?**
- **Should the patient have urgent radiographic imaging of her urinary tract?**

INTRODUCTION

Few symptoms are more alarming to patients than grossly red or brown urine. The first priority is to determine whether the discoloration is due to blood in the urine or another cause. Unless the symptoms are strongly suggestive, the diagnosis of gross hematuria, or visible blood in the urine, must be confirmed by centrifuging the urine specimen (Figure 41–1).

Microscopic hematuria is usually not noticed by the patient, but rather diagnosed on urinalysis performed after treatment for urinary tract infection or on routine urinalysis during insurance or employment screening. Neither the US Preventive Health Services Task Force nor the Canadian Task Force on Periodic Health recommends routine screening for microscopic hematuria.[1] The presence of microscopic hematuria has a low predictive value for bladder cancer, even in high-risk elderly patients, and there is currently no evidence that early detection improves prognosis.[1,2] In 5 studies examining prevalence, the percentage of patients with asymptomatic microscopic hematuria varied from 0.19% to 16.1%.[3] Some studies indicate the prevalence is higher in older people and higher among women than men.[1]

For purposes of the ensuing discussion, it is assumed that the diagnosis of true gross or microscopic hematuria has already been established. Although the prevalence of serious disease (eg, malignancy) is higher in patients with gross hematuria, microscopic hematuria may also indicate significant genitourinary pathology.[4,5] A careful history is essential in the evaluation of the patient with either condition.

KEY TERMS

Hematuria	Bleeding from the urinary tract.
Gross hematuria	The presence of blood in the urine in sufficient quantity to be visible to the naked eye. A recent study indicates that more than 95% of clinicians will only recognize gross hematuria when > 3500 red blood cells per high-power field are present.[6]
Microscopic hematuria	2–3 red blood cells per high-power field on urine microscopy. A lower cutoff results in more false-positive results (decreased specificity), whereas a higher cutoff results in more missed disease (decreased sensitivity).

ETIOLOGY

Both microscopic and gross hematuria can be manifestations of serious disease, including malignancy.

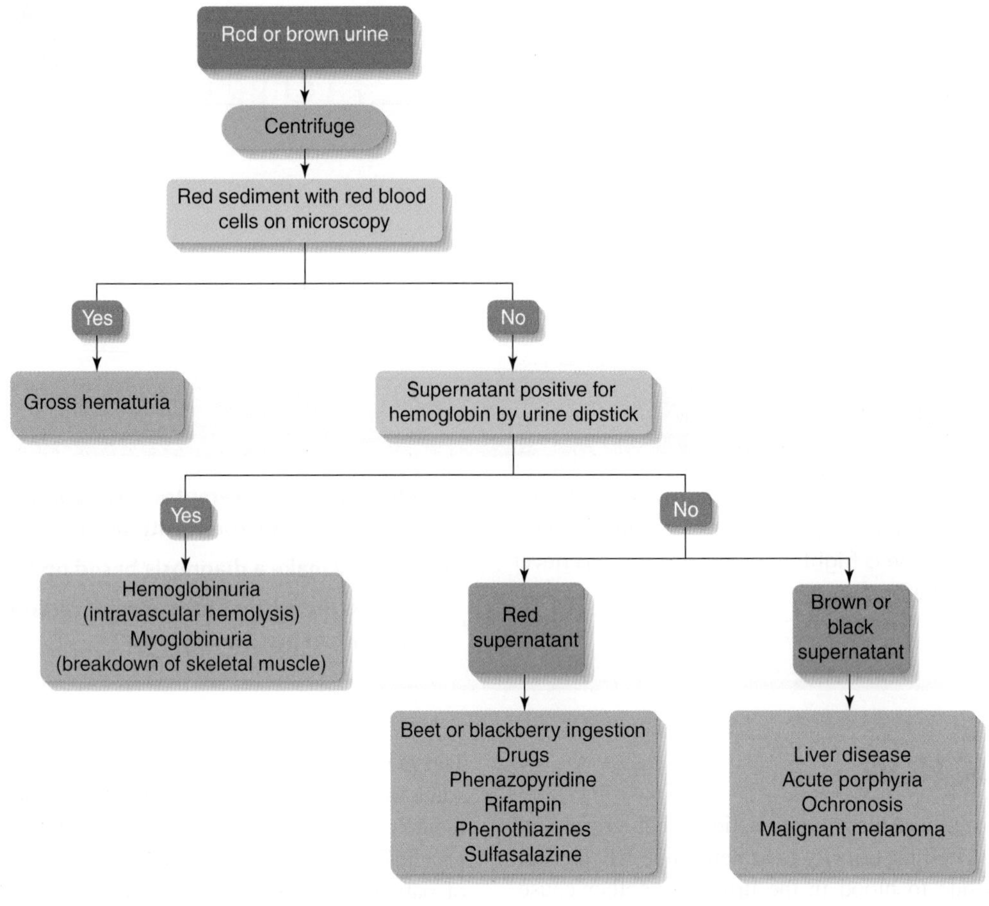

FIGURE 41–1 Diagnostic approach: Patient with suspected gross hematuria.

Common Causes of Microscopic and Gross Hematuria[4]

	Hematuria, No. (%) of Patients[a]	
	Microscopic (n = 1689)	**Gross (n = 1200)**
Urologic cancer	*86 (5.1)*	*270 (22.5)*
Bladder	63 (4.0)	178 (15.0)
Renal	9 (0.5)	45 (3.6)
Prostate	8 (0.5)	29 (2.4)
Ureteral	3 (0.2)	10 (0.8)
Other	3 (0.2)	8 (0.6)
Common benign lesions		
Nephrolithiasis	84 (5.0)	130 (11.0)
Renal disease	37 (2.2)	
Urinary tract infection	73 (4.3)	394 (33.0)
Prostatic hyperplasia	217 (13.0)	153 (13.0)
No source found	**717 (43.0)**	**101 (8.4)**

[a]Data are from multiple studies, so totals may not equal 100%.

Prevalence of Serious Disease in Patients With Hematuria

In a recent study of 578 consecutive patients referred for evaluation of gross hematuria who underwent complete urologic investigations, 18% were initially diagnosed with a urologic malignancy. After a mean follow-up of 6.9 years, in patients with recurrent hematuria, the likelihood of a urologic malignancy on repeat investigation was close to 10%.[7] Patients with gross hematuria have a higher likelihood (up to 4–7 times greater) of malignancy than those with microscopic hematuria.[4,5]

The prevalence of serious disease in patients with microscopic hematuria depends on the population studied. The general population has a lower prevalence of serious causes than patients referred to urologists or nephrologists. Older men with known risk factors (see Alarm Features) have a higher prevalence of serious disease than younger men or those with no risk factors.[1] Urologic malignancy has been identified in approximately 9% of men older than 50 years with asymptomatic microscopic hematuria.[5,8] By contrast, in a study of 636 young Israeli men, only 0.1% had neoplasia.[9] In a prospective study of 177 women ranging from 22 to

Nonglomerular and Glomerular Causes of Hematuria

Nonglomerular	*Think*
Lower urinary tract source	Urethritis, prostatitis Benign prostatic hypertrophy Cystitis Bladder carcinoma Prostate carcinoma Exercise induced
Upper urinary tract source	Ureteral calculus Renal calculus Hydronephrosis Pyelonephritis Polycystic kidney disease Hypercalciuria, hyperuricosuria, without stones Renal trauma Papillary necrosis Interstitial nephritis (drug-induced) Sickle cell trait or disease Renal infarct (embolic, eg, secondary to subacute bacterial endocarditis or atherosclerosis) Renal tuberculosis Infection with *Schistosoma haematobium* Renal vein thrombosis
Glomerular	***Think***
Primary glomerulonephritis	Immunoglobulin A (IgA) nephropathy Postinfectious Idiopathic (eg, focal glomerulosclerosis)
Secondary glomerulonephritis	Systemic lupus erythematosus Wegener's granulomatosis Other vasculitides
Familial	Thin basement membrane disease (benign familial hematuria) Hereditary nephritis (Alport syndrome)
Other	
Factitious	

87 years old with microscopic hematuria, no bladder malignancies were diagnosed, and only 2 patients had highly significant disease, defined as those conditions which could pose a clear threat to the patient's life or require a major surgical procedure.[10] In a population study of patients of all ages with microscopic hematuria in Rochester, Minnesota, 0.5% had highly significant disease.[11]

When considering a more exhaustive list of etiologies, it is useful to classify hematuria into nonglomerular or glomerular causes based on urinalysis (Figure 41–2). Because renal biopsy is not routinely performed to evaluate patients with hematuria, it is difficult to determine what percentage of patients has a glomerular source.[1] Estimates range from 0.1%[12] to 14%.[13]

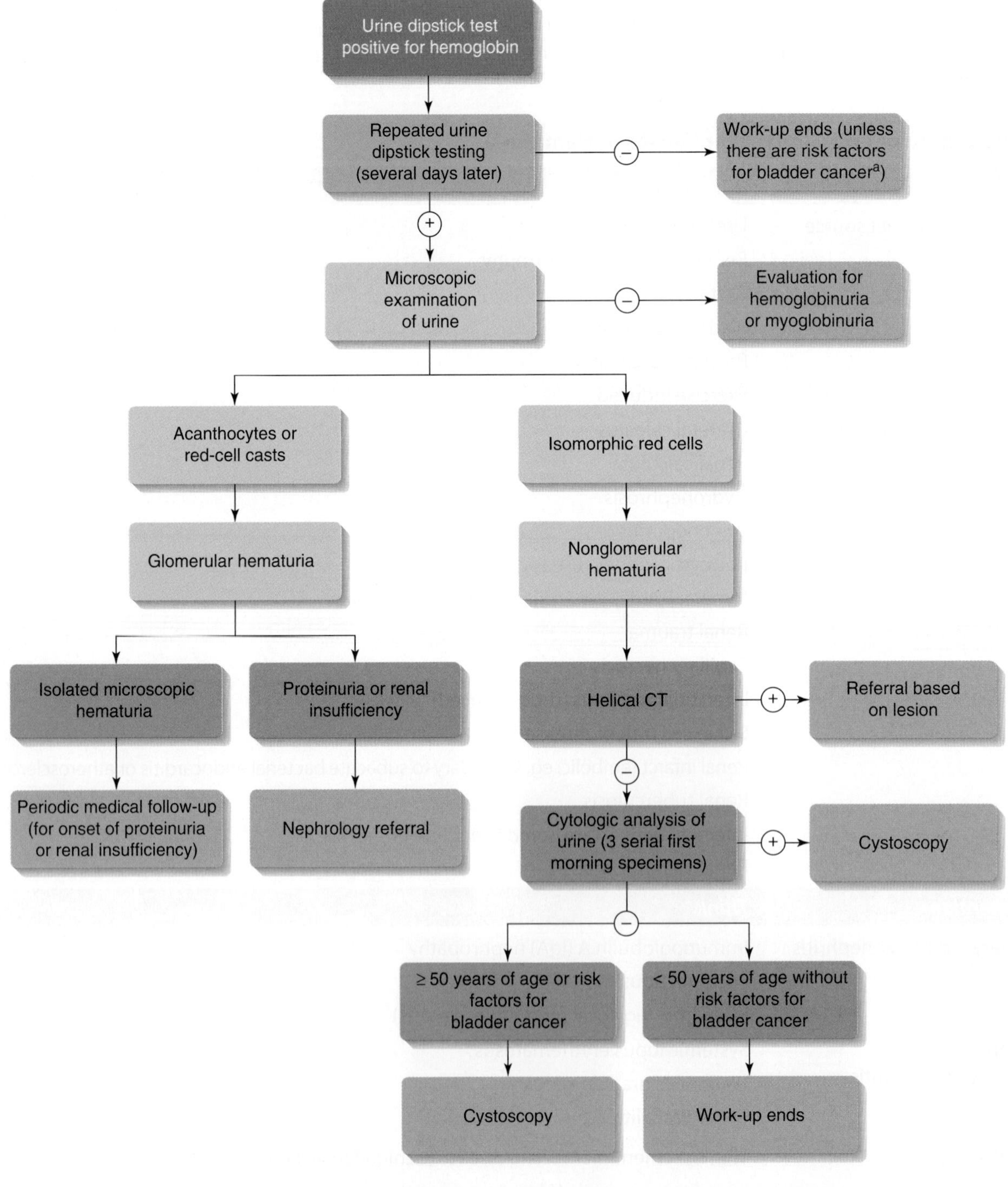

FIGURE 41–2 Diagnostic approach: Microscopic hematuria. CT, computed tomography.

[a]Risk factors for bladder cancer include cigarette smoking, occupational exposure to chemicals used in certain industries (leather, dye, and rubber or tire manufacturing), heavy phenacetin use, past treatment with high doses of cyclophosphamide, and ingestion of aristolochic acid found in some herbal weight-loss preparations. (Adapted with permission from Cohen RA, Brown RS. Microscopic hematuria. *N Engl J Med.* 2003;348:2330–2338.)

GETTING STARTED WITH THE HISTORY

Determine whether the patient is seeking medical attention because of an abnormal urinalysis without symptoms (asymptomatic microscopic hematuria) or if the patient has gross hematuria (see Figures 41–1 and 41–2).

Questions	Remember
Have you ever been told that there was blood in your urine?	A patient with microscopic hematuria may be asymptomatic.
Have you ever had diagnostic testing to further evaluate blood in your urine?	One study has documented a 10% incidence of urologic malignancy in patients with recurrent gross hematuria, even though initial evaluation was unrevealing.[7]
Describe an episode of seeing blood in your urine.	If the patient has gross hematuria, allow him or her to discuss the presentation and associated symptoms with minimal interruption.
	The presence of blood in the urine is frightening to most patients. Demonstrate concern and understanding, but do not reassure the patient until you have excluded "alarm features" (see below).

INTERVIEW FRAMEWORK

- First, determine whether there are predisposing factors suggesting a transient, self-limited cause:
  - Presence of menses
  - History of trauma (to flank or abdomen)
  - Recent genitourinary infection or instrumentation, including insertion of Foley (bladder) catheter
  - Recent extreme exercise (eg, running a marathon, intense cycling)
- Next, look for alarm symptoms or features of the family history or personal and social history suggesting the possibility of serious disease.
- Finally, ask focused questions about accompanying symptoms and characteristics of the hematuria, which may help pinpoint the lesion within the urinary tract.

IDENTIFYING ALARM FEATURES

- Increased age (particularly age older than 40–50 years) and male sex are associated with an increased incidence of neoplasm.
- Constitutional symptoms (weight loss, appetite loss, chronic malaise, or fatigue) suggest malignancy or chronic infection.
- A variety of factors in the personal and social history may increase the likelihood of a malignancy, including a heavy smoking history, exposure to aniline dyes in leather, tire, or rubber manufacturing industries; previous treatment with cyclophosphamide or pelvic irradiation; and ingestion of herbal weight loss preparations containing aristolochic acid.
- A positive family history of deafness or renal disease suggests familial disease.

Alarm Features or Symptoms	Serious Causes	Benign Causes
Increased age (> 40)	Cancer	
Male sex	Cancer	
Weight loss, chronic malaise	Cancer Chronic infection	
Appetite loss	Cancer Chronic infection	
Fever	Cancer (renal cell carcinoma), infection	Acute pyelonephritis

—*Continued next page*

Continued—		
Flank, back, or abdominal pain	Renal infarct Ureteral calculus Embolus from bacterial endocarditis Cyst rupture Neoplasm	Renal calculus Acute pyelonephritis
Recent sore throat, acute upper respiratory tract infection	Acute glomerulonephritis	
Swelling of eyelids and feet	Acute glomerulonephritis	
Nausea, vomiting	Uremia secondary to acute or chronic glomerulonephritis	Nephrolithiasis or pyelonephritis
Deafness	Alport's syndrome (hereditary nephritis)	
Hemoptysis	Wegener's granulomatosis Goodpasture's syndrome	
Recurrent sinusitis	Wegener's granulomatosis	
Joint pain or skin rash	Acute glomerulonephritis secondary to an underlying connective tissue disease (systemic lupus erythematosus, polyarteritis nodosa)	
Easy bruising, bleeding from gums	Bleeding disorder (eg, thrombocytopenia or excessive anticoagulation)	
Alarm features in past medical history, family history, and personal and social history		
Cigarette smoking	Bladder cancer	
Use of herbal weight loss preparations (containing aristolochic acid)	Genitourinary neoplasm	
Prior treatment with cyclophosphamide	Bladder cancer	
History of pelvic irradiation	Bladder cancer	
Prior treatment with analgesics containing phenacetin	Bladder cancer	
Medications including aspirin, antibiotics, and nonsteroidal anti-inflammatory drugs (NSAIDs)	Interstitial nephritis	
History of irregular heartbeat	Renal embolus from atrial fibrillation	
History of nephrotic syndrome	Renal vein thrombosis	
Family history of renal disease	Hereditary nephritis Polycystic kidney disease	
Occupation in the leather, dye, rubber, or tire manufacturing industries	Bladder cancer	
Travel to or immigration from North Africa, sub-Saharan Africa, Middle East, Turkey, India, or other third-world countries		Chronic Schistosoma haematobium infection or tuberculosis infection

FOCUSED QUESTIONS

After allowing the patient to describe the episode(s) of hematuria and asking about alarm symptoms or features, ask a more focused series of questions to narrow the differential diagnosis. These questions should also be asked in patients for whom microscopic hematuria has been discovered on urinalysis. First, determine whether the hematuria is transient (ie, self-limited), episodic, or persistent. Then, ask about the character of the urine. Finally, look for associated symptoms and other aspects of the medical history that suggest a more benign cause of hematuria.

QUESTIONS	THINK ABOUT...
Time course	
Is this the first episode of blood in your urine?	Transient or self-limited condition
Did you exercise vigorously prior to the hematuria?	Exercise-induced hematuria
Have you had a recent injury to your abdomen, back, or flank?	Trauma
Are you having your menstrual period?	Vaginal source or endometriosis
Have you recently had a urinary catheter in place, a urologic procedure, or a urinary tract infection?	Iatrogenic trauma or recurrent urinary tract infection
Have you had multiple episodes over months to years?	IgA nephropathy
When did the episodes first start?	IgA nephropathy (often seen in young adults)
Does anything seem to precipitate an episode?	IgA nephropathy (often preceded by a sore throat or upper respiratory infection symptoms)
Quality	
Does the urine contain clots?	Nonglomerular source
Do the clots look like pipes?	Bleeding from ureter
Are the clots bulky and look like balls?	Bleeding from bladder
Is blood present:	
• *At the beginning of the urine stream?*	A lesion in the urethra or a location distal to the bladder neck
• *At the end of voiding?*	A lesion in the posterior urethra, bladder neck, prostate, or bladder trigone
• *Throughout urination?*	Hemorrhagic cystitis Renal or ureteral source
Associated symptoms	
Had you had fevers or felt feverish?	Acute pyelonephritis Acute prostatitis Prostatic abscess
Do you have pain or burning on urination?	Urinary tract infection Hemorrhagic cystitis Passage of renal calculus Acute prostatitis
Do you have sharp pain in your lower abdomen above the groin?	Renal calculus

—Continued next page

Continued—

Do you have suprapubic pain?	Cystitis
Do you have flank pain or back pain?	Acute pyelonephritis Renal calculus Papillary necrosis
Do you have to urinate frequently at night, or have you noticed a decreased force of your urine stream?	Benign prostatic hypertrophy
Pertinent medical history	
Are you currently taking:	
• *A blood thinner (eg, warfarin)?*	Anticoagulation, especially excessive anticoagulation, which may unmask an underlying genitourinary lesion
• *Cyclophosphamide?*	Hemorrhagic cystitis. Occurs in a dose-dependent fashion in patients receiving intravenous (greater than oral) cyclophosphamide.
Have you ever had kidney stones?	Urinary calculus
Have you ever had gout?	Uric acid stones
Do you have sickle cell anemia?	Hematuria from sickling of red blood cells

DIAGNOSTIC APPROACH

All patients with even a single episode of gross hematuria should receive a thorough history and physical examination followed by urologic or nephrologic evaluation (see Figure 41–1) unless a self-limited, transient cause is identified (eg, trauma, infection, menses, exercise induced). Even in patients with transient causes, if there are significant risk factors for malignancy (see Alarm Features), further evaluation should be considered.

A careful history should also be performed in all patients with microscopic hematuria. Most experts recommend additional evaluation only if one or more repeated urinalyses confirm microscopic hematuria.[1,14] However, there is no evidence to suggest that an isolated episode is less serious than recurrent episodes.[1] Thus, some authors recommend that unless a self-limited cause is found, a complete evaluation (see Figure 41–2) should be undertaken, especially in men over the age of 40 and those with risk factors for significant disease.[3,6,15]

CAVEATS

- Hematuria in patients receiving anticoagulation therapy should not be attributed solely to the anticoagulant.[16]
- Blood in the urine can be an irritant and may cause dysuria, even in the absence of urinary tract infection or kidney stone disease.
- Because older men with microscopic or gross hematuria are more likely to have a genitourinary malignancy, diagnostic evaluation should be pursued even in the presence of nocturia, polyuria, and decreased force of urinary stream (symptoms suggestive of benign prostatic hypertrophy).

PROGNOSIS

The prognosis of hematuria depends on the etiology. Metastatic genitourinary malignancy is generally incurable. Localized malignancy is curable in a significant percentage of patients, depending on the site of the malignancy. An acute progressive glomerulonephritis occurs in approximately 10% of patients with IgA nephropathy, the most common cause of microscopic hematuria. In 20% to 30% of patients with IgA nephropathy, chronic kidney disease develops over 1 or 2 decades. The remaining patients continue to have gross or microscopic hematuria but do not develop progressive renal dysfunction. The majority of cases of acute postinfectious glomerulonephritis resolve in weeks to months, whereas other forms of acute glomerulonephritis (rapidly progressive, membranoproliferative) can progress rapidly to irreversible renal failure despite treatment with immunosuppressive agents.

CASE SCENARIO | Resolution

A previously healthy 18-year-old woman is seen in your office complaining of a 3-day episode of "red urine," which has now resolved. She is frightened because this has never happened to her before.

ADDITIONAL HISTORY

The patient also complains of severe pain and burning upon urination, and she is urinating more frequently than normal, up to 12 times per day. She and her boyfriend had sexual intercourse for the first time 1 week ago.

Question: What is the most likely diagnosis?

A. IgA nephropathy
B. Urinary tract infection (cystitis)
C. Bladder cancer
D. Ureteral calculus
E. Goodpasture's disease

Test Your Knowledge

1. A 75-year-old man with a negative past medical history comes to your office complaining of a 3-day history of painless "bloody urine," which has now resolved. He is frightened because he has never experienced bloody urine.
   Which of the following would be considered an alarm symptom or feature in this patient?
   A. Deafness
   B. Burning upon urination
   C. Smoking history
   D. Recent travel to the Ukraine
   E. History of ureteral calculus

2. A 30-year-old woman has recurrent episodes of "smoky" brownish urine and dysuria, usually preceded by a cough, nasal congestion, and feverishness. These episodes spontaneously resolve without treatment and then she feels well. She has smoked one-half pack of cigarettes per day for 5 years.
   What is the most likely diagnosis?
   A. Bladder cancer
   B. Urinary tract infection
   C. IgA nephropathy
   D. Renal infarct
   E. Renal calculus

3. A 30-year-old man complains of recurrent, self-limited episodes of "bloody" urine and abdominal pain. He has a 10-year history of smoking one-half pack of cigarettes per day. His grandfather died of kidney disease, and his paternal aunt and father are currently treated on the "kidney machine."
   What is the most likely diagnosis?
   A. Polycystic kidney disease
   B. Bladder cancer
   C. Ureteral calculus
   D. IgA nephropathy
   E. Urinary tract infection

References

1. Cohen RA, Brown RS. Microscopic hematuria. *N Engl J Med.* 2003;348:2330–2338.
2. Preventive Services Task Force. *Guide to Clinical Preventive Services: Report of the US Preventive Services Task Force.* 2nd ed. Philadelphia, PA: Williams & Wilkins, 1996.
3. Woolhandler S, Pels RJ, Bor DH, et al. Dipstick urinalysis screening of asymptomatic adults for urinary tract disorders. I. Hematuria and proteinuria. *JAMA.* 1989;262:1215–1224.
4. Sutton JM. Evaluation of hematuria in adults. *JAMA.* 1990;263:2475–2480.
5. Khadra MH, Pickard RS, Charlton M, et al. A prospective analysis of 1930 patients with hematuria to evaluate current diagnostic practice. *J Urol.* 2000;163:524–527.
6. Peacock PR, Souto HL, Benner GE, et al. What is gross hematuria? Correlation of subjective and objective assessment. *J Trauma.* 2001;50:1060–1062.
7. Mishriki SF, Grimsley SJS, Nabi G. Incidence of recurrent frank hematuria and urological cancers: prospective 6.9 years of followup. *J Urol.* 2009;182:1294–1298.
8. Messing EM, Young TB, Hunr VB, et al. Home screening for hematuria: results of a multi-clinic study. *J Urol.* 1992;148: 289–292.
9. Carson CC, Segura JW, Greene LF. Clinical importance of microhematuria. *JAMA.* 1979;241:149–150.
10. Bard RH. The significance of asymptomatic microhematuria and proteinuria in adult primary care. *CMAJ.* 2002;166: 348–353.

11. Greene LF, O'Shaughnessey JEJ, Hendricks ED. Study of five hundred patients with asymptomatic microscopic hematuria. *JAMA.* 1956;161:610–613.
12. Froom P, Ribak J, Benbassat J. Significance of microhematuria in young adults. *BMJ.* 1984;288:20–22.
13. Mohr DN, Offord KP, Melton LJ III. A symptomatic microhematuria and urologic disease. A population-based study. *JAMA.* 1986;256:224–229.
14. House AA, Cattran DC. Nephrology 2. Evaluation of asymptomatic hematuria and proteinuria in adult primary care. *CMAJ.* 2002;166:348–353.
15. Ritchie CD, Bevan EA, Collier SJ. Importance of occult hematuria found at screening. *BMJ.* 1986;292:681–683.
16. Van Savage JG, Fried FA. Anticoagulant associated hematuria: a prospective study. *J Urol.* 1995;153:1594–1596.

Chapter 42

Flank Pain

Paul Aronowitz, MD, and Aaron Falk, MD

CASE SCENARIO

A 36-year-old woman presents to the emergency department with left-sided flank pain. The pain is severe, located just below her left ribs, and has been constant for the past 12 hours. It does not radiate or change with position. She also reports a fever to 101°F and general malaise.

- **What additional questions will further characterize her flank pain and help narrow the differential diagnosis?**
- **What are the common diagnoses associated with flank pain?**

INTRODUCTION

Flank pain refers to pain occurring just below the 12th rib, encompassing the costovertebral angle and area lateral to that angle. Patients often describe flank pain as unilateral upper back pain. The initial differential diagnosis depends on the patient's age, gender, and comorbid illnesses. However, nephrolithiasis, pyelonephritis, and musculoskeletal strain account for most cases.

A careful history often suggests one of these possibilities or raises suspicion for a less common cause. For example, a history of chronic atrial fibrillation increases the likelihood of a renal vascular embolus. Splenic infarct as a cause of left flank pain is unusual but should be considered in patients with suspected endocarditis. If "red flags" arise in the history, life-threatening diagnoses such as rupturing abdominal aortic aneurysm (AAA) or retroperitoneal hemorrhage must also be considered.[1]

KEY TERMS

Dysuria	Difficulty urinating or pain with urination.
Gross hematuria	Bloody urine visible to the patient.
Renal colic	Pain caused by obstruction of the ureter as a result of increased hydrostatic pressure proximal to the obstruction.
	Considered to be one of the most painful conditions experienced by patients, just short of labor or childbirth.

ETIOLOGY

Unfortunately, few data exist on prevalence of the various causes of flank pain. Flank pain is often caused by sudden obstruction of a ureter by a renal calculus or renal colic. Renal colic tends to be sudden, severe, and debilitating. As the offending calculus descends through the collecting system, pain may also occur in the lower abdominal quadrants and genitalia, along with dysuria, frequency, urgency, and hematuria.[2]

Pyelonephritis commonly causes flank pain, particularly in women. Because women have shorter urethras than men, women have a greater incidence of lower urinary tract infections, which may ascend to one or both kidneys resulting in pyelonephritis. Pain is caused by inflammation of the kidney with stretching of the renal capsule; it may be less severe and more insidious than renal colic.[3] A history of fever or dysuria suggests pyelonephritis, although dysuria may not occur in patients with indwelling urinary catheters.[4,5] Occasionally, a kidney stone may obstruct the flow of urine, leading to the development of pyelonephritis.[6] Such patients have *both* pyelonephritis and nephrolithiasis, the 2 most common causes of flank pain.

Musculoskeletal causes of flank pain are often clinically obvious. The patient usually describes a precipitating event, such as swinging a baseball bat or lifting a heavy object.

It is helpful to think about the most common diagnoses first and then consider the less common or rare causes.

Differential Diagnosis

Nephrolithiasis	Common[3]
Pyelonephritis	Common[3]
Musculoskeletal (muscle strain)	Common
Herpes zoster	Common
Papillary necrosis	Uncommon
Renal abscess	Uncommon
Renal infarct (cardioembolic)	Uncommon (except with atrial fibrillation)
Renal vein thrombosis	Uncommon
Adult polycystic kidney disease (APKD) and its complications • Infected renal cyst • Rupturing renal cyst • Hemorrhage into renal cyst	Common cause of chronic kidney disease[7]
AAA	Uncommon[1]
Retroperitoneal hemorrhage	Uncommon; consider in patients receiving anticoagulants
Pulmonary embolism	Uncommon
Pneumonia (lower lobe)	Uncommon
Pleural effusion or empyema	Uncommon
Subphrenic abscess	Uncommon
Biliary tract (gallbladder) disease	Uncommon
Diverticulitis, appendicitis, psoas abscess	Uncommon
Vertebral compression fracture	Uncommon
Retroperitoneal malignancy (lymphoma, pancreatic cancer, metastatic cancer)	Uncommon
Malingering	Uncommon
Bacterial endocarditis with splenic infarct	Rare
Renal tuberculosis	Rare in the United States; more common in developing world
Retroperitoneal fibrosis	Rare

GETTING STARTED WITH THE HISTORY

- Characterize the onset, location, duration, quality, and associated features of the pain.
- Determine whether the patient has ever had similar pain before.
- Keep in mind the myriad medical conditions that predispose to renal stone formation—from hyperparathyroidism to myeloproliferative disorders to renal tubular acidosis.
- Obtain a careful occupational history and substance use or abuse history (eg, an intern on duty for long periods may not drink adequate fluids, putting her at higher risk for a kidney stone).

Open-Ended Questions	Tips for Effective Interviewing
Tell me about the pain you are having.	Listen.
Did the pain come on suddenly or gradually?	Don't interrupt.
Where in your body did you first notice the pain?	Don't jump to conclusions.
	Be empathic—the patient will often be in pain throughout the initial history.

INTERVIEW FRAMEWORK

- Further characterize the flank pain.
  - Onset
  - Duration
  - Frequency
  - Pain character
  - Location of pain
- Inquire about associated symptoms.
  - Nausea and/or vomiting
  - Fever
  - Hematuria

IDENTIFYING ALARM SYMPTOMS

- Flank pain associated with features such as pleuritic chest pain, cough, or drenching night sweats, requires urgent attention.
- Flank pain with a normal urinalysis should prompt consideration of pathology outside the kidney.[3]
- Consider a rupturing AAA or retroperitoneal hemorrhage in patients whose history suggests hypotension (ie, dizziness, fainting, or confusion). Mortality from ruptured AAA is 90% in all cases and ranges from 28% to 70% in patients who make it to the hospital and receive appropriate treatment.[8]

Serious Diagnoses

Serious causes of flank pain tend to be uncommon. Fortunately, the urinalysis rapidly narrows the initial differential diagnosis.

Alarm Symptoms	Serious Causes	Benign Causes
Confusion and fever	Pyelonephritis with sepsis (urosepsis) Cholecystitis Pneumonia	
Orthostatic dizziness	Shock from rupturing AAA or hemorrhage	Volume depletion from poor oral intake (easily corrects with intravenous fluids)
Concurrent use of anticoagulants	Retroperitoneal hemorrhage	
Pleuritic chest pain	Pulmonary embolism Pneumonia Subphrenic abscess	Pleurisy or muscle strain
Associated abdominal pain	AAA Subphrenic abscess Pancreatitis	
Weight loss	Malignancy	
Slow onset and failure to resolve	Malignancy Abscess	

—Continued next page

Continued—		
Prolonged fever with sudden-onset flank pain	Endocarditis with septic emboli	Viral syndrome
Pain associated with eating	Cholecystitis Bowel obstruction Pancreatitis	
Sudden onset of flank pain	AAA Nephrolithiasis Retroperitoneal hemorrhage Pulmonary embolism Renal infarct	

FOCUSED QUESTIONS

After letting the patient tell the story, focus on alarm symptoms or features suggestive of causes other than nephrolithiasis, pyelonephritis, or musculoskeletal disease.

QUESTIONS	THINK ABOUT...
Onset	
Tell me about how your symptoms started.	
• *Sudden onset*	Nephrolithiasis
• *Gradual onset*	Pyelonephritis
• *Onset associated with physical exertion*	Musculoskeletal strain
Duration	
How long have you been experiencing these symptoms?	
• *Hours to 1 week*	Pyelonephritis, nephrolithiasis
• *Weeks or months*	Malignancy, renal cyst
Pain character	
Can you describe in more detail what the pain feels like?	
• *Sharp, knife-like pain*	Nephrolithiasis
• *Colicky, intermittent spasm–like pain*	Nephrolithiasis
• *Tingling, numb sensation*	Herpes zoster
Associated symptoms	
What additional symptoms are you experiencing?	
• *Fever/malaise*	Pyelonephritis
• *Nausea and vomiting*	Pyelonephritis
• *Hematuria*	Nephrolithiasis, pyelonephritis

DIAGNOSTIC APPROACH (INCLUDING ALGORITHM)

Figure 42–1 shows the diagnostic approach algorithm for flank pain.

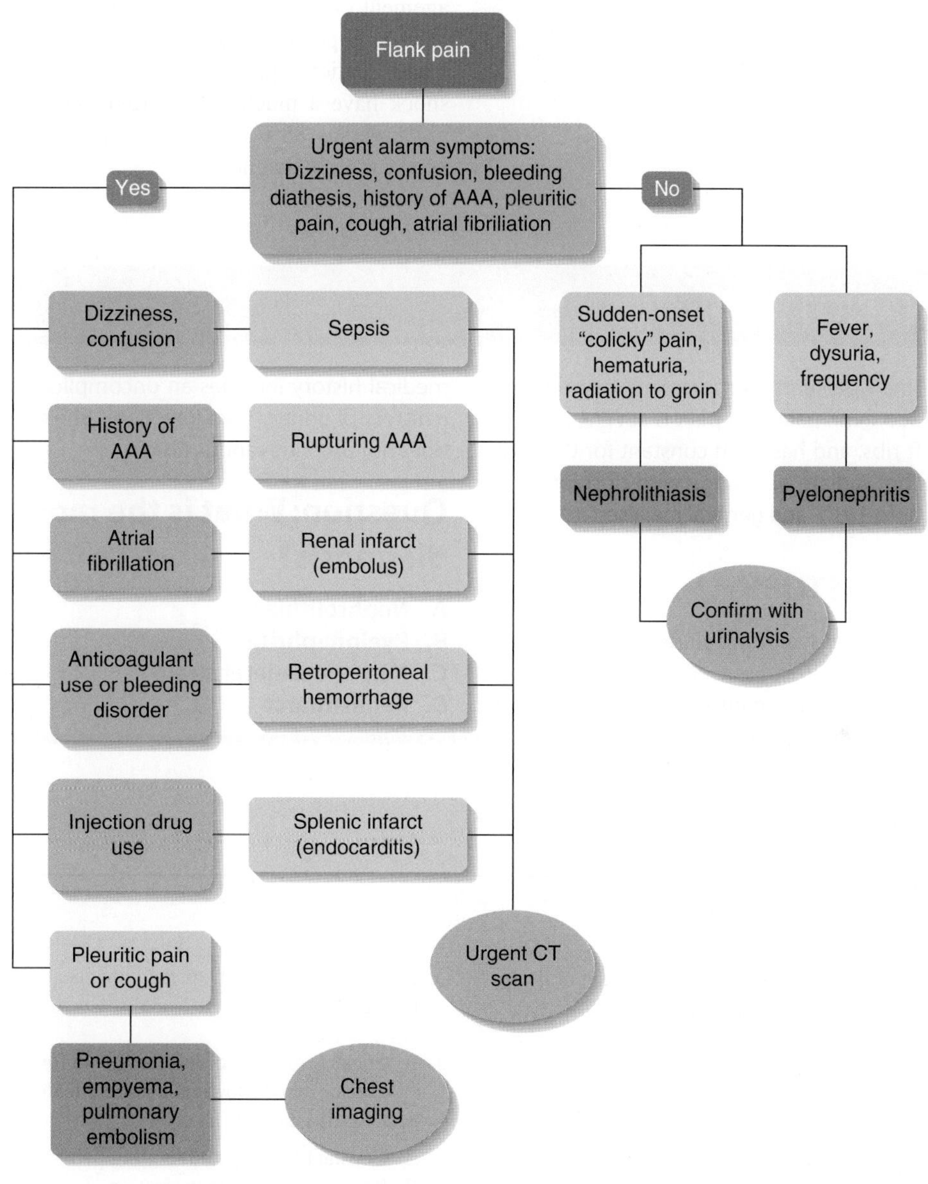

FIGURE 42–1 Diagnostic approach: Flank pain. AAA, abdominal aortic aneurysm; CT, computed tomography.

CAVEATS

- Age is important in establishing the initial differential diagnosis of flank pain. A young woman with flank pain is highly unlikely to have an AAA; however, AAA must be considered in an older man with peripheral vascular disease even if he has flank pain, fever, and dysuria.[1]
- Kidney stones may recur; often the patient will tell you the diagnosis because this pain tends to be unforgettable.[2]
- Always consider a rupturing AAA, which as an uncommon but potentially life-threatening diagnosis unless detected early.
- Injection drug abuse is a "red flag" in all patients with flank pain; such patients require a more careful evaluation for endocarditis.

- Attempt to differentiate pyelonephritis from nephrolithiasis because the latter usually requires a computed tomography scan or intravenous pyelogram.
- Listen to the patient's story; this will save time and prevent unnecessary testing.
- Remember that other common diseases (pneumonia, cholecystitis) can present in an uncommon fashion—namely, with flank pain.

PROGNOSIS

Prognosis depends on the underlying diagnosis. Patients with pyelonephritis generally do well with antibiotics. Patients with nephrolithiasis may do well with conservative management or sometimes need urologic intervention (eg, lithotripsy), depending on the size and location of the kidney stone.[2] Patients presenting with an enlarging AAA without shock have a much better prognosis than those with shock (22% versus 88% mortality, respectively),[1] highlighting the need for early diagnosis.

CASE SCENARIO | Resolution

A 36-year-old woman presents to the emergency department with left-sided flank pain. The pain is severe, located just below her left ribs, and has been constant for the past 12 hours. It does not radiate or change with position. She also reports a fever to 101°F and general malaise.

ADDITIONAL HISTORY

The patient reports that her symptoms started approximately 1 day after she noticed a burning sensation when urinating. Associated symptoms included nausea and vomiting. Past medical history includes an uncomplicated pregnancy and a history of urinary tract infections. She does not smoke and does not use intravenous drugs.

Question: What is the most likely diagnosis?

A. Nephrolithiasis
B. Pyelonephritis
C. Musculoskeletal strain
D. Renal infarct

Test Your Knowledge

1. In a patient with severe right-sided flank pain, which of the following lowers your suspicion for nephrolithiasis?

   A. Stabbing, severe pain
   B. Intermittent nature of pain
   C. Onset approximately 2 months ago
   D. Hematuria
   E. History of nephrolithiasis

2. You are evaluating a 65-year-old man in clinic for sudden onset of severe flank pain.
   Which of the following features is most alarming and should prompt an urgent evaluation?

   A. History of kidney stones
   B. Patient is taking warfarin (for stroke prevention due to atrial fibrillation)
   C. Radiation to the groin
   D. Pain started after he picked up a heavy box
   E. Hematuria

3. A patient complains of left flank pain for several days.
   Which of the following historical features suggests herpes zoster as the cause?

   A. Constant burning and tingling pain
   B. Recent cardiac catheterization
   C. Pain is worse after eating
   D. Radiation to the groin
   E. Association with nausea and vomiting

References

1. Lederle FA, Parenti CM, Chute EP. Ruptured abdominal aortic aneurysm: the internist as diagnostician. *Am J Med.* 1994;96: 163–167.
2. Teichman JMH. Acute renal colic from ureteral calculus. *N Engl J Med.* 2004;350:684–693.
3. Sobel JD, Kaye D. Urinary tract infections. In: *Mandell, Douglas, and Bennett's Principles and Practice of Infectious Diseases.* 6th ed. Vol. 1. Philadelphia, PA: Churchill Livingstone, 2005:875–905.
4. Tambyah PA, Maki DG. Catheter-associated urinary tract infection is rarely symptomatic. *Arch Intern Med.* 2000;160: 678–682.
5. Tolkoff-Rubin NE, Cotran RS, Rubin RH. Urinary tract infection, pyelonephritis, and reflux nephropathy. In: *Brenner and Rector's the Kidney.* 8th ed. Vol. 3. New York, NY: Saunders, 2007:1203–1238.
6. Weiss M, Liapis H, Tomaszewski JE, Arend LJ. Pyelonephritis and other infections, reflux nephropathy, hydronephrosis and nephrolithiasis. In: *Heptinstall's Pathology of the Kidney.* 6th ed. Vol. 2. New York, NY: Little, Brown, and Company, 2007:991–1081.
7. Grantham JJ. Clinical practice. Autosomal dominant polycystic kidney disease. *N Engl J Med.* 2008;359:1477–1485.
8. Davidovic L, Markovic M, Kostic D, et al. Ruptured abdominal aortic aneurysms: factors influencing early survival. *Ann Vasc Surg.* 2005;19:29–34.

Chapter 43

Erectile Dysfunction

Mary E. Harris, MD, and David R. Gutknecht, MD

CASE SCENARIO

A 65-year-old man comes to your office to ask about "ED" after seeing a television advertisement about potential treatments. For 3 years, he has noted progressive difficulty attaining erections adequate for sexual intercourse. He sheepishly tells his story and wonders if the medicines advertised on television would be right for him. He also asks about whether his blood pressure medication could be causing his symptoms and whether hormone treatments might help.

- **How do you make him feel more comfortable discussing his concerns?**
- **What organic disorders could be causing—or be associated with—his erectile dysfunction (ED)? How might those factors affect his treatment options?**
- **What effects do medications have on sexual function?**
- **How often are treatable hormone deficiencies responsible for ED?**

INTRODUCTION

Erectile dysfunction (ED) is the inability to attain and sustain an erection of sufficient rigidity for sexual activity. It affects nearly 1 in 5 men over 20 years of age, and the prevalence increases dramatically with advancing age. Seventy-eight percent of men over 75 years are affected and Hispanic men are more likely to report it.[1]

Although patients may be reluctant to discuss this problem it is important for physicians to inquire about it. Effective treatments based on improved understanding of the mechanisms of ED are now available. ED may be a sign of important comorbid cardiovascular disease. ED is a strong predictor of both coronary artery disease and peripheral artery disease as endothelial dysfunction contributes to all 3 conditions.

There are many associated or contributing conditions that should be explored, including urologic problems, diabetes, hormonal disturbances, depression, obstructive sleep apnea, neurologic disorders, and the use of medications.

KEY TERMS

Impotence	An outdated and potentially disparaging label for what we now call ED.
Loss of libido	Loss of sexual interest.
Premature ejaculation	A distinct sexual problem, sometimes confused with ED. An adequate erection is lost through early involuntary climax. More common than ED in patients under 50.
Positive likelihood ratio (LR^+)	The factor by which the odds of a diagnosis are multiplied if a given clinical factor is present. A $LR^+ > 10$ is usually considered diagnostically convincing.

ETIOLOGY AND PATHOPHYSIOLOGY

α-Adrenergic sympathetic tone limits blood flow to the penis and maintains the flaccid state. Erection occurs when erotic stimuli inhibit sympathetic tone and release nitric oxide and other vasoactive substances from nerve endings and endothelial cells in the penile arterioles. The cavernosal sinusoids become engorged with blood, and erection ensues. This is aided by a passive inhibition of venous outflow as the subtunical venous plexus is compressed between the expanding sinusoids and unyielding tunica albuginea. Forcible compression of the base of the penis by the ischiocavernous muscles then further increases the intracavernous pressure.

Any derangement in these events can cause ED, commonly the failure of nitric oxide release due to endothelial dysfunction. Improved understanding of these mechanisms has led to the development of drugs such as phosphodiesterase-5 inhibitors, which have revolutionized ED care.

Approximately 80% of ED has an organic cause, although concurrent psychological problems such as depression are quite common.[2]

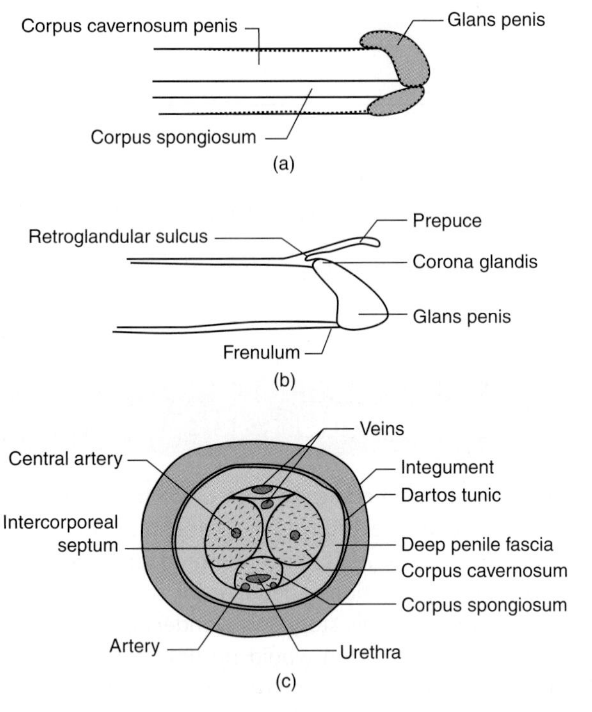

FIGURE 43–1 Structure of the penis. **A.** The shaft in its ventrolateral aspect, with integument removed. **B.** A sagittal section of the shaft with integument included. **C.** A cross-section of the shaft.

Differential Diagnosis

	Approximate Frequency
Psychogenic	20%[2]
Vascular	32% have overt vascular impairment distinct from diabetes.[3] Although not proven to be the cause, many patients over 60 with ED have high vascular disease risk (eg, 10-year coronary artery disease risk increased to 65%)[4]
Drug induced	12%–25%[3,5]
Hormonal (thyroid, pituitary, gonadal disease)	Variable reports, perhaps 3%–19% excluding diabetes.[3,6] There is no clear association between ED and low testosterone levels unless luteinizing hormone is elevated.[7]
Hormonal (diabetes)	5%–24%[3,8]
Neurogenic	4%[3]
Other	
• Urologic • Renal disease • Sickle cell disease • Sleep disorder[9] • Liver disease	5%[3]

GETTING STARTED WITH THE HISTORY

ED is a sensitive but very important topic, affecting the patient's sexual activity and self-image, as well as the patient's partner. Although now men are more open about this concern, healthcare providers should specifically ask all patients about ED. Routinely incorporate questions about ED into your review of systems. Differentiate ED from loss of libido, lack of orgasm, and premature ejaculation.

When seeking specific information, consider using a one-question approach, asking whether the patient always, usually, sometimes, or never is able to achieve and maintain a good erection. When responses to this inquiry were correlated with a "gold standard" clinical examination, the positive likelihood ratio was 8.57 for "sometimes" and 12.69 for "never."[10]

Questions	Remember
Many men have occasional problems getting or keeping an erection. Has this happened to you?	Use nonjudgmental, professional language. "Normalize" your questions by reminding patients how common ED is. Teach small bits of information ("it's common, treatable, and an appropriate topic to broach with your doctor") interspersed with questions. Overcome patient hesitance by asking direct questions first and later returning to open questions.
I always ask my patients some very personal questions related to their health. Do you ever have any problems with sexual intercourse? With erections?	
I'm glad you feel comfortable telling me about this. I'd like to ask you some specific questions about sexual function to figure out what we should do.	

INTERVIEW FRAMEWORK

- Determine the patient's agenda. For example, some want a prescription for a "cure-all," and others want an explanation.
- Differentiate psychogenic from physical (organic) causes of ED, but remember that patients often have a contribution from both.
- When considering physical (organic) causes, differentiate vascular, hormonal, neurologic, drug-induced, and other causes. It is common for patients to have more than one cause.
- Find unrecognized contributory conditions (see Focused Questions section).
- Pay particular attention to associated cardiovascular risk, which may influence treatment options.

IDENTIFYING ALARM SYMPTOMS

In patients with ED, systemic diseases such as diabetes, alcoholism, depression, or vascular diseases may occasionally go unrecognized without directed questioning. Serious diagnoses are rare, but cardiovascular risk is common.

Alarm Symptoms	If Present, Consider...	However, Less Serious Causes Include...
Concurrent hip and buttock cramps with walking	Abdominal aortic aneurysm	Intermittent claudication, spinal stenosis
Leg weakness or numbness, perineal numbness	Spinal cord compression or pelvic mass	Nerve root compression, peripheral neuropathy
Bowel or bladder incontinence	Spinal cord compression or pelvic mass	Bladder infection, fecal impaction, others
Galactorrhea (milk flow from the breast)	Pituitary tumor	
Abnormal secondary sexual characteristics (loss of beard, body hair, female body habitus)	Pituitary tumor	Normal variant, primary testicular failure
Visual field cuts (loss of portions of vision)	Pituitary tumor	Other eye disorders

FOCUSED QUESTIONS

QUESTIONS	THINK ABOUT...
If answered in the affirmative	
Do you have:	
• *History of depression, schizophrenia, or bipolar disorder?*	Psychogenic
• *Loss of interest, trouble concentrating, trouble with memory, or feelings of sadness?*	Psychogenic (depression)
• *Difficulties with relationship with partner?*	Psychogenic
• *Performance anxiety?*	Psychogenic
Do you smoke?	Vascular
Do you have high cholesterol, hypertension, chest pain, and/or leg claudication?	Vascular
Do you have a history of coronary artery disease? Do any members of your family? Is there any history of peripheral vascular disease?	Vascular Many ED patients will have cardiovascular risk, which should be addressed even if the ED is not due to overt vascular disease.[4]
Is there a past history of pelvic or spinal trauma, radiation, or surgery?	Neurologic (injury)
Have you had perineal numbness or bowel or bladder incontinence?	Neurologic (spinal cord or pelvic plexus)
Have you felt any foot or leg numbness or weakness?	Neurologic (diabetes; spinal cord, brain, or pelvic plexus lesion)
Are you taking medications known to cause ED (eg, antihypertensives, antidepressants, antiandrogenics, antihistamines, corticosteroids, digitalis)?	Drug induced Medications most likely to cause ED include hydrochlorothiazide and the selective serotonin reuptake inhibitor drugs. β-Blockers have uncertain effects, and angiotensin-converting enzyme inhibitors are usually not implicated.[4]
Do you ever drive under the influence? *Have you ever tried to cut down your alcohol intake? Do you get angry when others ask about your alcohol use? Do you feel guilty about your drinking? Do you drink a morning eye-opener? (CAGE questions)*	Alcoholism
Do you use alcohol, marijuana, or other drugs?	Drug induced Depression or other psychogenic cause
Do you have:	
• *History of thyroid disease?*	Hormonal (thyroid disease)
• *Heat/cold intolerance?*	Hormonal (thyroid disease)
• *Constipation/diarrhea?*	Hormonal (thyroid disease)
• *Weight gain/loss?*	Hormonal (thyroid disease)
• *Tremor?*	Hormonal (thyroid disease)

• *History of gonadal disease?*	Hormonal (gonadal disease)
• *Gynecomastia, loss of body hair, thinning of beard, or decreased testicular size?*	Hormonal (pituitary or gonadal)
• *History of pituitary disease?*	Hormonal (pituitary)
• *Visual field cuts or headache?*	Hormonal (pituitary mass)
• *Decreased libido?*	Hormonal (gonadal or pituitary) or psychogenic
• *A personal or family history of diabetes?*	Diabetes
• *Polyphagia, polyuria, or polydipsia?*	Diabetes
• *History of renal disease?*	Renal disease
• *Priapism or bone pains?*	Sickle cell disease
Do you snore or not feel refreshed on awakening? Do you have daytime somnolence?	Sleep disorder[8]
Do you have jaundice, pruritus, or nausea?	Liver disease
Quality	
Do erections take longer to achieve and have shorter duration and less rigidity?	Physical (organic) etiology
Is the problem severe (ie, preventing sexual activity) or more of a minor annoyance?	Impacts on patient's desire for treatment
Time course	
Was the onset:	
• *Sudden?*	Drug induced (if concurrent with medication start) or psychogenic
• *Gradual?*	Physical (organic) etiology
• *Intermittent?*	Psychogenic
Do you achieve normal erection but lose it too early?	Psychogenic
Is there a triggering psychological event (ie, discord with partner)?	Psychogenic
Associated symptoms	
Is there painful bending of penis with erection?	Peyronie disease (fibrous plaque, usually on dorsum of penis, which does not distend as normal skin does; with erection, failure to distend causes penis to bend toward side of plaque, causing pain and loss of erection)
Is there difficulty retracting foreskin?	Phimosis
Modifying symptoms	
Better with different partner?	Psychogenic
Better with masturbation or visual stimuli?	Psychogenic
Better with nocturnal or morning erections?	Psychogenic

DIAGNOSTIC APPROACH (INCLUDING ALGORITHM)

See Figure 43–2 for the diagnostic approach algorithm for ED.

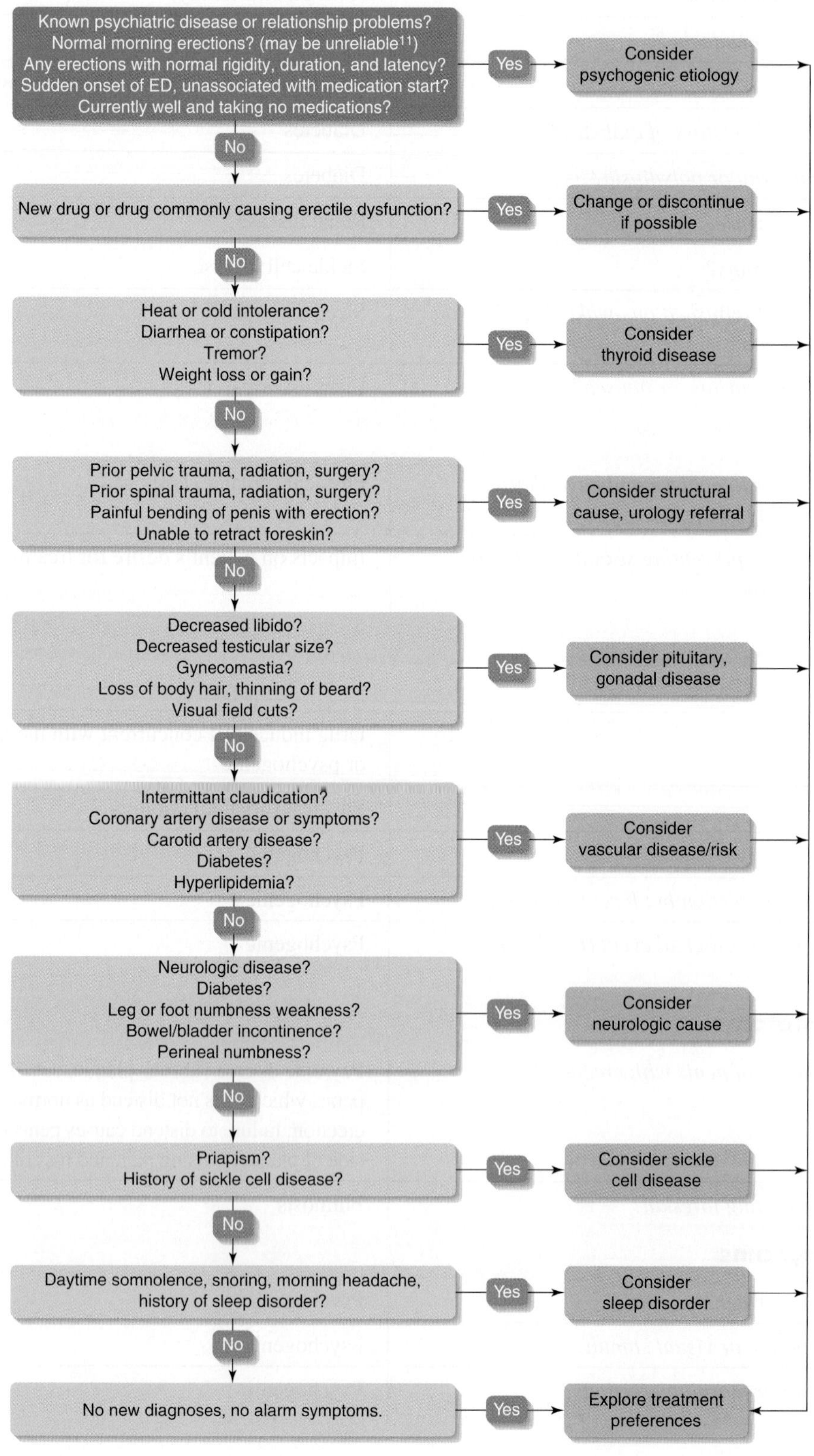

FIGURE 43–2 Diagnostic approach: Erectile dysfunction (ED). (Adapted from O'Keefe M, Hunt DK. Assessment and treatment of impotence. *Med Clin North Am*. 1995;79:415–434.)

CAVEATS

- ED with normal morning erections usually implies a psychogenic cause, but subjective reports may not be reliable.[11]
- A sudden onset of ED implicates a drug or psychogenic cause, unless there was recent urologic surgery.
- ED due to a drug, hormonal problem (other than diabetes), or psychogenic cause is eminently treatable. Be sure to look for these causes.
- ED may occasionally be the presenting symptom of a serious disorder (eg, vascular or neurologic disorder).

PROGNOSIS AND TREATMENT

- If a medication is causing ED, stopping the medication should be effective.
- Psychiatric therapy is effective in 50% to 80% of patients with psychogenic ED.
- Testosterone replacement may lead to improvement in severely hypogonadal patients, but benefit in others is less certain.[12]
- Medications or devices may improve ED in appropriately selected patients. Phosphodiesterase-5 inhibitors are effective in 70% of unselected patients with ED but are contraindicated or must be used with caution in patients with cardiovascular disease. This makes inquiry about associated cardiovascular disease especially important.

CASE SCENARIO | Resolution

A 65-year-old man comes to your office to ask about "ED" after seeing a television advertisement about potential treatments. For 3 years, he has noted progressive difficulty attaining erections adequate for sexual intercourse. He sheepishly tells his story and wonders if the medicines advertised on television would be right for him. He also asks about whether his blood pressure medication could be causing his symptoms and whether hormone treatments might help.

ADDITIONAL HISTORY

The patient reports only "sometimes" getting a good erection and that morning erections are unusual. He is not diabetic, denies chest pain or claudication, and has no neurologic symptoms. He has no headaches, breast enlargement, or change in his body habitus. He does have a family history of heart disease, has "borderline" cholesterol, and takes an angiotensin-converting enzyme inhibitor for hypertension. He is frustrated by his problem but appears neither anxious nor depressed. He reports his partner is supportive.

Question: What is the most likely diagnosis?

A. Psychogenic ED
B. Testosterone deficiency
C. Organic ED with modifiable cardiovascular risk factors
D. Drug-induced ED

Test Your Knowledge

1. Among older men with organic (physical) causes of ED, which of the following problems is most frequent?

   A. Diabetes
   B. Vascular disease
   C. Drug effect
   D. Neurologic disease

2. A 55-year-old man complains of ED but also reports frontal headaches, trouble with peripheral vision, and occasional breast discharge.

   Which of the following conditions is the most serious possible cause of his complaints?

   A. Primary testicular failure
   B. Drug effect
   C. Pituitary tumor
   D. Migraine

3. A 70-year-old widower in a new relationship complains of sudden loss of erectile function. He reports no previous erectile difficulty, but ever since a recent and disappointing encounter, he has been unable to achieve satisfactory erections. Morning erections do seem better than those occurring during intercourse. He denies starting any new medications or prior urologic problems. He is saddened by his problem and appears visibly depressed. He has no known cardiovascular disease.

   Which element of his history *most* supports a psychogenic cause for his ED?

   A. Sudden onset
   B. Depressed affect
   C. Persistence of morning erections
   D. Absence of cardiovascular symptoms

References

1. Saigal CS, Wessells H, Pace J, et al. Predictors and prevalence of erectile dysfunction in a racially diverse population. *Arch Intern Med.* 2006;166:207–212.
2. Levine LA. Diagnosis and treatment of erectile dysfunction. *Am J Med.* 2000;109:S3–S12.
3. Burnett AL. Erectile dysfunction. *J Urol.* 2006;175:S25–S31.
4. Miner MM, Kurltzky L. Erectile dysfunction: a sentinel marker for cardiovascular disease in primary care. *Cleve Clin J Med.* 2007;74(Suppl 3):S30–S37.
5. Derby CA, Barbour MM, Hume AL, McKinley JB. Drug therapy and prevalence of erectile dysfunction in the Massachusetts Male Aging Study cohort. *Pharmacotherapy.* 2001;21:676–683.
6. Johnson AR, Jarow JP. Is routine endocrine testing of impotent men necessary? *J Urol.* 1992;147:1542–1543.
7. Kupelian V, Shabsigh R, Travison TG, et al. Is there a relationship between sex hormones and erectile dysfunction? Results from the Massachusetts Male Aging Study. *J Urol.* 2006;176:2584–2588.
8. Sairam K, Kulinskaya GB, Hanbury DC, McNicholas TA. Prevalence of undiagnosed diabetes mellitus in male erectile dysfunction. *BJU Int.* 2001;88:68–71.
9. Jankowski JT, Seftel AD, Strohl KP. Erectile dysfunction and sleep related disorders. *J Urol.* 2008;179:837–841.
10. O'Donnell AB, Araujo AB, Goldstein I, et al. The validity of a single-question self-report of erectile dysfunction. Results from the Massachusetts Male Aging Study. *J Gen Intern Med.* 2005; 20:515–519.
11. McMahon CG, Touma K. Predictive value of patient history and correlation of nocturnal penile tumescence, colour duplex Doppler ultrasonography and dynamic cavernosometry and cavernosography in the evaluation of erectile dysfunction. *Int J Impot Res.* 1999;11:47–51.
12. Bolona ER, Uraga MV, Haddad RM, et al. Testosterone use in men with sexual dysfunction: a systematic review and meta-analysis of randomized placebo-controlled trials. *Mayo Clin Proc.* 2007;82:20–28.

Suggested Reading

Ellsworth P, Kirshenbaum EM. Current concepts in the evaluation and management of erectile dysfunction. *Urol Nurs.* 2008;28:357–369.

Mcvary KT. Erectile dysfunction. *N Engl J Med.* 2007;357: 2472–2481.

Qaseem A, Snow V, Denberg TD, et al.; Clinical Efficacy Assessment Subcommittee of the American College of Physicians. Hormonal testing and pharmacologic treatment of erectile dysfunction: a clinical practice guideline from the American College of Physicians. *Ann Intern Med.* 2009;151:639–649.

Chapter 44

Urinary Incontinence

Calvin H. Hirsch, MD

CASE SCENARIO

A healthy 51-year-old stockbroker comes to the clinic for an annual checkup. She states that over the past year she has gained 25 lbs and attributes the weight gain to giving up jogging and jazzercise classes. She relates that running and jumping sometimes cause her to leak urine, which is uncomfortable and embarrassing. She now uses a heavy panty liner at all times to avoid wetting herself. She is upset that she is "developing a bladder like my 80-year-old mother."

- **What is the most likely cause of her urinary incontinence?**
- **What additional questions should you ask her to better characterize her incontinence?**
- **What are the risk factors for the exercise-induced incontinence that she describes?**
- **What are the differences in the prevalence of the different types of incontinence between younger and older patients and between men and women?**

INTRODUCTION

Occasional involuntary leakage of urine is common, affecting approximately 5% of men age 19 to 44 and 21% of men over age 65.[1] At least monthly urinary leakage is reported by 13% to 25% of women over age 18, 40% of women over age 64, and 55% of women over age 80.[2,3] When urinary incontinence (UI) is severe, it can result in social isolation, depression, and even institutionalization. In the United States, the average annual out-of-pocket cost of UI for women has been estimated at greater than $250 (2005 dollars).[4]

KEY TERMS

Incontinence	The involuntary leakage of urine. There are several types: urge, detrusor disinhibition, stress, overflow (includes detrusor hyperactivity with impaired contractility and detrusor-sphincter dyssynergy), functional, and mixed.
Urge	Involuntary detrusor contractions cause an urgent need to void. After a variable latency period (seconds to minutes), the contractions exceed bladder outlet resistance (normally produced by the internal sphincter), resulting in incontinence (Figure 44–1). Also called detrusor hyperreflexia and idiopathic overactive bladder with incontinence.

—Continued next page

Continued—

Detrusor disinhibition	Spontaneous triggering of the spinal reflex voiding mechanism when the bladder reaches a threshold volume and there is inadequate inhibition of bladder contractions by the central nervous system. Urine loss may occur with or without warning. Also called neurogenic detrusor overactivity.
Stress	Leakage caused by an increase in intra-abdominal pressure, as produced by a cough, sneeze, laughing, standing up, or heavy lifting (Figure 44–2). Also called sphincter incompetence.
Overflow	Due to urinary retention, pressure in the bladder exceeds outlet (sphincter) resistance, causing leakage until the bladder pressure drops below outlet resistance.
Detrusor hyperactivity with impaired contractility (DHIC)	Found mainly in debilitated older persons. Despite an overactive bladder, detrusor contractions are ineffective, resulting in bladder distention and overflow incontinence.
Detrusor-sphincter dyssynergy	Failure to synchronize bladder contractions with release of sphincter, due to multiple sclerosis or other conditions causing suprasacral spinal cord lesions.
Functional	Incontinence despite a normally functioning bladder due to the inability to reach a toilet in time.
Mixed	Incontinence from multiple etiologies, most commonly stress and urge.
Idiopathic overactive bladder	Involuntary detrusor contractions that occur before the bladder is full, creating a sensation of urgently needing to void. May occur with or without incontinence.

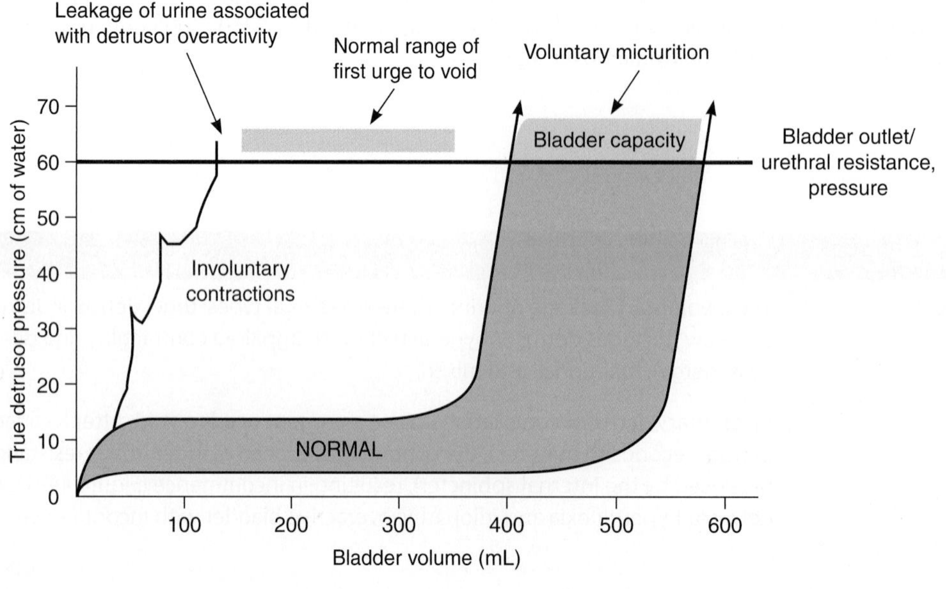

FIGURE 44–1 Mechanism of urge incontinence. (Adapted from Kane RL, Ouslander JG, Abrass IB. *Essentials of Clinical Geriatrics*. 3rd ed. New York, NY: McGraw-Hill, 1994.)

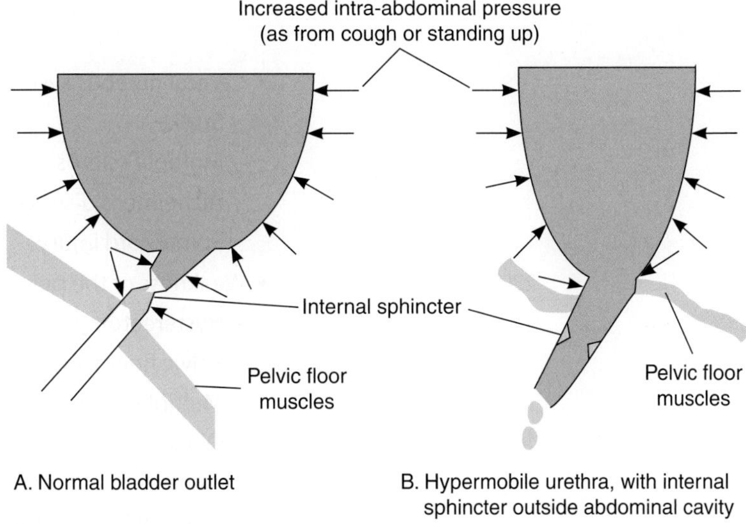

FIGURE 44–2 With a normal bladder outlet **(A)**, increased intra-abdominal pressure ("stress") is applied equally to outside of bladder and sphincter, keeping the bladder pressure–sphincter pressure ratio unchanged. When the sphincter drops below the pelvic diaphragm because of pelvic floor laxity **(B)**, all of the increased intra-abdominal pressure is applied above the sphincter, causing the bladder pressure to exceed the sphincter pressure and resulting in loss of sphincter competence and leakage. Damage to the internal sphincter itself, as might occur from prior instrumentation, can also lead to sphincter incompetence. (Adapted from Kane RL, Ouslander JG, Abrass IB. *Essentials of Clinical Geriatrics*. 3rd ed. New York, NY: McGraw-Hill, 1994.)

ETIOLOGY

The prevalence of the various incontinence types depends on age and gender. An overactive bladder (with or without incontinence) affects approximately 9% of women and 3% of men in their early 40s, but after age 74, more men than women report symptoms of an overactive bladder (approximately 40% versus 30%, respectively).[5] Because the prevalence of UI due to an overactive bladder increases more rapidly with age in women than in men, nearly all women over age 74 with an overactive bladder experience urge incontinence, compared to roughly 75% of men with an overactive bladder. As a result, the prevalence of urge incontinence reaches approximately 30% in both sexes by the eighth decade.[6] Stress incontinence occurs predominantly in women because of pelvic floor laxity; however, it may occur in men who have damage to the internal sphincter resulting from instrumentation or prostate surgery. Incontinence in older women is more likely to have an urge component, compared with younger women. Among women free of stress incontinence, those 70 and older are much less likely to develop new stress incontinence than women age 54 to 59.[7] However, in a survey of 647 currently incontinent women age 48 to 79 years, over 80% described symptoms suggesting a mixed etiology that included urgency and stress.[8]

Differential Diagnosis

	Reported Prevalence[a,b]	Associated Conditions
Urge	24%–29%	• Idiopathic overactive bladder • Benign prostatic hypertrophy • Local bladder or urethral irritation - Infection - Nonbacterial cystitis - Atrophic urethritis - Bladder stones - Fecal impaction - Other bladder irritants

—*Continued next page*

Continued—

Detrusor disinhibition		• Central nervous system disorder – Stroke – Multiple sclerosis – Alzheimer's disease and other dementias – Spinal cord injury
Stress	23%–29%	• Weakness of the pelvic floor – Hysterectomy – Pelvic floor surgery or injury – Multiple vaginal births9 – Obesity[8,9] • Incompetent sphincter – Urethral instrumentation – Transurethral resection of the prostate
Overflow	5%–10%[c]	• Bladder outlet obstruction – Benign prostatic hypertrophy – Urethral stricture – Surgical overcorrection of stress incontinence – Cystocele – Fecal impaction • Ineffective detrusor contractions – Pelvic irradiation – Autonomic dysfunction • Diabetic neuropathy • Spinal stenosis • Neurodegenerative diseases • DHIC
Functional		• Conditions causing immobility • Environmental barriers (eg, restraints or bedrails) • Excessive sedation • Psychological disorder – Refusal to go to toilet – Indifference to wetting self • Diuretics • Metabolic disorders causing polyuria – Hyperglycemia – Hypercalcemia
Mixed	23%–33%	

[a]The range in which the reported prevalence falls in most surveys of incontinent middle-aged and older adults.

[b]Empty cells indicate the prevalence is not available.

[c]Among older patients.

GETTING STARTED WITH THE HISTORY

Many patients are embarrassed by UI and may not report it unless asked. The history is the most cost-effective diagnostic tool for detecting UI, although its sensitivity and specificity vary according to the way questions are asked and by the age-specific prevalence of incontinence subtypes. A 7-day voiding diary can provide information about the frequency and circumstances of incontinent episodes, which can be especially helpful when ascertaining the dominant type in a patient reporting mixed symptoms (Figure 44–3). The voiding diary also can be used to track the effectiveness of interventions.

VOIDING DIARY

Name ____________________

Day ____________________

Date____/____/____
Mo Day Year

Instructions:
For **each** time period,

1. In the first column, mark how many times you urinated in the toilet.
2. In the second column, check the box if you had an accident during that time period, then check whether it was a leak (small amount) or a large amount (soaking clothing or pad).
3. In the third column, write down the **reason** for the accident or **the situation in which it occurred.**
   For example,
   If you leaked after coughing, write down, "Coughed."
   If you had an accident after having a strong urge to urinate, write "Urge."
4. In the fourth column, write down about how much time passed in minutes between feeling a strong need to urinate and the time you had the accident. If it was instantaneous, write,"0."

Column #	1	2	3	4
Time period	Times urinated in toilet	Check if accident happened	Reason or situation	Time between urge and accident
6–8 AM		Accident ☐ Leak ☐ Large ☐		
8–10 AM		Accident ☐ Leak ☐ Largc ☐		
10–12 N		Accident ☐ Leak ☐ Large ☐		
12–2 PM		Accident ☐ Leak ☐ Large ☐		
2–4 PM		Accident ☐ Leak ☐ Large ☐		
4–6 PM		Accident ☐ Leak ☐ Large ☐		
6–8 PM		Accident ☐ Leak ☐ Large ☐		
8–10 PM		Accident ☐ Leak ☐ Large ☐		
10–12 MN		Accident ☐ Leak ☐ Large ☐		
Overnight		Accident ☐ Leak ☐ Large ☐		

FIGURE 44–3 Sample voiding diary.

Establishing the Presence of UI

Questions	Remember
Tell me about any troubles you're having with your bladder.	Use simple, easily understood terminology. The first open-ended request encourages the patient to report other bladder symptoms that may be related to the UI.
Tell me about any trouble you're having holding your urine (water).	Specific questions can be used as part of a previsit screening questionnaire.
In the last 6 months, have you lost your urine when you didn't want to? (How often?)	An odor of urine helps establish the presence of UI but may also be a clue to self-neglect and unmet care needs.
In the last 6 months, have you had to wear a pad or a protective undergarment to catch your urine?	
In the last 6 months, have you awoken in the morning with a damp nightgown (pajamas) or bedclothes?	

INTERVIEW FRAMEWORK

Incontinence is a symptom, not a diagnosis. The goal of the interview is to classify the UI in order to focus the physical examination, laboratory testing, and management. The following steps should be performed in most patients presenting with UI:

- CHARACTERISTICS: Assess the basic characteristics of the UI.
  - When does it occur? (Are there associated activities, movements, or circumstances related to the urinary accidents?)
  - Are there warning signs? (Is the UI instantaneous, or is it preceded by an urge to void? If there is urgency, how long between the first urge and the involuntary loss of urine?)
  - How long has it been occurring, and has it been getting worse?
  - What is the frequency, severity, and diurnal pattern of UI? Severity can be measured indirectly by having the patient estimate the number of pads, incontinence briefs, or other protective devices used per day.
  - For patients with a prior history of incontinence:
    - Note *changes* in the frequency, severity, and diurnal pattern.
    - Note previous treatments for UI, their effectiveness, and side effects.
- CAUSES: Assess potentially etiologic or contributing factors.
  - Previous pelvic conditions:
    - Pelvic surgery or radiation therapy
    - Known vaginal prolapse, cystocele, or rectocele
    - Obstetric history (especially number of vaginal deliveries)
    - History of prostate surgery or disease
    - History of pelvic trauma
  - Other lower urinary tract and perineal symptoms (eg, frequency, nocturia, dysuria, hesitancy, dribbling, straining, hematuria, suprapubic or perineal pain).
  - Quantity and timing of fluid intake, especially of caffeine-containing beverages.
  - Presence of conditions that may affect urine output (eg, congestive heart failure, diabetes mellitus).
  - Obtain a list of all prescription and nonprescription drugs and food supplements, because many common medications can affect bladder function (eg, diuretics).
  - Ask about alterations in bowel habits or sexual function.
  - For older patients with new or worsening UI, assess the patient's functional and mental status (eg, mobility, recent falls, confusion).
- CONSEQUENCES AND COPING: Assess the impact of the UI and current management strategies.
  - Ascertain how the patient is currently managing the UI (eg, use of pads and diapers, making sure that a bathroom is always nearby, stopping aerobic exercise).
  - Ask about how the UI is affecting other health-related concerns (eg, sleep, adherence to prescribed medications that may affect bladder function).
  - Determine how the UI is affecting the patient's social functioning. UI is a major cause of social isolation and depression. Because it is an important factor in the decision to institutionalize an older person, assess the reaction of the caregiver (if there is one).
- COLLABORATION: Ask about the patient's goals and expectations for treatment.

IDENTIFYING ALARM SYMPTOMS

- In developmentally disabled and older adults, new or worsening UI may herald acute illness remote from the urinary tract (eg, pneumonia).
- In these patients, UI may be one of several recent changes in the patient's functional status, some of which may be serious (eg, falls, delirium).

Alarm Symptoms	If Present, Consider...
In older or developmentally disabled patients: new or worsening UI with or without other acute changes in the patient's functional or cognitive status	Urinary tract or other infection Acute metabolic disturbance Stroke, myocardial infarction, or other acute medical condition
Continuous leakage (every few minutes) with inability to urinate or sensation of full bladder	Severe urinary retention with overflow Postvoid residual measurement is mandatory to confirm retention.
UI with dysuria	Bacterial cystitis, urethritis from a sexually transmitted disease, atrophic urethritis from estrogen deficiency, nonbacterial cystitis
UI with gross hematuria	Hemorrhagic cystitis, bladder or urethral cancer
UI with polyuria	Metabolic disturbance (eg, hyperglycemia, hypercalcemia)
UI with fecal matter or large air bubbles excreted during urination	Vesicorectal (or vesicosigmoid) fistula resulting from pelvic carcinoma, inflammatory bowel disease, or previous pelvic irradiation
Consistent loss of urine in upright posture or with any action that produces a minimal increase in intra-abdominal pressure, despite bladder not feeling full	Incompetent urethral sphincter or severe pelvic floor collapse

FOCUSED QUESTIONS

These questions help you identify the type(s) of UI and contributing factors. The frequency of symptoms can help determine the relative contribution of each type in cases of mixed incontinence.

QUESTIONS	THINK ABOUT...
For questions marked by an asterisk (*), also ask about frequency: *Never, rarely, once in a while, often, most of the time, all of the time.*[10]	
Quality	
Do you leak urine (even small drops), wet yourself, or wet your pads or undergarments... * *When you cough or sneeze?* * *When you bend down or lift something up?* * *When you walk quickly, jog, or exercise?*	Stress incontinence

—Continued next page

Continued—	
* *While you are undressing to use the toilet?* * *When you delay going to the toilet immediately after first feeling the need to urinate?*	Urge incontinence
Do you get such a strong and uncomfortable need to urinate that you leak (even small drops) or wet yourself before reaching the toilet?	
Do you have to rush to the bathroom because you feel a sudden, strong need to urinate? *Do you experience a warning (urge to urinate)? Is the warning at least 1 minute before you leak urine?*	
• *Yes to both questions*	Urge incontinence
• *No to both questions: urine just comes out*	Detrusor disinhibition Overflow incontinence
• *Yes to first and no to second question: experience a warning, but the urine comes out within a few seconds*	Detrusor disinhibition Urge incontinence with short latency
Do you ever leak urine while seated or lying without realizing it until later?	Detrusor disinhibition Overflow incontinence
Are you unable to feel your bladder getting full before you experience a leakage of urine?	Autonomic neuropathy, causing urinary retention with overflow Detrusor disinhibition
When you leak urine, how large is the amount?	
• *Moderate to large*	Urge incontinence or detrusor disinhibition
• *Small*	Stress or overflow incontinence
Time course	
Did the difficulty controlling your urine start or significantly worsen fairly suddenly, over hours to days? • *Describe any symptoms that accompanied or immediately preceded the start or worsening of your urine leakage.*	
∘ *Symptoms of urge incontinence; see above*	Acute urinary tract infection or urethritis producing urge incontinence
∘ *Sudden onset of weakness or paralysis, suggesting a stroke*	Detrusor disinhibition
∘ *Difficulty starting stream, dribbling (men), sensation of incomplete emptying of bladder*	Urinary retention with overflow
• *Describe any recent procedures that immediately preceded the start or significant worsening of your urine leakage.*	
∘ *Vaginal delivery* ∘ *Transurethral prostatectomy, other urethral instrumentation*	Stress incontinence
∘ *Bladder catheter*	Acute urinary tract infection producing urge incontinence
Did the difficulty controlling your urine come on gradually, over weeks to months?	Any incontinence subtype

Associated symptoms	
Is it painful to urinate?	Urinary tract infection Urethritis from a sexually transmitted disease (STD; eg, chlamydia, gonococcus) Atrophic urethritis (in women, associated with vaginal dryness, painful intercourse, sensitive labia)
Do you need to go frequently (urinary frequency)?	Overactive bladder Urinary tract infection STD with urethritis Atrophic urethritis Diuretics or conditions causing polyuria (eg, diabetes, hypercalcemia)
On average, how long is the interval between leakages?	
• *At least 1 hour*	Urge or detrusor disinhibition
• *Minutes or nearly continuous*	Overflow incontinence
• *Variable (depends on bladder volume plus maneuvers that increase intra-abdominal pressure)*	Stress incontinence
Do you have constipation (eg, last bowel movement 3 or more days ago)?	Fecal impaction, which may cause urge incontinence or urinary retention with overflow
In the past month, have you wet the bed at night, or needed to use a pad or protective cover beneath you because of leaking while asleep?	Detrusor disinhibition Urge incontinence with short latency Functional incontinence (major difficulty getting to the toilet)
Do you need to strain or push to begin your stream? *Is there a significant delay between trying to urinate and the urine starting to flow?*	Obstructive uropathy (eg, from an enlarged prostate), which may cause a hyperactive bladder or urinary retention with overflow
(Men) *Is your stream weak or do you dribble?*	
When you urinate, do you feel that you are unable to completely empty your bladder?	Urinary retention with overflow DHIC in frail, older person
(Women) *How many children have you had by vaginal delivery?*	Stress incontinence due to pelvic floor laxity (the greater the number, the higher the risk)
Pelvic floor disorders (women)[11]	
• *Do you usually experience pressure in the lower abdomen?*	Stress incontinence due to uterine, rectal, or bladder prolapse
• *Do you usually experience pain in the lower abdomen or genital area?*	
• *Do you usually experience heaviness or dullness in the pelvic area?*	
• *Do you usually have a sensation of bulging or protrusion from the vaginal area?*	

—Continued next page

Continued—	
After finishing urinating, do you need to return to the toilet in a few minutes because you feel the need to void again? If yes and you void again, what is the amount?	
• *None to a few drops*	Urethritis or cystitis
• *Small*	Urinary retention with overflow
• *Moderate to large*	Large cystocele[a] Diuretics, conditions causing polyuria (eg, diabetes)
Directed to family member or caregiver: Has the patient been confused?	Delirium or dementia causing detrusor disinhibition (in older patients, delirium and UI may signal an infection or metabolic disturbance; urinary retention may also cause delirium)
Have you been depressed or lost interest in things? *To family member or caregiver: Has the patient seemed very depressed or lost interest in things?*	Detrusor disinhibition Functional incontinence (patient indifferent to self-soiling)
Do you require assistance to go to the toilet?	Functional incontinence
Do you have moderate or severe pain?	Overflow incontinence due to inhibition of sphincter relaxation (from elevated serum catecholamines)
Modifying symptoms	
Is the incontinence worse at night?	Excessive consumption of fluids or caffeinated beverages in the late afternoon or evening Taking diuretics in the evening
Is the incontinence worse during the day?	Excessive consumption of fluids or caffeinated beverages, use of diuretics or drugs that promote diuresis (eg, alcohol, theophylline)
Do you have a chronic cough that makes the incontinence worse?	Stress incontinence
Have you started a new medication or increased the dose?	
• *A diuretic*	Urge or functional incontinence
• *α-Adrenergic blocker (terazosin, others)*	Stress incontinence due to sphincter relaxation
• *Anticholinergic drug (amitriptyline, diphenhydramine, oxybutynin, others)*	Overflow incontinence due to impaired bladder contractility (usually in presence of pre-existing bladder outlet obstruction or detrusor dysfunction)
• *α-Adrenergic agonist (pseudoephedrine, others)*	Overflow incontinence due to inadequate relaxation of sphincter (usually in presence of pre-existing bladder outlet obstruction or detrusor dysfunction)
Have you been spending most of your time in bed?	Overflow incontinence from urinary retention due to prolonged bed rest

[a]*A moderate amount of urine may be trapped inside a large cystocele during toileting but flows back into the main bladder cavity when the patient lies down, causing the patient to re-experience bladder fullness.*

DIAGNOSTIC APPROACH (INCLUDING ALGORITHM)

See Figure 44–4 for the diagnostic approach algorithm for urinary incontinence.

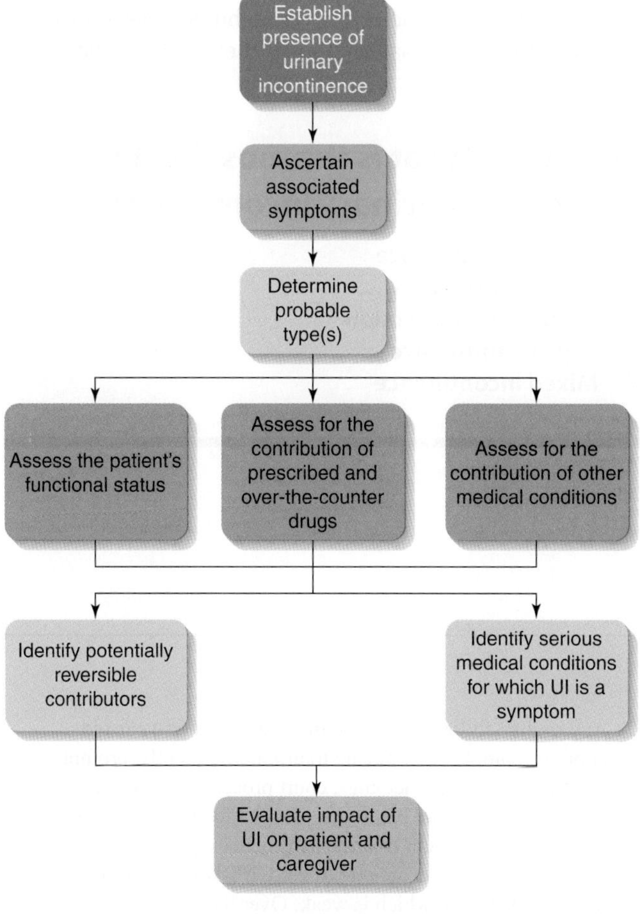

FIGURE 44–4 Diagnostic approach to the patient with urinary incontinence (UI).

CAVEATS

- Because UI is a symptom, a diagnostic approach aimed solely at identifying the type may preclude identification of serious underlying conditions or iatrogenic contributors.
- In elderly and disabled persons, UI may herald other functional impairments. Evaluation of UI should include an assessment of the patient's cognitive and physical functioning.
- Urge incontinence and detrusor disinhibition in elderly and disabled persons often persist as a chronic condition, which may have a negative impact on the patient's and caregiver's quality of life. Periodic reassessment of intervention strategies and patient and caregiver coping is an essential part of the ongoing management of UI.

PROGNOSIS

Approximately one-third of middle-aged and older women with infrequent leakage (once per month) will progress to weekly or more frequent UI over the course of 2 years. Conversely, fewer than 10% of women with frequent leakage report a reduction in UI to once a month or less 2 years later.[7]

- Acute UI related to reversible causes generally has a good prognosis.
- Both urge and stress UI can improve with bladder retraining exercises, which may be as effective as medication.
- Topical estrogens may improve mild stress and urge UI.
- Anticholinergic medication for urge UI (oxybutynin, darifenacin, and others) may increase the latency between urge and leakage and thus reduce the frequency of incontinent episodes.
- Newer surgical techniques and artificial sphincters have improved the prognosis for patients with severe UI due to pelvic floor dysfunction or sphincter incompetence.

CASE SCENARIO | Resolution

A healthy 51-year-old stockbroker comes to clinic for an annual checkup. She states that over the past year she has gained 25 lbs and attributes the weight gain to giving up jogging and jazzercise classes. She relates that running and jumping sometimes cause her to leak urine, which is uncomfortable and embarrassing. She now uses a heavy panty liner at all times to avoid wetting herself. She is upset that she is "developing a bladder like my 80-year-old mother."

ADDITIONAL HISTORY

The patient, the mother of 2 teenage sons by vaginal delivery, still menstruates, although her periods have become irregular. She began wearing the panty liners as protection for those times that she might have to wait more than a few minutes after feeling an urge to void. In recent months, she has noticed that when her bladder is full, the urge to void can be sudden and intense. By squeezing her pelvic muscles, she is able to keep from involuntarily emptying her bladder before she reaches the toilet, but she has noticed that she still leaks a small amount at the very beginning of the voiding urge.

Question: What is the most likely cause of her urinary incontinence?

A. Stress incontinence
B. Pelvic prolapse
C. Urinary tract infection
D. Urge incontinence
E. Mixed incontinence

Test Your Knowledge

1. A 74-year-old woman with a history of hypertension (treated with a thiazide diuretic) and well-controlled diabetes mellitus comes to your clinic with the youngest of her 4 children for follow-up of a sprained left ankle sustained after tripping and falling 6 days ago. After the fall, she went to the emergency department, where a fracture was ruled out and she was prescribed a narcotic analgesic and given a cane. She reports moderate pain when she bears weight on her left ankle. Since the fall, she complains of 1 to 2 episodes of urinary incontinence per day, often while in bed, soaking her underwear and bed sheets. Before the ankle sprain, she had experienced occasional episodes of slight moistening of her panties when she got up from her seat after a long movie or plane ride, but otherwise was able to get to the bathroom in time. She denies dysuria or frequent urination, and states that she has cut back on liquids to avoid having to go to the bathroom as often.

   What is the most likely explanation for her worsened urinary incontinence?

   A. Progression of stress incontinence
   B. Urinary tract infection
   C. Side effect of the diuretic medication
   D. Functional incontinence
   E. Overflow incontinence resulting from diabetic autonomic neuropathy

2. At a routine follow-up appointment, Mr. S, a 64-year-old attorney, complains of having to urinate frequently, prompting him to interrupt meetings, court proceedings, and social activities to go to the bathroom. Despite feeling a strong need to urinate, the amount of urine he produces is small—"just a few ounces." Despite an urge to void, it takes several seconds to start the stream, which is weak. Over the past 2 months, he has noticed that the urge to void can come on suddenly and intensely, sometimes accompanied by leakage of a small amount of urine that visibly wets his pants (which he finds extremely embarrassing). If he zips up his trousers promptly after emptying his bladder, he often finds a small wet mark on the front of his pants when he leaves the washroom. Because of his long work hours, Mr. S admits to a long-standing habit of drinking an espresso in the morning and 2 to 3 cups of regular coffee over the course of the day.

   What is the most likely etiology of his incontinence?

   A. Idiopathic overactive bladder
   B. Incompetent urethral sphincter
   C. Bladder outlet obstruction with overflow
   D. Excessive caffeine intake
   E. Detrusor hyperactivity due to prostatic hyperplasia

3. An 87-year-old woman is brought from her assisted living facility for evaluation of urinary incontinence. She is wheelchair-bound and has early Alzheimer's disease. She has required diapers since her admission 3 months ago. The patient complains of a constant need to urinate and that her diapers are always wet. Her aide confirms that she has to change the patient's diapers at least 6 times a day. The patient informs the staff when she has to urinate, but involuntarily voids into the diaper if not brought to the toilet within 2 to 3 minutes. The aide notes that after changing a diaper, the new one becomes damp within 1 hour and saturated within 4 hours.

   This pattern of incontinence is most consistent with which of the following types?

   A. Detrusor disinhibition
   B. Detrusor hyperactivity with incomplete contraction (DHIC)
   C. Functional incontinence
   D. Outflow tract obstruction with overflow
   E. Urge incontinence

References

1. Shamliyan TA, Wyman JF, Ping R, Wilt TJ, Kane RL. Male urinary incontinence: prevalence, risk factors, and preventive interventions. *Rev Urol.* 2009;11:145–165.
2. Melville JL, Katon W, Delaney K, Newton K. Urinary incontinence in US women: a population-based study. *Arch Intern Med.* 2005;165:537–542.
3. Sung VW, Hampton BS. Epidemiology of pelvic floor dysfunction. *Obstet Gynecol Clin North Am.* 2009;36:421–443.
4. Subak L, Van Den Eeden S, Thom D, Creasman JM, Brown JS. Urinary incontinence in women: direct costs of routine care. *Am J Obstet Gynecol.* 2007;197:596.e591–599.
5. Tyagi S, Thomas CA, Hayashi Y, Chancellor MB. The overactive bladder: epidemiology and morbidity. *Urol Clin North Am.* 2006;33:433–438.
6. Nuotio M, Jylha M, Luukkaala T, Tammela TL. Urgency, urge incontinence and voiding symptoms in men and women aged 70 years and over. *BJU Int.* 2002;89:350–355.
7. Lifford KL, Townsend MK, Curhan GC, Resnick NM, Grodstein F. The epidemiology of urinary incontinence in older women: incidence, progression, and remission. *J Am Geriatr Soc.* 2008;56:1191–1198.
8. Miller YD, Brown WJ, Russell A, Chiarelli P. Urinary incontinence across the lifespan. *Neurourol Urodyn.* 2003;22: 550–557.
9. Parazzini F, Chiaffarino F, Lavezzari M, Giambanco V. Risk factors for stress, urge or mixed urinary incontinence in Italy. *BJOG.* 2003;110:927–933.
10. Bradley CS, Rovner ES, Morgan MA, et al. A new questionnaire for urinary incontinence diagnosis in women: development and testing. *Am J Obstet Gynecol.* 2005;192:66–73.
11. Barber MD, Kuchibhatla MN, Pieper CF, Bump RC. Psychometric evaluation of 2 comprehensive condition-specific quality of life instruments for women with pelvic floor disorders. *Am J Obstet Gynecol.* 2001;185:1388–1395.

Suggested Reading

Abed H, Rogers RG. Urinary incontinence and pelvic organ prolapse: diagnosis and treatment for the primary care physician. *Med Clin North Am.* 2008;92:1273–1293.

Gibbs CF, Johnson TM 2nd, Ouslander JG. Office management of geriatric urinary incontinence. *Am J Med.* 2007;120: 211–220.

Holroyd-Leduc JM, Tannenbaum C, Thorpe KE, Straus SE. What type of urinary incontinence does this woman have? *JAMA.* 2008;299:1446–1456.

Smith PP, McCrery RJ, Appell RA. Current trends in the evaluation and management of female urinary incontinence. *CMAJ.* 2006;175:1233–1240.

Chapter 45

Scrotal Pain

Mysti D.W. Schott, MD

CASE SCENARIO

A 10-year-old boy comes to the emergency department with right-sided scrotal pain that began 27 hours earlier.

- **What additional questions would you ask to learn more about the pain?**
- **How do you differentiate the various causes of scrotal pain?**
- **What features suggest an alarming or urgent problem?**
- **Can you make a definite diagnosis through an open-ended history followed by focused questions?**

INTRODUCTION

Scrotal pain is a relatively common complaint in multiple settings, including primary care and the emergency department (accounting for 0.5% of total emergency department visits each year[1]). It occurs in all age groups, from childhood to late adulthood. Scrotal pain can result from a variety of causes, including emergencies that can lead to testicular morbidity and benign conditions requiring no intervention.

Although the patient's history may suggest the cause of scrotal pain, a focused physical examination is required to confirm the diagnosis. A careful history can help narrow the diagnosis and identify alarm symptoms that require urgent evaluation and treatment. In addition, it will suggest the appropriate diagnostic testing for more chronic and benign causes of pain.

KEY TERMS

Testicular appendage	Remnants of müllerian duct system located on the testicle or epididymis.
Orchitis	Inflammation/infection of the testicle.
Varicocele	Dilation and engorgement of the pampiniform plexus of spermatic veins.
Epididymal cyst	Cyst at the head of the epididymis.
Spermatocele	Large epididymal cyst (> 2 cm).
Hydrocele	Collection of fluid in the tunica vaginalis that surrounds the testicle and spermatic cord.
Epididymitis	Infection and/or inflammation of the epididymis.
Testicular torsion	Twisting and strangulation of the testicle on the spermatic cord. Due to a congenital poor fixation of the testicle to the tunica vaginalis.
Fournier's gangrene	Severe subcutaneous tissue bacterial infection of the perineum spreading from skin to muscle and underlying structures, causing death of infected tissue.
Referred pain	Pain at a site removed from the actual disease.

ETIOLOGY

The key to understanding the different etiologies of scrotal pain requires an understanding of scrotal anatomy (Figures 45–1 and 45–2). In addition to the testicle, the scrotum contains the epididymis, which sits posteriorly on the testicle connected at its base to the spermatic cord. Within the spermatic cord are the vas deferens, testicular artery, and spermatic veins. A large portion of the testicle and spermatic cord is surrounded by the tunica vaginalis, which has a parietal and a visceral layer. Additionally there are 4 testicular appendages: the appendix testes, appendix epididymis, vas aberrans, and paradidymis. These are embryologic remnants of the müllerian duct system.

Scrotal pain should be characterized as either acute or chronic. The age of the patient helps determine the cause. The most common causes of acute scrotal pain are testicular torsion, torsion of one of the testicular appendages, and epididymitis.[2–5] Older studies found testicular torsion to have the highest incidence, but these studies may have oversampled hospitalized and postoperative patients and missed patients discharged from the emergency department or physicians' offices after having torsion clinically ruled out. More recent studies of emergency department patients show a higher incidence of epididymitis and torsion of the testicular appendage, with testicular torsion occurring an average of 17% to 25% of the time.[3,4]

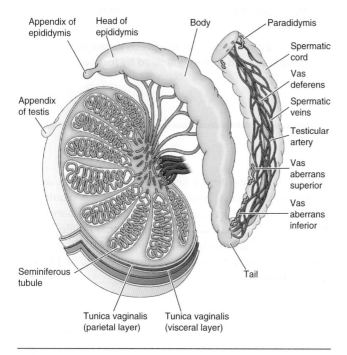

FIGURE 45–1 Normal scrotal anatomy.

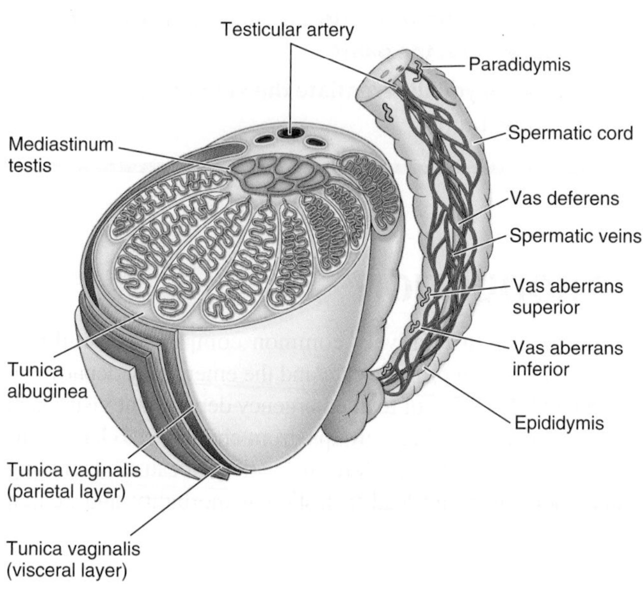

FIGURE 45–2 Cross section of normal scrotal anatomy.

Differential Diagnosis of Acute Scrotal Pain

Differential Diagnosis	Prevalence Among Patients Presenting to the Emergency Department With Scrotal Pain[a]
Testicular torsion	16%–42%[2–5]
Epididymitis-orchitis	10%–36%[2–5]
Torsion of testicular appendage	30%–45%[2–5]
Prostatitis	
Traumatic testicular rupture	

Traumatic hematoma	
Fournier's gangrene	
Strangulated inguinal hernia	8%[3]
Hemorrhage/edema into previously undiagnosed testicular cancer	
Henoch-Schönlein purpura	
Orchitis (mumps, etc)	
Scrotal abscess	
Urolithiasis	
Appendicitis and other causes of peritonitis	
Abdominal aortic aneurysm rupture	
Constipation	

[a]Empty cells indicate that the prevalence is unknown.

Differential Diagnosis of Nonacute Scrotal Pain[a]

Varicocele
Hydrocele
Epididymal cyst/spermatocele
Inguinal hernia
Testicular cancer
Epididymitis
Postvasectomy
Retroperitoneal tumor
Neurogenic causes (pudendal nerve entrapment, vertebral disease with sacral nerve root impingement)
Chronic scrotal pain syndrome (idiopathic)

[a]Empty cells indicate that the prevalence is unknown.

The differential diagnosis of acute scrotal pain can be narrowed by considering the patient's age, although no cause can reliably be ruled out based solely on age.[6] Testicular torsion and torsion of the testicular appendage occur predominately in patients under age 20 but can occur at any age. There have even been case reports of men in their 60s and 70s with testicular torsion.

Testicular torsion occurs when the testicle is not properly fixed to the scrotal wall (see Figure 45–2). Incidence peaks in 2 age groups: neonate and pubescence, which are ages of high testicular movement or growth. Testicular appendages, pedunculated remnants of the müllerian duct system, may also undergo torsion typically in the prepubescent and early teen years.[2,3,5,6]

Testicular cancer occurs in men age 18 to 40. Similarly, abdominal aortic aneurysm, Fournier's gangrene, or retroperitoneal tumor would present in an adult male over age 50. Epididymitis occurs in all ages.[6]

GETTING STARTED WITH THE HISTORY

- Let the patient tell the story in his own words before asking more directed and focused questions.
- With scrotal pain, the history directs your physical examination and any subsequent diagnostic testing or procedures.

Questions	Remember
Tell me more about your scrotal pain.	Listen to the story.
When did this pain first start?	Do not interrupt or focus the history too soon.
Have you ever had this pain before? Tell me about that.	

INTERVIEW FRAMEWORK

- Inquire about the scrotal pain using the cardinal symptom features:
  - Timing
    - Onset: Gradual or sudden?
    - Duration: Hours, days, or weeks?
    - Frequency: Constant or intermittent? (Any prior episodes that spontaneously resolved?)
  - Pain character: Sharp or dull?
  - Location of pain: Focal scrotal, diffuse scrotal, generalized to the lower pelvic area, or radiating even further?
  - Pain severity: Mild, moderate, or severe?
  - Setting in which pain has occurred:
    - After physical or sexual activity?
    - During the night while asleep?
    - Trauma?
    - Recent genitourinary instrumentation or surgery?
  - Associated features:
    - Fever, dysuria, nausea, vomiting, urethral discharge, or penile lesions?
- Additionally, the patient's sexual history plays a key role by identifying potential infectious causes of the patient's symptoms.
  - Sexually active? Recently?
  - Number of partners?
  - Sexual orientation?

IDENTIFYING ALARM SYMPTOMS

- Acute spontaneous pain in a young male is most worrisome for testicular torsion, which may lead to testicular infarction and loss if not treated in a timely manner.
- The more acute, diffuse, and severe the scrotal pain is, the more likely it is due to a serious cause requiring urgent evaluation.

Serious Causes of Scrotal Pain

There are serious causes of both acute and nonacute scrotal pain. Untreated, testicular morbidity is high in both testicular torsion and traumatic testicular rupture. There is also high mortality in Fournier's gangrene and ruptured abdominal aortic aneurysm. Appendicitis and other causes of peritonitis are also serious causes.

Testicular cancer is often thought of as a "painless mass." However, Wilson and Cooksey reviewed 115 patients with testicular cancer and found that 23.5% presented with pain alone or pain with swelling.[7] The pain can be acute or nonacute.

Alarm Symptoms	If Present, Consider Serious Causes...	Positive Likelihood Ratio (LR+) for Predicting Serious Cause	However, Benign Causes Include...
Sharp/severe pain	Testicular torsion		
Recurrent episodes of pain	Testicular torsion	3.82[5]	
Awakening during the night or morning with severe pain	Testicular torsion		
Pain unrelieved with elevation of scrotal contents	Testicular torsion		
Pain after physical or sexual activity	Testicular torsion		

Pain after trauma	Testicular rupture Testicular torsion	3.57[5,a]	Testicular hematoma
Nausea/vomiting	Testicular torsion Appendicitis Peritonitis	9.86[5,a]	Epididymitis
Sudden pain and swelling	Testicular torsion Testicular cancer (hemorrhage or edema into a mass)		
Abdominal pain	Aortic aneurysm rupture Peritonitis Appendicitis Testicular torsion Fournier's gangrene		Nephrolithiasis Prostatitis
Fever	Fournier's gangrene Appendicitis		Epididymitis Prostatitis

[a]LR for testicular torsion as cause.

FOCUSED QUESTIONS

After asking open-ended questions and considering possible alarm symptoms, ask the following questions to narrow the differential diagnosis.

QUESTIONS	THINK ABOUT...
Onset	
Is the onset:	
• *Acute (sudden onset)?*	Testicular torsion
• *Subacute (up to a few days)?*	Torsion of testicular appendage Epididymitis Orchitis Fournier's gangrene Aortic aneurysm rupture Appendicitis/peritonitis
• *Nonacute (chronic)?*	Varicocele Hydrocele Testicular cancer Epididymal cyst
Duration	
• *Is the duration < 12 hours?*	Testicular torsion

—Continued next page

Continued—

Question	Differential diagnosis
Frequency	
Do you have recurrent episodes that resolve spontaneously?	Testicular torsion
Pain character	
Is the scrotal pain:	
• *Sharp?*	Testicular torsion Torsion of testicular appendage
• *Dull, aching?*	Varicocele Hydrocele
How severe is the pain?	
• *Severe*	Testicular torsion Strangulated inguinal hernia Fournier's gangrene
• *Moderate*	Torsion of testicular appendage Epididymitis
Location of pain	
Where is the pain located in your scrotum?	
• *Diffuse*	Testicular torsion Varicocele Hydrocele
• *Upper pole of testis*	Torsion of testicular appendage
• *Epididymis*	Epididymitis Epididymal cyst Postvasectomy pain
• *Left sided*	Varicocele
Associated features	
Do you have:	
• *Fever?*	Epididymitis Testicular torsion Trauma Appendicitis Fournier's gangrene
• *Hematuria?*	Epididymitis
• *Hematospermia?*	Prostatitis
• *Infertility?*	Varicocele
• *Nausea/vomiting?*	Testicular torsion Trauma Appendicitis Peritonitis

• *Testicular atrophy?*	Varicocele
• *Scrotal swelling?*	Epididymitis Testicular torsion Torsion of testicular appendage Trauma Hydrocele Varicocele (swelling resolves when in recumbent position; feels like "bag of worms") Epididymal cyst Inguinal hernia Mumps
• *Gynecomastia?*	Testicular cancer
• *Arthralgia?*	Henoch-Schönlein purpura
• *Abdominal pain?*	Testicular torsion Torsion of testicular appendage Fournier's gangrene Henoch-Schönlein purpura
• *Gastrointestinal bleeding?*	Henoch-Schönlein purpura
• *Dysuria?*	Epididymitis Trauma
Setting	
What occurred prior to the onset of this pain?	
• *Sexual activity*	Testicular torsion Torsion of testicular appendage
• *Physical activity*	Testicular torsion Torsion of testicular appendage
• *Vasectomy*	Epididymitis Postvasectomy referred pain
• *Prolonged sitting*	Epididymitis (inflammatory)
• *Trauma*	Testicular rupture Testicular torsion Testicular hematoma
• *Recent urinary catheter or procedure*	Prostatitis Epididymitis

DIAGNOSTIC APPROACH (INCLUDING ALGORITHM)

The first step is to distinguish between acute and nonacute scrotal pain. In evaluating acute pain, clinicians must pay particular attention to the presence of alarm features. Timely diagnosis of serious acute causes of scrotal pain will prevent morbidity and mortality. Figure 45–3 presents the algorithm for evaluating patients with scrotal pain.

Unfortunately, no historical features have been shown to reliably differentiate between the top 3 causes of acute scrotal pain in children.[2,5] Nonetheless, the following features are more worrisome for testicular torsion: presentation at < 12 hours of pain,[3,5] severe pain, abrupt onset of pain, prior episodes of pain, nausea/vomiting, and lack of dysuria.

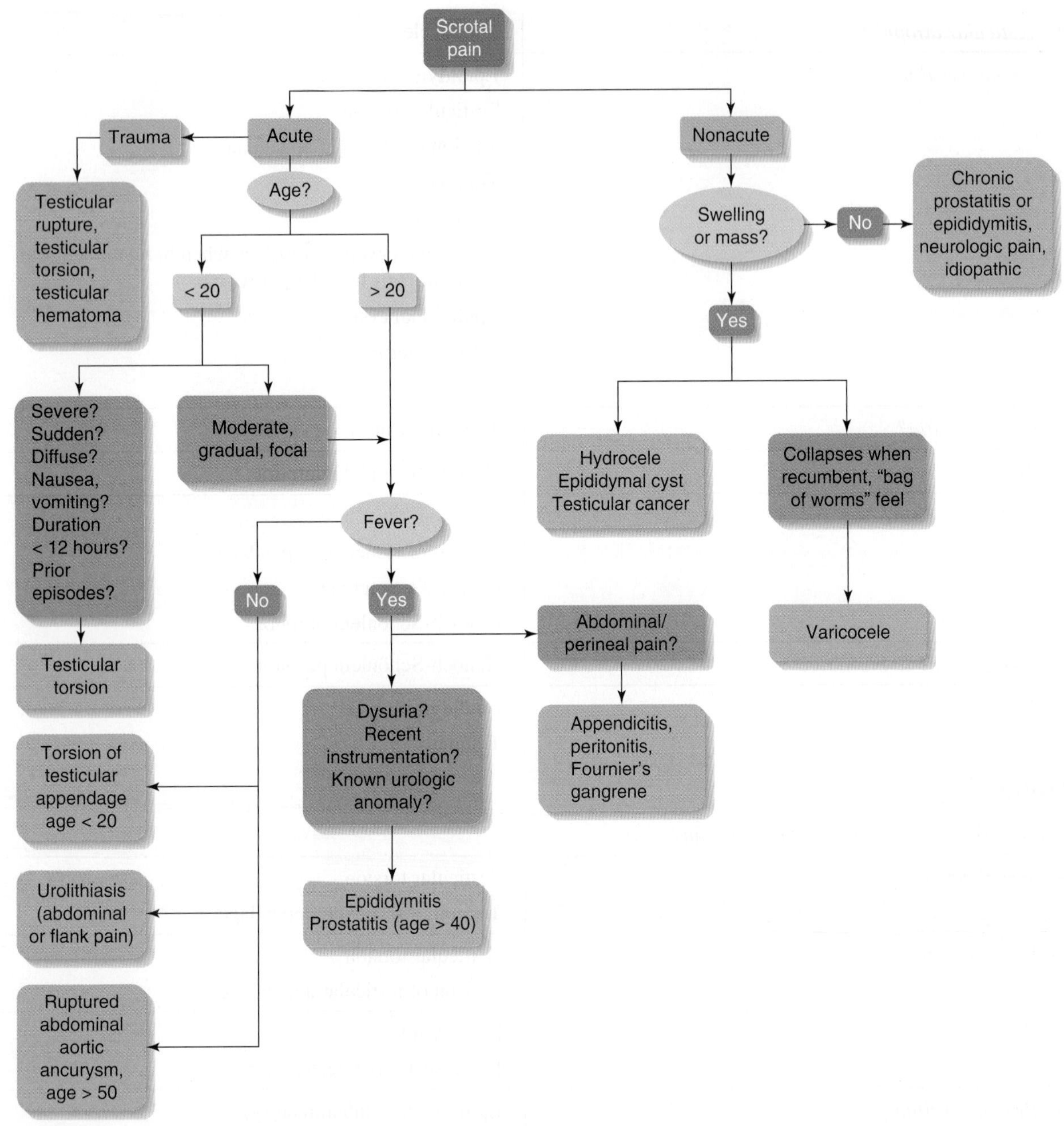

FIGURE 45–3 Algorithm for evaluating patients with scrotal pain.

Feature	LR+ for the Diagnosis of Testicular Torsion Compared to Epididymitis or Torsion of Testicular Appendage	LR– for the Diagnosis of Testicular Torsion Compared to Epididymitis or Torsion of Testicular Appendage
Prior episode(s) of pain	3.4[2]	0.87[2]
Nausea/vomiting	9[2]	0.40[2]
Abdominal pain	2.85[2]	0.87[2]
Dysuria	0.28[10]	1.45[10]

CAVEATS

- The scrotal pain history must always be followed by a physical examination. If there is any doubt about the diagnosis, an appropriate imaging study, usually ultrasonography, should be obtained.
- Testicular torsion is most likely in patients under 20 but may occur in older patients.
- Patients with acute testicular torsion present earlier in their course than patients with torsion of the testicular appendage or epididymitis.
- If no scrotal pathology is found, consider referred pain.

PROGNOSIS

The prognosis for testicular torsion is poor, especially if not recognized (and treated) in a timely manner. Epididymitis and torsion of a testicular appendage will not cause significant morbidity. There are several other potentially fatal causes of scrotal pain, including Fournier's gangrene and abdominal aortic aneurysm rupture, that must be recognized and treated immediately. Chronic causes of scrotal pain are typically benign with treatment based on the patient's level of discomfort from the symptoms.

CASE SCENARIO | Resolution

A 10-year-old boy comes to the emergency department with right-sided scrotal pain that began 27 hours earlier.

ADDITIONAL HISTORY

The pain is described as a gradual-onset, moderately severe, constant pain. When asked to localize the pain, the patient points to the anterior superior pole of his testicle. He denies fever, dysuria, nausea, or vomiting. He has never had anything like this previously and denies recent trauma.

Question: What is the most likely diagnosis?

A. Torsion of testicular appendage
B. Epididymitis
C. Testicular torsion
D. Testicular rupture

Test Your Knowledge

1. A 46-year-old man presents complaining of dull, left-sided scrotal pain and swelling. The swelling goes away when he lays down. The patient reports that he isn't really sure when his symptoms started, but they have been present and slowly progressive for several years. With further questioning, he admits to infertility.

   Which is the most likely diagnosis?

   A. Testicular torsion
   B. Prostatitis
   C. Varicocele
   D. Hydrocele
   E. Epididymitis

2. A 15-year-old boy presents for his routine annual checkup with his pediatrician. He reluctantly admits to 2 recent episodes of pain in his left testicle. The pain was quite intense but subsided in 15 minutes and 60 minutes, respectively.

   Which of the following is the most likely cause of recurrent episodes of testicular pain that resolve spontaneously?

   A. Acute appendicitis
   B. Testicular torsion
   C. Epididymitis
   D. Torsion of the testicular appendage

3. A 78-year-old man presents to your clinic with gradual onset of perineal and scrotal pain and fever over the past 36 hours. He was recently hospitalized with pneumonia and discharged 7 days ago. With further questioning, he reports dysuria since hospital discharge, which he relates to the removal of a bladder catheter he had in place while in the hospital.

   Which of the following is the most likely cause of his pain?

   A. Urolithiasis
   B. Abdominal aortic aneurysm
   C. Testicular torsion
   D. Inguinal hernia
   E. Prostatitis

References

1. Lewis AG, Bukowski TP, Jarvie PD, et al. Evaluation of the acute scrotum in the emergency department. *J Pediatr Surg*. 1995;30:277–281.
2. Lyronis ID, Ploumis N, Vlahakis I, Chjarissis G. Acute scrotum: etiology, clinical presentation and seasonal variation. *Indian J Pediatr*. 2009;76:407–410.
3. Makela E, Lahdes-Vasama T, Rajakorpi H, Wikstrom S. A 19-year review of paediatric patients with acute scrotum. *Scand J Surg*. 2007;96:62–66.
4. Burgher S. Acute scrotal pain. *Emerg Med Clin North Am*. 1998;16:781–809.
5. Ciftci AO, Senocak ME, Tanyel FC, Buyukpamukcu N. Clinical predictors for the differential diagnosis of acute scrotum. *Eur J Pediatr Surg*. 2004;14:333–338.
6. Marcozzi D, Suner S. The nontraumatic, acute scrotum. *Emerg Med Clin North Am*. 2001;19:547–568.
7. Wilson JP, Cooksey G. Testicular pain as the initial presentation of testicular neoplasms. *Ann R Coll Surg Engl*. 2004;86:284–288.

Suggested Reading

Cole F, Vogler R. The acute, nontraumatic scrotum: assessment, diagnosis, and management. *J Am Acad Nurse Pract*. 2004;16:54–60.

McGee S. Referred scrotal pain. *J Gen Intern Med*. 1993;8:694–701.

Trojian T, Lishnak T, Heiman D. Epididymitis and orchitis: an overview. *Am Fam Physician*. 2009;79:583–587.

SECTION

IX

WOMEN'S HEALTH

Chapter 46

Amenorrhea

Stephany Sanchez, MD, Steven Gelber, MD, MPH, and Tonya Fancher, MD, MPH, FACP

CASE SCENARIO

A 26 year-old woman comes to clinic for evaluation of abnormal menses. After having previously irregular menses, she now reports a 9-month history of amenorrhea. She and her husband are now interested in having a child.

- **What additional questions would you ask to characterize her abnormal menstrual cycles?**
- **Which questions will help you diagnose the major causes of amenorrhea?**
- **What clues would you look for on physical examination?**

INTRODUCTION

Amenorrhea, the absence of menses, is a common problem in the primary care setting. This condition may be transient, intermittent, or permanent, and usually results from congenital, neuroendocrine, or anatomic abnormalities. The first diagnostic step is determining whether amenorrhea is primary (before menarche) or secondary (after menarche).

Primary amenorrhea is the absence of menses by age 16 in the presence of otherwise normal secondary sexual characteristics or by age 14 if secondary sexual development has not occurred. Secondary amenorrhea is the absence of menses for 3 months in a woman with previously normal menses or 9 months in a woman with oligomenorrhea (light or infrequent menses).[1]

A thorough history and physical examination helps narrow the differential diagnosis prior to ordering any laboratory tests or studies.

KEY TERMS

Asherman's syndrome	Intrauterine adhesions usually resulting from uterine instrumentation (eg, curettage or scraping of the uterine cavity to remove tissue).
Follicle-stimulating hormone (FSH) and luteinizing hormone (LH)	Pituitary hormones that stimulate the follicles of the ovary and assist in follicular maturation.
Gonadal dysgenesis (Turner syndrome)	The failure of the gonads to develop in the presence of an abnormal karyotype. Gonadal failure in the presence of a normal karyotype is termed gonadal agenesis.
Gonadotropin-releasing hormone (GnRH)	A hormone secreted by the hypothalamus that stimulates FSH and LH release.
Hypothalamic or functional amenorrhea	Disorder of GnRH release resulting in loss of the LH surge and anovulation.
Hypothalamic-pituitary-ovarian (HPO) axis	The hormonal regulatory system that controls the menstrual/reproductive cycle.

—Continued next page

Continued—	
Müllerian agenesis	The absence of the fallopian tubes, uterus, and internal portion of the vagina. Patients have normal female genotype, normal secondary sex characteristics (phenotype), and amenorrhea.
Polycystic ovarian syndrome (PCOS)	Syndrome characterized by hirsutism (excessive body and facial hair), obesity, menstrual abnormalities, infertility, and enlarged ovaries.
Postpill amenorrhea	Failure to resume ovulation 6 months after discontinuing hormonal contraception.
Premature ovarian failure	Depletion of oocytes and surrounding follicles before age 40. Causes include chemotherapy, radiation, and autoimmune disease.
Primary amenorrhea	The absence of menses by age 16 if otherwise normal development of secondary sexual characteristics, or by age 14 if secondary sexual development has not occurred.
Secondary amenorrhea	The absence of menses for 3 months in a woman with a previously normal menses or for 9 months in a woman with oligomenorrhea.

ETIOLOGY

Primary amenorrhea in the United States has a prevalence of 0.3%. Secondary amenorrhea is much more common, with a prevalence of 3.3% (excluding pregnancy).[2] Once pregnancy has been ruled out, the causes of secondary amenorrhea include ovarian disease (40%), hypothalamic dysfunction (35%), pituitary disease (19%), uterine disease (5%), and other (1%).[3]

The Normal Menstrual Cycle

Understanding the normal menstrual cycle is fundamental to determining the etiology of amenorrhea. Menstruation results from a complex interaction between the hypothalamic-pituitary axis, the ovaries, and the outflow tract (Figure 46–1).[4] An intact and functioning hypothalamus secretes gonadotropin-releasing hormone (GnRH) in a pulsatile fashion, causing the anterior pituitary to release follicle-stimulating hormone (FSH) and luteinizing hormone (LH). The released FSH and LH then act on the ovary to release estradiol and progesterone. These hormones, in turn, downregulate the production of GnRH, LH, and FSH through negative feedback to the hypothalamus and pituitary. FSH causes a dominant follicle to develop. A midcycle peak in estrogen secretion stimulates an LH surge that triggers ovulation. Following ovulation, a corpus luteum cyst develops, which produces progesterone and stimulates growth of the endometrium. If fertilization does not occur, the corpus luteum involutes and menses occurs. Any disruption in this complex pathway can result in abnormal menses.[1]

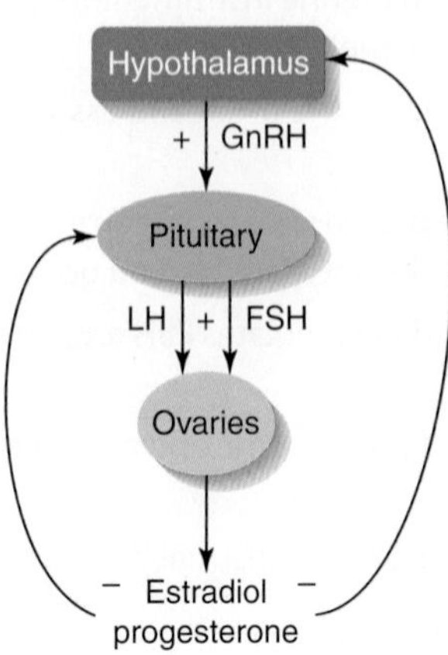

FIGURE 46–1 The hypothalamic-pituitary axis. FSH, follicle-stimulating hormone; GnRH, gonadotropin-releasing hormone; LH, luteinizing hormone.

Differential Diagnosis

Once pregnancy has been ruled out, the most common causes of amenorrhea are diseases of the ovaries, hypothalamic-pituitary-ovarian (HPO) axis, and uterus. Ovarian diseases include ovarian failure and hyperandrogenism (eg, polycystic ovarian syndrome [PCOS]). Disruption of the HPO axis, such as decreased GnRH secretion from an eating disorder, exercise, or stress, can also cause amenorrhea. Uterine causes should be considered in a woman with a history of uterine infection or prior instrumentation with resultant scarring of the endometrium. If the history and physical suggest primary amenorrhea, congenital and anatomic abnormalities must also be considered.

Causes and Prevalence of Primary and Secondary Amenorrhea

Primary amenorrhea	*Prevalence*[4,5]
Pregnancy	Most common
Gonadal dysgenesis (Turner syndrome)	40%
Constitutional delay	18%
Müllerian agenesis	10%
Androgen insensitivity	9%
Prolactin-secreting tumor	5%
Stress, weight loss, anorexia (hypothalamic amenorrhea)	3%
Congenital adrenal hyperplasia	3%
Obstructed outflow tract (transverse vaginal septum, imperforate hymen)	3%
Kallmann syndrome	2%
Other	1%
Secondary amenorrhea	***Prevalence***[2,4]
Pregnancy	Most common
Ovarian disease	40%
• PCOS	• 30%
• Premature ovarian failure	• 10%
Hypothalamic dysfunction	35%
• Stress	• 10%–21%
• Weight loss/anorexia/bulimia	• 15%–54%
• Infiltrative lesions or tumors (lymphoma, sarcoidosis)	• < 0.1%
Pituitary disease	19%
• Prolactin-secreting tumor	• 17%
• Empty sella syndrome	• 1%
• Sheehan syndrome	• 1%
• Adrenocorticotropic hormone-secreting tumor	• < 1%
• Growth hormone secreting tumor	
Uterine	7%
• Asherman's syndrome	• 7%
Other	1%
• Nonclassic adrenal hyperplasia	
• Drug induced	
• Postpill amenorrhea	

Reversible Versus Irreversible Causes of Amenorrhea	
Reversible Causes[3,5]	*Irreversible Causes*[6]
• Imperforate hymen • Asherman's syndrome • Polycystic ovarian syndrome • Hyperprolactinemia • Postpill amenorrhea • Drug induced • Exercise, stress, or weight loss induced • Systemic illness	• Empty sella syndrome • Cushing's syndrome • Kallmann syndrome • Gonadal dysgenesis • Müllerian defects • Androgen insensitivity syndrome

GETTING STARTED WITH THE HISTORY

- Let the patient tell the story in her own words without interruption, before asking more direct and focused questions.
- Try to assess the patient's overall health status. Poor overall health can cause amenorrhea.
- If the patient is not alone, set aside time to speak with her privately. Patients may be uncomfortable discussing certain issues with friends or family members present.
- Although a history is essential, keep in mind that laboratory tests and imaging will often be required to make the diagnosis.

Pertinent Questions
Tell me about your periods.
At what age did your periods begin?
When did your last period begin?
Do you have regular periods?
What is your usual cycle length?
Could you be pregnant?

INTERVIEW FRAMEWORK

- Explore the possibility of pregnancy first.
- Assess for alarm symptoms that may require urgent evaluation.
- Classify whether the patient has primary or secondary amenorrhea, which narrows the differential diagnosis and informs subsequent diagnostic testing.
- If the patient has primary amenorrhea, consider congenital or genetic disorders.
- Be sure to ask about other developmental problems. Remember that development will be normal in patients with outflow tract defects.
- Secondary amenorrhea is more likely to be due to a neuroendocrine disorder. The interview should include a detailed menstrual history from menarche to present.

IDENTIFYING ALARM SYMPTOMS

Amenorrhea is rarely a medical emergency, but some causes require prompt diagnosis and treatment.

Alarm Signs and Symptoms	Consider
Recent unprotected intercourse	Pregnancy
Headaches, galactorrhea, loss of peripheral vision	Pituitary tumor
Body weight 15% below ideal and impaired body image	Anorexia

FOCUSED QUESTIONS

After asking the open-ended questions and listening to the patient's story, ask more focused questions to narrow the differential diagnosis.

QUESTIONS	THINK ABOUT...
Have you had unprotected intercourse?	Pregnancy
Have you had morning nausea?	Pregnancy
Have you noticed that most of your friends developed breasts and pubic hair before you?	Hypogonadism Turner syndrome
Are most of your friends (of similar age) taller than you?	Hypogonadism Turner syndrome
Have you recently gained weight?	PCOS Thyroid disease
Have you recently lost weight?	Hypothalamic dysfunction Occult malignancy
Have you ever been told that you exercise too much?	Hypothalamic dysfunction
Have you been under greater than usual psychosocial stress?	Hypothalamic dysfunction
Do you have an impaired sense of smell?	Kallmann syndrome
Have you ever been diagnosed with chronic kidney disease, thyroid disease, sarcoidosis, lymphoma, histiocytosis X, or juvenile rheumatoid arthritis?	Many systemic illnesses cause amenorrhea
What medications are you taking?	Medications such as oral contraceptives, dopamine antagonists (haloperidol, risperidone, metoclopramide, domperidone), antihypertensive drugs that raise serum prolactin levels (methyldopa, reserpine), GnRH antagonists (danazol), and high-dose progestins may cause amenorrhea
Have you taken oral contraceptives in the past year?	Postpill amenorrhea
Have you ever had a uterine surgical procedure, infection, or abortion?	Asherman's syndrome
Have you been pregnant recently?	Postpartum amenorrhea
If you recently gave birth, were there any complications?	Sheehan syndrome
Have you ever been exposed to high doses of radiation (eg, for treatment of cancer)?	Premature ovarian failure
Have you ever received chemotherapy for cancer?	Premature ovarian failure
Have you recently experienced hot flashes, night sweats, mood changes, or vaginal dryness?	Premature ovarian failure
Have you noticed excessive facial hair or acne?	PCOS
Have you noticed heat or cold intolerance, a change in energy level, weight loss or gain, diarrhea or constipation, heart palpitations, or a change in skin or hair texture?	Thyroid disease
Have you had headaches or changes in your mood or personality?	Hypothalamic dysfunction due to infiltrative lesions

—Continued next page

Continued—

Have you experienced fatigue, anorexia, weight loss, or fever?	Lymphoma Sarcoidosis
Do you have a chronic cough or difficulty breathing?	Sarcoidosis
Have you had weakness, weight loss, arthritis, or a change in skin color?	Hemochromatosis
Do you have a depressed mood, change in appetite, alteration of sleep patterns, or a lack of interest in things you normally enjoy?	Depression
Do you have recurring intrusive thoughts that cause you to engage in repetitive behaviors?	Obsessive-compulsive disorder and associated medications
Do you see or hear things that others do not?	Schizophrenia and associated medications

DIAGNOSTIC APPROACH (INCLUDING ALGORITHMS)

- Once again, the first step is to rule out pregnancy. Then establish if amenorrhea is primary or secondary and follow the appropriate algorithms shown in Figures 46–2 and 46–3 for primary and secondary amenorrhea, respectively.
- The history should specifically include a detailed gynecologic history, medication history, and assessment for signs and symptoms of estrogen deficiency (eg, hot flashes, decreased libido), excess prolactin (eg, galactorrhea), or hyperandrogenism (eg, hirsutism, excessive acne).

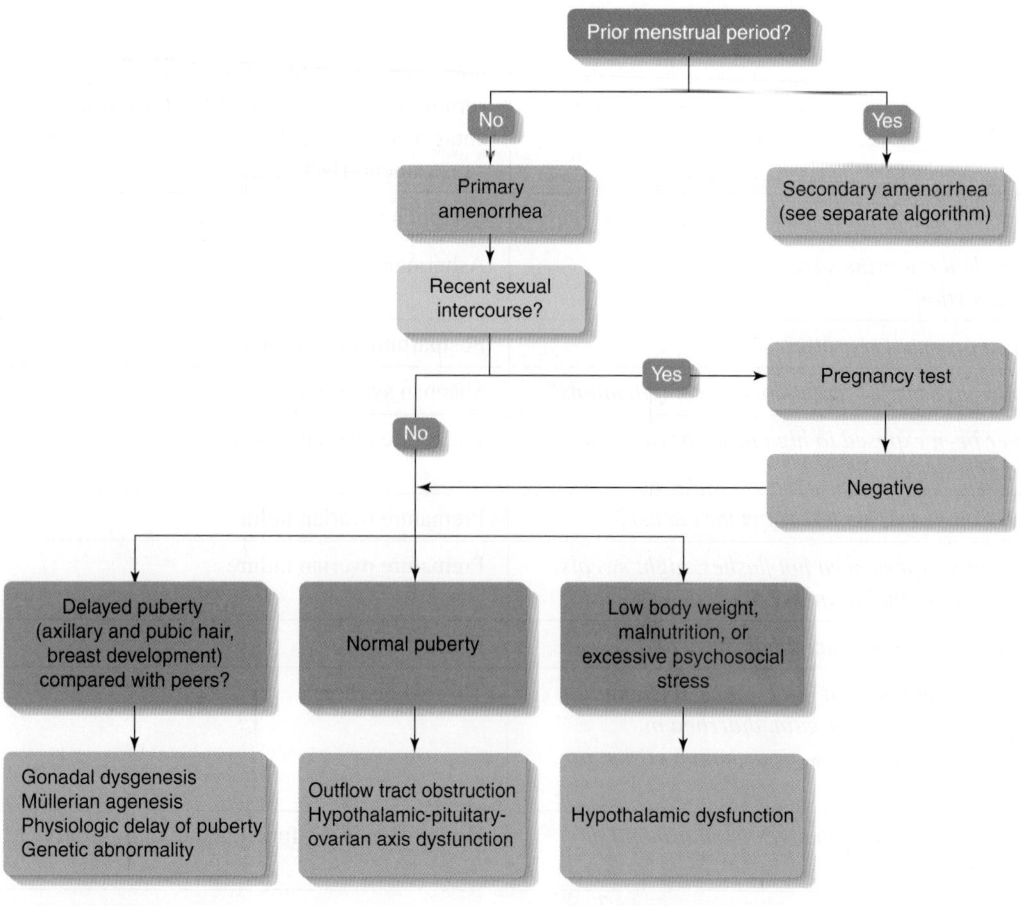

FIGURE 46–2 Diagnostic approach: Primary amenorrhea.

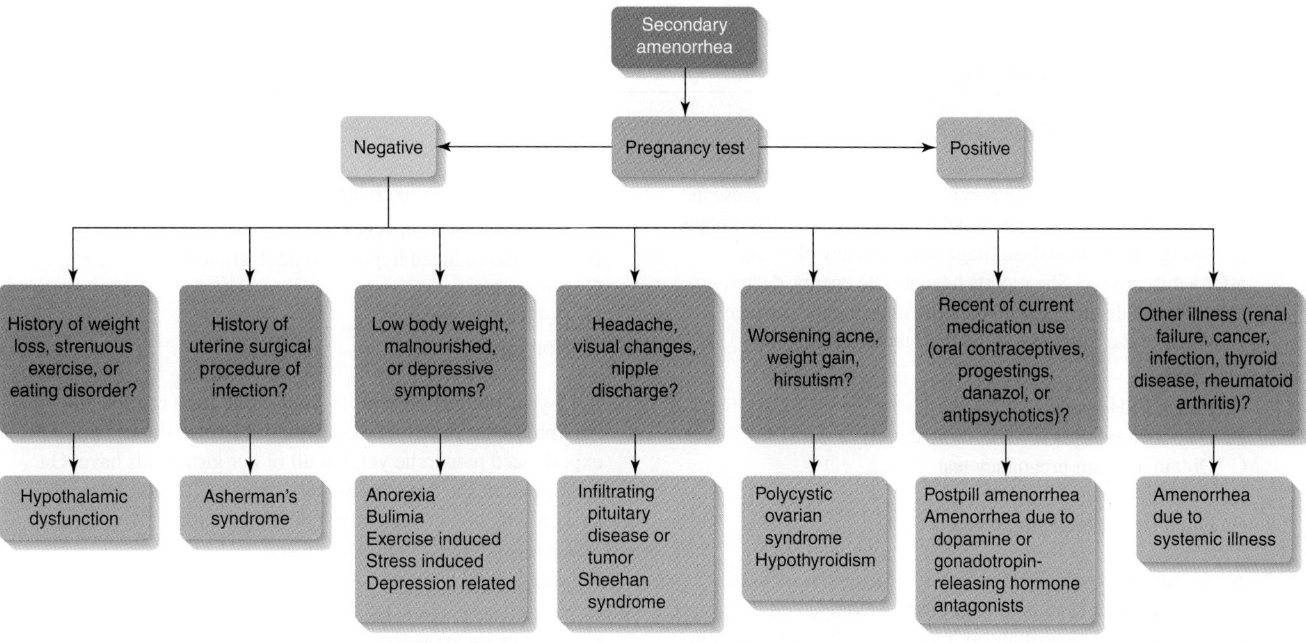

FIGURE 46–3 Diagnostic approach: Secondary amenorrhea.

- The physical examination should include assessment of body mass index and signs of secondary sexual development or hyperandrogenism.
- Subsequent laboratory testing and imaging should be dictated by the history and physical examination findings.

PROGNOSIS

Patients with amenorrhea often seek medical attention because they are concerned about future fertility. Recovery of normal menstrual cycles and reproductive ability depends on the etiology of amenorrhea. Women with Turner syndrome and other genetic abnormalities are usually infertile, and in those women who are able to conceive, there are high rates of miscarriage, stillbirth, and birth defects. Anatomic defects such as imperforate hymen and Asherman's syndrome are often amenable to surgical correction. Amenorrhea associated with PCOS and pituitary tumors may be corrected with medical therapy alone (if hormone levels normalize) or in conjunction with surgery. Amenorrhea due to systemic illness and hypothalamic amenorrhea often resolve with treatment of the underlying condition.

CASE SCENARIO | Resolution

A 26-year-old woman comes to clinic for evaluation of abnormal menses. After having previously irregular menses, she now reports a 9-month history of amenorrhea. She and her husband are now interested in having a child.

ADDITIONAL HISTORY

The patient underwent menarche at age 13 and has always had irregular periods. In the last 3 years, her periods have become increasingly irregular with several episodes of heavy bleeding. She has also gained a significant amount of weight over this period. She denies headaches, vision changes, cold intolerance, changes in her hair or nails, hot flashes, or change in libido. She takes no medications.

On physical examination, the patient is overweight with a body mass index of 29. Blood pressure is 122/68 mm Hg, and pulse 70 bpm. She has coarse hair noted on her upper lip and a few terminal hairs on her chin. Her abdomen is obese. Reflexes are normal. Pelvic examination reveals a normal-sized uterus, and bimanual examination reveals that the ovaries are not palpable. A rapid pregnancy test is negative.

Questions: What is the most likely diagnosis?

A. Premature ovarian failure
B. Pituitary tumor
C. Cushing's syndrome
D. Polycystic ovarian syndrome
E. Hypothyroidism

Test Your Knowledge

1. A 30-year-old woman with previously normal menses presents to your clinic concerned about not having a period for 4 months following a dilation and curettage to treat heavy bleeding after a miscarriage. She reports having little energy, decreased appetite, and disturbed sleep patterns since the miscarriage.
   Which of the following is the first step in making the diagnosis?
   A. Check FSH levels
   B. Discuss her stress level in more detail
   C. Obtain a serum pregnancy test
   D. Perform hysteroscopy
   E. Order thyroid function levels

2. A 19-year-old woman with a history of irregular menses since menarche presents to your clinic accompanied by her mother for evaluation of absent menses for the past 9 months. She has never had an evaluation of her abnormal menses. She is on the gymnastics team at her university, and her body mass index is 17. On physical examination, she has no hirsutism or acne. A serum pregnancy test is negative.
   What is the most likely diagnosis?
   A. Polycystic ovarian syndrome
   B. Exercise-induced hypothalamic dysfunction
   C. Pregnancy
   D. Delayed puberty
   E. Nothing is wrong

3. A 15-year-old girl presents to your clinic for a routine annual physical. She expresses concern because she has not experienced menarche yet, but all of her girlfriends have. On examination, she has a body mass index of 21, normal pubic hair growth, and normal breast development.
   What is the most likely diagnosis?
   A. Primary amenorrhea
   B. Secondary amenorrhea
   C. Normal development
   D. Premature ovarian failure
   E. Polycystic ovarian syndrome

References

1. Heiman DL. Amenorrhea. *Prim Care*. 2009;36:1–17.
2. Wilson GR, Haddad JE, Haddad CJ. Amenorrhea: common causes and evaluation. *Compr Ther*. 2005;31:270–278.
3. The Practice Committee of the American Society for Reproductive Medicine. Current evaluation of amenorrhea. *Fertil Steril*. 2008;90:S219–S225.
4. Homburg R. The mechanism of ovulation. Global Library of Women's Medicine. October 2008. DOI 10.3843/GLOWM.10290. Available at: http://glowm.com. Accessed October 26, 2011.
5. Reindollar RH, Novak M, Tho SPT, McDonough PG. Adult-onset amenorrhea: a study of 262 patients. *Am J Obstet Gynecol*. 1986;155:531–543.
6. Ledger WL, Skull J. Amenorrhea: investigation and treatment. *Curr Obset Gynaecol*. 2004;14:254–260.

Suggested Reading

Hamilton-Fairly D, Taylor A. ABC of subfertility: anovulation. *BMJ*. 2003;327:546–549.

Heiman DL. Amenorrhea. *Prim Care*. 2009;36:1–17.

Chapter 47

Breast Complaints

Helen K. Chew, MD

CASE SCENARIO

A 40-year-old woman sees you for "lumps" in her breasts. She describes a history of fibrocystic disease and lumpy breasts but thinks that her lumps are becoming more noticeable. She is worried because her maternal aunt was recently diagnosed with breast cancer at age 68.

- **What additional questions would you ask regarding her breast lumps?**
- **What are the historical risk factors for breast cancer?**
- **How can the patient history distinguish between benign breast disease and breast cancer?**

INTRODUCTION

The 3 most common breast complaints are breast lumps, breast pain, and nipple discharge.[1–3] Although most of these concerns prove to be due to a benign cause, the greatest fear among patients is the diagnosis of breast cancer. A delay in the diagnosis of breast cancer remains a leading cause of medical malpractice suits.[4] Therefore, it is important to elicit features of the history that suggest a malignant process. The purpose of the physician evaluation is to rule out breast cancer and to address the underlying cause of the breast complaint.

KEY TERMS

Breast cancer	Cancerous growth beginning in the ductal/lobular unit of the breast. If the cancer is confined to the ductal/lobular unit, it is referred to as ductal carcinoma in situ. If the cancer disrupts the basement membrane, it is referred to as invasive or infiltrating carcinoma.
Duct ectasia	The benign distention of subareolar ducts associated with breast discharge.
Fibroadenoma	A benign solid tumor with glandular and fibrous tissue, which is well defined and mobile.
Fibrocystic changes	An increased number of cysts or fibrous tissue in an otherwise normal breast. When these changes are accompanied by symptoms such as pain, nipple discharge, or lump(s), the condition is referred to as fibrocystic disease.
Mastalgia	Breast pain.
Papilloma	The growth of papillary cells from the wall of a duct or cyst into the lumen. This lesion is usually benign.
Proliferative breast disease	Premalignant changes in the breast including ductal hyperplasia, atypical ductal hyperplasia, and atypical lobular hyperplasia.

ETIOLOGY

Most breast complaints prove to be due to a benign condition. However, the cause varies based on the particular symptom, the patient's age, and menopausal status. For example, fibroadenoma is more common in younger, premenopausal women. In contrast, the incidence of breast cancer increases with age.

Differential Diagnosis

	Comments	Prevalence[a]
Fibrocystic disease	The most common cause of breast lumpiness and pain	Accounts for 20% of breast complaints in primary care clinic[1]
Fibroadenoma		The cause in 7%–13% of breast lumps in a specialty clinic
Mastitis/breast abscess		Occurs in up to 13% of lactating postpartum women[5]
Stretching of Cooper ligaments	Cyclical breast pain in women with large, pendulous breasts	
Papilloma	The most common cause of a bloody nipple discharge	50% of patients have nipple discharge without a palpable mass[6]
Breast cancer	The risk of developing breast cancer increases with age. For women up to age 39 years, the risk is 1 in 228; for women age 40–59 years, the risk is 1 in 24; for women age 60–79 years, the risk is 1 in 14.[7]	Found in < 10% of biopsies for lumps, pain, or discharge in primary care clinics[1,3]

[a]Prevalence is unknown when not indicated.

GETTING STARTED WITH THE HISTORY

- Review medication list prior to evaluation and confirm with patient.
- Determine whether patient is menopausal.

Questions	Remember
Tell me about your breast problem.	Allow patient to use her (or his) own words.
How long have you had this breast problem?	Determine the patient's anxiety level regarding breast cancer.
Is this problem in one or both breasts?	
Is there any relationship of this problem to your periods (if patient is premenopausal)?	
Is there any relationship of this problem to new medicines, including oral contraceptives or hormone replacement therapy?	
Are you worried about breast cancer?	

INTERVIEW FRAMEWORK

For any breast problem, a thorough history should focus on:

- The patient's breast cancer risk factors
- Medications
- Other medical problems
- Relationship to the menstrual cycle

Breast cancer risk factors include[8]:

- Increasing age
- Early age at menarche (< 11 years)
- Older age at menopause (> 55 years)
- Nulliparity or age at first live birth > 35 years
- Family history of breast cancer, particularly in first-degree relatives
- Known *BRCA1* and *BRCA2* mutation carrier
- Prior breast biopsies, especially showing atypia
- Prior breast cancer
- Prior neck or chest radiation
- Exogenous estrogen use in postmenopausal women

The Gail Model is a commonly used tool to calculate a woman's risk for developing breast cancer (www.cancer.gov/bcrisktool/). Factors that contribute to the model include current age, age at first menarche, age at first live birth, number of first-degree relatives with breast cancer, number of prior breast biopsies, and any biopsy with atypia.[8] The Gail Model was developed from the Breast Cancer Detection Demonstration Project, a mammogram screening program in the general population. Despite these established risk factors, 70% of women who develop breast cancer have no identifiable risk factor except for age.[9]

Five to 10% of patients will have a family history suggestive of hereditary breast cancer. It is important to ask about both the maternal and paternal sides of the family history. Clues to hereditary breast cancer syndromes include individuals diagnosed at a young age (< 40 years), bilateral breast cancers, history of ovarian cancer or male breast cancer, and multiple affected family members in each generation.

Inquire about recent medications, even if already discontinued. Ask specifically about oral contraceptive pills (OCPs), transdermal estrogen formulations, and hormone replacement therapy (HRT) because the patient may overlook these. Exogenous estrogens may contribute to breast symptoms, including breast tenderness or breast lumps. In the Women's Health Initiative, HRT conferred an increase in breast cancer, but the effect was modest (8 more cases of invasive breast cancer per 10,000 patient-years).[10]

Ask about other medical problems, particularly hypothyroidism, pituitary problems, and the possibility of pregnancy or recent lactation. Also inquire about accompanying symptoms such as headaches or visual changes, which may be associated with less common causes such as hypothyroidism or pituitary adenomas.

Many breast complaints are cyclical and worse prior to menstruation. Ask about menstrual irregularities and infertility.

If a patient is over 35 years of age, determine whether she had breast imaging such as a mammogram.

IDENTIFYING ALARM SYMPTOMS

In the absence of a breast mass or radiographic abnormalities, the majority of breast complaints prove to be due to a benign cause.[3] If the patient describes breast pain or discharge, ask directly about whether she feels a mass or if there are accompanying changes in the skin overlying the breast.

The prevalence of breast cancer in patients with breast complaints has not been well established. However, breast cancer is the ultimate diagnosis in less than 10% of women undergoing breast biopsy in primary care clinics.[1,3]

Serious Diagnoses

- Breast cancer

Alarm Symptoms	If Present, Consider Serious Causes...	Positive Likelihood Ratio (LR+) for Predicting Any Serious Cause	However, Benign Causes for This Feature Include...
Breast mass	Breast cancer	15 (11.7–19.3)[3]	Fibrocystic disease Fibroadenoma
Skin ulceration, thickening	Inflammatory breast cancer Breast abscess		Mastitis
Axillary mass	Breast cancer		Benign adenopathy

—*Continued next page*

Continued—			
Bloody nipple discharge	Breast cancer	3.1 (1.2–8.4), for any nipple complaint[3]	Papilloma Physiologic conditions
Strong family history of breast and/or ovarian cancer	Hereditary breast cancer		Sporadic cancer history
Systemic symptoms, including new respiratory symptoms, bone pain, headaches	Metastatic breast cancer		Unrelated symptoms (eg, respiratory infection, arthritis, migraines, etc)

FOCUSED QUESTIONS

QUESTIONS	THINK ABOUT...
Breast lump or skin changes	
How quickly did this change come on? Did it begin gradually or all of a sudden?	Chronic lumpiness may be due to fibrocystic breasts. A long-standing breast mass in a young woman may be a fibroadenoma.
Is this lump movable?	Cancer is more likely if the mass is immobile or fixed to surrounding structures. However, nearly all early-stage breast cancers are mobile.
Is this the only lump, or are there many?	Cancer is more of a concern when nodules are discrete and solitary. Diffuse lumpiness is usually benign.
Is this lumpiness in one breast or both?	Bilateral breast cancer is extremely rare and accounts for 1% of all breast cancers. Bilateral breast lumpiness is usually due to fibrocystic changes.
Are you taking hormones for any reason?	Hormonal changes in the breast are common and associated with OCPs and HRT.
Does this lump change with your periods?	Cyclical lumps are usually due to hormonal surges prior to menstruation.
Nipple inversion	
Has the inversion been gradual or sudden?	Gradual inversion over a few years is usually benign. More acute inversion may be due to duct ectasia, mastitis, breast surgery, or malignancy.
Breast pain, sensitivity, or soreness	
Can you feel a mass or lump in the area of pain?	Breast cancer or fibroadenoma
Does the pain change with your periods?	Cyclical breast sensitivity is usually due to hormonal surges prior to menstruation. Chronic pain may be due to large, pendulous breasts and the stretching of Cooper ligaments.
Did the pain begin suddenly?	Mastitis, cellulitis, or other infection. Thrombosis of the lateral thoracic vein (Mondor disease) is extremely rare.

Have you hurt yourself in the chest, been in an automobile accident, or had recent surgery?	Trauma. Chest wall pain may also be due to costochondritis (Tietze syndrome) or radicular pain from the thoracic spine.
Have you had a fever, or is the skin warm?	Mastitis, cellulitis, or other infection
Does caffeine make it worse?	Fibrocystic breasts may be more sensitive to caffeine.
Is the pain severe, interfering with life?	Reassure if other work-up negative and consider treatment for mastalgia.[8]
Breast discharge[11,12]	
Can you feel a mass or lump in the breast?	Breast cancer
Is the discharge in one breast or both?	Bilateral discharge is almost always due to physiologic or endocrine etiologies.
If in one breast, is the discharge from one part of the nipple (one duct) or from all parts of the nipple?	Discharge from one duct is more likely due to a problem with a specific duct such as papilloma or, less commonly, in situ cancer. Discharge from multiple ducts is more likely due to a physiologic cause, such as medications or lactation, or, less commonly, to duct ectasia.
Does the discharge come out by itself, or do you have to express it?	Cancer is more of a concern when discharge is spontaneous. Discharge only with breast stimulation is less worrisome.
Describe the color of your discharge.	Cancer or papilloma is more of a concern when discharge is bloody serosanguineous. Green, black, brown, or other colored discharge is usually due to a benign problem such as duct ectasia or normal physiologic discharge.
Does this discharge change with your period?	Physiologic discharge may be due to hormonal surges prior to menstruation.
Is there a recent change in bra?	Constrictive clothing may stimulate breast discharge.
Do you have headaches or changes in your vision?	Pituitary adenoma may cause galactorrhea.
Time course	
Is the lump/pain/discharge associated with your period?	Most causes of benign breast disease are cyclical in nature.
Did you notice this symptom after starting a new medication?	Hormonal therapy may increase lumpiness or tenderness and cause discharge. Dopamine antagonists (eg, phenothiazines, haloperidol) and other medications may cause discharge.
Have you recently stopped/started nursing?	Discharge may last for up to several months after prior lactation.
Associated and modifying symptoms	
Do you have headaches, nausea and vomiting, or vision changes?	Pituitary pathology
Have you had fevers?	Infection may lead to skin changes
Have you had prior breast surgery?	Scar tissue, recent trauma

DIAGNOSTIC APPROACH (INCLUDING ALGORITHM)

- Determine whether there is an underlying mass. Most complaints of pain or discharge without a palpable mass or radiographic abnormality are due to benign conditions, and the patient can be reassured.[13]
- What is the patient's risk of breast malignancy? Is this an older postmenopausal woman with a new lump or skin changes (more likely to have cancer) or a young woman with cyclical lumpiness (more likely to be fibrocystic disease)?
- If the patient is over age 35 years and has not had a mammogram, imaging should be considered to evaluate a new breast complaint.
- A persistent mass requires a thorough evaluation even if radiography is unremarkable.
- See Figure 47–1 for the diagnostic approach algorithm for breast complaints.

CAVEATS

- Although breast cancer risk assessment may help to stratify patients, most patients in whom breast cancer develops do not have these risk factors.
- If a patient notes a discrete mass, this requires a complete work-up (eg, breast biopsy) even with a "normal" or unremarkable mammogram.
- Breast pain or discharge in the absence of a mass or radiographic abnormality is unlikely to be due to cancer.
- Increase your suspicion of breast cancer in patients who are postmenopausal or have had prior breast cancer or a prior breast biopsy showing atypia.
- Male breast cancer is rare. However, a history of a breast mass should prompt appropriate work-up.[14]

PROGNOSIS

- Fibrocystic disease does not increase the risk of developing breast cancer.
- Cyclical breast pain is more likely to respond to medical treatment than noncyclical mastalgia.[15]
- The prognosis for breast cancer varies with stage. Five-year survival is 97% for patients with localized disease, 79% for patients with regional involvement, and only 23% for patients who have distant (metastatic) disease. Fortunately, only 10% of patients have distant disease at presentation, according to the American Cancer Society and Surveillance, Epidemiology, and End Results database (www.cancer.org).

CASE SCENARIO | Resolution

A 40-year-old woman sees you for "lumps" in her breasts. She describes a history of fibrocystic disease and lumpy breasts but thinks that her lumps are becoming more noticeable. She is worried because her maternal aunt was recently diagnosed with breast cancer at age 68.

ADDITIONAL HISTORY

The patient reveals that she has had bilateral, diffuse, lumpy breasts since her 20s. These lumps are more prominent and tender just before her menses. She has not noticed any discrete breast mass and is not taking any new medications. She has no other alarm symptoms, including skin changes, nipple complaints, or systemic complaints. She has no significant medical problems and has not had a prior breast biopsy. Her reproductive history includes menarche at age 12; she has never been pregnant. She has taken the same oral contraceptive for the last 10 years. Her family history is limited to her maternal aunt. She had a baseline mammogram 6 months ago, which was normal.

Question: What is the most likely diagnosis?

A. Breast cancer
B. Papilloma
C. Fibrocystic disease
D. Mastitis

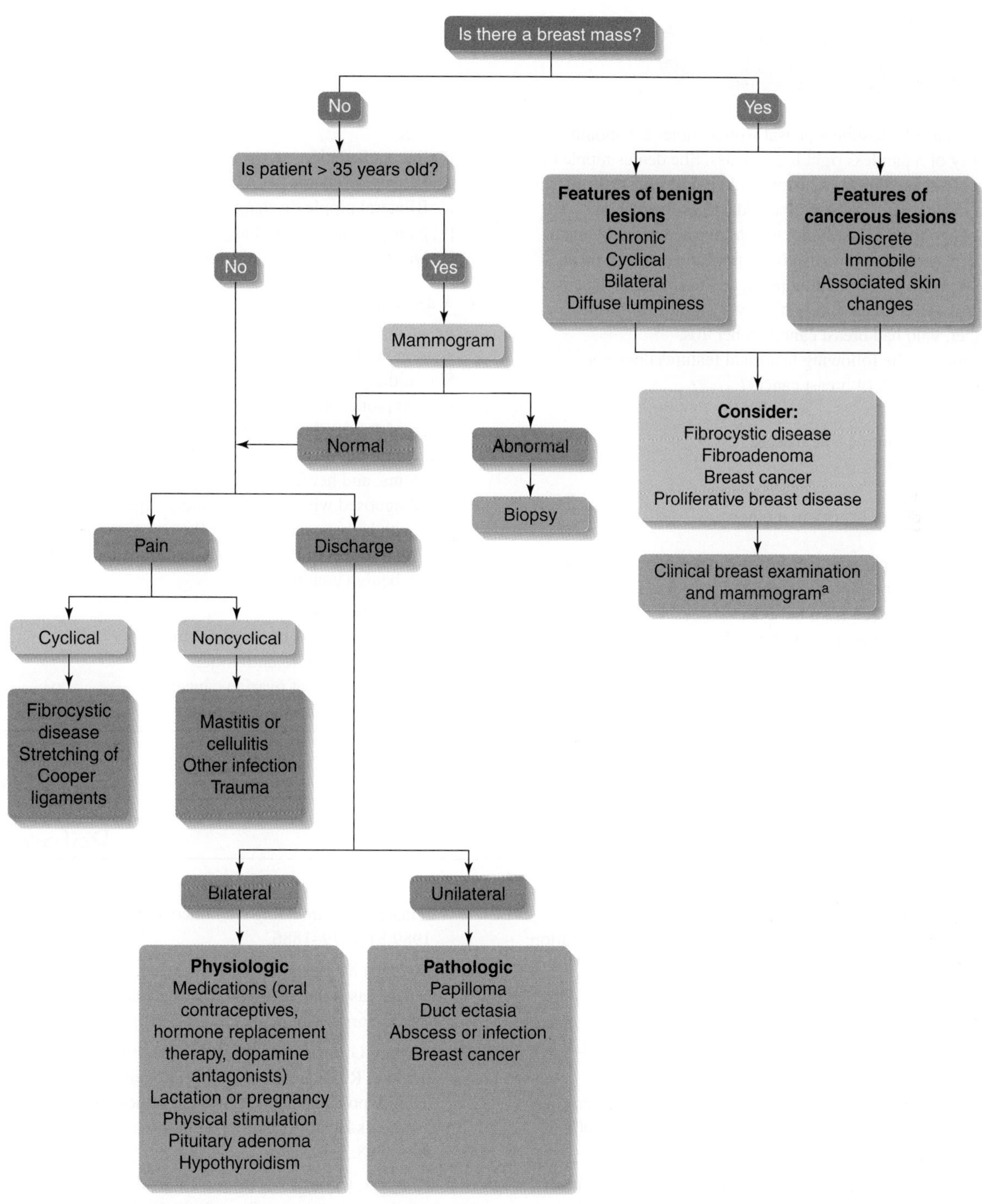

FIGURE 47–1. Diagnostic approach: Breast complaints.
[a]Physical examination and radiographic features are imperative in the diagnostic evaluation.

Test Your Knowledge

1. A 65-year-old postmenopausal woman notes a 1-month history of a painless right breast mass. She denies nipple or skin changes. She has a history of hypertension, arthritis, and fibrocystic breast disease. She had a right breast biopsy 10 years ago for a breast lump, which revealed atypical ductal hyperplasia but no invasive or in situ cancer. She is on an antihypertensive, acetaminophen, and hormone replacement therapy (HRT). Her family history is significant for her mother, who had breast cancer in her 70s.

   Which of the following historical features does *not* increase the risk of breast cancer?

   A. Age
   B. History of fibrocystic disease
   C. Prior breast biopsy
   D. HRT use
   E. Breast cancer history in mother

2. A 38-year-old premenopausal woman sees you for blood-tinged bilateral nipple discharge for 2 weeks. The discharge has to be expressed from her breasts, does not appear spontaneously, and appears from several ducts. She is concerned because she stopped lactating 6 months ago.

   Which is the most worrisome feature of this patient's history?

   A. Age
   B. Recent lactation
   C. Bloody discharge
   D. Bilateral nipple discharge
   E. Nonspontaneous discharge
   F. Discharge from multiple ducts

3. A 45-year-old woman has made an appointment to see you for an 8-week history of redness and thickening overlying the skin on her left breast. She stopped nursing 3 months ago. She initially received a course of antibiotics for mastitis, but the symptoms only partially improved. A diagnostic mammogram 4 weeks ago revealed dense breast tissue and skin thickening but no obvious mass. She has no other medical problems, and her family history is significant for a sister who was diagnosed with ovarian cancer at age 50 and a paternal aunt with breast cancer in her 60s.

   Which aspect of this patient's history is most consistent with a benign condition?

   A. Recent lactation
   B. Absence of mass on mammogram
   C. Partial response to antibiotics
   D. Family history of ovarian cancer

References

1. Barton MB, Elmore JG, Fletcher SW. Breast symptoms among women enrolled in a health maintenance organization: frequency, evaluation, and outcome. *Ann Intern Med.* 1999; 130:651–657.
2. Williams RS, Brook D, Monypenny IJ, et al. The relevance of reported symptoms in a breast screening programme. *Clin Radiol.* 2002;57:725–729.
3. Eberl MM, Phillips RL Jr, Lamberts H, et al. Characterizing breast symptoms in family practice. *Ann Fam Med.* 2008;6: 528–533.
4. Singh H, Sethi S, Raber M, et al. Errors in cancer diagnosis: current understanding and future directions. *J Clin Oncol.* 2007;25:5009–5018.
5. Foxman B, D'Arcy H, Gillespie B, et al. Lactation mastitis: occurrence and medical management among 946 breastfeeding women in the United States. *Am J Epidemiol.* 2002;155: 103–114.
6. Florio MG, Manganaro T, Pollicino A, et al. Surgical approach to nipple discharge: a ten-year experience. *J Surg Oncol.* 1999;71:235–238.
7. Jemal A, Siegel R, Ward E, et al. Cancer statistics, 2009. *CA Cancer J Clin.* 2009;59:225–249.
8. Gail MH, Brinton LA, Byar DP, et al. Projecting individualized probabilities of developing breast cancer for white females who are being examined annually. *J Natl Cancer Inst.* 1989;81:1879–1886.
9. Madigan MP, Ziegler RG, Benichou J, et al. Proportion of breast cancer cases in the United States explained by well-established risk factors. *J Natl Cancer Inst.* 1995;87:1681–1685.
10. Writing Group for the Women's Health Initiative Investigators. Risks and benefits of estrogen plus progestin in healthy postmenopausal women: principal results from the Women's Health Initiative randomized controlled trial. *JAMA.* 2002;288:321–333.
11. King TA, Carter KM, Bolton JS, et al. A simple approach to nipple discharge. *Am Surg.* 2000;66:960–965.
12. Montroni I, Santini D, Zucchini G, et al. Nipple discharge: is its significance as a risk factor for breast cancer fully understood? Observational study including 915 consecutive patients who underwent selective duct excision. *Breast Cancer Res Treat.* 2010;123:895–900.
13. Morrow M. The evaluation of common breast problems. *Am Fam Physician.* 2000;61:2371–2378, 2385.
14. Ottini L, Palli D, Rizzo S, et al. Male breast cancer. *Crit Rev Oncol Hematol.* 2010;73:141–155.
15. Gateley CA, Miers M, Mansel RE, et al. Drug treatments for mastalgia: 17 years experience in the Cardiff Mastalgia Clinic. *J R Soc Med.* 1992;85:12–15.

Suggested Reading

Armstrong K, Eisen A, Weber B. Assessing the risk of breast cancer. *N Engl J Med.* 2000;342:564–571.

Morrow M. The evaluation of common breast problems. *Am Fam Physician.* 2000;61:2371–2378, 2385.

Santen RJ, Mansel R. Benign breast disorders. *N Engl J Med.* 2005;353:275–285.

Chapter 48

Pelvic Pain

Francesca C. Dwamena, MD, MS

CASE SCENARIO

A 24-year-old woman presents to her primary care physician complaining of a deep, achy pain in her lower abdomen. When the pain began just over 3 months ago, she thought it was her usual menstrual cramps. She has had menstrual cramps since menarche at age 12. On several occasions, they were so severe that she had to miss school. Previously, the pain usually lasted for 3 to 4 days and was sometimes improved with ibuprofen. She decided to see the doctor because of persistence of the pain.

- **What additional questions would you ask to learn more about her pelvic pain?**
- **How would you classify the pelvic pain?**
- **Can you narrow the differential through an effective history?**
- **How can you use the history to decide on the appropriate diagnostic tests?**

INTRODUCTION

Pelvic pain is a common problem plaguing 39% of women in primary care,[1] and it accounts for 10% to 40% of gynecologic visits.[2] Worldwide, the rate of dysmenorrhea is 16.8% to 81%, that of dyspareunia is 8% to 21.8%, and that of chronic pelvic pain (CPP) is 2.1% to 24%.[3] In a study of nearly 300,000 women age 12 to 70 years, the annual prevalence of CPP was similar to that of migraine, asthma, and back pain.[4] CPP is the primary reason for 10% to 35% of laparoscopies and 10% to 12% of hysterectomies performed in the United States at an estimated cost of more than $2 billion annually.[2]

KEY TERMS

Acute pelvic pain (APP)	Pain symptoms below the umbilicus that have been present for < 3 months.
Chronic pelvic pain (CPP)	Nonmenstrual pain below the umbilicus of at least 3 months in duration.
Cyclic pelvic pain	Pain below the umbilicus that is exacerbated before and during menses.
Dysmenorrhea	Recurrent crampy, lower abdominal pain during menses.
Dyspareunia	A deep pain below the umbilicus that occurs with sexual intercourse.
Positive likelihood ratio (LR+)	The likelihood of a particular diagnosis if a factor is present.
Negative likelihood ratio (LR–)	The likelihood of a particular diagnosis if a factor is absent.

ETIOLOGY

The most serious causes of pelvic pain present acutely (< 3 months) and can be classified as pregnancy-related causes, gynecologic disorders, and nonreproductive disorders.[5] The relative frequencies of these disorders in patients with acute pelvic pain (APP) have not been elucidated, and clinical diagnosis has been notoriously difficult. For example, laparoscopy confirmed pelvic inflammatory disease (PID) in only 46% of cases clinically diagnosed as PID,[6] and only 37.8% of cases with a clinical diagnosis of adnexal torsion were confirmed by surgery in another series.[7] Diagnosis of CPP is even more challenging. Although pelvic adhesions and endometriosis are frequently found with laparoscopy,[8] controlled studies suggest that they may be incidental rather than causal.[9] In many patients, CPP may be functional (eg, myofascial pain, irritable bowel syndrome) or psychogenic (eg, depression, anxiety, somatization).[9]

Differential Diagnoses of APP

Pregnancy related	**Nongynecologic, gastrointestinal**
Ectopic pregnancy	Acute appendicitis
Abortion	Inflammatory bowel disease
Intrauterine pregnancy with corpus luteum bleeding	Mesenteric adenitis
Gynecologic	Irritable bowel syndrome
Acute PID	Diverticulitis
Endometriosis	**Nongynecologic, urinary tract**
Ovarian cyst (hemorrhage or rupture)	Urinary tract infection
Adnexal torsion	Renal calculus
Uterine leiomyoma (degeneration or torsion)	**Medically unexplained**
Tumor	

Differential Diagnosis of CPP

	Prevalence
Cyclic or recurrent pelvic pain	
Primary dysmenorrhea	16.8%–81%[3]
Mittelschmerz	
Endometriosis	1.4%–50% in fertile women; 2.1%–77% in infertile women[10]
Adnexal torsion	
Obstruction müllerian duct anomalies	
Noncyclic CPP (laparoscopic findings)[b]	
Endometriosis	37%
Pelvic adhesions	26%
Cystic ovaries	1%
Normal laparoscopy	36%

[a]Prevalence is unknown when not indicated.

[b]CPP may also be functional or psychogenic.

GETTING STARTED WITH THE HISTORY

- Let the patient tell the pelvic pain story in her own words before asking more directed and focused questions.
- Be sure to elicit the patient's personal and emotional story to establish rapport and to assess whether there is primary or comorbid psychological disease.
- Understand the patient's agenda. Patients often seek medical care due to concern about a serious cause.

Open-Ended Questions	Remember
Tell me about your pelvic pain	Listen to the story.
Is this pain the same pelvic pain you've had before, or is it different in some way?	Don't try to rush the interview by interrupting and focusing the history too soon. Reassure the patient when possible.
When did the pelvic pain first start?	This question determines whether pain is acute, chronic, or both. CPP is usually benign.
Give me an example of your most recent pelvic pain; tell me what you experienced from beginning to end.	
Why did you choose to see me for the pelvic pain today?	Determine the patient's primary agenda for the visit and most concerning feature.

INTERVIEW FRAMEWORK

- The first goal is to determine whether the pelvic pain is acute or chronic and cyclic or noncyclic.
- Inquire about pain characteristics using the cardinal symptom features:
  - Onset
  - Duration
  - Frequency
  - Pain character
  - Location of pain
  - Associated features
  - Precipitating and alleviating factors
  - Change in frequency or character over time

IDENTIFYING ALARM SYMPTOMS

Serious Diagnoses

Serious diagnoses in patients with pelvic pain are rare. The relative frequencies of the following conditions in patients with pelvic pain are unknown but are likely to be lower than reported.

After the open-ended portion of the history, determine whether pelvic pain is acute (< 3 months) or chronic (≥ 3 months). If not clear, then specifically ask about the presence of the alarm symptoms to assess for the possibility of a serious cause.

Serious Diagnosis	Population	Frequency
Acute PID	Age 15–39	1%–1.3%[11]
	Age 20–24	2%[11] (incidence)
Ectopic pregnancy	All reported pregnancies in the United States (in 1992)	2%[a] (prevalence)
Adnexal torsion	Gynecologic surgical emergencies	2.7%[7] (prevalence)
Acute appendicitis	Patients suspected of acute appendicitis	0.84%[12] (incidence)

[a]From Centers for Disease Control and Prevention. Available at: http://www.cdc.gov/mmwr/preview/mmwrhtml/00035709.htm.

Alarm Symptoms	If Present, Consider...	LR+[a]	LR–[a]
Duration of pain < 15 days	Appendicitis Acute PID		
Sexual contact with known gonorrhea carrier	PID	2.22[13]	0.73[13]
Fever or chills	PID	1.36, 2.05[13]	0.88, 0.74[13]
Abnormal vaginal bleeding	PID Endometriosis Ectopic pregnancy Acute appendicitis Endometrial cancer in postmenopausal women		
Delayed menstruation in a woman of childbearing age	Pregnancy-related condition such as ectopic pregnancy		
Intense, progressive pain that started as a repetitive transitory pain	Adnexal torsion		

[a]Likelihood ratios are unknown when not indicated.

FOCUSED QUESTIONS

After hearing the patient's story and considering possible alarm symptoms, ask the following questions to begin to narrow the differential diagnosis.

QUESTIONS	THINK ABOUT...
How old are you?	Young age (15–25 years) is a risk factor for PID.
Menstrual history	
• *How old were you when you first started your periods?*	
• *How long do your periods last?*	
• *What is the length of your cycle?*	
• *How heavy are your periods? How many times do you have to change your pads or tampons?*	Excessive bleeding suggests uterine fibroids or adenomyosis.
Obstetric history	
• *Have you ever been pregnant?* • *Have you had any problem becoming pregnant?*	A history of infertility and dysmenorrhea suggests endometriosis.
Have you been sexually involved with a partner in the past 6 months? *If yes, ask the following questions:*	Sexual abstinence rules out pregnancy-related disorders, although a pregnancy test is suggested in all patients.
• *With women, men, or both?*	A male sexual partner with symptoms of urethritis increases the risk for PID.

• *Have you had more than 5 sexual partners in your lifetime?*	Multiple sexual partners increase the risk of PID.
• *When did you last have sex with a partner?*	A woman who has been sexually abstinent in the months preceding the onset of pain is unlikely to have a pregnancy-related etiology.
• *What is your method of contraception?*	Use of an intrauterine contraceptive device (IUD) is a risk factor for PID and ectopic pregnancy. Conversely, risk for PID is reduced by 50% in patients taking oral contraceptive pills (OCPs) or using a barrier method, and reliable use of combined OCPs decreases risk for ectopic pregnancy and complications of functional ovarian cysts. Pregnancy in a woman who has undergone tubal ligation has a 30-fold risk of being ectopic.[5]
• *Do you have pain with intercourse?*	Deep dyspareunia suggests endometriosis.[5]
Has anyone ever hit you or forced you to have sex? How old were you?	Childhood sexual abuse is associated with the later development of CPP (combined odds ratio from 10 studies, 2.73; 95% confidence interval, 1.73–4.30).[14]
Quality	
What does the pain feel like?	
• *Constant and burning*	Neuropathic pain such as pudendal neuralgia (pain in area supplied by the pudendal nerve such as external genitalia, urethra, anus, and perineum)
Where is the pain located?	
• *It started in the epigastrium or periumbilical area and migrated to right lower quadrant.*	Appendicitis
• *Pain is unilateral.*	Adnexal torsion
• *Pain is bilateral.*	PID, ruptured or hemorrhagic ovarian cyst
• *Colicky flank pain that radiates to the anterior abdomen*	Urinary stone disease
On a scale of 1 to 10, with 10 being the worst pain you ever had in your life, how severe is your pain?	
Time course	
Tell me about how the pain started and progressed.	Symptoms associated with infection (eg, PID) usually develop progressively over a few days. Pain occurs suddenly with rupture or torsion, and the patient can usually tell precisely at what time symptoms began.[15]
Associated symptoms	
Have you noticed any urgency or increased frequency of urination?	Patients with interstitial cystitis report urgency and increased frequency as the most distressing symptoms.
Have you noticed any blood in your stool?	Bloody diarrhea suggests inflammatory bowel disease.
Modifying factors	
Have you found that anything in particular worsens or improves your pelvic pain?	
• *Rest makes it better.*	Musculoskeletal or adnexal torsion

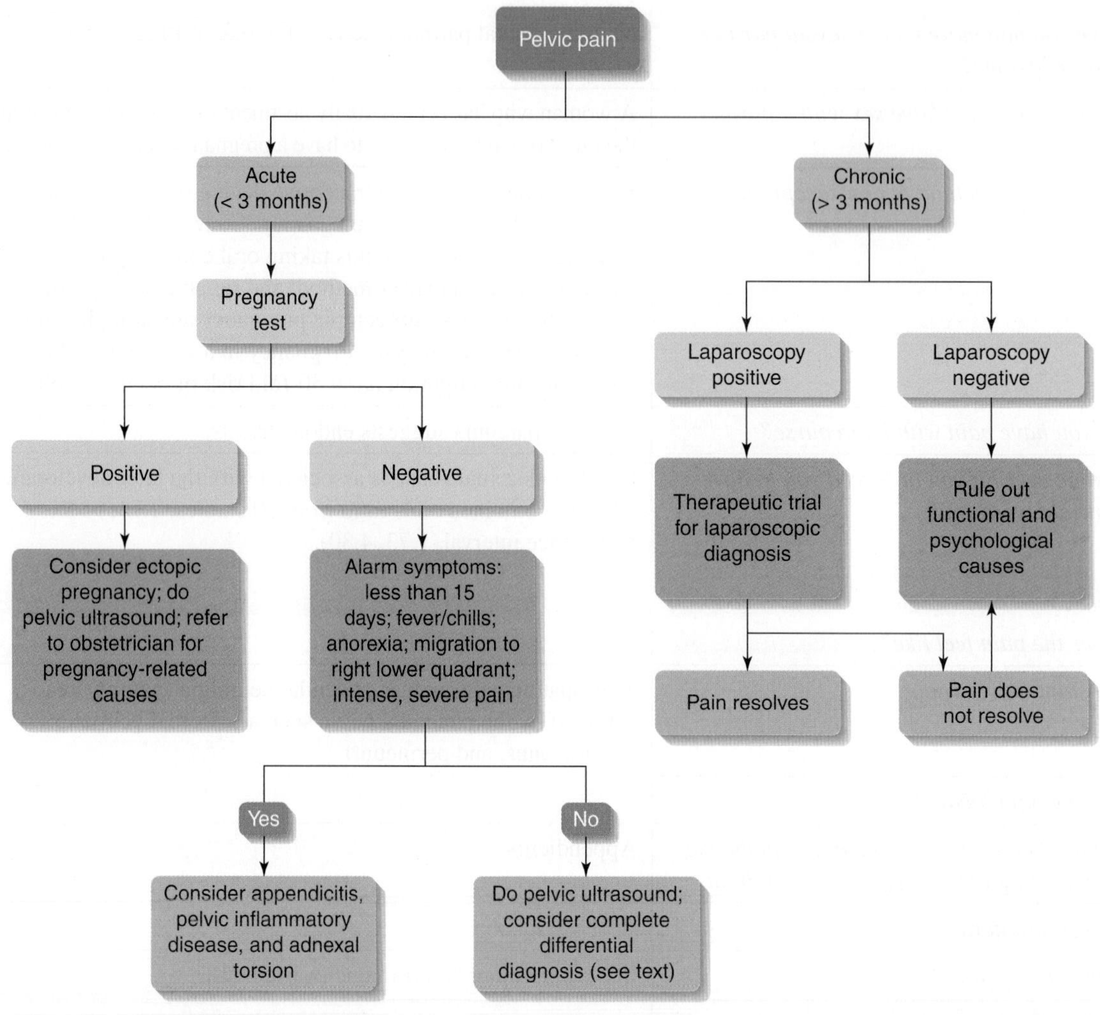

FIGURE 48–1 Diagnostic approach: Pelvic pain.

DIAGNOSTIC APPROACH (INCLUDING ALGORITHM)

The first step is to determine whether pelvic pain is acute or chronic and to distinguish old from new pain. The history should include a thorough review of the gynecologic, gastrointestinal, urologic, and psychological systems. See Figure 48–1 for the diagnostic approach algorithm for a patient with pelvic pain.

PROGNOSIS

The prognosis of pelvic pain is excellent in most patients. In a retrospective cohort study of 86 females with pelvic pain and negative ultrasound, 77% of patients reported improvement or resolution of symptoms after a mean follow-up period of 15 months.[2] In that study, those with APP were more likely to report improvement than those with CPP (86% versus 50%), and only 4 of 11 patients who had subsequent laparoscopies were found to have significant abnormality (eg, endometriosis, adenomyosis, pelvic adhesions). Similarly, Baker et al[16] reported improved pain scores after 6 months in 58 of 60 patients with CPP and negative laparoscopy. However, many women with CPP suffer from anxiety, depression, physical worries, and marital problems despite modest improvement of pain.[17] This emphasizes the importance of a multidisciplinary approach to these patients.

CASE SCENARIO | Resolution

A 24-year-old woman presents to her primary care physician complaining of a deep, achy pain in her lower abdomen. When the pain began just over 3 months ago, she thought it was her usual menstrual cramps. She has had menstrual cramps since menarche at age 12. On several occasions, they were so severe that she had to miss school. Previously, the pain usually lasted for 3 to 4 days and was sometimes improved with ibuprofen. She decided to see the doctor because of persistence of the pain.

ADDITIONAL HISTORY

Her pain is similar in quality and severity to her usual menstrual cramping; however, over the last 3 months, she has had cramps even when she is not menstruating. You learn that her periods have been getting steadily heavier over the last 5 years to the point that she now soaks through a pad every hour for the first 3 days of her periods. She has a 3-year-old daughter and had a normal vaginal delivery of another child a year ago. She has not been sexually active since her divorce 10 months ago. She denies pain with intercourse when she was sexually active. She does not have any fever or chills. On further questioning, you find out she recently remembered being abused sexually as a teenager and has just started seeing a counselor for therapy.

Question: What is the most likely diagnosis?

A. Pelvic inflammatory disease
B. Endometriosis
C. Uterine fibroids
D. Somatization

Test Your Knowledge

1. A 25-year-old woman with a history of 3 miscarriages and no live births presents with worsening pelvic pain over the last 4 months. Her last pregnancy was 2 years ago. She has had dysmenorrhea since she began her periods at 15 years. She has noticed dyspareunia over the last year. Her menstrual periods are irregular, but her flow is normal. Her last period was 1 week ago. She has been taking fluoxetine for depression and anxiety for 3 months. She denies any fever, chills, or vaginal discharge.
   What is the most likely diagnosis?
   A. Pelvic inflammatory disease
   B. Ectopic pregnancy
   C. Adnexal torsion
   D. Endometriosis

2. A 30-year-old mother of 2 healthy children presents with acute pelvic pain.
   Which of the following symptoms is most suggestive of a surgical emergency?
   A. Fever or chills
   B. Crampy abdominal pain
   C. Intense, progressive pain that started as repetitive transitory pain
   D. Deep dyspareunia

3. A 60-year-old woman presents with 2 months of progressive, crampy, lower abdominal pain and cyclical diarrhea.
   Which of the following features, if present, would be most concerning for endometrial cancer?
   A. Fever or chills
   B. Abnormal vaginal bleeding
   C. Dyspareunia
   D. Multiple sexual contacts

References

1. Jamieson DJ, Steege JF. The prevalence of dysmenorrhea, dyspareunia, pelvic pain, and irritable bowel syndrome in primary care practices. *Obstet Gynecol.* 1996;87:55–58.
2. Harris RD, Holtzman SR, Poppe AM. Clinical outcome in female patients with pelvic pain and normal pelvic US findings. *Radiology.* 2000;216:440–443.
3. Latthe P, Latthe M, Say L, Gulmezoglu M, Khan KS. WHO systematic review of prevalence of chronic pelvic pain: a neglected reproductive health morbidity. *BMC Public Health.* 2006;6:177.
4. Zondervan KT, Yudkin PL, Vessey MP, Dawes MG, Barlow DH, Kennedy SH. Prevalence and incidence of chronic pelvic pain in primary care: evidence from a national general practice database. *Br J Obstet Gynaecol.* 1999;106:1149–1155.
5. Quan M. Diagnosis of acute pelvic pain. *J Fam Pract.* 1992;35:422–432.
6. Chaparro MV, Ghosh S, Nashed A, Poliak A. Laparoscopy for the confirmation and prognostic evaluation of pelvic inflammatory disease. *Int J Gynaecol Obstet.* 1978;15:307–309.
7. Hibbard LT. Adnexal torsion. *Am J Obstet Gynecol.* 1985;152:456–461.
8. Kresch AJ, Seifer DB, Sachs LB, Barrese I. Laparoscopy in 100 women with chronic pelvic pain. *Obstet Gynecol.* 1984;64:672–674.
9. Walker E, Katon W, Harrop-Griffiths J, Holm L, Russo J, Hickok LR. Relationship of chronic pelvic pain to psychiatric diagnoses and childhood sexual abuse. *Am J Psychiatry.* 1988; 145:75–80.
10. Guo SW, Wang Y. The prevalence of endometriosis in women with chronic pelvic pain. *Gynecol Obstet Invest.* 2006;62: 121–130.
11. Westrom L. Incidence, prevalence, and trends of acute pelvic inflammatory disease and its consequences in industrialized countries. *Am J Obstet Gynecol.* 1980;138:880–892.
12. Korner H, Soreide JA, Pedersen EJ, Bru T, Sondenaa K, Vatten L. Stability in incidence of acute appendicitis. A population-based longitudinal study. *Dig Surg.* 2001;18: 61–66.
13. Kahn JG, Walker CK, Washington AE, Landers DV, Sweet RL. Diagnosing pelvic inflammatory disease. A comprehensive analysis and considerations for developing a new model. *JAMA.* 1991;266:2594–2604.
14. Paras ML, Murad MH, Chen LP, et al. Sexual abuse and lifetime diagnosis of somatic disorders: a systematic review and meta-analysis. *JAMA.* 2009;302:550–561.
15. Goldstein DP. Acute and chronic pelvic pain. *Pediatr Clin North Am.* 1989;36:573–580.
16. Baker PN, Symonds EM. The resolution of chronic pelvic pain after normal laparoscopy findings. *Am J Obstet Gynecol.* 1992;166:835–836.
17. Richter HE, Holley RL, Chandraiah S, Varner RE. Laparoscopic and psychologic evaluation of women with chronic pelvic pain. *Int J Psychiatry Med.* 1998;28:243–253.

Suggested Reading

Fall M, Baranowski AP, Elneil S, et al. EAU Guidelines on chronic pelvic pain. *Eur Urol.* 2010;57:35–48.

Hewitt GD, Brown RT. Acute and chronic pelvic pain in female adolescents. *Med Clin North Am.* 2000;84:1009–1025.

Lifford KL, Barbieri RL. Diagnosis and management of chronic pelvic pain. *Urol Clin North Am.* 2002;29:637–647.

Quan M. Diagnosis of acute pelvic pain. *J Fam Pract.* 1992;35:422–432.

Chapter 49

Vaginitis

Carol K. Bates, MD

CASE SCENARIO

A 21-year-old woman is upset to report vaginal discharge. The discharge has been present for the past 10 days. She has never had this before and appears to be very anxious.

- **What additional questions would you ask to learn more about her discharge?**
- **Why do you think that she is anxious, and how will you explore that with her?**
- **What associated symptoms might she have?**
- **What will you need to know about her sexual history?**

INTRODUCTION

Vulvovaginal symptoms are among the most common reasons that patients consult a primary care physician. It is difficult to assess the actual prevalence of vulvovaginitis because many patients treat their own symptoms with over-the-counter medications and never seek medical advice.

Although not usually life threatening, recurrent or chronic vulvovaginal complaints often involve significant discomfort, sexual dysfunction, and emotional distress. Most patients will ultimately prove to have a benign cause of vaginitis, but vaginal symptoms may indicate more serious upper genital tract disease requiring urgent evaluation and treatment. Clinicians should not rely on history alone and should confirm the suspected diagnosis with pelvic examination and microscopy.

KEY TERMS

Vaginitis — Inflammation of the vagina characterized by vaginal soreness and/or itching, usually but not always accompanied by vaginal discharge. A summative term used to describe a variety of vaginal complaints.

Vaginal discharge — Vaginal fluid composed of cervical mucus, exfoliated epithelial cells, bacteria, and vaginal secretions. Normally, it is odorless and white or clear in appearance. The appearance and amount of vaginal discharge vary with estrogen and progesterone levels, irritation, and infection.

Vulvitis — Symptoms of irritation felt externally in the vulva. The irritation is not always accompanied by an increase or change in vaginal discharge.

Vulvovaginitis — Irritation felt externally in the vulva and internally in the vagina.

Cervicitis — Irritation or infection that primarily involves the cervix and can cause vaginal discharge. Usually the vulva is spared.

Dyspareunia — Discomfort during intercourse. The discomfort may be superficial (pain on initial penetration or with attempted penetration) or deep (related to deep penetration only).

—Continued next page

Continued—

Dysuria	Pain or burning with urination.
Pruritus	Itching.
Upper genital tract	The upper genital tract includes the ovaries, fallopian tubes, and uterus.
Lower genital tract	The lower genital tract includes the vagina, vulva, and other external structures. The cervix is in the lower tract but is the portal to the upper tract and so may be involved in upper tract processes.
Sexually transmitted infection (STI)	Infection anywhere in the genital tract transmitted via interpersonal genital contact. Includes infection with chlamydia, gonorrhea, syphilis, herpes simplex, and *Trichomonas*.
Pelvic inflammatory disease (PID)	Infection involving the uterus, fallopian tubes, and ovaries, which can lead to peritonitis.
Toxic shock syndrome (TSS)	Life-threatening syndrome of fever, hypotension, multiorgan failure, and rash caused by enterotoxins produced by *Staphylococcus aureus* or group A *Streptococcus*. Associated with the use of highly absorbent tampons or foreign bodies left in the vagina for prolonged periods.

ETIOLOGY

Approximately 90% of all vulvovaginitis is infectious and is due to candidiasis, trichomoniasis, or bacterial vaginosis.[1–4] The remaining 10% of vulvovaginitis results from noninfectious causes such as irritants, low estrogen states, and dermatologic disorders. Up to 26% of women with a complaint of vaginitis will have no diagnosable disorder.[5]

Differential Diagnosis

	Prevalence[a]
Infections	
Candidiasis	17%–39%[4,5]
Bacterial vaginosis	20%–58%[4,5]
Trichomoniasis	4%–35%[4,5]
Cervicitis	20%–25% in urban STI clinic[3]
Others	
Atrophic vaginitis	7%–63% of postmenopausal women[6,7]
Dermatologic disorders	
Irritant vaginitis (ie, latex, chemical vaginitis from douche)	
Physiologic discharge	Up to 26%[5]

[a]Empty cells indicate that the prevalence is unknown.

GETTING STARTED WITH THE HISTORY

- Vaginal complaints can be very difficult for women to discuss. Be patient and let the patient tell the story in her own words before asking more directed and focused questions.
- Taking a detailed sexual history is paramount. Remember to obtain the history in an open and nonjudgmental manner. Patients may be concerned about sexually transmitted diseases and about their partners' fidelity.
- Many women do not examine their vulvas or vaginas and so cannot pinpoint the location of their symptoms. Gently encourage the patient to be specific about symptoms. Vaginitis is common in adolescent and young adult women who may be particularly embarrassed to discuss vaginal complaints and their sexual history.
- Small amounts of vaginal discharge are normal. Between 1 and 4 mL of fluid is produced daily. Normal vaginal discharge may be colorless, white, or pale yellow. Vaginal discharge increases normally at ovulation when the thick and viscid cervical mucus plug is expelled.

Questions	Remember
Tell me what the discharge looks and feels like.	Elucidate the color, consistency, odor, and amount of the discharge.
Is there discomfort or itching? If so, where?	
Are you currently involved in a sexual relationship?	

INTERVIEW FRAMEWORK

- First, ask about prior episodes of vaginitis, their treatment, and the degree to which current symptoms resemble any prior symptoms.
- You must understand the patient's risk of STI. Ask about prior STIs, condom use, number of sexual partners, and specific sexual practices (see Focused Questions).
- Several underlying medical disorders and steroid use can increase the risk of candidiasis, and several dermatologic problems can affect the vagina and vulva. Take a medication history focused on steroids and immunosuppressives. Inquire about history of systemic illness, particularly human immunodeficiency virus (HIV), diabetes, and dermatologic problems.
- Explore the use of any vaginal topical or douching products because these can modify flora and/or cause irritation.
- Although not a strong predictor of etiology of vaginitis, take a menstrual history, because *Candida* and bacterial vaginosis have varying prevalence in different phases of menses.

IDENTIFYING ALARM SYMPTOMS

Although vulvovaginitis causes discomfort and irritation, it does not cause acute systemic illness. Serious symptoms (eg, fever, abdominal pain, dizziness, fainting) warrant consideration of upper genital tract disease or toxic shock syndrome (TSS). If fever and abdominal pain predominate, consider pelvic inflammatory disease (PID).

Serious Diagnoses

Diagnosis	Prevalence
PID	55% of adolescents in one series with laparoscopically confirmed PID reported vaginal discharge[8]
TSS	Relative risk of 2.1 of TSS in women with antecedent vaginitis[9]
Erythema multiforme major	Rare
Urinary tract infection	Common
Malignancy (vulvar, vaginal, cervical)	Rare; relative risk of 6.1 of vaginal cancer in women with prior vaginitis[10]
Foreign body (ie, retained tampon)	Common
Rectovaginal fistula	Rare

After the open-ended questions, ask about the presence of the following alarm symptoms to assess for the possibility of a serious cause and to determine the pace of subsequent evaluation or "triage." With the exception of fetid discharge indicative of fistula, all of the alarm symptoms fall into the category of associated symptoms and are not really features of the primary symptom of vaginitis.

Alarm Symptoms	If Present, Consider Serious Causes...	However, Benign Causes for This Symptom Include...
Always indicates a serious cause for vaginitis		
Confusion, lethargy	TSS	
Fetid or feculent discharge	Rectovaginal fistula	

—Continued next page

Continued—		
Urinary frequency, hematuria	Urinary tract infection, renal stone	
Lower abdominal pain	PID, urinary tract infection	
May indicate a serious cause for vaginitis		
Bleeding	Trauma, malignancy, foreign body	Menses
Fever	PID, TSS, urinary tract infection, erythema multiforme major	Coincident viral syndrome
Dizziness or near syncope	TSS	Vasovagal syncope
Rash	TSS, erythema multiforme major	Psoriasis, other dermatoses
Nausea and vomiting	TSS, pregnancy, PID	Coincident gastroenteritis
Vaginal sores	Herpes infection, Behçet syndrome, dermatoses (pemphigus, pemphigoid, erythema multiforme major)	Local trauma from scratching

FOCUSED QUESTIONS

After hearing the history in the patient's own words and considering possible alarm symptoms, ask the following questions to narrow the differential diagnosis.

QUESTIONS	THINK ABOUT...
Do you have sex with men, women, or both?	Penile vaginal penetration increases the risk of trichomoniasis, *Chlamydia*, gonorrhea, and bacterial vaginosis.
In women sexually active only with other women, consider asking about sex toy and digital insertion.	Recent evidence suggests that bacterial vaginosis is associated with vaginal penetration, including digital and sex toy use.
Do you engage in oral sex?	Candidiasis
Have you tried over-the-counter yeast preparations, and if so, do they help?	Candidiasis
Are you postmenopausal?	Atrophic vaginitis
If postmenopausal, are you using estrogen products (orally or vaginally)?	Candidiasis
Discharge characteristics	
Do you notice an odor?	Bacterial vaginosis, trichomoniasis, foreign body
What color is the discharge?	
• *White*	Candidiasis

• *Gray*	Bacterial vaginosis
• *Yellow or green*	Trichomoniasis
What is the consistency of the discharge?	
• *Clumped*	Candidiasis
• *Thin*	Bacterial vaginosis, trichomoniasis
Timing	
When did the discharge occur in relation to your menstrual cycle?	
• *Premenstrual*	Candidiasis
• *Postmenstrual*	Trichomoniasis
Have you recently been treated with antibiotics?	Candidiasis
Does the discharge occur after condom use?	Latex allergy, other irritant (nonoxynol-9, propylene glycol)
Associated symptoms	
Do you notice itching? Is it internal, external, or both?	
• *Internal or both*	Candidiasis
• *External only*	Lichen sclerosis, lichen planus, lichen simplex chronicus, psoriasis
Do you experience burning with urination? If so, is it internal or external?	
• *Internal*	Urinary tract infection
• *External*	Vulvar candidiasis, dermatosis
Do you have pain with intercourse?	
• *With initial penetration*	Atrophic vaginitis
• *With deeper thrusting*	Upper track problem (PID, endometriosis, fibroids, etc)
Are there blisters in the vagina or vulva?	Herpes infection, pemphigus, cicatricial pemphigoid, Behçet syndrome, erythema multiforme major

DIAGNOSTIC APPROACH (INCLUDING ALGORITHM)

The first step is to rule out serious upper genital tract disease. Fever, abdominal pain, deep dyspareunia, or weight loss suggest a serious diagnosis.

Certain historical features change the likelihood of candidiasis and bacterial vaginosis. If, for example, a patient describes an odor associated with discharge, the likelihood of bacterial vaginosis increases by 60%, whereas the likelihood of candidiasis decreases by about 40%. No symptoms are clearly predictive for trichomoniasis. See Figure 49–1 for the diagnostic approach to vaginitis.

Feature	LR+ for the Diagnosis of Candidiasis	LR– for the Diagnosis of Candidiasis	LR+ for the Diagnosis of Bacterial Vaginosis	LR– for the Diagnosis of Bacterial Vaginosis
Cheesy	2.4	0.48		
Watery	0.12	1.5		
Odor	0.35–0.48	1.6–2.1	1.6	0.07
Itching	1.7–1.8	0.18–0.38		
Redness	2.0	0.84		
"Another yeast infection"	3.3	0.72		

Adapted from Anderson MR, Klink K, Cohrssen A. Evaluation of vaginal complaints. JAMA. 2004;291:1368–1379.

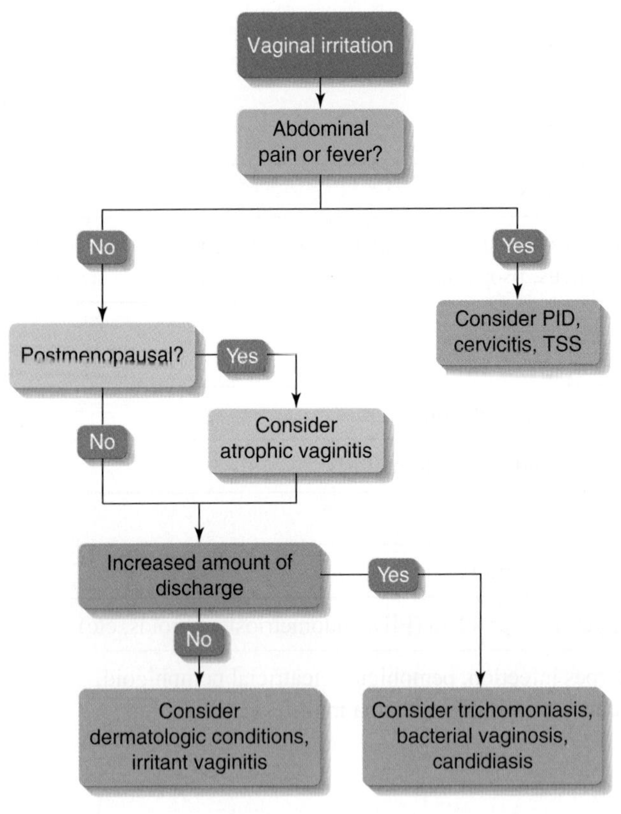

FIGURE 49–1 Diagnostic approach: Vaginitis. PID, pelvic inflammatory disease; TSS, toxic shock syndrome.

CAVEATS

- Differentiate between lower and upper tract symptoms.
- Not all vaginal discharge is pathologic or due to infection.
- The diagnosis of any STI should prompt investigation for other STIs and patient education about measures to prevent new infections.
- Vulvar edema only occurs in candidiasis, trichomoniasis, or dermatologic disorders.
- Deep dyspareunia most often occurs with conditions other than vaginitis, implying pain with movement of deeper structures such as the uterus, ovaries, fallopian tubes, or bladder.
- Distinguish external dysuria (pain experienced in the vulva as urine passes over the skin) from internal dysuria (pain felt deeper in the pelvis in the area of the bladder or urethra). External dysuria most often results from a vulvovaginal problem. Internal dysuria is often accompanied by other lower urinary tract symptoms including urgency and frequency.
- Be aware that mixed genital infections occur frequently.
- In the postmenopausal or postpartum woman, strongly consider atrophic vaginitis as the etiology of discharge. However, infectious causes remain common after menopause.
- Refine all diagnostic impressions based on history with a careful genital examination, wet preparation, and potassium hydroxide (KOH) microscopy of vaginal secretions.

PROGNOSIS

Infectious causes of vulvovaginitis are easily treated. Recurrent infections with *Candida* and bacterial vaginosis are very common. Atrophic vaginitis may be a chronic problem but generally responds well to topical estrogen therapy. Dermatologic disorders of the vulva (eg, lichen sclerosis) may be more difficult to manage and require prolonged courses of treatment. Recognition of upper tract infections is important because these infections may cause significant morbidity and require urgent systemic antibiotic therapy.

CASE SCENARIO | Resolution

A 21-year-old woman is upset to report vaginal discharge. The discharge has been present for the past 10 days. She has never had this before and appears to be very anxious.

ADDITIONAL HISTORY

She has also noted an odor that is particularly embarrassing; she hesitated to share this information. Her first intercourse was 3 weeks ago, and she is very worried about a sexually transmitted infection. She has been with only one partner who is male. She generally uses condoms, but on one occasion, the condom broke. The discharge is thin in consistency; she denies clumped discharge or itching. She has no dysuria.

Question: What is the most likely diagnosis?

A. Candidiasis
B. Bacterial vaginosis
C. Trichomoniasis
D. Psoriasis

Test Your Knowledge

1. A 20-year-old woman has just been diagnosed with bacterial vaginosis. She wants to know if this is a sexually transmitted infection.

   What do you tell her?

   A. All forms of vaginitis are sexually transmitted.
   B. Bacterial vaginosis implies that her partner has been intimate with someone else.
   C. Bacterial vaginosis occurs in women who have had sex, but it is not considered to be a sexually transmitted infection.

2. Your 22-year-old patient has her fourth episode of yeast vaginitis in 3 months.

   You recommend that she be tested for which of the following?

   A. Hypothyroidism
   B. Trichomoniasis
   C. HIV
   D. Uterine fibroids

3. A 55-year-old woman is in your office with dyspareunia and vaginal discharge. She is widowed and just recently started a new relationship with a 60-year-old man.

   A possible cause of her symptoms includes which of the following?

   A. Atrophic vaginitis
   B. Trichomoniasis
   C. *Candida* vaginitis
   D. All of the above

References

1. Schaaf M, Perez-Stable E, Borchardt K. The limited value of symptoms and signs in the diagnosis of vaginal infections. *Arch Intern Med.* 1990;150:1929–1933.
2. Kent H. Epidemiology of vaginitis. *Am J Obstet Gynecol.* 1991;165:1168–1176.
3. Fleury F. Adult vaginitis. *Clin Obstet Gynecol.* 1981;24:407–438.
4. Anderson MR, Klink K, Cohrssen A. Evaluation of vaginal complaints. *JAMA*. 2004;291:1368–1379.
5. Lowe NK, Neal JL, Ryan-Wenger NA. Accuracy of the clinical diagnosis of vaginitis compared with a DNA probe laboratory standard. *Obstet Gynecol.* 2009;113:89–95.

6. Spinillo A, Bernuzzi AM, Cevini C, et al. The relationship of bacterial vaginosis, Candida and Trichomonas infection to symptomatic vaginitis in postmenopausal women attending a vaginitis clinic. *Maturitas.* 1997;27:253–260.
7. Mac Bride MB, Rhodes, DJ, Shuster LT. Vulvovaginal atrophy. *Mayo Clin Proc*. 2010;85:87–94.
8. Freij B. Acute pelvic inflammatory disease. *Semin Adolesc Med.* 1986;2:143–153.
9. Lanes S, Poole C, Dreyer NA, Lanza LL. Toxic shock syndrome, contraceptive methods and vaginitis. *Am J Obstet Gynecol.* 1986;154:989–991.
10. Brinton L, Nasca PC, Mallin K, et al. Case-control study of in situ and invasive carcinoma of the vagina. *Gynecol Oncol.* 1990;38:49–59.

Suggested Reading

Centers for Disease Control and Prevention. Sexually transmitted diseases treatment guidelines. 2010. *MMWR Recomm Rep.* 2010;59:RR-12.

Egan M, Lipsky M. Diagnosis of vaginitis. *Am Fam Physician.* 2000;62:1095–1104.

Fisher B, Margesson L. *Genital Skin Disorders*. St. Louis, MO: Mosby, 1998.

Sobel J. Vaginitis. *N Engl J Med.* 1997;337:1896–1903.

Stewart E. *The V Book*. New York, NY: Bantam, 2002.

Wilson JF. In the clinic. Vaginitis and cervicitis. *Ann Intern Med.* 2009;151:ITC3-1–ITC3-15.

Chapter 50

Abnormal Vaginal Bleeding

Amy N. Ship, MD

CASE SCENARIO

A 46-year-old woman comes to your office because she is concerned about heavy vaginal bleeding. Her menstrual cycle has not changed, but over the past year, she has noticed increasingly heavy periods, requiring many more pads than she previously used, and the passage of blood clots. Over the past 3 months, she has become very tired as well, prompting her visit today.

- **What additional questions would you ask to learn more about her bleeding?**
- **What questions would you use to classify her bleeding?**
- **How can you determine whether her bleeding is ovulatory or anovulatory?**
- **Can you narrow the diagnosis using specific questions about her history?**
- **How can you use the patient history to distinguish between worrisome and nonworrisome sources of bleeding?**

INTRODUCTION

Abnormal vaginal bleeding is one of the most common clinical problems in women's health. Statistics regarding the frequency of various causes of abnormal vaginal bleeding are not available. Abnormal vaginal bleeding may be categorized as independent of or related to hormonal cycles. Normal menstrual bleeding lasts an average of 4 days (ranging from 2 to 7 days) and involves loss of about 30 to 60 mL of blood. Vaginal bleeding related to the menstrual cycle is considered abnormal if it varies from normal menstrual bleeding in volume, frequency, or timing. Otherwise, abnormal vaginal bleeding may result from hormonal abnormalities or structural abnormalities anywhere along the genital tract. The likely source depends on the age and reproductive status of the woman.

KEY TERMS

Dysfunctional uterine bleeding (DUB)	Abnormal uterine bleeding that is hormonal in nature and not due to structural or systemic disease.
Menometrorrhagia	Irregular or excessive bleeding during menstruation and between periods.
Menorrhagia	Bleeding of excessive flow and duration that occurs at regular intervals.
Metrorrhagia	Bleeding that occurs at irregular intervals.
Oligomenorrhea	Bleeding that occurs at intervals > 35 days.
Ovulation bleeding	A single episode of spotting between regular menstrual periods.
Polymenorrhea	Bleeding that occurs at intervals < 21 days.
Positive likelihood ratio (LR+)	The increase in the odds of a particular diagnosis if a given factor is present.

ETIOLOGY

The etiology of abnormal vaginal bleeding depends on the age and reproductive status of the patient. Although the vast majority of abnormal bleeding is dysfunctional uterine bleeding, this is a diagnosis of exclusion. Pregnancy, abnormalities of the reproductive tract, systemic diseases, and medications (eg, oral contraceptive pills [OCPs]) may all cause abnormal vaginal bleeding; clinicians must consider these diagnoses before assigning a diagnosis of DUB.

Differential Diagnosis

	Prevalence[a]
Complications related to pregnancy	
Normal intrauterine pregnancy	
Ectopic pregnancy	
Gestational trophoblastic disease	
Spontaneous abortion (threatened, incomplete, or missed)	
Placenta previa	
Retained products of conception after therapeutic abortion	
Abnormalities of the reproductive tract	***67% of women referred for hysteroscopy***[1]
Benign lesions (cervical, endometrial, adenomyosis)	
Malignant lesions (cervical, endometrial)	5% of postmenopausal women[2]
Infection (cervicitis, endometritis)	
Trauma (laceration, abrasion, foreign body)	
Systemic disease	
Endocrinopathy (hypothyroidism, hyperprolactinemia, Cushing's disease, polycystic ovarian syndrome, adrenal dysfunction/tumor)	19% of adolescent patients; 11% of patients[3] age 18–45 years[4]
Coagulopathy	
• von Willebrand disease	
• Thrombocytopenia	
• Leukemia	
Renal disease	
Hepatic disease	
Iatrogenic factors/medications	
Anticoagulation therapy	
Intrauterine device	
Hormone therapy (oral, topical, or injection contraceptives; estrogen replacement therapy; selective estrogen receptor modulators)	
Psychotropic agents	
DUB	

[a]Among women with abnormal menstrual bleeding in the specific population described; prevalence is unknown when not indicated.

GETTING STARTED WITH THE HISTORY

- Establish how long the abnormal bleeding has been present and how excessive it is.
- Consider pregnancy in any woman of reproductive age.
- Remember that although worrisome to patients, abnormal vaginal bleeding does not indicate serious disease in the vast majority of patients.

Questions	Remember
Tell me more about your bleeding.	Listen to the story.
Do you have any other symptoms?	Don't rush the interview by interrupting and focusing the history too soon.
What are you most worried about?	Reassure the patient when appropriate.

INTERVIEW FRAMEWORK

- After determining the patient's age, focus questions based on bleeding issues common in the appropriate age group.
- Assess whether bleeding has normal intervals and volume or is erratic and excessive.
- If the patient is premenopausal, establish her normal menstrual pattern. If she is postmenopausal, obtain a brief menstrual history, including when cycles stopped and previous intervals.
- Establish that the source of bleeding is vaginal rather than from the gastrointestinal or urinary tract.
- Inquire about bleeding characteristics, including the following:
  - Onset
  - Precipitating factors
  - Nature of bleeding (temporal pattern, duration, postcoital, quantity)
  - Associated symptoms
  - Patient's medical history
  - Medication use and history
  - Personal or family history of bleeding disorder.

IDENTIFYING ALARM SYMPTOMS

Although abnormal vaginal bleeding may be due to worrisome diseases, only 2 life-threatening conditions must be considered: ectopic pregnancy and intrauterine hemorrhage from various causes. Women with life-threatening vaginal hemorrhage will usually seek medical attention at urgent care settings and appear ill due to marked, dramatic blood loss with tachycardia, hypotension, light-headedness, dizziness, or syncope. Patients with ectopic pregnancy may have the classic symptoms of severe abdominal pain and bleeding in the setting of a known pregnancy or more subtle clinical features such as mild abdominal discomfort and light bleeding.

Serious Diagnoses

- Ectopic pregnancy
- Gynecologic cancer
- Severe bleeding diathesis
- Vaginal hemorrhage

Alarm Features	Serious Causes	LR+	Benign Causes
Dizziness, light-headedness, syncope, palpitations, tachycardia	Hemorrhage		Anxiety Arrhythmia
Abdominal pain and known pregnancy	Ectopic pregnancy	1.4–6.1[5]	Normal pregnancy Fibroid Benign gastrointestinal source
Weight loss	Endometrial cancer		Lifestyle change Thyroid abnormality
Bloating, increasing abdominal girth	Ovarian cancer		Hormonal change Thyroid abnormality Inactivity

FOCUSED QUESTIONS

QUESTIONS	THINK ABOUT...
Are your menstrual cycles regular?	Provides a baseline against which bleeding can be assessed
What is the usual interval between periods?	DUB if interval does not fall between 25 and 31 days
What was the first day of your last period?	Establishing baseline for irregular bleeding
Is your period late?	Pregnancy
Do you have bleeding occurring:	
• *Irregularly between menstrual cycles?*	OCPs Breakthrough bleeding Uterine lesions Cervicitis
• *After sexual intercourse?*	Irritation Cervical mass or lesion
• *Midway between periods? Associated with dull aching pain?*	Midcycle bleeding (mittelschmerz) associated with ovulation
• *A few days before the onset of your normal cycle?*	Premenstrual spotting, a variant of metrorrhagia
Does the bleeding occur irregularly? Is it unpredictable as to amount and duration?	DUB Perimenopause (if patient is 45–55 years old) Stress Illness Polycystic ovarian syndrome Breakthrough bleeding
Duration of menses	
What is the duration of flow?	
• *2–7 days*	Normal
• *> 7 days*	Menorrhagia Uterine lesions
• *Prolonged and with irregular intermenstrual bleeding*	Menometrorrhagia Chronic anovulation
Amount of blood loss	
What is the amount of menstrual blood loss?	
• *Increased? Excessive?*	Hypermenorrhea Abnormality of reproductive tract Bleeding diathesis
• *Spotty? Light? With regular predictable menstruation?*	Hypomenorrhea Obstruction of outflow tract Scarring
How many tampons or pads do you use daily?	A poor estimate of blood loss; normal use varies widely
Are you passing any clots?	Heavy bleeding

Accompanying symptoms	
Do you have:	
• *The following symptoms a few days before the onset of menstrual flow: breast fullness or tenderness, abdominal bloating, low back pain, weight gain, or mood changes?*	Premenstrual symptoms suggestive of ovulatory bleeding
• *Abdominal cramping with or just prior to your menstruations?*	Dysmenorrhea; more common during ovulatory cycles
• *Dull aching pain at midcycle?*	Ovulatory bleeding (mittelschmerz)
• *Chronic pain in the lower abdomen that increases during menstruation?*	Fibroids Infection Pelvic inflammatory disease (PID) Endometriosis
• *Fever?*	PID
• *Vaginal discharge or itching?*	Vaginal infection
• *Milky nipple discharge?*	Pregnancy Hyperprolactinemia
• *Easy bruising or bleeding from other sites?*	Bleeding diathesis or clotting disorder
• *Hot flashes or night sweats?*	Vasomotor instability associated with menopause in patient of appropriate age
• *Heat or cold intolerance?*	Thyroid disorder
Additional issues	
What medications are you taking?	Medication-associated bleeding (ie, warfarin, enoxaparin, OCPs, hormone preparations)
Do you use OCPs? Have you recently started OCPs? Have you missed a pill?	Inadequate dosing or a missed pill may cause "breakthrough bleeding."
Are you having sexual intercourse?	Pregnancy PID Trauma
Have you had any recent change in weight, chronic illness, or stress?	DUB
Have you recently stopped taking hormonal therapy?	In postmenopausal woman, estrogen withdrawal bleeding
Are you pregnant?	Implantation bleeding Ectopic pregnancy Abortion (threatened or incomplete)
Have you had a previous ectopic pregnancy or PID?	Ectopic pregnancy
Have you had a recent pregnancy or a recent abortion?	Retention of gestational products
Have you been forced to have sexual relations, or have you had sex that was rough or painful?	Trauma
Are you having abnormal bleeding from any other site? Have you bruised easily recently?	Bleeding diathesis

DIAGNOSTIC APPROACH (INCLUDING ALGORITHM)

Once alarm symptoms have been excluded, the first step is to determine whether the patient is premenopausal or postmenopausal. In any woman of reproductive age, consider bleeding to be a possible complication of pregnancy until proven otherwise. If the patient is premenopausal and not likely to be pregnant, determine whether a specific source for the bleeding is suggested by the history (trauma, infection, medication use, or systemic disease) or whether DUB is likely. In the postmenopausal population, inquire about the use of hormone replacement therapy before considering an anatomic source. See Figure 50–1 for the diagnostic approach algorithm for abnormal vaginal bleeding.

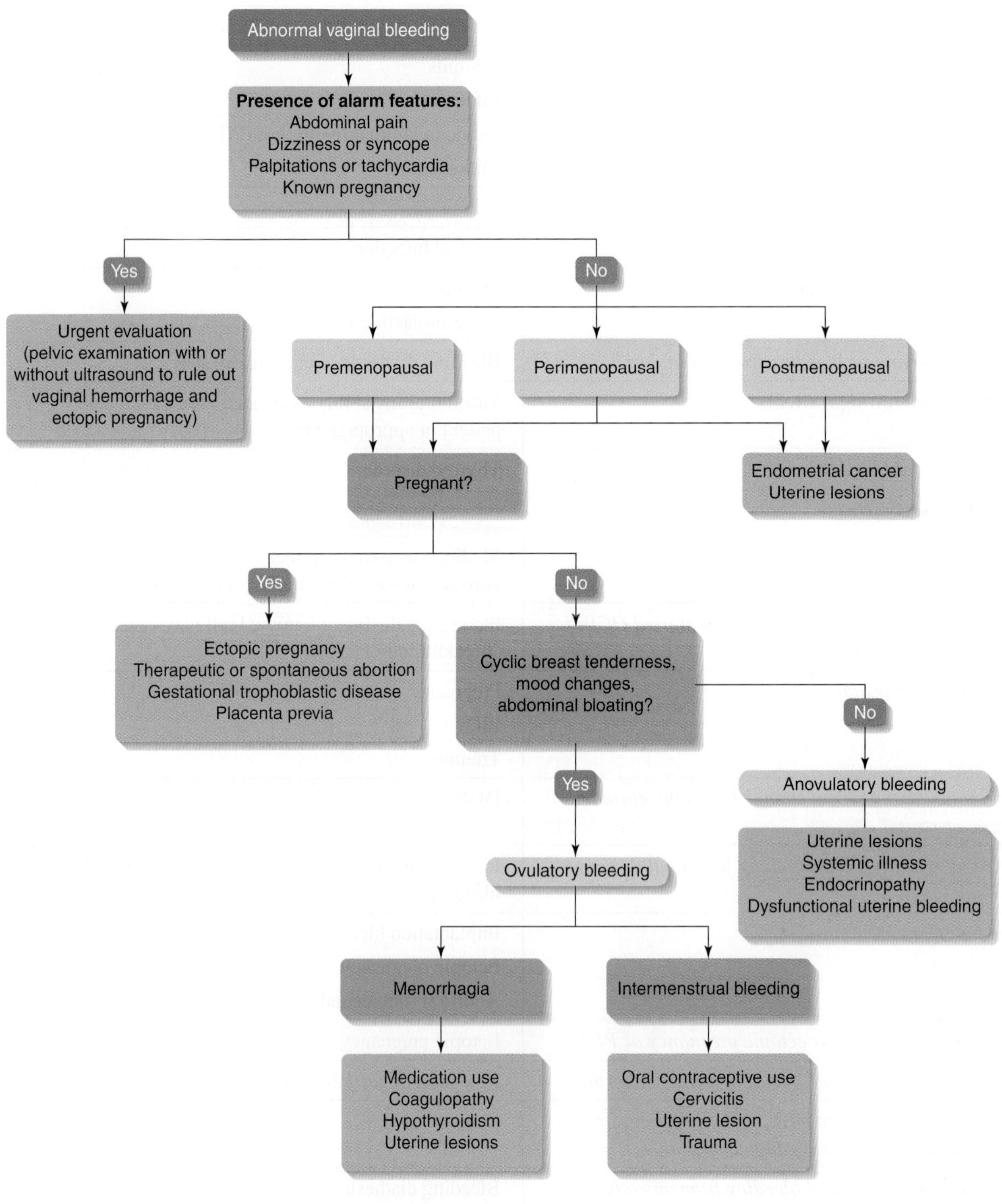

FIGURE 50–1 Diagnostic approach: Abnormal vaginal bleeding.

CAVEATS

- Establish the patient's age and menopausal status in order to move correctly through the diagnostic algorithm.
- Consider pregnancy in any woman of reproductive age. Unless the woman is not sexually active with men, pregnancy must be excluded.
- Make sure to establish the patient's sexual history, including recent sexual intercourse, potential for sexual trauma, history of sexually transmitted diseases, and prior pregnancy history.
- Irregular bleeding is acceptable during the first 6 months of hormone replacement therapy; if bleeding persists after 6 months, it should be investigated further.
- Consider the less likely causes of abnormal vaginal bleeding (eg, hepatic and renal disease) in women with risk factors or other suggestive symptoms.
- Consider coagulopathy in adolescent females with heavy abnormal vaginal bleeding.
- Consider pelvic lesions in women without other sources of bleeding whose history suggests ovulatory bleeding (cyclic symptoms including breast tenderness, moodiness, and abdominal bloating).
- Remember that DUB is a diagnosis of exclusion, which is most often due to anovulation. It is more common at the extremes of reproductive age (postmenarchal and perimenopausal periods).

PROGNOSIS

In the absence of vaginal hemorrhage or ruptured ectopic pregnancy, abnormal vaginal bleeding has a favorable prognosis in the vast majority of cases. Although postmenopausal vaginal bleeding may suggest a gynecologic cancer, vaginal atrophy is 6 times more likely, and cancers identified are often at an early treatable stage.

CASE SCENARIO | Resolution

A 46-year-old woman comes to your office because she is concerned about heavy vaginal bleeding. Her menstrual cycle has not changed, but over the past year, she has noticed increasingly heavy periods, requiring many more pads than she previously used, and the passage of blood clots. Over the past 3 months, she has become very tired as well, prompting her visit today.

ADDITIONAL HISTORY

The interval between her periods has not changed, nor has she had a month without bleeding. She describes increased pelvic discomfort and menstrual cramps with her menses. She is sexually active and monogamous with her husband who has had a vasectomy. She has had no abnormal vaginal discharge. She denies increased sweating, cold intolerance, and constipation but, as stated, endorses significant fatigue. Her only medications are vitamin D and calcium. She has noticed no other bleeding sites and no easy bruising. She has no "alarm" symptoms, such as acute abdominal pain, dizziness, syncope, or palpitations. Office staff obtains a pregnancy test, which is negative.

Question: What is the most likely diagnosis?

A. Endometrial cancer
B. Uterine fibroids
C. Coagulopathy
D. Hypothyroidism

Test Your Knowledge

1. A 19-year-old woman presents with one isolated episode of light spotting between her periods.
   Which of the following is *not* a likely cause of her bleeding?
   A. Cervicitis
   B. Traumatic intercourse
   C. Coagulopathy
   D. Oral contraceptive use

2. A 35-year-old woman with a negative pregnancy test is concerned about her menstrual bleeding.
   Which of the following symptoms associated with the bleeding is *not* suggestive that her bleeding is ovulatory in nature?
   A. Bloating
   B. Cold intolerance
   C. Breast tenderness
   D. Moodiness

3. A 56-year-old woman presents with vaginal bleeding and intermittent abdominal cramping. She does not track her menstrual cycle but states that her periods are very irregular. She thinks she last bled more than 9 months ago.
   Which of the following diagnoses should you exclude first?
   A. Menopause
   B. Dysfunctional uterine bleeding
   C. Hormonal effect
   D. Pregnancy

References

1. Motashaw ND, Dave S. Diagnostic and therapeutic hysteroscopy in the management of abnormal uterine bleeding. *J Reprod Med.* 1990;35:616–620.
2. MacMahon B. Overview of studies on endometrial cancer and other types of cancer in humans: perspectives of an epidemiologist. *Semin Oncol.* 1997;24(suppl 1):S1–S122.
3. Claessens EA, Cowell CA. Acute adolescent menorrhagia. *Am J Obstet Gynecol.* 1981;139:277–280.
4. Dilley A, Drews C, Miller C, et al. von Willebrand disease and other inherited bleeding disorders in women with diagnosed menorrhagia. *Obstet Gynecol.* 2001;97:630–636.
5. Buckley RG, King KJ, Disney JD, et al. History and physical examination to estimate the risk of ectopic pregnancy: validation of a clinical prediction model. *Ann Emerg Med.* 1999;34: 664–667.

Suggested Reading

Fazio SB, Ship AN. Abnormal uterine bleeding. *South Med J.* 2007;100:376–382.

Goodman AK. Terminology and differential diagnosis of genital tract bleeding in women. UpToDate online, 2003. Available at: http://www.uptodateonline.com. Accessed October 26, 2011.

Kilbourn CL, Richards CS. Abnormal uterine bleeding; diagnostic considerations, management options. *Postgrad Med.* 2001;109:137–138, 141–144, 147–150.

Oriel KA, Schrager, SA. Abnormal uterine bleeding. *Am Fam Physician.* 1999;60:1371–1382.

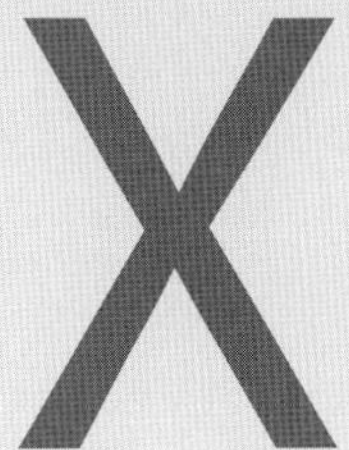

SECTION

X

MUSCULOSKELETAL SYSTEM

Chapter 51

Neck Pain

John D. Goodson, MD

CASE SCENARIO

A 57-year-old science teacher presents with right-sided neck pain. He describes intense discomfort in the back of his neck and upper back along the medial aspect of his right scapula. The pain has been present for 10 days and began after he had installed new overhead lighting in his basement workshop.

- **What repetitive positions are most likely to aggravate the neck?**
- **What is the pattern of referred pain from cervical radicular root irritation?**
- **Which muscle groups are affected by cervical nerve root impingement?**
- **What symptoms require urgent imaging and/or surgical consultation?**

INTRODUCTION

Neck pain can be categorized by location and onset. Most neck pain originates in the back (posterior) portion of the neck in the muscular, neurologic, or bony structures. Patients may also describe pain as most intense in the neck or shoulders or the upper extremities along the distribution of a cervical nerve root.[1,2] Pain in the back of the neck is generally *axial*, meaning along the midline or the paraspinous region, or *radicular*, meaning radiating to the shoulder or arm on one side or both sides.

Pain arising from muscular, vascular, and glandular structures, as well as the trachea and esophagus, commonly refers to the front (anterior portion) of the neck. Finally, pain may be referred from other parts of the body such as the chest, heart, and esophagus.

KEY TERMS

Anterior neck pain	Pain in the front of the neck. May originate from cervical lymph nodes, sternoclavicular muscles, trachea, pharynx, carotid arteries, thyroid, or esophagus. Referred pain from the heart, lungs, or pericardium generally occurs in the anterior neck.
Carotidynia	Pain in the anterior neck overlying the carotid artery. The pulsation of the artery can generally be felt.
Cervical radiculopathy	Pain or numbness in the distribution of one or more of the cervical nerve roots (see Figure 51–1 and box titled "Motor Function for Select Cervical Spine Myotomes"). Patients may report little or no neck pain per se. Focal weakness may also occur. Impingement can result from disk herniation or from nerve root entrapment due to degenerative arthritis of the facet joints.
Complex regional pain syndrome	A combination of pain, swelling, and dysautonomic symptoms such as flushing or warmth in an anatomic region such as an extremity or part of an extremity (see Chapter 53).

—*Continued next page*

Continued—

Dermatome	The cutaneous sensory distribution of an individual spinal nerve bundle or root.
Neck stiffness	A generalized decrease in neck mobility. This usually results from facet joint arthritis or neck injury with associated neck muscle or trapezius muscle spasm from nerve root irritation. Other causes include polymyalgia rheumatica, localized infection, and meningitis.
Occipital neuralgia	Pain located at the base of the skull at the juncture of the occiput and the first cervical vertebral body (atlas). Pain may radiate to the back of the head in the distribution of the second cervical nerve root. Pain is commonly referred to the vertex (top) of the head and even to the forehead.
Axial or radicular neck pain	Axial pain is located in the paraspinous muscle(s) of the neck, the trapezius muscle(s), or the paraspinous muscle(s) of the upper back. Radicular pain radiates to one or both shoulders or arms; see cervical radiculopathy entry above. Causes include cervical disk herniation, nerve root impingement, hypertrophy or thickening of the facet joints, and congenital spinal stenosis.
Thoracic outlet syndrome	Mechanical compromise of the neurovascular bundle to an upper extremity by bone or soft tissue structures (eg, neck or shoulder muscles). The classic symptom triad is numbness, weakness, and swelling in one extremity.
Whiplash	A rapid acceleration/deceleration injury to the soft tissue or bony structures of the neck.

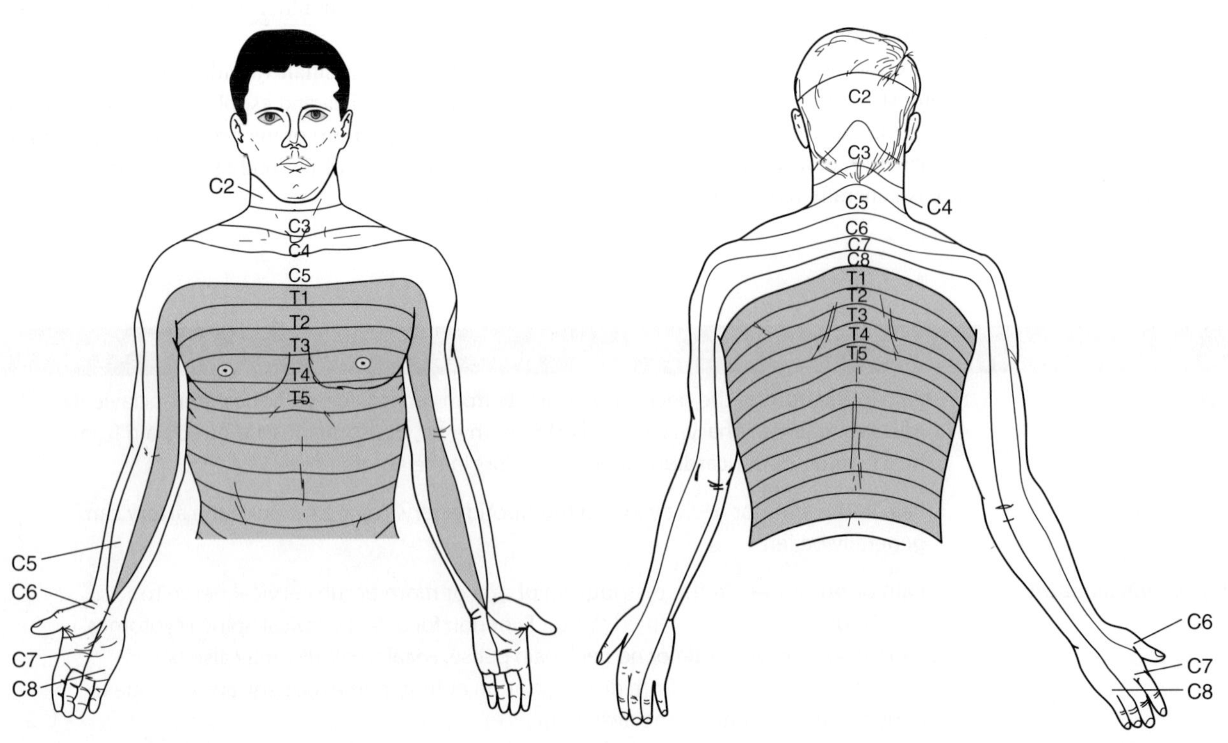

FIGURE 51–1 Dermatome distribution for cervical and high thoracic spine. (Reprinted from Nakano KK. Neck pain. In: McCullough K, Burton C, eds. *Textbook of Rheumatology*. 3rd ed. Philadelphia, PA: WB Saunders Company, 1989:475.)

ETIOLOGY

Many acute and chronic illnesses cause neck pain. Generally, neck pain is due to chronic and repetitive use combined with genetic and environmental factors such as smoking. Many occupations are particularly stressful to the neck. These usually require repetitive activities that demand looking upward, such as working on ceilings.

Acute severe trauma can cause immediate neck pain due to bone fracture, disk protrusion, or soft tissue strain. More often, trauma triggers pain in a neck vulnerable due to aging or previous repetitive injury.

Posterior axial and/or radicular neck pain is common and is the only type that has been well studied from an epidemiologic standpoint. For example, in a UK survey of 5752 adults in 3 general practices, the prevalence of posterior neck pain was 18%, of which roughly 5% was intense, disabling, and chronic.[3]

Differential Diagnosis

	Prevalence[a]
Axial and/or radicular neck pain	18% in a primary care setting[2]
Cervical radiculopathy with or without neck pain	0.5% in patients with traumatic neck pain in an emergency department[3]
Anterior neck pain	
Neck stiffness	
Occipital neuralgia	

[a]Prevalence is unknown when not indicated.

GETTING STARTED WITH THE HISTORY

- Determine whether a life-threatening or disabling condition is present. If the neck is mechanically stable and no immediate risk of cord injury or airway compromise exists, stratify the pain based on location (eg, anterior or posterior neck pain).
- Patients often localize anterior neck pain to a specific part of the neck. If the patient cannot localize the pain, consider the possibility of referred pain from the lungs, upper chest, heart, or mediastinum.
- Inquire about daily activities that can cause repetitive neck injury. This is an opportunity to explore the patient's routine. Ask for details. For example, have the patient demonstrate to you how he or she sits at work. A secretary might spend hours sitting at a reception desk looking upward to greet clients.

Questions	Remember
Describe your neck pain.	Allow the patient to describe the nature and location of the pain. Ask the patient to point to the area(s) of pain. Ask the patient to point on your body to the area where the pain is worse. Specifically ask about pain referred to the shoulder(s), upper back, and arm(s).
How did the pain start? What were you doing when you first noticed your neck pain?	Ask about positions or repetitive motions that provoke the pain. Inquire about all aspects of daily routine, asking the patient to demonstrate as appropriate
How severe is the pain on a scale from 1 to 10, where 10 is severe pain?	Observe the patient's neck movement to determine the extent of limitation and severity.

INTERVIEW FRAMEWORK

Encourage the patient to identify the location by pointing to the site of the neck pain. It is helpful to have patients point out on your body where they feel the pain on their body.

Ask about:

- Onset of the pain, including the time and date of onset and the circumstances
- Repetitive activities that strain the neck
  - Twisting
  - Bending the neck to the side or cradling
  - Protraction or leaning forward with the chin extended
  - Neck hyperextension or looking upward
- History of recent and past neck trauma
- Duration of pain
- Frequency of pain
- Radiation of the pain to the:
  - Paraspinous muscles of the upper back/scapular region
  - Shoulder(s)
  - Arm(s), specifically to the thumb (sixth cervical nerve root), middle finger (seventh cervical nerve root), or little finger (eighth cervical nerve root)
- Positions or postures that both worsen and improve the symptoms
- Fever
- Headache
- Upper body, torso, or arm stiffness

Review the patient record to determine whether the patient has a history of neck complaints or problems.

IDENTIFYING ALARM SYMPTOMS

First determine whether there is any threat to the integrity of the spinal cord. This is most concerning in the context of acute severe trauma but should be considered after minor trauma in the elderly or in those with pre-existing chronic neck pain. Next, determine whether there is any concern for an acute infectious process such as meningitis or osteomyelitis. Finally, symptoms of airway obstruction require immediate diagnosis and treatment.

Consider spinal cord impingement in patients with the following features:

- Acute injury such as whiplash
- Acute worsening of chronic neck pain
- Weakness or clumsiness in an extremity
- Gait instability
- Change in bowel or bladder function

In a large multicenter study of patients seeking medical attention at an emergency department with blunt neck injury, the following combination of features had a 99.9% negative predictive value for cervical spine injury[4,5]:

- Absence of midline cervical tenderness
- Absence of focal neurologic deficit
- Normal alertness
- No evidence of intoxication
- No other clinically apparent pain that might distract the patient from the pain of the neck injury per se

Among certain patients, such as the elderly and those with connective tissue diseases (eg, rheumatoid arthritis, ankylosing spondylitis) or cervical spinal stenosis, even minor trauma can cause bony and soft tissue shifts, putting the cervical spinal cord at risk for injury. These patients usually have an extensive prior history of neck pain. Take a comprehensive history with such patients in order to understand the nature and extent of disease. If there is uncertainty, then seek corroborating information from records and previous providers.

In patients with acute injury or recent deterioration of chronic neck pain, assess for peripheral nerve damage and loss of sensory or motor function in the distribution of one or more cervical nerve roots. The sensory distribution and the motor effects of damage to different cervical nerve roots are shown in Figure 51–1 and in the box titled "Motor Function for Select Cervical Spine Myotomes."

Serious Diagnoses

	Prevalence[a]
Airway obstruction	
Cervical spinal cord injury	
Peripheral motor or sensory nerve injury	< 0.5%[4]
Cervical spine fracture	2.4%–2.6%[4,5]
Neck pain following motor vehicle accident	26%[6]

[a]Among patients presenting to an emergency department with neck pain; prevalence is unknown when not indicated.

Alarm Symptoms	Serious Causes	Benign Causes
Dyspnea	Airway obstruction	Anxiety
	Aspiration of a foreign body	Gastroesophageal reflux disease (GERD)
Sensation of having something stuck in throat	Airway obstruction Aspiration of a foreign body	Anxiety GERD
Inability to talk	Airway obstruction Aspiration of a foreign body	Anxiety GERD
Weakness in arms or legs Tingling in hands or feet Tingling up and down spine when neck is flexed or extended (Lhermitte sign)	Myelopathy due to: • Central cervical disk herniation • Vertebral osteomyelitis • Epidural abscess • Cervical spinal stenosis • Multiple sclerosis	
Weakness in shoulders, arms, or hands	Impingement or entrapment of one or more cervical nerve roots	Carpal tunnel syndrome Cubital fossa syndrome
Loss of sensation in arms or hands (see Figure 51–1)	Impingement or entrapment of one or more cervical nerve roots	Carpal tunnel syndrome Cubital fossa syndrome
Dropping things	Impingement or entrapment of one or more cervical nerve roots	Carpal tunnel syndrome Cubital fossa syndrome
Intense pain (following an injury) Neck pain and fever	Cervical spine fracture Meningitis, epidural abscess, osteomyelitis	Paraspinous muscle spasm Benign viral infection

Motor Function for Select Cervical Spine Myotomes

	Motor	Reflex
C5	Arm elevation (deltoid) Elbow flexion (biceps)	Biceps
C6	Wrist extension (extensor carpi)	Forearm
C7	Elbow extension (triceps) Finger extension	Triceps

FOCUSED QUESTIONS

Direct questions toward the most likely anatomic location of the neck symptoms.

QUESTIONS	THINK ABOUT...
Is the pain located in the back of the neck or in the muscles between your neck and shoulder (trapezius)?	Mild whiplash Chronic overuse Polymyalgia rheumatica
Does the pain spread from your neck (or trapezius) to the upper back, shoulder, or arm?	Cervical radicular pain Complex regional pain syndrome Thoracic outlet syndrome
Is the pain exclusively located in the shoulder or arm?	Cervical radicular pain Complex regional pain syndrome Thoracic outlet syndrome
Is the pain located on the side or the front of the neck?	Painful lymphadenopathy Spasm or pain in the sternoclavicular muscle Temporomandibular joint pain Carotidynia Carotid artery dissection Acute or chronic pharyngitis Acute or chronic tracheitis Acute or chronic esophagitis Foreign body in airway Inflammation of thyroid cartilage Polychondritis Painful thyroiditis Herpes zoster Pericarditis Aortic dissection Angina
Associated symptoms	
Do you have numbness or tingling in the arms, shoulders, or hands?	Cervical radiculopathy Complex regional pain syndrome Thoracic outlet syndrome
Can you reproduce the pain by touching or pressing on parts of your neck?	
• *Front of the neck (anterior cervical lymph nodes)?*	Lymphadenitis
• *The area of your jaw in front of the ears (parotid gland)?*	Parotitis Temporomandibular joint disorder
• *The neck artery pulsation?*	Carotidynia Carotid dissection

Question	Diagnosis
• *The low front of the neck (the thyroid cartilage and thyroid gland)?*	Relapsing polychondritis Rheumatoid arthritis Painful thyroiditis
Is the pain associated with chewing?	Parotitis Temporomandibular joint disorder Temporal arteritis
Have you had fever?	Acute pharyngitis Epiglottitis Meningitis Osteomyelitis Diskitis
Do you have a painful rash?	Herpes zoster
Have you noticed any neck lumps?	Malignancy, usually lymphoma or squamous cell carcinoma
Is the pain at the base of the occiput?	Occipital neuralgia Migraine
Is there fever, cognitive change, or photophobia?	Meningitis
Quality	
Is the pain intense, 6 or greater (on a scale of 1 to 10)?	Acute whiplash Acute exacerbation of a chronic neck arthritis Acute exacerbation of a chronic neck overuse syndrome
Is the pain mild, 3 or less (on a scale of 1 to 10)?	Chronic neck arthritis Chronic overuse syndrome
Is the neck stiff?	Chronic neck arthritis Chronic overuse syndrome
Where does the pain radiate?	See Figure 51–1 for the sensory distribution of the cervical nerve roots.
Time course	
Did the pain occur after an acute injury?	Acute whiplash Acute exacerbation of chronic neck arthritis
Did the pain occur after a minor injury or event such as falling asleep in an unusual posture?	Chronic neck arthritis Chronic overuse syndrome
Has the pain been intermittent for weeks or months?	Chronic neck arthritis Chronic overuse syndrome
Modifying symptoms	
Does the pain worsen with neck movement?	Chronic neck arthritis Chronic overuse syndrome Polymyalgia rheumatica

—Continued next page

Continued—

Does the pain worsen with activity or exertion?	Angina
Are there radicular symptoms that occur with neck movement, such as numbness or pain over one of the cervical nerve root dermatomes?	Whiplash Chronic neck arthritis Chronic overuse syndrome
Does the pain occur with swallowing?	Pharyngitis Esophagitis Relapsing polychondritis Rheumatoid arthritis

DIAGNOSTIC APPROACH (INCLUDING ALGORITHM)

The first step is to localize the pain to the front or back of the neck. Next, determine if the pain is *axial*, along the midline or paraspinous region(s), or *radicular*, radiating to the upper back, shoulder, or arm on one side or both. If axial, ask if the pain is at the base of the skull or is dominant on one side.

Next, inquire about trauma, and then determine the relationship of symptoms to a specific event or to specific repetitive activities. Ask about motions or positions that worsen the pain. Encourage the patient to point and describe the pain to determine what mechanical activities worsen the pain. Inquire about the radiation of pain and any localized weakness such as clumsiness in the hands or gait instability. Don't forget to ask about relevant work or leisure activities that might cause chronic irritation of bony or soft tissue structures in the neck.

Associated symptoms such as fever or dysphagia may be important elements of the history. See Figure 51–2 for the diagnostic approach algorithm for neck pain.

CAVEATS

- Nearly all adults have wear and tear changes of the neck structures resulting from the normal aging process and the twisting, turning, and bending of modern life. Ten-year follow-up studies of initially asymptomatic men and women showed that 80% demonstrated magnetic resonance imaging progression of degenerative disease findings such as disk protrusion and ligamentous thickening.
- Hyperreflexia in all 4 extremities suggests cervical spinal cord compression and myelopathy. This is an alarm finding.
- Chronic neck problems frequently result from overuse. Examples include chronic neck hyperextension, such as when individuals work above their heads repeatedly or hyperextend their necks in order to bring reading glasses into focus. People who cradle phones between the shrugged shoulder and the angle of the jaw are also at risk for mechanical nerve root impingement.
- When evaluating a whiplash-type injury, recognize that significant injury to the bony and soft tissue structures may not be readily apparent. Muscle spasm in the neck is protective. In an English cohort of patients followed after a motor vehicle accident, the following 8 factors were associated with recurrent pain. Recurrent pain was low for those with only 2 or fewer risk factors and was over 60% for those with 5 or more risk factors.
    - Younger age
    - Female gender
    - History of neck pain
    - Collision from behind
    - Vehicle stationary at impact
    - More severe collision
    - Not being at fault
    - Monotonous work
- Neck manipulation by chiropractors and physical therapists can create rather significant additional morbidity, including carotid artery dissection and exacerbation of underlying arthritis.[7]
- Neck pain may be the presenting feature of shoulder joint impingement syndromes.[8]
- *Polymyalgia rheumatica* is a subtle inflammatory condition that causes pain and stiffness in the neck and shoulders. It may also be associated with a more worrisome inflammatory condition involving the arteries, giant cell arteritis (GCA). GCA is a medical emergency that can lead to stroke or blindness.
- Torticollis is a tonic contraction of the neck muscles that causes the head to turn uncontrollably. It is a sign of an underlying neuromuscular disorder, such as dystonia or cervical nerve root damage.
- An upper extremity *complex regional pain syndrome*, formally known as reflex sympathetic dystrophy, is an inflammatory condition that can affect the arm, usually after mechanical trauma. Symptoms include severe pain with swelling, erythema, and skin temperature changes.

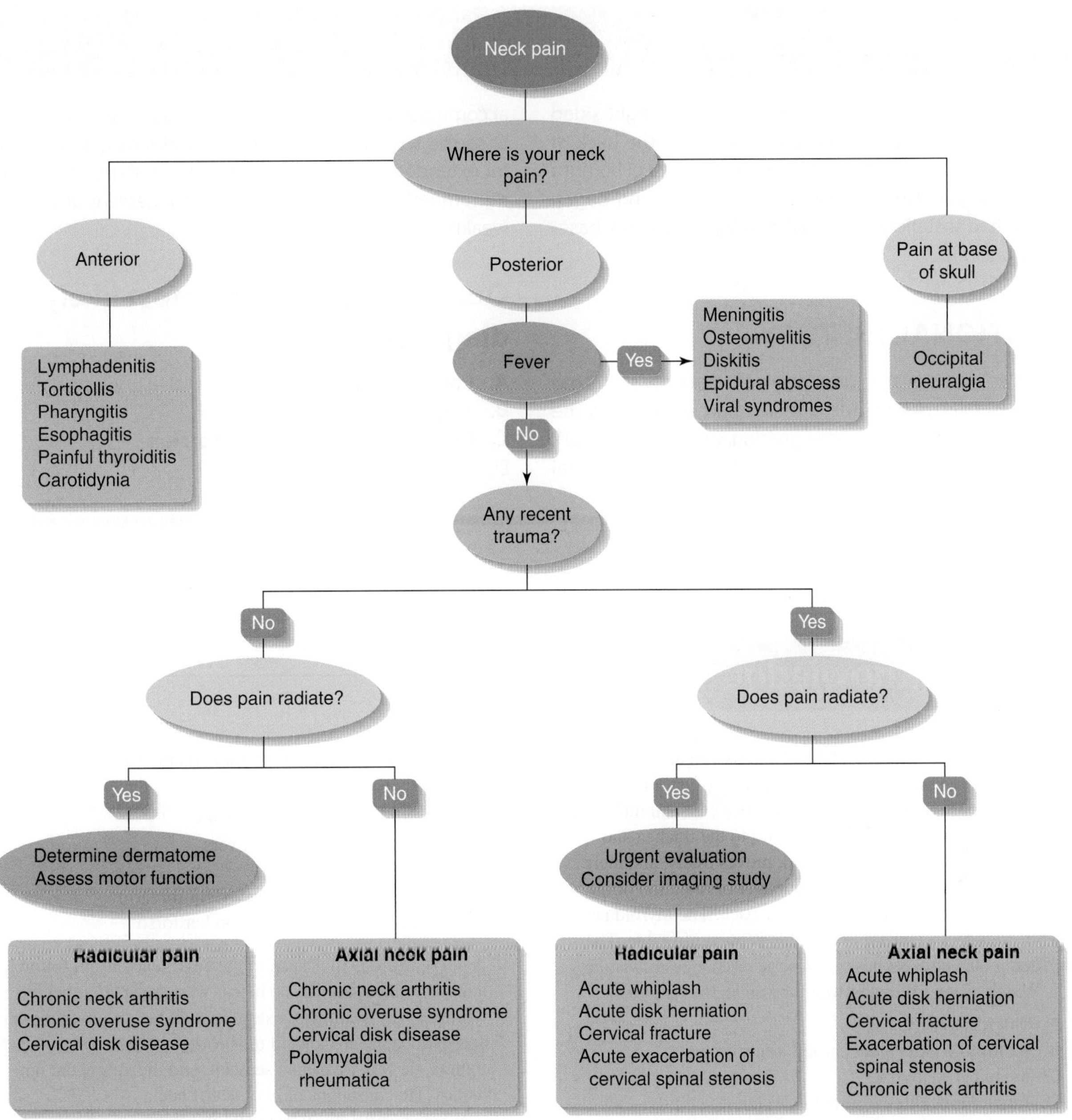

FIGURE 51–2 Diagnostic approach: Neck pain.

PROGNOSIS

Most patients with acute or chronic neck pain from soft tissue and/or bony abnormalities improve with time as long as the neck is protected from further injury or damage. The most common impediment to recovery is the continued irritation of the neck by repeated misuse, especially flexion, extension, or lateral bending. The prognosis of an unrecognized and untreated cervical spine fracture is poor.

Even patients with significant nerve root compression with resultant motor and sensory loss will usually improve over time. Patient reassurance is helpful but should always include an expected time prognosis for recovery; a review of alarm signs such as weakness, extremity clumsiness, or new radicular symptoms; and specific instructions on how to protect the neck, especially the avoidance of repetitive overuse habits that compromise the neck. Neck protection applies while conscious and unconscious. This can best be accomplished during sleep with "pillowing," the use of multiple pillows to stabilize the neck.

CASE SCENARIO | Resolution

A 57-year-old science teacher presents with right-sided neck pain. He describes intense discomfort in the back of his neck and upper back along the medial aspect of his right scapula. The pain has been present for 10 days and began after he had installed new overhead lighting in his basement workshop.

ADDITIONAL HISTORY

The patient has never injured his neck in accident and has not had similar pain in the past. As part of his work, he spends about 2 hours per day grading student homework at his home computer. Unfortunately, he has lost his visual accommodation due to his age and now must use bifocals to see his screen clearly. Sometimes, after he has been online for extended periods, he notes an unusual dull feeling in his right thumb and forefinger. He has not had any arm or hand weakness.

Question: What is the most likely diagnosis?

A. Carotidynia
B. Thyroiditis
C. Cervical nerve root compression
D. Thoracic outlet syndrome

Test Your Knowledge

1. A colleague asks you for advice. He tells you about a 63-year-old woman with a 1-week history of anterior neck pain. The pain came on suddenly and is a constant dull ache on the left side of her neck just lateral to the trachea and under the line of the jaw. The neck moves freely, and there is no pain with any evocative maneuver or radiation of the discomfiture to the shoulder, arm, or back. The thyroid is not tender. He feels a pulsatile area that is uncomfortable. The patient notes no weakness, dizziness, or changes in vision.
   Which of the following would be an alarm symptom?
   A. Gait instability
   B. A pulsatile and tender carotid artery
   C. Asymmetric thyroid
   D. Temporomandibular joint (TMJ) pain
   E. Asymmetric neck pain

2. An 85-year-old woman sees you for intense pain in the right shoulder and arm. The pain began slowly over a few days and then intensified. She has never had any previous neck pain; she has not had any injury or trauma. She describes a burning sensation and a cluster of red bumps on her forearm.
   What findings would you immediately look for on physical examination?
   A. Hyperreflexia in her extremities
   B. Pain with evocative maneuvers
   C. Weakness in the biceps
   D. A vesicular eruption on her right forearm
   E. A diffuse eczematous rash on her torso

3. A 45-year-old man is seen in the emergency room following a motor vehicle accident. His car was struck from behind while he was waiting at a stop light. He was thrown forward and then backward toward his headrest. There was no head trauma, he was wearing a seatbelt, and the airbag did not deploy. He complains only of a stiff neck.
   What specific question would you ask?
   A. How severe was the accident?
   B. What sort of work do you do?
   C. Have you had a prior history of neck pain?
   D. Does the pain radiate?
   E. Point to the area on my neck where you have pain?
   F. All of the above.

References

1. Isaac Z, Anderson BC. Evaluation of the patient with neck pain and cervical spine disorders. In: UpToDate. Available at: http://uptodateonline.com/application/topic/print. Accessed January 2010.
2. Guzman J, Haldeman DC, Carroll L, et al. Clinical practice implications of the bone and joint decade 2000-2010 task force on neck pain and its associated disorders. *Spine*. 2008;33: S199–S213.
3. Webb R, Brammah T, Lunt M, et al. Prevalence and predictors of intense, chronic, and disabling neck and back pain in the UK general population. *Spine.* 2003;28:1195–1202.
4. Stiell IG, Clement CM, McKnight RD, et al. The Canadian C-spine rule versus the NEXUS low-risk criteria in patients with trauma. *N Engl J Med.* 2003;349:2510–2518.
5. Hoffman JR, Mower WR, Wolfson AB, et al. Validity of a set of clinical criteria to rule out injury to the cervical spine in patients with blunt trauma. *N Engl J Med.* 2003;343:94–99.
6. Wiles NJ, Jones GT, Silman AJ, MacFarlane GJ. Onset of neck pain after a motor vehicle accident: a case-control study. *J Rheumatol*. 2005;32:1576–1583.
7. Smith WS, Johnston SC, Skalabrin EJ, et al. Spinal manipulative therapy is an independent risk factor for vertebral artery dissection. *Neurology.* 2003;60:1424–1428.
8. Devereaux MW. Neck and lower back pain. *Med Clin North Am.* 2003;87:643–662.

Suggested Reading

Barnsley L. Neck pain. In: Klippel JH, Dieppe PA, eds. *Rheumatology*. 2nd ed. London, UK: Mosby International, 1998:4.1–4.12.

Glazer PA, Taft K. The cervical spine. In: Gates SJ, Mooar PA, eds. *Musculoskeletal Primary Care*. Philadelphia, PA: Lippincott Williams & Wilkins, 1999:48–74.

Hoppenfeld S. *Physical Examination of the Spine and Extremities.* New York, NY: Appleton-Century-Crofts, 1976.

Nakano KK. Neck pain. In: McCullough K, Burton C, eds. *Textbook of Rheumatology*. 3rd ed. Philadelphia, PA: WB Saunders Company, 1989:471–490.

Okada E, Matsumoto M, Ichihara D, et al. Aging of the cervical spine in healthy volunteers: a 10-year longitudinal study. *Spine*. 2009;34:706–712.

Chapter 52

Shoulder Pain

Craig R. Keenan, MD, and John Wolfe Blotzer, MD

CASE SCENARIO

A 62-year-old man comes to your office to discuss his self-diagnosed right "shoulder bursitis" of over 6 months. The aching pain began insidiously and has worsened over time. The pain is exacerbated by painting (on an easel) and not relieved by acetaminophen or ibuprofen.

- **What additional questions would you ask to learn more about his shoulder pain?**
- **How do you classify causes of shoulder pain?**
- **How can you use the patient history to distinguish between benign and serious causes requiring urgent attention?**

INTRODUCTION

Shoulder pain is a common reason for seeking medical attention. In Great Britain, shoulder pain is the third most common musculoskeletal complaint, representing 5% of musculoskeletal general practice visits. The incidence of shoulder pain reaches a peak in the fourth to sixth decades of life.

Although patients often think of the shoulder as an anatomic region, the clinician must not automatically equate shoulder pain with shoulder joint pain or, more narrowly, glenohumeral joint pain. Many nonmusculoskeletal disorders refer pain to the shoulder. Furthermore, shoulder range of motion involves 4 articulations—glenohumeral, acromioclavicular, sternoclavicular, and scapulothoracic—as well as the associated ligaments, tendons, bursae, muscles, and neurovascular bundles. Disorders in any of these structures can lead to shoulder discomfort.

Evidence-based literature on history in the diagnosis of specific shoulder disorders is limited. Nevertheless, most shoulder pain can be diagnosed by history and physical examination. Imaging is then often used to confirm the diagnosis or assess the severity of a given condition. Figure 52–1 shows the shoulder anatomy.

KEY TERMS

Rotator cuff	Musculotendinous structure blending into the glenohumeral joint capsule providing range of motion and strength. It is composed of the insertions of the supraspinatus, infraspinatus, teres minor, and subscapularis tendons.
Intrinsic pain (also called moving parts pain)	Pain related to structures in the shoulder, including bones, joints, muscles, bursae, tendons, and ligaments. Typically exacerbated by shoulder movement.
Extrinsic pain (also called referred shoulder pain)	Pain from a process in a nonshoulder area or organ perceived as shoulder discomfort. Typically, pain is unrelated to shoulder movement.
Impingement syndrome	Collection of symptoms and signs resulting from compression of the rotator cuff tendons and subacromial bursa between the humeral head and lateral acromion process. Occurs in many different shoulder conditions. See Figure 52–2.

—Continued next page

Continued—

Subacromial bursitis	Inflammation of the subacromial bursa. Usually causes symptoms of impingement syndrome, and often coexists with rotator cuff tendinopathy.
Rotator cuff tendinopathy	Degenerative changes within the rotator cuff tendons leading to pathology ranging from simple inflammation to fibrosis with resultant rotator cuff tears. Patients usually have the impingement syndrome.
Calcific tendinitis	Calcification of a rotator cuff tendon, usually the supraspinatus, proposed to be part of the degenerative process of rotator cuff tendinopathy.
Biceps tendinitis	Overuse syndrome of the long head of the biceps tendon, usually producing anterior shoulder pain.
Acromioclavicular arthritis	Osteoarthritis in the joint between the acromion and clavicle. Usually develops in people who do repetitive overhead work or lots of overhead lifting (eg, bodybuilders). Usually produces focal pain over the acromioclavicular joint and pain when reaching across the body.
Acromioclavicular joint separation	Disruption of the ligaments that attach the acromion to the clavicle, resulting in "separation" of the acromioclavicular joint. Usually caused by fall or blow to tip of the shoulder or fall on an outstretched hand.
Adhesive capsulitis (also called frozen shoulder)	Painful restriction of both active and passive range of motion of the glenohumeral joint in all planes of motion. Usually the end result of other shoulder disorders.

ETIOLOGY[1–7]

Although most shoulder pain arises from articular and periarticular structures (ie, intrinsic pain), the shoulder is also a common location for referred pain from other structures (ie, extrinsic pain). Many causes of extrinsic pain are life threatening. Table 52–1 outlines the myriad causes of referred pain, which can be subdivided into neurologic disorders or visceral conditions that refer pain to the shoulder. Cervical spine disease is the most common cause of pain referred to the shoulder.

The etiology of intrinsic shoulder pain will vary depending on age, vocation, recreational activities, and history of trauma. Often the cause of shoulder pain is multifactorial. Most intrinsic shoulder pain involves the rotator cuff apparatus, including subacromial bursitis and rotator cuff tendinopathy (tendinitis or rotator cuff tears). These conditions usually produce the impingement syndrome. Less common causes include glenohumeral disorders (mainly adhesive capsulitis and glenohumeral osteoarthritis), biceps tendinitis, acromioclavicular (AC) joint osteoarthritis, AC joint separation, and tears of the labrum.

Much less commonly, inflammatory disorders such as rheumatoid arthritis (RA) can affect the shoulder. RA typically causes symmetrical hand and wrist arthritis but occasionally presents first in the glenohumeral joint. Gout and pseudogout can involve both the glenohumeral and sternoclavicular joints, but such patients typically have a long history of the disease or polyarticular disease at presentation. Septic arthritis uncommonly occurs in the shoulder but must always be considered. Polymyalgia rheumatica may present with shoulder pain and occasionally be difficult to distinguish from early frozen shoulder or capsulitis. Shoulder symptoms are rarely the first manifestation of primary or metastatic tumors.

The age of the patient is often helpful. Adolescents and adults younger than 30 often develop overuse injuries to the rotator cuff, AC joint separations, and glenohumeral dislocations. Impingement syndrome and rotator cuff tears are rare in this age group. Middle-aged and older adults frequently get the impingement syndrome related to subacromial bursitis (mild disease) or rotator cuff tendinopathy (moderate or severe disease). This group may also develop rotator cuff tears, osteoarthritis, and adhesive capsulitis.

Lastly, recent trauma, such as blunt force injury, falling onto the shoulder, or falling onto an outstretched arm, is an important clue. Patients with trauma are much more likely to develop clavicle, scapula, or humerus fractures; AC joint separation; labral or rotator cuff tears; or diaphragmatic irritation from splenic rupture. Burning pain that radiates down the arm after a blow to the neck and shoulder may indicate a transient brachial plexus injury, also called a "stinger."

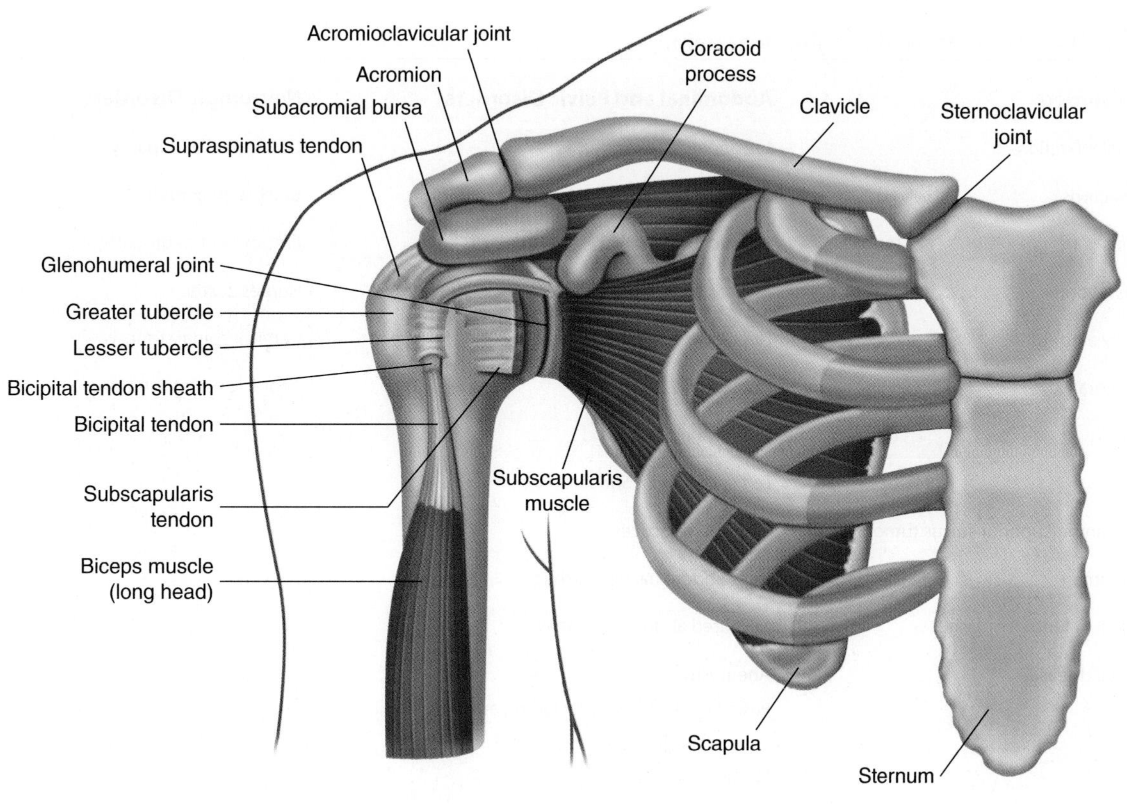

FIGURE 52–1 Shoulder anatomy.

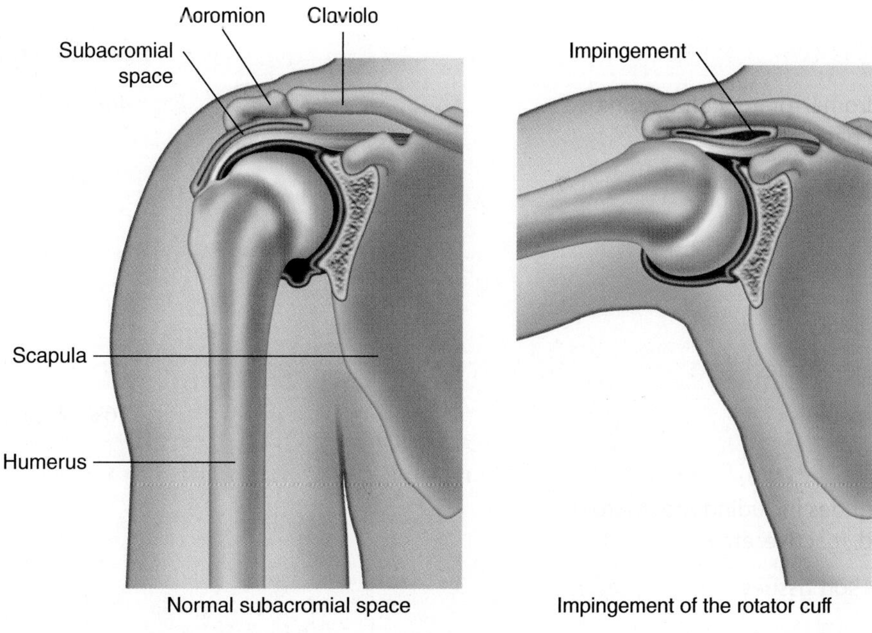

FIGURE 52–2 Impingement syndrome.

Table **52–1.** **Causes of extrinsic shoulder pain.**

Chest Disorders	Abdominal and Pelvic Disorders	Neurologic Disorders
Myocardial infarction	*Left Shoulder Pain*	Cervical radiculopathy
Angina pectoris	Splenic infarction	Brachial plexopathy
Pericarditis	Splenic rupture	Entrapment neuropathy
Aortic dissection	*Right Shoulder Pain*	Herpes zoster
Pulmonary embolism	Hepatic abscess	Cervical spinal stenosis
Pneumothorax	Cholecystitis	Thoracic outlet syndrome
Pneumonia	Hepatic hematoma	
Pleuritis	*Left and/or Right Shoulder Pain*	
Pancoast tumor (superior sulcus tumor)	Subphrenic abscess	
Mesothelioma	Intra-abdominal hemorrhage	
Mediastinal or lung neoplasm	Ruptured abdominal viscus	
Esophageal disease	Aneurysm Vascular insufficiency including arteritis Venous thrombosis Peptic ulcer Pancreatitis Abdominal neoplasms Ectopic pregnancy	

Causes of Intrinsic Shoulder Pain

Cause	Prevalence[a]
Impingement syndrome/rotator cuff tendinitis (includes full and partial tears)	48%–85%
Calcific tendinitis	6%
Rotator cuff tear	
Biceps tendinitis	
Glenohumeral instability	
Acromioclavicular syndromes	
Frozen shoulder/capsulitis	16%–22%
Glenoid labrum tear	
Inflammatory arthritides including rheumatoid, crystal-associated, reactive, etc	
Infection of joint or soft tissues	
Osteoarthritis	
Polymyalgia rheumatica	
Osteonecrosis	

[a]Prevalence in primary care setting[1–7]; prevalence is unknown when not indicated. In one study, 77% of patients had more than one diagnosis.[6]

GETTING STARTED WITH THE HISTORY

- Let patients tell their story in their own words without interruption before resorting to focused questions. An excellent opening is, "Tell me about your shoulder pain, starting from when you very first felt it."

INTERVIEW FRAMEWORK[8]

- Detail the nature of the onset of the shoulder pain, particularly if there was any preceding trauma.
- Determine the key features of the shoulder pain, including:
  - Location (Localizing pain is very helpful in narrowing the differential diagnosis.)
  - Pain character
  - Duration
  - Frequency
  - Exacerbating factors, especially movement of the shoulder
  - Alleviating factors
- Ask about occupational or recreational activities that predispose to shoulder disorders. Frequent overhead work or play (eg, carpentry, painting, throwing) predisposes to impingement syndrome or rotator cuff tendinopathy.
- Ask about pain in other joints, which may indicate a systemic condition.
- Obtain a past medical history, concentrating on injuries or prior surgery involving the shoulder, and history of arthritis (eg, RA, gout, pseudogout, osteoarthritis) or diabetes (predisposes to development of adhesive capsulitis).
- Determine the effect of the shoulder pain on the patient's function.
- The most helpful historical features include preceding trauma, location of the pain, and exacerbating movements.

FOCUSED QUESTIONS

QUESTIONS	THINK ABOUT...
Did the pain come on suddenly, or was it more gradual?	Sudden onset suggests trauma, tendon tears, infection, or serious acute referred pain (eg, ruptured viscus, acute cardiac disease, ectopic pregnancy). Gradual onset suggests a more chronic condition such as osteoarthritis or impingement syndrome.
Did you injure your shoulder recently or fall?	Fracture (glenohumeral, clavicular, scapular) AC joint separation Rotator cuff tear Labral tear Transient brachial plexopathy ("stinger")
Point to the location of pain in your shoulder.	Anterolateral or lateral shoulder pain most commonly is due to impingement syndrome, which may be due to subacromial bursitis, rotator cuff tendinopathy, rotator cuff tear, frozen shoulder, or a combination of these. Anterior pain that is very localized to either the AC joint or the bicipital groove highly suggests AC joint disease or biceps tendinitis, respectively. Posterior shoulder pain is less common and often refers to osteoarthritis or rotator cuff tendinopathy involving the teres minor or infraspinatus. Superior pain (in the trapezius area) is often referred from the neck (ie, cervical strain or radiculopathy). AC joint disease can also cause pain on the top of the shoulder. Poorly localized pain often is due to extrinsic causes, but labral tears sometimes have deep poorly localized pain.
Does the pain radiate?	Pain radiating down the arm suggests cervical radiculopathy.

—Continued next page

Continued—

What does the pain feel like?	Dull aching suggests impingement or rotator cuff tendinopathy. Tingling numbness, sharp shooting pain, or burning pain suggests neuropathic pain from cervical disease.
What movements make the pain worse? Is it all motions or only certain directions?	Anterolateral or deltoid pain exacerbated by forward elevation of the shoulder suggests impingement/rotator cuff tendinopathy. Pain in all planes of motion suggests frozen shoulder, glenohumeral osteoarthritis, infection, or polymyalgia rheumatica. Pain with flexion of the biceps (eg, lifting a bag of groceries) or supination of the wrist suggests biceps tendonitis. Pain with flexion of arm across the front of the body suggests AC joint disease. If the pain is not associated with movement, strongly consider referred pain.
Does reaching over your head aggravate your pain?	Worsening with this motion suggests impingement syndrome.
Do you have night pain or difficulty sleeping on the affected side?	Impingement syndrome, frozen shoulder, major rotator cuff tear, or infection.
What other joints are involved?	Bilateral shoulder pain and stiffness are seen in polymyalgia rheumatica. Multiple joint involvement suggests osteoarthritis or systemic arthritis (eg, RA, crystal arthropathy, or diffuse osteoarthritis).
Do you notice any associated symptoms such as fever, night sweats, or weight loss?	Referred pain from the chest or abdomen A systemic disorder, especially polymyalgia rheumatica or neoplasm Septic arthritis
Do you have stiffness relieved by activity and worsened by rest? (gelling)	Polymyalgia rheumatica or RA
Do you have stiffness in the morning lasting greater than 60 minutes that improves with activity? (morning stiffness)	Polymyalgia rheumatica or RA
Is your shoulder constantly stiff?	Frozen shoulder
Have you taken high doses of glucocorticoids?	Osteonecrosis
Is your shoulder weak?	Large rotator cuff tear Cervical radiculopathy or brachial plexopathy
Do your arms feel weak? Do you notice numbness, tingling, a sensation of burning, or a pins and needles sensation?	Cervical radiculopathy or brachial plexopathy
What kind of work do you do? What kind of recreations do you pursue?	Impingement syndrome, tendinitis, and tendon and muscle tears are associated with activities that involve frequently lifting the arms. Examples include welding, pitching, painting, conducting a symphony orchestra, and tennis.
Is your shoulder unstable? Does it slip or "pop out"?	Glenohumeral instability

Does your shoulder catch or lock?	Labral tear Loose body in glenohumeral joint
Do you have any other health problems?	Frozen shoulder is common in diabetics. Gout and pseudogout may manifest in the shoulder, but this typically occurs later in their course.

It is also important to assess the patient's function. The 12 questions outlined in Table 52–2 can help determine severity and demonstrate concern for the repercussions of the patient's problem.[9] Alternatively, ask whether patients can comb their hair, brush their teeth, fasten a bra, put on a sweater, get their arm into a blouse or shirt, or pull a wallet out of a back pocket.

Table **52–2. Questions to determine effect on function.**

1. Is your arm comfortable with your arm at rest by your side?
2. Does your shoulder allow you to sleep comfortably?
3. Can you reach the small of your back to tuck in your shirt/blouse with your hand?
4. Can you place your hand behind your head with the elbow straight out to the side?
5. Can you place a coin on a shelf at the level of your shoulder without bending your elbow?
6. Can you lift 1 lb (a full pint container) to the level of the top of your head without bending your elbow?
7. Can you lift an 8-lb (a full gallon) container to the level of the top of your head without bending your elbow?
8. Can you carry 20 lb at your side with the affected extremity?
9. Do you think you can throw a softball underhand 10 yards with the affected extremity?
10. Do you think you can throw a softball overhand 20 yards with the affected extremity?
11. Can you wash the back of your opposite shoulder with the affected extremity?
12. Would your shoulder allow you to work full time at your usual job?

IDENTIFYING ALARM SYMPTOMS

Alarm symptoms generally suggest a dangerous extrinsic cause, serious traumatic injury, or infection within the shoulder joint.

Alarm Symptoms	Consider
Visible swelling or deformity	Septic arthritis Fracture Dislocation AC joint separation Malignant tumors Amyloidosis

—Continued next page

Continued—

Fever and chills	Infection (septic arthritis, soft tissue abscess) Polymyalgia rheumatica (low-grade fever)
Constant and progressive pain	Referred pain Infection Tumor
Axillary pain	Referred pain from the mediastinum
Night pain	Infection Fracture Major rotator cuff tear Neoplasm
Numbness or tingling in upper extremity	Radiculopathy Neuropathy Myelopathy Thoracic outlet obstruction
Inability to abduct or maintain abduction	Rotator cuff tear
Shoulder pain aggravated by neck motion	Cervical radiculopathy
Shoulder pain unrelated to arm movement	Referred pain
Weight loss	Neoplasm Infection Polymyalgia rheumatica
Dyspnea	Heart disease (cardiac ischemia) Pulmonary embolism Pulmonary disease
Trauma with loss of normal shape	Dislocation
Trauma or acute disabling pain/weakness	Fracture Dislocation AC joint separation Major rotator cuff tear
Headache or visual changes	Polymyalgia rheumatica

DIAGNOSTIC APPROACH (INCLUDING ALGORITHM)

The first step is to assess for intrinsic versus extrinsic causes, based on the presence of pain worsening with shoulder and arm movement. If extrinsic causes are suggested, focused questions are used to assess for neurologic (usually cervical), abdominal, or thoracic processes.

If intrinsic causes are suspected, determine whether trauma preceded the pain, which suggests fracture, dislocation, or rotator cuff or labral tears. If there is no antecedent trauma, the patient should be questioned about alarm symptoms.

Next, determine whether the pain occurs with only active range of motion (which stresses the muscles, tendons, and ligaments) or with *both* active and passive range of motion. Pain with both active and passive motions suggests involvement of the glenohumeral joint (eg, osteoarthritis, frozen shoulder, gout, osteonecrosis) or AC joint disease (eg, separation or osteoarthritis). Pain with active but not passive motion suggests soft tissue disorders such as rotator cuff or biceps tendonitis, rotator cuff tendinopathy or tears, or subacromial bursitis. Pain with elevation of arm above the head suggests impingement syndrome. Pain on lifting items with the biceps or pain with wrist supination suggests biceps tendinitis.

Once the history is completed, the physical examination offers valuable information to confirm or refute disorders suggested by the history. Imaging is sometimes helpful and should be guided by the history and physical examination findings. See Figure 52–3 for the diagnostic approach algorithm for shoulder pain.

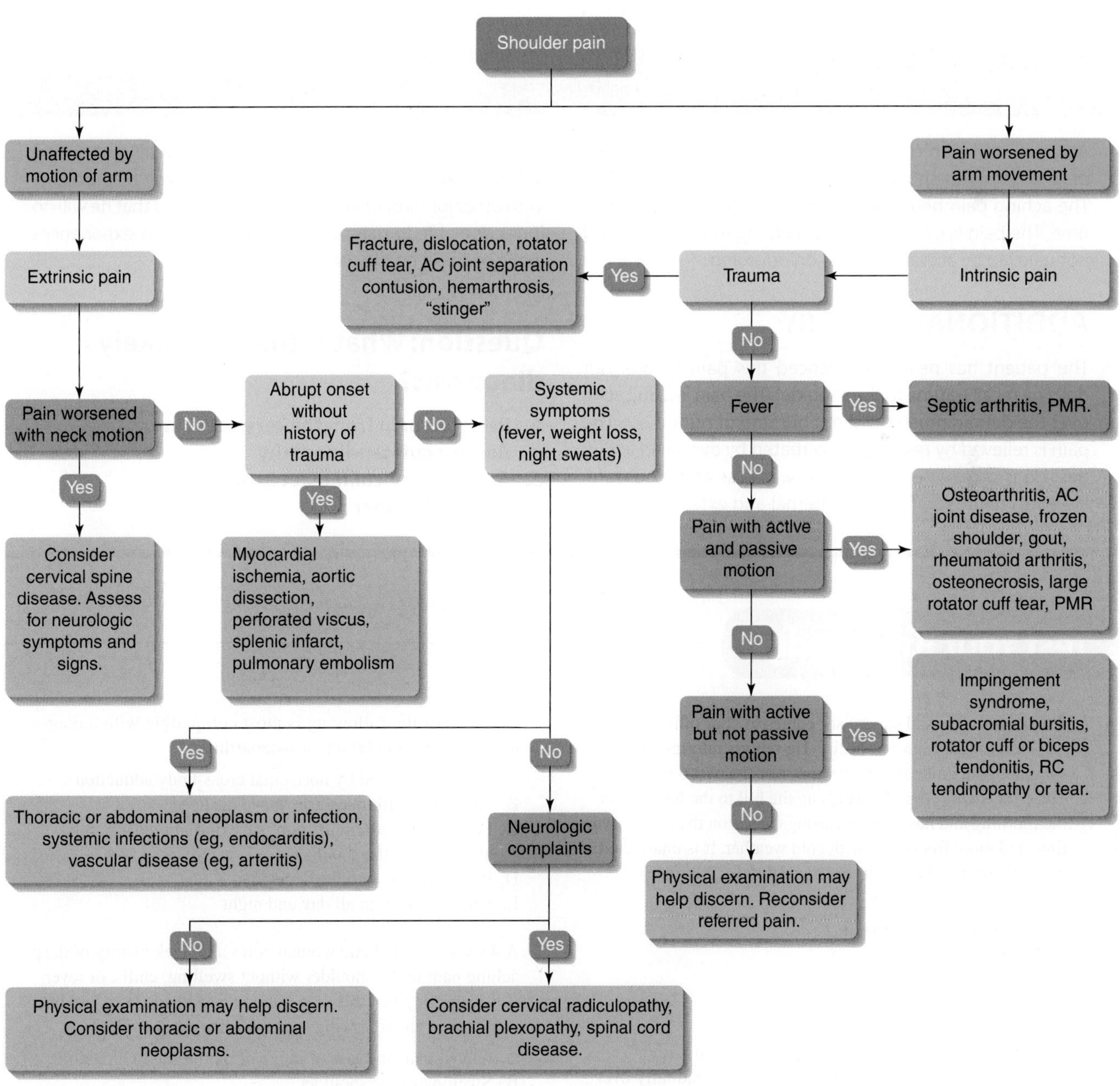

FIGURE 52–3 Diagnostic approach: Shoulder pain. AC, acromioclavicular; PMR, polymyalgia rheumatica; RC, rotator cuff.

CAVEATS

- Early RA and polymyalgia rheumatica can be difficult to distinguish from impingement in older patients.
- Referred pain to the shoulder is uncommon and most often due to cervical radiculopathy; however, it may represent serious thoracic, cardiac, or abdominal disease.
- The hallmark of rotator cuff tears is weakness. The history, however, is often inadequate for distinguishing weakness secondary to pain from true weakness. Physical examination and strength testing after local anesthetic injection into the joint may be required to make this distinction.

PROGNOSIS

The prognosis of shoulder pain depends on the nature of the specific problem. Periarticular disorders, such as impingement, may be self-limited and respond to rest, analgesics, and range of motion and strengthening exercises. Impingement syndrome can be chronic and recurrent, leading to rotator cuff tendinopathy. This can ultimately progress to full-thickness rotator cuff tears and secondary glenohumeral osteoarthritis. By middle age, asymptomatic rotator cuff tears are common. Large tears can often lead to loss of abduction and decreased strength and function; these patients should be referred to a specialist.

CASE SCENARIO | Resolution

A 62-year-old man comes to your office to discuss his self-diagnosed right "shoulder bursitis" of 6 months' duration. The aching pain began insidiously and has worsened over time. The pain is exacerbated by painting (on an easel) and not relieved by acetaminophen or ibuprofen.

ADDITIONAL HISTORY

The patient has never experienced this pain before, nor does he recall trauma to the shoulder. The pain is a dull ache over the deltoid muscle without burning or numbness. The pain is relieved by rest and exacerbated by overhead activities. He is otherwise healthy and works as an accountant. He notes no discomfort with internal and external rotation or adduction of the shoulder. He denies swelling, morning stiffness, fever, chills, weight loss, or a history of problems with other joints or of arthritis. He is concerned that he will no longer be able to paint because of the pain he experiences while painting on the easel.

Question: What is the most likely diagnosis?

A. Referred pain from the cervical spine
B. Rotator cuff tendinopathy
C. Acromioclavicular osteoarthritis
D. Frozen shoulder

Test Your Knowledge

1. A 67-year-old postal supervisor comes to your office saying, "Doctor, I think I have arthritis." He reports intermittent left shoulder pain gradually worsening over the past 6 months. The pain occurs when he walks up the hill to the bus stop in the morning and has been occurring earlier on the ascent over time and more frequently with cold weather. It is unaffected by arm movement and relieved by resting for 5 minutes.

   What is the most likely diagnosis?

   A. Rotator cuff tendinopathy
   B. Frozen shoulder
   C. Referred pain
   D. Osteoarthritis

2. A 50-year-old chief financial officer comes in with a refractory shoulder pain that has worsened gradually over the past year. He points to his anterior shoulder to localize the pain. He is an avid weightlifter, and the pain occurs with any motion of the shoulder.

   Which of the following is most compatible with a diagnosis of acromioclavicular osteoarthritis?

   A. Pain exacerbated by horizontal cross-body adduction
   B. Pain when lifting his arm above his head
   C. Fear the shoulder will "pop" on external rotation and abduction of the shoulder
   D. Pain radiating into the neck
   E. Unrelenting pain all day and night

3. A 48-year-old diabetic woman notes a 3-week history of deep aching pain in the shoulder without swelling, chills, or fever. It is restricting her ability to put on a jacket and hook her bra.

   Which of the following suggests a frozen shoulder?

   A. Global pain and loss of range of motion in all directions
   B. Swelling of the shoulder
   C. Morning stiffness lasting 60 minutes
   D. Pain mainly with overhead activities
   E. Swelling and pitting edema of the ipsilateral hand

References

1. Unwin M, Symmons D, Allison T, et al. Estimating the burden of musculoskeletal disorders in the community: the comparative prevalence of symptoms at different anatomical sites, and the relation to social deprivation. *Ann Rheum Dis.* 1998;57:649–655.
2. Winter de AF, Jans MP, Scholten RJPM, et al. Diagnostic classification of shoulder disorders: interobserver agreement and determinants of disagreement. *Ann Rheum Dis.* 1999;58:272–277.
3. van der Windt DAWM, Koes BW, Jong de BA, Bouter LM. Shoulder disorders in general practice: incidence, patient characteristics, and management. *Ann Rheum Dis.* 1995;54: 959–964.
3. Luime JJ, Koes BW, Hendrikson IJM, et al. Prevalence and incidence of shoulder pain in the general population: a systematic review. *Scand J Rheumatol.* 2004;33:73–81.
4. Walker-Bone KE, Palmer KT, Reading I, Cooper C. Soft-tissue rheumatic disorders of the neck and upper limbs: prevalence and risk factors. *Semin Arthritis Rheum.* 2003;33:185–203.
5. Mitchell C, Adebajo A, Hay E, Carr A. Shoulder pain: diagnosis and management in primary care. *BMJ.* 2005;331:1124–1128.
6. Oster AJ, Richards CA, Prevost AT, Speed CA, Hazelman BI. Diagnosis and relation in general health of shoulder disorders presenting to primary care. *Rheumatology.* 2005;44: 800–805.
7. Linsell L, Dawson, Zondervan K, et al. Prevalence and incidence of adults consulting for shoulder conditions in UK primary care: patterns of diagnosis and referral. *Rheumatology.* 2006;45:215–221.
8. Burbank KM, Stevenson JH, Czarnecki GR, Dorfman J. Chronic shoulder pain. Part I. Evaluation and diagnosis. *Am Fam Phys.* 2008;77:454–460.
9. Matsen FA III, Lippitt SB, Sidles JA, Harryman DT II. *Practical Evaluation and Management of the Shoulder.* New York, NY: Saunders, 1994:6–15.

Suggested Reading

Griffin LY, ed. *Essentials of Musculoskeletal Care.* 3rd ed. Chicago, IL: American Academy of Orthopedic Surgeons, 2005.

Lottke PA, Abboud JA, Ende J, eds. *Lippincott's Primary Care Orthopedics.* Philadelphia, PA: Wolters Kluwer/Lippincott Williams & Wilkins, 2008.

Martin SD, Thornhill TS. Shoulder pain. In: Firestein GS, Budd RC, Harris ED Jr, McInnes IB, Ruddy S, Sergent JS, eds. *Kelley's Textbook of Rheumatology.* 8th ed. New York, NY: Saunders, 2009:587–615.

Chapter 53

Arm and Hand Pain

Christopher M. Wittich, MD, PharmD, and Robert D. Ficalora, MD

CASE SCENARIO

A 33-year-old right-handed man presents to your clinic with upper extremity pain that started 2 weeks ago. The pain is worse with movement and relieved with ibuprofen. He denies antecedent trauma but began taking tennis lessons 3 weeks earlier. The pain only occurs in his serving arm and has recently progressed, prompting his visit today.

- **What additional questions would you ask to learn more about his upper extremity pain?**
- **How would localizing the pain help in generating a differential diagnosis?**
- **What activities put the patient at risk for specific upper extremity problems?**
- **How can you use the history to identify serious diagnoses?**

INTRODUCTION

Pain in the upper extremities most commonly arises from musculoskeletal sources. However, pain may also result from soft tissue infection or diseases of blood vessels or peripheral nerves or be referred from embryologically linked structures in the chest. Deep pain, arising from vessels, fascia, joints, tendons, periosteum, and supporting structures, is often poorly localized and dull and may be accompanied by the perception of joint stiffness and deep tenderness. Pain arising from adjacent or supporting structures may be attributed to the joints in the absence of true joint pathology. Pain from disorders of proximal joints (elbow and wrist) is usually related to local inflammation from overuse syndromes or work-related activities (1% of work-related injuries affect the forearm, and 55% of work-related injuries affect the wrist). Pain in the hand joints is often a consequence of degenerative or inflammatory disease.

Painful intermittent vasospasm in the hands (Raynaud's phenomenon) is often attributable to digital artery vascular instability in young women but occurs in all age groups. It occurs less commonly in men. A variety of medications have been implicated as exacerbating this phenomenon. Atherosclerotic narrowing of vessels occurs rarely in the upper extremity, usually in the setting of systemic vascular disease. Pain from peripheral nerve disease or entrapment neuropathies, such as carpal or ulnar tunnel entrapment, is accompanied by motor (weakness), reflex, and other sensory changes (burning or tingling).

Rarely, neuropathic pain in the upper extremity results from reflex sympathetic dystrophy/chronic regional pain syndrome (RSD/CRPS), a poorly understood condition that follows local trauma, stroke, or spinal cord injury. Irritation of the cervical nerve roots (herniated nucleus pulposus, osteoarthritis) can cause upper extremity pain. Upper extremity pain caused by compression of the nerves and blood vessels as they exit the thorax (thoracic outlet syndrome) is frequently associated with evidence of vascular compression. Referred pain, originating from structures of the chest, such as thoracic outlet syndrome, ischemic heart disease, or gastroesophageal reflux disease (GERD), may radiate to the inner surfaces of the arm.

KEY TERMS

Bursitis	Pain and inflammation of the structure containing the fluid that lubricates a joint or tendon sheath.
Degenerative joint disease	Painful, noninflammatory changes in a joint that result from "wear and tear" of chronic use and abuse.
Entrapment neuropathy	Pain and loss of function resulting from a nerve passing through a physiologic space that is narrowed secondary to acute or chronic trauma or inflammation.
Epicondylitis	Pain and inflammation of the area where bone and tendon connect.
Neuropathic pain	Pain in a region as a result of nerve inflammation, trauma, or neurologic disease.
Overuse syndrome	Pain and inflammation resulting from intense or repetitive use of regional anatomic structures in the course of occupational or recreational activities.
Referred pain	Pain originating in one structure that is perceived in the area of another, usually because of physiologic or embryologic links between the 2 structures.
Tendinitis	Pain and inflammation of a tendon or tendon sheath.
Vasospasm	Spontaneous contraction or closure of a blood vessel.

ETIOLOGY

Differential Diagnosis: Forearm and Elbow Pain

Diagnosis	Explanation	Prevalence
Lateral epicondylitis (tennis elbow)	A strain of the wrist extensor attachments at the humerus, usually in tennis players with poor technique.	1%–3% of the general population 40%–50% of tennis players, especially those over age 30[1]
Medial epicondylitis (golfer's elbow)	Any strain of the common flexor tendon can cause this injury. Involvement of the nearby ulnar nerve may result in tingling.	2.5% of workers[2]
Olecranon bursitis	Inflammatory fluid accumulating in the bursa often following local trauma; may be spontaneous in patients with gout, pseudogout, or rheumatoid arthritis. When resulting from infection within the bursa, this is called septic olecranon bursitis.	0.718% of the mentally retarded Up to 1% of rheumatoid arthritis patients[3]
Ulnar tunnel syndrome or Guyon tunnel syndrome	The ulnar (Guyon) tunnel is a space at the elbow between the bones of the joint through which the ulnar nerve travels surrounded by a ligament. If this ligament hardens, the nerve is compressed into the ulnar groove or "entrapped," causing pain and tingling in the arm between the elbow and fingers.	1.7%–2.5% of industrial workers; 25% of patients with carpal tunnel syndrome also have ulnar tunnel syndrome[4]

Referred pain from chest structures	Ischemic or irritative pain from the organs adjacent to the diaphragm (heart, stomach); structures in and near the diaphragmatic hiatus (hiatus hernia, esophagus) refer pain to the lateral forearm and elbow.	0.6% of general population; 20% of angina patients have pain referred to their left arm[5]
Cubital tunnel syndrome	Ulnar nerve is compressed as it enters the cubital tunnel at the elbow, resulting in pain that is like "hitting your funny bone." Persons who perform repetitive bending of the elbow by pulling levers, reaching, or lifting are at risk.	9% of musicians[6]
RSD/CRPS	A chronic progressive neurologic condition that affects a region, such as an arm or a leg. May occur after a major injury, but in some cases, there is no precipitating event. Pain begins in one area or limb and then spreads. RSD/CRPS is characterized by burning pain, excessive sweating, swelling, and sensitivity to touch. Marked osteopenia is noted in bones within the nerve distribution.	2%–5% of peripheral nerve injury patients 12%–21% of patients with hemiplegia (paralysis on one side of the body) 1%–2% of bone fracture patients[2]

Differential Diagnosis: Wrist Pain

Diagnosis	Explanation	Prevalence
Carpal tunnel syndrome	Compression of the median nerve inside of the carpal tunnel of the wrist with pain and loss of function of the first 2 or 3 digits of the hand. May be related to overuse, pregnancy, or hypothyroidism.	2.7% of the general population[6]
de Quervain tenosynovitis	The abductor pollicis longus and extensor pollicis longus run in a tunnel along the side of the wrist above the thumb. Repeatedly grasping, pinching, squeezing, or wringing may lead to a tenosynovitis. This causes swelling, which further hampers the smooth gliding action of the tendons within the tunnel. Soreness on the thumb side of the forearm is the initial symptom. Pain spreads up the forearm or down into the wrist and thumb. The tendons may actually squeak as they move through the constricted tunnel.	0.46% of working adults[7]
Intersection syndrome (tenosynovitis at the wrist)	Tendinitis in the first and second dorsal compartments of the wrist. The tendons cross at a 60-degree angle proximal to the wrist joint on the dorsal aspect. It has also been described as a stenosing tenosynovitis of the tendon sheath where it crosses the bellies of the abductor pollicis longus and extensor pollicis brevis muscles.	12% of Alpine skiers[8]

Differential Diagnosis: Hand Pain

Diagnosis	Explanation	Prevalence
Trigger finger	Irritation from the tendon sliding through the pulley causes the tendon to swell and create a nodule. Pain at the bottom of the digit and a clicking sensation occur when the digit is bent and straightened. Can be a complication of diabetes.	2.6% in nondiabetic patients over 30 years of age 16%–42% in diabetics[9]
Hand osteoarthritis	Hand pain, aching, or stiffness and 3 or 4 of the following features: • Enlargement of 2 or more of 10 joints • Enlargement of 2 or more distal interphalangeal joints • Fewer than 3 swollen metacarpophalangeal joints • Deformity of at least 1 of 10 joints	Symptomatic disease in persons over 70 years: women, 26.2%; men, 13.4% Radiographic evidence in persons over 70 years: 36%[10]
Rheumatoid arthritis	The cause is unknown. Hand involvement can be particularly debilitating. Synovial tissue and joint destruction occur early in the disease often before classic deformities develop.	2% in persons older than 60 years[11]
Raynaud's disorder	Vasospasm of the digital vessels causes the characteristic 3-color changes of the digits—blanching (white), cyanosis (blue), and numbness and rubor (red)—after cold exposure and rewarming.	15% of the general population[12]
Thoracic outlet syndrome	Compression of the nerves and vessels to the arm at the shoulder associated with repetitive motion of the arms held overhead or extended forward. Pain, weakness, numbness and tingling, swelling, fatigue, or coldness of the arm and hand can mimic a herniated cervical disk or ulnar tunnel or carpal tunnel syndromes.	0.1% of the general population[13]

GETTING STARTED WITH THE HISTORY

- Upper extremity complaints are usually localized and commonly follow an injury, inciting event, or recreational or occupational overuse.
- Basic questions about the onset, location, quality, and aggravating or ameliorating factors are most helpful.
- An occupational and leisure time history is essential.

Questions	Remember
Where is the pain?	• Most patients will not be able to adequately describe the precise location of the pain, so pointing is helpful. • Physical demonstrations of typical activities may be valuable adjuncts to the history. • Trying to be helpful, patients often group unrelated symptoms. Make sure that you understand each individual symptom or sign completely before moving on.
When did it start?	
Can you describe it for me? Is it dull? Sharp? Burning? Does it ever change?	
Is there swelling?	
Is there a rash or discoloration?	
What makes it better or worse?	
Show me how you use your arms at work.	
Tell me about your leisure time activities.	

INTERVIEW FRAMEWORK

- Assess for alarm symptoms.
- Identify activities that put the patient at risk.
- Systematically identify complaints as they relate to the following structures or diagnoses: joints, soft tissues, nerves and neuropathic disorders, and cervical and thoracic structures that refer pain to the upper extremity.

IDENTIFYING ALARM SYMPTOMS

Serious Diagnoses

- Septic olecranon bursitis
- Ischemic heart disease
- Cervical nerve root or spinal cord disorders
- Deep venous thrombosis

Alarm Symptoms	Serious Causes	Benign Causes
Arm complaints (especially on the left side) associated with dyspnea, chest pain, dizziness, or palpitations	Ischemic heart disease or other cardiopulmonary conditions	Fatigue Anxiety GERD
Persistent sensory abnormalities, such as numbness, burning, or tingling, especially with associated neck complaints	Acute cervical nerve root or spinal cord disorders	Muscle strain Anxiety GERD Entrapment neuropathy
Painful redness, swelling, weeping, or draining lesions with fever, fatigue, or malaise (especially related to trauma)	Septic olecranon bursitis or other soft tissue infections	Crystalline arthropathies (eg, gout or pseudogout)

FOCUSED QUESTIONS

After listening to the patient's complaint, put the description in a context of related risks and activities. Patients may have an idea of the cause of their symptoms from the media, friends, or the Internet, but often will not be able to put all the pieces together.

Because most upper extremity disorders are not primary physiologic derangements but rather the effects of overuse or injury, narrowing down the differential diagnosis begins with defining the patient's activities.

QUESTIONS	THINK ABOUT...
What is your occupation?	
• *Work on an assembly line or keyboard operation*	Thoracic outlet syndrome from repetitive shoulder movements
• *Sewing, operating computers*	Carpal tunnel syndrome due to repetitive wrist motion
• *Chain saw or pneumatic drill operator*	Raynaud's syndrome from chronic exposure to vibration
• *Hammer, saw, or screwdriver use*	de Quervain tendinitis Trigger finger
Tell me about your leisure time activities.	
• *Do you play golf or tennis?*	Medial epicondylitis Lateral epicondylitis
• *Are you a home improvement enthusiast who uses hammers and screwdrivers only on the weekends?*	Medial epicondylitis de Quervain tendinitis Trigger finger
• *Do you drink? If so, how much?*	Olecranon bursitis (drinker's elbow) from repeated trauma secondary to leaning on a curb or bar
• *Are you a professional musician?*	Cubital tunnel syndrome (especially saxophone playing)
• *Are you a skier?*	Intersection syndrome
• *Do you lead a sedentary lifestyle? Do you smoke?*	Coronary artery disease
Quality	
Is the pain:	
• *Steady?*	Rheumatoid arthritis Osteoarthritis Infection
• *Aching?*	Overuse syndrome or referred pain
• *Shooting? Sharp?*	Entrapment neuropathy
• *Burning?*	Neuropathic pain
• *Severe?*	Arthritis (at rest) Osteomyelitis (with motion) Gout Infection Trauma
• *Throbbing?*	Inflammatory or vascular disorder

Location

Where do you have pain?	
• *In or around what joint?*	Pain resulting from an articular disorder is perceived as coming directly from the joint not from the bones around the joints.
• *Elbows?*	Septic arthritis Crystalline arthropathies (eg, pseudogout, gout) Trauma Neuropathic pain from entrapment neuropathy Medial epicondylitis Lateral epicondylitis
• *Wrists?*	Entrapment neuropathy (median nerve or tendinitis)
• *Metacarpophalangeal joints?*	Rheumatoid arthritis Occasionally in gout
• *Proximal interphalangeal joints?*	Rheumatoid arthritis (nontender Bouchard nodes in osteoarthritis)
• *Distal interphalangeal joints?*	Osteoarthritis (Heberden nodes; often painless) Psoriatic arthritis
• *Carpometacarpal joint of thumb?*	Osteoarthritis
• *In an area adjacent to a joint?*	Periarticular structures (tendinitis, bursitis, bone)
• *In the first 3 fingers?*	Carpal tunnel syndrome: compression of the median nerve at the wrist
• *At the ulnar aspect of the hand?*	Ulnar nerve lesion (commonly at the elbow) or lesion of the brachial plexus
• *In the fingers or at the finger tips? (on exposure to cold)*	Raynaud's phenomenon or disease
• *Along the limb spanning joint and muscle areas?*	Lesion of nerve or blood vessels Nerve root compression Thoracic outlet syndrome Peripheral nerve lesion Referred pain Ischemic heart disease

Time course

Is the pain related to an activity?	Overuse syndromes may come on after hours, days, or weeks of a repetitive activity or after resumption of an activity after some time away from it.

—*Continued next page*

Continued—

Does the pain wax and wane?	Overuse syndromes are often better on weekends and worse on Fridays. Carpal tunnel syndrome may be most painful at night. Epicondylitis can be most symptomatic the day after the activity.
Was the onset of pain:	
• *Sudden? (minutes to hours)*	Acute infectious process Trauma Crystalline arthropathies Vascular processes Referred pain Inflammatory processes (eg, rheumatoid arthritis)
• *Gradual?*	Arthritis Tendinitis Bursitis Rheumatoid arthritis Neuropathic pain

Associated symptoms

Is there swelling:	
• *In the area of the pain?* • *Around or near it?*	In rheumatoid and crystalline arthritis, the joints are painful and swollen. In RSD/CRPS, the entire region may be swollen. In carpal tunnel syndrome, the wrist swelling may be hard to appreciate, but more distal swelling is often obvious.
Is the skin red?	Tendinitis may have erythema (redness) over the affected tendon. Infected structures often have surrounding erythema.
Does the skin change colors?	Vasomotor processes (Raynaud's), although the classic 3-color changes may not always be present

Modifying factors

Is joint pain:	
• *Present only with movements?*	Suggests effusion, such as in osteoarthritis
• *Present at rest?*	Inflammation (eg, rheumatoid arthritis)
• *Increased by motion? Activity?*	Abnormalities of the tendons or bursae Typical of overuse syndromes
Is your arm pain induced or made worse:	
• *By sneezing? Coughing? Hyperextension of the neck? Shaving under the chin?*	Cervical radiculopathy or cervical nerve root involvement

• *Upon rotating the head? Or upon laterally flexing the neck?*	Cervical spine lesion
• *When elevating the arm above the head? With exertion?*	Referred pain: ischemic heart disease Thoracic outlet syndrome
• *After a meal?*	GERD
• *By light touch?*	Neuropathic pain (eg, entrapment neuropathy)
Does the pain occur:	
• *When grasping an object for a prolonged time?*	Carpal tunnel syndrome Intersection syndrome
• *At night?*	Carpal tunnel syndrome
• *After activity is over?*	Epicondylitis Tendinitis
• *With exposure to cold?*	Raynaud's phenomenon
Arm function and related symptoms	
Are you unable to remove a ring? Wear a watch? Slip the hand into an old glove?	Diffuse swelling of the hand may indicate an inflammatory disorder (eg, rheumatoid arthritis, Raynaud's disease, neurovascular compression syndrome).
Are you unable to drive a car? To dress? Eat?	Related to pain, rather than restricted motion at the elbow (the shoulder is able to compensate for most limitation of elbow motion)
Are you unable to lift with the hands? Shave? Sew? Open jars?	Disability related to disorders of the wrist or hand
Is the pain:	
• *Greatest in the morning?*	Rheumatoid arthritis, also referred to as "morning gel"
• *Worse with prolonged use of the joint?*	Osteoarthritis
Do you have:	
• *Fever? Chills?*	Septic arthritis or bursitis
• *Numbness, tingling, or burning in the arm?*	Neuropathic pain such as entrapment neuropathy, thoracic outlet syndrome, peripheral neuropathy
• *Chest pain on exertion?*	Ischemic heart disease with referred pain to the arm

DIAGNOSTIC APPROACH (INCLUDING ALGORITHM)

- Characterize the pain, including type, onset, and associated complaints.
- Localize the pain to joints, tendons, and soft tissue.
- Assess for hints that the pain is referred or neuropathic.
- Consider the functional anatomy of the region, including specific movements that cause, exacerbate, or relieve the pain.
- Identify potential causes such as occupation, activity, habits, and lifestyle.

See Figure 53–1 for the diagnostic approach algorithm for arm and hand pain.

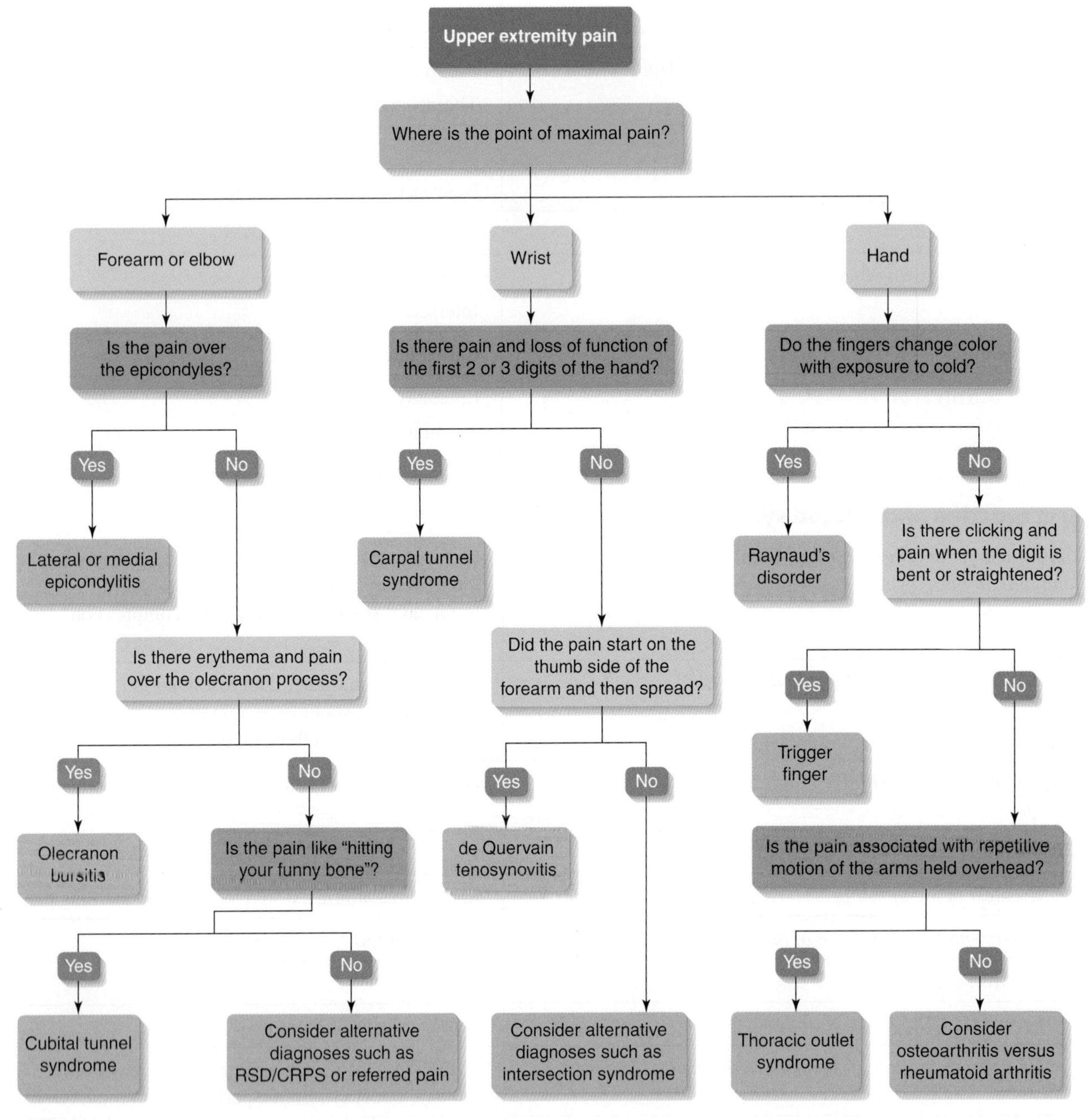

FIGURE 53–1 Diagnostic approach: Arm and hand pain. No, no; RSD/CRPS, reflex sympathetic dystrophy/chronic regional pain syndrome; Y, yes.

CAVEATS

Significant morbidity from upper extremity musculoskeletal disorders is rare. However, life- or limb-threatening disease can result from joint or soft tissue infection and cardiopulmonary diseases presenting as upper limb discomfort. These entities should always be considered.

Neuropathic pain is the great mimicker. Although investigation of the painful structure is necessary, also consider inflamed nerves, nerve roots, or pain referred from other structures.

Descriptions are helpful when considering upper extremity pain, but there is no substitute for pointing to the area in question and performing the movement that causes the pain or demonstrating the inducing work-related activity.

PROGNOSIS

Most primary causes of upper extremity pain resolve spontaneously or with cessation of the inciting activity. Physical therapy helps many patients. More aggressive treatment is reserved for patients in whom conservative treatment fails. Learning ergonomically safe ways to accomplish a task, such as perfecting a tennis swing, limits recurrences. Permanent disability is unusual.

CASE SCENARIO | Resolution

A 33-year-old right-handed man presents to your clinic with upper extremity pain that started 2 weeks ago. The pain is worse with movement and relieved with ibuprofen. He denies antecedent trauma but began taking tennis lessons 3 weeks earlier. The pain only occurs in his serving arm and has recently progressed, prompting his visit today.

ADDITIONAL HISTORY

When asked to point to the location of the pain, he points over his lateral epicondyle of his right arm. He denies swelling or erythema of the elbow. There is no pain in his wrist or fingers. He was told by his tennis coach that his technique still needs a lot of work.

Question: What is the most likely diagnosis?

A. Medial epicondylitis
B. Olecranon bursitis
C. Lateral epicondylitis
D. de Quervain tenosynovitis

Test Your Knowledge

1. A 42-year-old woman presents to your clinic with 1 year of progressive weakness and numbness in the hand and wrist. The pain has progressed to include her forearm, elbow, and upper arm. She was in a car accident about 18 months ago. She describes the pain as burning, and touching the arm makes the pain much worse.
   What is the most likely cause of her upper extremity pain?
   A. Cubital tunnel syndrome
   B. Carpal tunnel syndrome
   C. Intersection syndrome
   D. Olecranon bursitis
   E. Reflex sympathetic dystrophy

2. A 35-year-old woman describes periodic pain in her fingers and hands. The pain has been present for more than 3 years and is worse in the winter. She notes that when the pain is present, her fingers turn white, then blue, and then red.
   What is the most likely diagnosis?
   A. Thoracic outlet syndrome
   B. Cubital tunnel syndrome
   C. de Quervain tenosynovitis
   D. Carpel tunnel syndrome
   E. Raynaud's disorder

3. A 55-year-old man presents to your clinic with elbow pain. He recently retired and has started to play golf more frequently. The pain improves with rest. There is no swelling or erythema of the elbow. The pain is worse with wrist flexion.
   What is the most likely diagnosis?
   A. Medial epicondylitis
   B. Lateral epicondylitis
   C. Referred pain from chest structures
   D. Reflex sympathetic dystrophy
   E. Olecranon bursitis

References

1. Cooke AJ, Roussopoulos K, Pallis JM, Haake S. Correlation between racquet design and arm injuries. 4th International Conference of the Engineering of Sport. September 2002.
2. National Institute for Occupational Safety and Health (NIOSH). Report. Cincinnati, OH: NIOSH, 1997.
3. National Institute for Occupational Safety and Health (NIOSH). *A Critical Review of Epidemiologic Evidence for Work-Related Musculoskeletal Disorders of the Neck, Upper Extremity, and Low Back*. Cincinnati, OH: Public Health Service, Centers for Disease Control and Prevention, NIOSH, 1997.
4. Gibbons RJ, Chatterjee K, Daley J, et al. ACC/AHA/ACP-ASIM guidelines for the management of patients with chronic stable angina: a report of the American College of Cardiology/American Heart Association Task Force on Practice Guidelines (Committee on Management of Patients With Chronic Stable Angina). *J Am Coll Cardiol.* 1999;33:2092–2197.
5. Brandfonbrener AG. Musicians with focal dystonia. *Med Probl Perform Art.* 1991;6:132–136.
6. Atroshi I, Gummesson C, Johnsson R, et al. Prevalence of carpal tunnel syndrome in a general population. *JAMA.* 1999;282:153–158.

7. Tanaka S, Petersen M, Cameron L. Prevalence and risk factors of tendinitis and related disorders of the distal upper extremity along U.S. workers: comparison to carpal tunnel syndrome. *Am J Ind Med.* 2001;39:328–335.
8. Servi JT. Wrist pain from overuse: detecting and relieving intersection syndrome. *Phys Sportsmed.* 1997;25:41–44.
9. Gorsche R, Wiley JP, Renger R, et al. Prevalence and incidence of stenosing flexor tenosynovitis (trigger finger) in a meat-packing plant. *J Occup Environ Med.* 1998;40:556–560.
10. Altman R, Alarcon G, Appelrouth D, et al. The American College of Rheumatology criteria for the classification and reporting of osteoarthritis of the hand. *Arthritis Rheum.* 1990;33:1601–1610.
11. Rasch EK, Hirsch R, Paulose-Ram R, Hochberg MC. Prevalence of rheumatoid arthritis in persons 60 years of age and older in the United States: effect of different methods of case classification. *Arthritis Rheum.* 2003;48:917–926.
12. Zhang Y, Niu J, Kelly-Hayes M, et al. Prevalence of symptomatic hand osteoarthritis and its impact on functional status among the elderly: the Framingham Study. *Am J Epidemiol.* 2002;156:1021–1027.
13. Edwards DP, Mulkern E, Raja AN, Barker P. Trans-axillary first ribs excision for thoracic outlet syndrome. *J R Coll Surg Edinb.* 1999;44:362–365.

Suggested Reading

Greene WB, ed. *Essentials of Musculoskeletal Care.* 2nd ed. Chicago, IL: American Academy of Orthopaedic Surgeons, American Academy of Pediatrics, 2001.

McCue FC III. *The Injured Athlete.* 2nd ed. Philadelphia, PA: JB Lippincott Co., 1992.

Miller MD, Hart JA, MacKnight JM, eds. *Essential Orthopaedics.* New York, NY: Elsevier, Inc., 2010.

Chapter 54

Low Back Pain

M.E. Beth Smith, DO, Roger Chou, MD, and Richard A. Deyo, MD, MPH

CASE SCENARIO

A 51-year-old woman presents to your clinic with a complaint of low back pain, which began acutely 2 weeks earlier, 1 day after a 10-km run. The pain is described as achy, intermittent, and located in the central region of her low back. It is associated with an occasional electrical sensation shooting down her left leg. The pain is aggravated by rolling over in bed, prolonged sitting, and running; it is relieved by rest, changing positions, and ibuprofen.

- **What additional questions would you ask to learn more about her low back pain?**
- **How do you classify low back pain?**
- **How do you determine whether her symptoms are worrisome for a serious neurologic, systemic, or nonspinal condition?**
- **What features suggest a better or worse prognosis for developing a chronic disabling condition?**
- **How do you determine whether further diagnostic or therapeutic intervention in indicated?**

INTRODUCTION

Low back pain (LBP) is a common reason for office appointments in the United States, accounting for 2% of all visits.[1] Approximately 70% of adults will have an episode of LBP during their lifetime, and 25% to 40% will have multiple episodes.[1,2] It is also one of the most costly conditions in terms of time lost from work and decreased productivity while at work.[2,3] Additionally, the prevalence of chronic LBP seems to be increasing. In North Carolina, the prevalence of persistent back pain that interfered with function increased from 3.9% in 1992 to 10.2% in 2006.[3] A small minority of patients with chronic disabling LBP account for a disproportionate share of the healthcare costs. Fortunately, most cases of acute LBP follow a benign, self-limited course with substantial improvement or resolution within the first 4 to 8 weeks.[4] The practitioner must identify worrisome features suggesting a serious etiology or risk of developing a chronic disabling condition.

KEY TERMS

Acute LBP	An episode of back pain lasting < 3 months in duration, most commonly < 2 weeks.
Ankylosing spondylitis	Inflammatory disorder affecting primarily the axial skeleton with symptoms usually beginning in late adolescence or early adulthood, the hallmark being sacroiliitis.
Cauda equina syndrome	Acute compressive radiculopathy of the sacral nerve roots that comprise the cauda equina. Symptoms include severe back pain, urinary retention or urinary and fecal incontinence, saddle anesthesia, and leg weakness. Arises most commonly from a large midline disk herniation but can complicate any process that leads to spinal canal narrowing at the level of the cauda equina (eg, tumor, spinal stenosis).
Chronic LBP	An episode of back pain lasting > 3 months in duration.

—Continued next page

Continued—	
Myelopathy	Pathologic disturbance of spinal cord function manifested by peripheral muscle weakness, increased muscle tone, spasticity, and hyperreflexia.
Radiculopathy	A nonspecific term referring to the compression or irritation of a nerve root and manifesting in symptoms of pain, weakness, or sensory loss in the distribution of the nerve.
Neurogenic claudication (pseudoclaudication)	Pain typically located in the low back, buttocks, and proximal thighs associated with spinal stenosis. Pain is aggravated by exercise and improves with rest, sitting, or leaning forward.
Sciatica	Most common symptom of radiculopathy, characterized by pain radiating down the leg in the distribution of the sciatic nerve. It is most commonly due to compression of the L4, L5, or S1 nerve roots.
Spinal stenosis	Narrowing of the spinal canal leading to compression of the spinal cord or cauda equina. It is most commonly seen in older patients with severe degenerative changes of the spine.
Spondylolisthesis	Occurs when one vertebra slips anteriorly over the vertebra below. May be caused by a congenital defect in the pars interarticularis, although the most common cause in adults is degenerative changes of the facet joints, often associated with spinal stenosis. Posterior displacement is far less common and is usually called retrolisthesis.
Positive likelihood ratio (LR+)	The increase in odds of a diagnosis if a given clinical factor is present.
Negative likelihood ratio (LR–)	The decrease in odds of a diagnosis if a given clinical factor is absent.
Odds ratio	A measure of the odds of an event occurring in one group compared to the odds of the same event occurring in another group.

ETIOLOGY

The etiology of most cases of LBP remains elusive. Although specific structures such as muscle, ligaments, or skeletal components may be responsible for the patient's symptoms, the ability to accurately identify the specific cause remains limited.[5–7] Imaging results frequently do not correlate with examination findings, limiting their utility in terms of reaching a definitive diagnosis. Furthermore, ascribing LBP to a specific etiology often does not affect treatment decisions or improve patient outcomes.[7] It is clinically more useful to classify LBP into 1 of 3 categories:

1. Back pain without radiculopathy
2. Back pain associated with radiculopathy
3. Back pain associated with a systemic disease, organ system, or other specific cause.[7]

Differential Diagnosis

		Prevalence[1,2,6–8]
Back pain without radiculopathy	Nonspecific	~75%–80%
	Degenerative	10%
	Spondylolisthesis	3%
	Vertebral fracture	1%–4%
Back pain associated with radiculopathy	Disk herniation requiring surgical intervention	2%
	Spinal stenosis	3%
	Cauda equina	0.0004 (1%–2% of disk herniations)

Visceral and other specific causes	Cancer/tumor	0.7%
	Spinal infection	0.01%
	Ankylosing spondylitis	0.3%
	Osteoporotic compression fracture	4%
	Abdominal aortic aneurysm	
	Renal: pyelonephritis, nephrolithiasis, perinephric abscess	
	Gastrointestinal: pancreatitis, cholecystitis or cholelithiasis, perforating peptic ulcer	
	Urogenital: endometriosis, pelvic inflammatory disease, prostatitis	

GETTING STARTED WITH THE HISTORY

When evaluating a patient with LBP, the following objectives should guide your approach:

1. Understand the chronology and the nature of the symptoms, including a description of the pain and associated triggers.
2. Determine the functional impact of the condition on the patient.
3. Identify patients with worrisome or alarming features.
4. Identify patients at heightened risk of developing a chronic disabling condition.

Start with an open-ended question and listen to the patient's story. Much can be learned about the impact of the symptoms by active listening and observation.

Questions	Remember
Tell me about your back pain?	Listen to the whole story without interruptions.
When did it first start? How has it changed?	Reassure the patient when appropriate. Appreciate the impact that it is having on the patient's life and well-being.

INTERVIEW FRAMEWORK

Because 90% of LBP patients seen in a primary care setting will have a mechanical or nonspecific etiology, focus your inquiry on identifying those with a more serious or specific pathology. If an injury occurred, the mechanics of that injury may be helpful. The following characteristics may help direct treatment options and identify those at risk of developing a more disabling condition:

- Location
- Description (allow patients to describe in their own words before offering options)
- Duration and frequency (ie, transient versus unremitting, constant versus occasional)
- Aggravating and relieving factors
- Change in character over time

IDENTIFYING ALARM SYMPTOMS

Alarm symptoms are symptoms associated with a greater likelihood of serious underlying disease. Their presence increases the probability of serious disease, although their absence may not preclude it. Fortunately, serious causes of LBP are uncommon.

Is There Evidence of Neurologic Compromise?

Neurologic compromise in LBP occurs by some form of compression or entrapment either on the spinal canal itself, the cauda equina, or the nerve root. This is manifested by sensory, motor, or reflex pathway dysfunction, usually causing lower extremity symptoms. Sciatica or leg pain without weakness or reflex changes is the most common symptom of radiculopathy and generally does not constitute an emergent or urgent concern. Typical symptoms of sciatica have moderate sensitivity but poor specificity for clinically significant nerve compression including disk herniation (sensitivity and specificity ranges, 0.74–0.99 and 0.14–0.58, respectfully).[9,10] Weakness, however, is considered a more specific symptom of nerve compression causing neurologic compromise. Whether occurring from disk herniation, spinal stenosis, tumor, or infection, motor weakness must be fully evaluated to determine the degree of urgency. Patients with isolated sciatica but no motor or reflex changes can be monitored conservatively. Symptoms persisting with no improvement for more than 1 month may warrant imaging. Plain x-ray may be appropriate for most, but for surgical candidates, magnetic resonance imaging is generally preferred over computed tomography.[7] Multilevel, profound, or progressive weakness requires urgent investigation and referral. Myelopathy is typically characterized by leg weakness and spasticity resulting from tumor, infection, or severe degenerative changes affecting the spinal cord. It often results from cord compression above the lumbar spine because the spinal cord ends at the L1 or L2 level. Cauda equina syndrome is usually caused by a massive midline disk herniation. Although the prevalence of cauda equina syndrome and myelopathy in patients with LBP is quite low, both are considered spinal emergencies because delayed treatment may lead to irreversible neurologic damage.

Differential Diagnosis		Presence of Symptom or Risk Factor	Absence of Symptom or Risk Factor	Quality of the Evidence
Disk herniation[6,9] (mean age, 30–55 years)	Typical symptoms of sciatica	LR+ ~1.28	LR– ~0.67	Fair to good
	No relief with rest	LR+ 1.1 (1.0–1.3)	LR– 0.59 (0.35–1.0)	Fair
Spinal stenosis[7] (mean age, 55 years)	Neurogenic claudication[a]	LR+ 1.2		Fair
	Typical symptoms of sciatica	LR+ 2.2		
	Age > 65 years	LR+ 2.5	LR– 0.33	Good
Cauda equina[6] (usually due to a massive midline disk herniation)	Urinary retention (often manifested as overflow incontinence)	Sensitivity 0.90	Probability 1 in 10,000	Fair
	Saddle anesthesia	Sensitivity 0.75		Fair
Myelopathy (due to lumbar spinal cord compression)	Weakness Hypertonicity Spasticity Hyperreflexia	No data	No data	No evidence

[a]Pain with or without neurologic deficit in the legs most often seen in walking, standing, and/or coughing.

Is There Evidence of a Specific Condition Causing the Symptoms but Without Evidence of Neurologic Compromise?

When considering whether the patient's symptoms are caused by an underlying disease process or being referred from a visceral structure, consider the patient's age, comorbid characteristics, and associated symptoms. The most common systemic diseases causing LBP include cancer, osteoporosis causing compression fracture, infection causing osteomyelitis or abscess, and ankylosing spondylitis. Cancer or infection must be diagnosed and treated expeditiously because, if untreated, it may result in irreversible neurologic sequelae, pathologic fractures, or progressive disease that is more difficult to manage. Constant and nocturnal pain not improved with rest is more often associated with a systemic disease process such as cancer.[6] The most significant risk factor for malignancy causing LBP is a personal history of cancer (excluding nonmelanoma skin cancer).[7] Any patient with new back pain and a prior history of cancer should undergo imaging of the spine. Based on the estimated positive likelihood ratio, such a history increases a patient's probability of cancer from less than 1% in a primary care setting to nearly 9%.[7] Other risk factors such as age greater than 50 years, unexplained weight loss, and failure to improve within 1 month are weaker predictors of cancer, increasing the probability to just over 1%.[7] In such patients, it may be reasonable to forego immediate imaging while treating for nonspecific LBP, unless there are additional features suggestive of malignancy.

Back pain may also be referred from a visceral structure, often suggested by additional symptoms and underlying medical conditions. For instance, one must consider abdominal aortic aneurysm in a white male smoker older than age 65 with a history of hypertension. Although evidence on historical features of back pain referred from a visceral organ is sparse, isolated LBP seems to be rare. Rather, associated symptoms such as fever, nausea, vomiting, and gastrointestinal symptoms are usually present. Visceral pain may have an intermittent colicky nature when referred from an abdominal or pelvic source.

Differential Diagnosis		Presence/Absence of Symptom or Risk Factor	Quality of the Evidence
Cancer[6,7]	History of cancer	LR+ 14.7	Good
	Age > 50 years	LR+ 2.7	Good
	Unexplained weight loss	LR+ 2.7	Good
	Failure to improve in 1 month	LR+ 3.0	Good
	Nocturnal pain	LR+ 1.7 LR– 0.17	Fair
Compression fracture[6,8]	Age ≥ 70 years	LR+ 5.5–11.2 LR– 0.81–0.52	Good
	Significant trauma	LR+ 2.0–10.1 LR– 0.02–0.77	Fair
	Corticosteroid use	LR+ 6.0–48.5 LR– 0.95–0.75	Fair
Infection[6]	Injection drug use, urinary tract infection, or skin infection	Sensitivity 0.40	Poor
Ankylosing spondylitis[6]	Age at onset ≤ 40 years	LR+ 1.08 LR– 0.01	Fair
	Pain not relieved supine	LR+ 1.57 LR– 0.41	Fair
	Morning back stiffness	LR+ 1.56 LR– 0.61	Fair
	Pain duration ≥ 3 months	LR+ 1.54 LR– 0.54	Fair
	4 of 5 positive responses[a]	LR+ 1.28 LR– 0.94	Fair

[a]Five screening questions: 1. Onset of back discomfort before age 40? 2. Did the problem begin slowly? 3. Persistence for at least 3 months? 4. Morning stiffness? 5. Improved by exercise?

Differential Diagnosis		Features
Vascular[11]	Abdominal aortic aneurysm	Current or former smoker: OR 3.40 (95% CI, 2.97–3.89), P < .0001 Male gender: OR 1.96 (95% CI, 1.71–2.23), P < .0001 Age > 65: OR 1.07 (95% CI, 1.06–10.7), P < .0001 White: OR 1.46 (95% CI, 1.28–1.66), P < .0001 HTN: OR 1.29 (95% CI, 1.13–1.48), P < .0006 Diabetes mellitus: OR 0.59 (95% CI, 0.52–0.66), P < .0001
Renal	Pyelonephritis	Nausea, fever, dysuria
	Nephrolithiasis	Colicky abdominal pain
	Perinephric abscess	Nausea, fever, abdominal pain
Gastrointestinal	Pancreatitis	Nausea, vomiting, periumbilical abdominal pain
	Cholecystitis or lithiasis	Right upper quadrant abdominal pain, nausea
	Peptic ulcer disease	Epigastric abdominal pain, nausea, vomiting, eased with eating
Urogenital	Endometriosis	Associated with menstrual cycle
	Pelvic inflammatory disease	Fever, abdominal pain, vaginal discharge

HTN, hypertension; OR, odds ratio.

FOCUSED QUESTIONS

QUESTIONS	THINK ABOUT...
History	
Do you have a personal history of cancer?	Malignancy: In patients with a personal history of cancer, new back pain should be considered malignant until proven otherwise (LR+ 14.7).
Age?	> 50: malignancy LR+ 2.7 > 65: abdominal aortic aneurysm in a male current or former smoker > 70: compression fracture with or without trauma < 40: ankylosing spondylitis, sensitivity 1.0 but low specificity
Have you been treated with corticosteroids for more than 1 month?	Compression fracture: Although insensitive, the specificity of prior steroid use is 0.99 for a compression fracture.
Do you use injection drugs or have a current infection?	Osteomyelitis or paraspinal abscess: although sensitivity is low at 0.40
Location	
Is the pain localized to the back, or does it go elsewhere?	Pain remaining above the knee: hip pathology Pain radiating down the leg below the knee: sciatica (irritation or compression of the L4–5, S1 nerve roots usually from a disk herniation) Pain in the abdomen or pelvis: visceral source

Description/quality	
Is the pain electrical or shock-like?	Disk herniation
Is the pain constant and nocturnal?	Malignancy when worse with rest Mechanical when improved with rest
Is the pain colicky?	Referred pain from a visceral organ
Does the pain have a tearing or ripping quality?	Aortic dissection
Duration/frequency	
Was the onset abrupt?	Fracture or injury induced
Has the pain been persistent and progressive?	> 1 month: malignancy in older patient (sensitivity 0.50, specificity 0.81) > 3 months: ankylosing spondylitis in younger patient; sensitivity 1.0 but nonspecific (specificity 0.07)
Is the pain cyclical?	Endometriosis
Aggravating and relieving factors	
Is the pain worse in the morning and associated with morning stiffness?	Ankylosing spondylitis (sensitivity 0.64, specificity 0.59)
Is there pain in the legs with standing that increases with cough or walking?	Neurogenic claudication from spinal stenosis
How does the pain change with forward bending or sitting?	Improves: spinal stenosis or spondylolisthesis Worsens: disk herniation (if promotes sciatica)
Does the pain improve with exercise?	Ankylosing spondylitis or nonspecific etiology
Does the pain change in intensity with eating?	Improves: peptic ulcer disease Worsens: pancreatitis, gallbladder disease, or other visceral organ
Associated symptoms	
Abdominal pain	Visceral etiology
Nausea or vomiting	Pancreatitis, peptic ulcer disease, appendicitis
Fever	Osteomyelitis, malignancy, or infection related to intra-abdominal or pelvic etiology

PREDICTORS OF CHRONIC DISABLING BACK PAIN

Although most patients with nonspecific back pain have resolution of their symptoms within 6 weeks, 30% to 40% will have recurrences over time, and approximately 7% will develop chronic LBP that affects their ability to function normally.[4,12] A recent systematic review for the Rational Clinical Examination Series in the *Journal of the American Medical Association* identified features that place an individual at increased risk of developing a chronic disabling condition.[13] By identifying such individuals early, a more proactive approach to management with closer follow-up may help to optimize their care.

Predictors of Worse Outcome at 1 Year	Median LR (Range)	Quality of the Evidence
Nonorganic signs (higher somatization scores suggesting a strong psychological component to pain or intentionally false or exaggerated symptoms)	LR+ 3.0 (1.7–4.6) LR– 0.71 (0.31–0.76)	Fair
Maladaptive pain coping behaviors (avoiding work and other activities due to fear of worsening symptoms and excessively negative thoughts and statements about the future)	LR+ 2.5 (2.2–2.8) LR– 0.39 (0.38–0.40)	Fair-good
High baseline functional impairment (as determined by a measure such as the Roland-Morris disability questionnaire)[14]	LR+ 2.1 (1.2–2.7) LR– 0.40 (0.10–0.52)	Good
Psychiatric comorbidities	LR+ 2.2 (1.9–2.3)	Good
Low general health status	LR+ 1.8 (1.1–2.0)	Fair-good

DIAGNOSTIC APPROACH (INCLUDING ALGORITHM)

When gathering the history from a patient with acute LBP, remember the context. Most LBP is nonspecific and self-limited, so the clinician must identify individuals with a more worrisome etiology. Serious causes should be considered if there are features suggesting neurologic compromise, a systemic disease, or referred pain from a visceral organ. Equally important is to identify features that place patients at increased risk of developing a more chronic and disabling condition, because early intervention may preserve long-term function. See Figure 54–1 for the diagnostic approach algorithm for low back pain.

CAVEATS

- Greater than 90% of acute LBP seen in the primary care setting has a nonspecific, mechanical etiology and will be self-limited.
- Neurologic symptoms require assessment for motor or reflex deficits, which, if present, necessitate an urgent or emergent investigation.
- Cauda equina syndrome and myelopathy are rare complications that require urgent evaluation. In the absence of urinary retention (often manifested as overflow incontinence), the likelihood of cauda equina syndrome is about 1 in 10,000. Lumbar myelopathy is suggested by lower extremity weakness, increased tone, spasticity, and hyperreflexia.
- Increasing age, history of cancer, known vascular disease, and associated features such as abdominal symptoms, fever, weight loss, and blood pressure abnormalities suggest a systemic process or referred pain from a visceral organ.
- Patients at heightened risk of developing a chronic and disabling condition may benefit from a multifaceted management approach.

CASE SCENARIO | Resolution

A 51-year-old woman presents to your clinic with a complaint of low back pain, which began acutely 2 weeks earlier, 1 day after a 10-km run. The pain is as achy, intermittent, and located in the central region of her low back. It is associated with an occasional electrical sensation shooting down her left leg. The pain is aggravated by rolling over in bed, prolonged sitting, and running; it is relieved by rest, changing positions, and ibuprofen.

ADDITIONAL HISTORY

Although it disturbs her training routine, the pain is occasional and dull, allowing her to function normally at work. Her pain is easily relieved by changing positions. The shooting pain in her left leg has been improving, no longer occurs daily, and lasts only seconds. She denies any weakness or numbness, which is confirmed by neurologic examination. Ibuprofen and ice have helped, but primarily she avoids backward bending, running, and lying prone.

Question: What is the most likely diagnosis?

A. Spinal stenosis
B. Disk herniation
C. Nonspecific low back pain (LBP)
D. Compression fracture
E. Abdominal aortic aneurysm

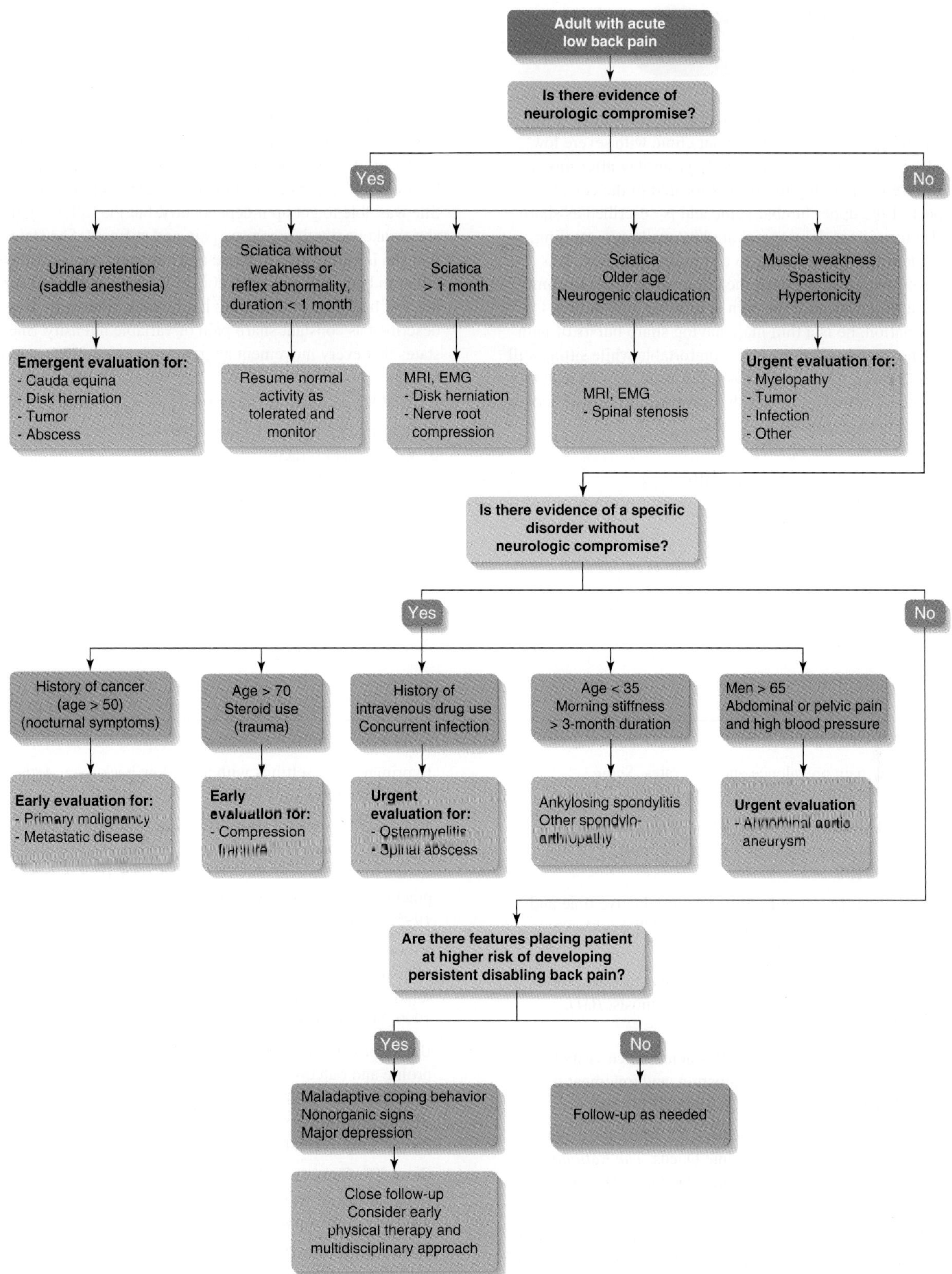

FIGURE 54–1 Diagnostic approach: Low back pain. EMG, electromyography; MRI, magnetic resonance imaging.

Test Your Knowledge

1. A 72-year-old male smoker with chronic obstructive pulmonary disease presents to your clinic with severe low back pain. The pain began acutely yesterday after moving furniture in his living room. It is located in the central aspect of the upper lumbar spine and is described as sharp and intermittent. It is aggravated by walking, standing, and moving from a sitting to a standing position. It is relieved with rest. He used the clinic wheelchair to come to your office because the pain is limiting ambulation. On examination, he is a thin male having sharp bursts of pain with movement, although he is comfortable while sitting still between these episodes. He has severe tenderness to palpation over the L1 spinal process with milder pain to palpation over the paraspinous muscles.
   What is your leading diagnosis?
   A. Nonspecific low back pain (LBP)
   B. Compression fracture
   C. Spinal stenosis
   D. Abdominal aortic aneurysm
   E. Disk herniation

2. A 34-year-old female real estate agent presents to your office with low back pain that began 6 days ago when she slipped in the foyer of a new condominium building. She fell onto her buttocks and experienced immediate pain over her tailbone. She was able to get up independently, but the following day, she awakened with increased pain and stiffness. She states that she is barely able to move and has spent the last 5 days either in bed or lying on her couch. Her pain is located across her low back and radiates into her buttock bilaterally. It is described as constant sharp pain of variable intensity. She states that every movement aggravates it and nothing seems to help.
   What is your leading diagnosis?
   A. Nonspecific low back pain (LBP)
   B. Compression fracture
   C. Spinal stenosis
   D. Abdominal aortic aneurysm
   E. Disk herniation

References

1. Deyo R. Back pain prevalence and visit rates. *Spine*. 2006;31:2724–2727.
2. Freburger J, Holmes GM, Agans RP, et al. The rising prevalence of chronic low back pain. *Arch Intern Med*. 2009;169:251–258
3. Stewart W, Ricci JA, Chee E, et al. Lost productive time and cost due to common pain conditions in the US workforce. *JAMA*. 2003;290:2443–2454.
4. Pengel LH, Herbert RD, Maher CG, Refshauge KM. Acute low back pain: systematic review of its prognosis. *BMJ*. 2003;327:323.
5. Hart LG, Deyo RA, Cherkin DC. Physician office visits for low back pain: frequency, clinical evaluation, and treatment patterns from a U.S. national survey. *Spine*. 1995;20:11–19.
6. Stern B, Deyo RA, Rainville J, Bedlack RS. Make the diagnosis: low back pain. In: Simel DL, Rennie D, eds. *The Rational Clinical Examination: Evidence-Based Clinical Diagnosis*. New York, NY: McGraw Hill, 2009.
7. Chou R, Qaseem A, Snow V, et al. Diagnosis and treatment of low back pain: a joint clinical practice guideline from the American College of Physicians and the American Pain Society. *Ann Intern Med*. 2007;147:478–491.
8. Henschke N, Maher CG, Refshauge KM, et al. Prevalence of and screening for serious spinal pathology in patients presenting to primary care settings with acute low back pain. *Arthritis Rheum*. 2009;60:3072–3080.
9. Van den Hoogen HM, Koes BW, van Eijk JT, Bouter LM. On the accuracy of history, physical examination, and erythrocyte sedimentation rate in diagnosing low back pain in general practice. A criteria-based review of the literature. *Spine*. 1995;20:318–327.
10. Vroomen PC, de Krom MC, Knottnerus JA. Diagnostic value of history and physical examination in patients suspected of sciatica due to disc herniation: a systematic review. *J Neurol*. 1999;246:899–906.
11. Baumgartner I, Hirsch AT, Abola MT, et al. Cardiovascular risk profile and outcome of patients with abdominal aortic aneurysm in out-patients with atherothrombosis: data from the Reduction of Atherothrombosis for Continued Health (REACH) registry. *J Vasc Surg*. 2008;48:808–814.
12. Carey TS, Garrett JM, Jackman AM. Beyond the good prognosis. Examination of an inception cohort of patients with chronic low back pain. *Spine*. 2000;25: 115–120.
13. Chou R, Shekelle P. Will this patient develop persistent disabling low back pain? *JAMA*. 2010;303:1295–1302.
14. Roland Morris Disability Questionnaire. Available at: http://www.rmdq.org/index.htm. Accessed October 28, 2011.

Suggested Reading

Chou R, Qaseem A, Snow V, et al. Diagnosis and treatment of low back pain: a joint clinical practice guideline from the American College of Physicians and the American Pain Society. *Ann Intern Med*. 2007;147:478–491.

Chou R, Shekelle P. Will this patient develop persistent disabling low back pain? *JAMA*. 2010;303:1295–1302.

Stern B, Deyo RA, Rainville J, Bedlack RS. Make the diagnosis: low back pain. In: Simel DL, Rennie D, eds. *The Rational Clinical Examination: Evidence-Based Clinical Diagnosis*. New York, NY: McGraw Hill, 2009.

Chapter 55

Buttock, Hip, and Thigh Pain

Christopher M. Wittich, MD, PharmD, and Robert D. Ficalora, MD

CASE SCENARIO

A 72-year-old woman presents to your clinic complaining of left hip pain. She denies antecedent trauma and localizes the pain to the lateral hip. It radiates down her left lateral thigh but not to her groin. The pain is exacerbated when she lays on it at night. The pain has progressed, prompting her visit today.

- **What additional questions would you ask to learn more about her lower extremity pain?**
- **How does localizing the pain help in generating a differential diagnosis?**
- **How can you use the patient history to identify serious diagnoses?**

INTRODUCTION

Pain in the proximal lower extremities may result from diseases of blood vessels or peripheral nerves or local infection, or it may be referred from local structures, such as hip pain referred to the ipsilateral knee. Disorders of use and abuse, particularly sports-related disorders, predominate in this area.

Deep pain arising from vessels, fascia, joints, tendons, periosteum, and supporting structures is often poorly localized and dull; it may be accompanied by joint stiffness and deep tenderness. The close proximity of structures and complicated functional anatomy of the region make localization of the pain and identification of the affected structure even more difficult. Pain that arises from adjacent or supporting structures may be attributed to the joints in the absence of any true joint pathology.

Pain arising from disorders of the tendons, muscles, and bursae of the buttock and thigh commonly results from inflammation due to athletic injuries. Hip pain is often a consequence of degenerative or inflammatory conditions. Pain caused by diseases of the peripheral nerves or by entrapment neuropathies, such as meralgia paresthetica, can be difficult to sort out by history. Neuropathic pain may result from reflex sympathetic dystrophy/chronic regional pain syndrome (RSD/CRPS), a poorly understood condition that occasionally follows local trauma, stroke, or spinal cord injury. Irritation of the lumbar nerve roots (herniated nucleus pulposus, osteoarthritis) can cause lower extremity pain and may complicate the diagnosis of more localized disorders such as trochanteric bursitis and peripheral sciatic nerve inflammation.

Complex functional relationships may obscure primary and secondary etiologies of pain. Gait abnormalities are a common consequence and occasional cause of disorders in this region. Degenerative hip joint disease may result in a gait disturbance that causes piriformis syndrome or trochanteric bursitis. Atherosclerotic complications usually occur in the setting of extensive or systemic vascular disease. Deep venous thrombosis (DVT) requires immediate identification and action.

KEY TERMS

Bursitis	Pain and inflammation of the structure containing the fluid that lubricates a joint or tendon sheath.
Degenerative joint disease	Characteristic painful, noninflammatory changes in a joint that result from "wear and tear" of chronic use and abuse.
Entrapment neuropathy	Pain and loss of function resulting from a nerve passing through a physiologic space that is narrowed secondary to acute or chronic trauma or inflammation.

—Continued next page

Continued—

Neuropathic pain	Pain in a region as a result of nerve inflammation, trauma, or neurologic disease.
Overuse syndrome	Pain and inflammation resulting from intense or repetitive use of regional anatomic structures in the course of occupational or recreational activities.
Radiculopathy	Pain caused by irritation or compression of a nerve in or near the spinal column. It produces symptoms in the area of innervation.
Referred pain	Pain originating in one structure that is perceived in the area of another, usually because of physiologic or embryologic links between the 2 structures.
Strain	Micro-tears of muscle fibers; can be indistinguishable from muscle tear, and the terms are often used interchangeably.
Tendinitis	Pain and inflammation of a tendon or tendon sheath.

ETIOLOGY

Differential Diagnosis: Buttock Pain

Diagnosis	Explanation	Prevalence
Coccydynia	Pain at the base of the spine that represents a variety of conditions with different causes ranging from hypermobility of the sacral vertebra to neuropathic pain as a result of multiple traumatic events. Coccydynia can follow falls, childbirth, repetitive strain, or surgery.	Up to 20% of women after difficult deliveries[1]
Sciatica	Pain, weakness, numbness, and other discomfort along the path of the sciatic nerve; often accompanies low back pain. It indicates a problem at some point along the sciatic nerve, such as herniated disk, spinal stenosis, obturator foramen stenosis or hernia, or piriformis syndrome.	5.7% of workers with low back pain[2]
Hamstring/ischial tuberosity syndrome	Pain in the posterior thigh, particularly during and following activities like running. Hamstring injuries occur in sports that require bursts of speed or rapid acceleration, such as track, soccer, and football. Predisposing factors include improper warm-up, fatigue, previous injury, strength imbalance, and poor flexibility.	2%–11% of all injuries in athletes annually[3,4]
Piriformis syndrome	Spasm of a small buttock muscle through which the sciatic nerve runs. Pain and leg symptoms are attributed to entrapment of the sciatic nerve. Occurs primarily in individuals with gait abnormalities, weakness of postural muscles, and pregnancy. May occur concurrently with trochanteric bursitis.	Up to 13% of patients with symptoms of sciatica[5]
RSD/CRPS	A chronic progressive neurologic condition that affects a region, such as an arm or a leg. May occur after a minor injury or sprain, but in some cases, there is no precipitating event. Pain begins in one area or limb and then spreads. RSD/CRPS is characterized by burning pain, excessive sweating, swelling, and sensitivity to touch. Marked osteopenia is noted in bones within the nerve distribution.	2%–5% of peripheral nerve injury patients 12%–21% of patients with hemiplegia (paralysis on one side of the body) 1%–2% of bone fracture patients[6]

Differential Diagnosis: Hip and Thigh Pain

Diagnosis	Explanation	Prevalence
Lateral femoral cutaneous nerve (LFCN) syndrome or meralgia paresthetica	Damage to the LFCN from: surgery on the iliac crest, hysterectomy, laparoscopic herniorrhaphy, aortic valve surgery, or coronary artery bypass surgery; diabetic neuropathy; restrictive clothing; or tightly worn, wide weightlifting belts.	Varies widely but has been reported in up to 20% of some surgical procedures[7]
Quadriceps muscle strain or tear	The quadriceps muscles consist of the vastus lateralis, vastus medialis, vastus intermedius, and the rectus femoris. Any of these muscles can strain (or tear), but the most common is the rectus femoris. Occurs in football/soccer players, skaters, runners, and older athletes whose exercise program is primarily walking.	US Military Academy at West Point prevalence data on causative activity: rugby, 4.7%; karate and judo, 2.3%; football, 1.6%; all other sports, < 1%[8]
Hamstring strain	Hamstrings are long muscles that extend down the back of the thigh. Because hamstrings work to pull back the leg and bend the knee, they can be injured during running, kicking, or jumping. Patients may feel a "pop," usually at the back of the thigh, when the muscle tears.	Unknown[9]
Trochanteric bursitis	Inflammation of one or more of the 4 bursae usually present around the greater trochanter; 3 are constant—2 major and 1 minor. These bursae function as a gliding mechanism for the anterior portion of the gluteus maximus tendon as it passes over the greater trochanter to insert into the iliotibial band (ITB). Any inflammation or irritation of these bursae can result in symptoms of trochanteric bursitis. Seen typically with disorders of gait due to hip, knee, or low back problems; obesity; or pregnancy.	Unknown[10]
Lumbar radiculopathy (L2, L3), lumbar facet syndrome	A sensory or motor nerve exiting the spinal column may be irritated or entrapped by arthritis of the foramina or facet or compressed by a herniated disk, with pain referring to the lateral thigh.	2% of the population. Of these, 10%–25% develop symptoms that persist for > 6 weeks[2]
Iliopsoas bursitis/ tendinitis, iliopsoas syndrome ("snapping hip syndrome")	Pain and snapping in medial groin or thigh. Acute injury and overuse are the 2 main causes. The acute injury involves an eccentric contraction of the iliopsoas muscle or direct trauma. Overuse injury occurs in activities involving repeated hip flexion or external rotation of the thigh. Seen in dancers, gymnasts, cheerleaders, and runners.	43.8% of ballet dancers with hip pain[11]
Hip adductor strain or "groin pull," also called "gracilis strain," which is a misnomer because all the hip adductor muscles can be involved	A bruise or strain of the muscles that run from the front of the hip bone to the inside of the thigh. These muscles stabilize the hip and leg during all sporting activities that involve running. Pain and stiffness in the groin region occur in the morning and at the beginning of athletic activity. May abate after warming up but often recurs after athletic activity.	62% of groin injuries; accounts for 5% of all soccer injuries and 2.5% of karate injuries[12]

—Continued next page

Continued—

ITB syndrome ("runner's knee")	Lateral hip, thigh, or knee pain or snapping as ITB passes over the greater trochanter. It is caused by repetitive friction of the ITB on the lateral femoral condyle during flexion-extension, resulting in an inflammatory reaction.	Unknown; occurs mainly in athletes, especially runners and cyclists[13]
DVT of the thigh	Characterized by unilateral warmth, erythema, swelling, and tenderness of the calf and thigh, in which a large vein is occluded by thrombus.	5% of patients with lower limb orthopedic conditions (especially surgery) without prophylaxis; can be significantly increased in persons with hypercoagulable states[14]
Entrapment neuropathies involving the subcostal and the lateral cutaneous branches of the iliohypogastric nerves	Cause pain in the proximal anterior thigh and occur after abdominal surgical procedures (eg, appendectomy, herniorrhaphy).	Unknown[15]
Avascular necrosis of the femoral head	Vascular supply to the femoral head is precarious and easily compromised. A large portion of the total surface is covered with articular cartilage through which vessels do not penetrate. The blood supply enters through a restricted space, and there is limited collateral circulation. Risk factors include fracture, corticosteroid therapy, alcohol, gout, diabetes, sickle cell anemia, and Gaucher disease.	0.72% of general population; corticosteroids increase risk significantly[13]
Hip fracture	A fracture of the femur above a point 5 cm below the distal part of the lesser trochanter. An intracapsular fracture occurs proximal to the point at which the hip joint capsule attaches to the femur. Subtrochanteric fractures occur in the most distal part of the proximal femoral segment (below the lesser trochanter). Extracapsular fractures occur distal to the hip joint capsule.	0.11% of the general population; prevalence increases from about 3 per 100 women age 65–74 to 12.6 per 100 women age 85 or older[16]
Hip osteoarthritis	Osteoarthritis is a mechanically stimulated, chemically mediated process in which attempted repair of microtrauma results in abnormal bone structure. Risk factors include aging, obesity, occupation, and gender.	70% of the general population over 65 years[17]
Rheumatoid arthritis	Inflammatory, destructive arthritis of unknown cause. Hip involvement, because it compromises mobility, can be particularly debilitating. Synovial tissue and joint destruction can occur early in the disease process, before classic deformities develop.	2% in persons older than 60[18]

INTERVIEW FRAMEWORK

- Assess for alarm symptoms.
- Identify predisposing conditions.
- Systematically identify complaints as they relate to the following structures or diagnoses: joints; soft tissues, including tendons, bursae, and muscle groups; nerves and neuropathic disorders; and lumbar structures that refer pain to the lower extremity.

GETTING STARTED WITH THE HISTORY

- Lower extremity complaints are usually localized and commonly follow an inciting event, injury, or recreational or occupational overuse.
- Anatomic and functional relationships are complex and require careful investigation.
- Basic questions including the onset, location, qualities, and aggravating or ameliorating factors are most useful.
- An occupational and leisure time (especially athletic) history is essential.

Questions	Remember
Where is the pain?	Most patients will not be able to adequately describe the precise location of the pain, so pointing is helpful.
When did it start?	Physical demonstrations of typical activities or descriptions of sports-related movements may be valuable adjuncts to the history.
Can you describe it for me? Is it dull, sharp, or burning? Does it ever change?	Trying to be helpful, patients often group unrelated symptoms. Make sure that each individual symptom or sign is understood completely before moving on.
Is there swelling?	
Is there a rash or discoloration?	
What activity makes it better or worse?	
Can you bear weight?	
Can you show me how you use your legs at work, or when you play?	
Tell me about your leisure time activities.	

IDENTIFYING ALARM SYMPTOMS

Serious Diagnoses

- Acute disk herniation
- Hip fracture
- Aseptic necrosis of the femoral head
- DVT
- Primary or metastatic tumor

Alarm Symptoms	Serious Causes	Benign Causes
Loss of bowel or bladder control or persistent sensory abnormalities (eg, numbness, burning, or tingling), especially if associated with back complaints	Lumbar nerve root or spinal cord disorders, especially acute lumbar disk herniation Epidural metastasis	Anxiety (may be a side effect of medications)
Inability to bear weight	Hip fracture or aseptic necrosis of the femoral head	Pain from tendinitis, bursitis, or degenerative joint disease may be so intense that patients refuse to bear weight.
Painful redness and swelling of the thigh, particularly over the common femoral vein	Thigh DVT is associated with a high risk for pulmonary embolism and cardiopulmonary complications.	Local trauma or skin infection

FOCUSED QUESTIONS

After listening to the patient's complaint, put the description in a context of related risks and activities. Patients may have an idea of the cause of their symptoms from the media, friends, or the Internet, but often will not be able to put all the pieces together.

Because most disorders of the lower extremity are not primary physiologic derangements but rather effects of overuse or injury (work related or athletic), narrowing down the differential diagnosis begins with defining the patient's activities.

QUESTIONS	THINK ABOUT...
Tell me about your work.	
Do you perform repetitive activities such as unloading trucks or work on an assembly line?	Repetitive motion of the hip and lower back, as well as lifting, increases the risk of several forms of tendinitis or bursitis, lumbar radiculopathy, and disk herniation.
Do you wear a lumbar support belt, weightlifting belt, or other constrictive clothing?	Meralgia paresthetica or LFCN syndrome is an entrapment neuropathy that can result from tight, restrictive clothing.
Do you jump off trucks, platforms, or heavy equipment?	Osteoarthritis results from chronic minor trauma to the hip.
Tell me about your leisure time activities.	
Do you play football or soccer? Run track?	Hamstring/ischial tuberosity syndrome from improper or inadequate stretching or warm-up
Do you play football or soccer? Skate? Run?	Quadriceps muscle strain or tear
Do you practice judo or karate? Do you walk (in older patients)?	Hip adductor strain
Do you participate in gymnastics or football?	Hamstring tear, from kicking or jumping, after feeling a "pop" in the back of the thigh
Have you taken any long car rides or airplane trips?	Inactivity without hourly stretching or movement of the legs is a risk factor for DVT.
Quality	
Is the pain:	
• *Steady?*	Rheumatoid arthritis Osteoarthritis Infection
• *Aching?*	Overuse syndrome or referred pain
• *Shooting? Sharp?*	Entrapment neuropathy
• *Burning?*	Neuropathic pain
• *Severe?*	Arthritis (at rest) Gout Infection Trauma Tumor
• *Throbbing?*	Inflammatory or vascular (DVT)
• *Related to activity?*	Tendinitis or bursitis

Location

Where do you have pain?	
• *In or around what joint?*	Pain resulting from an articular disorder is perceived as coming directly from the joint, not from the bones between the joints. Pain from true hip pathology is felt in the groin. Patients describe lateral thigh pain as "hip" pain, which is usually a soft tissue problem.
• *Buttock?*	Coccydynia, sciatica (with radiation down leg), piriformis syndrome
• *Hip?*	Osteoarthritis Hip fracture or aseptic necrosis Rheumatoid arthritis
• *Anterior thigh?*	Entrapment neuropathies Meralgia paresthetica (LFCN syndrome) Lumbar (L2/L3) radiculopathy Quadriceps muscle strain/tear Hip adductor strain
• *Lateral thigh?*	Trochanteric bursitis Entrapment neuropathies
• *Medial thigh*	DVT Iliopsoas bursitis or tendinitis
• *Posterior thigh?*	Hamstring strain Ischial tuberosity syndrome
• *Along the limb spanning joint and muscle?*	Lesion of blood vessels such as DVT Nerve root compression

Time course

Is the pain related to an activity?	Overuse syndromes may come on after hours, days, or weeks of a repetitive activity or after resumption of an activity after some time away from it.
Does the pain wax and wane?	Work-related overuse syndromes are often better on weekends and worse on Fridays. Sports-related overuse syndromes may have the reverse (worse on Mondays) or a variable pattern. Bursitis is most painful at night.
Was the onset of pain:	
• *Sudden? (minutes to hours)*	Acute infectious process Trauma Vascular processes Referred pain
• *Gradual?*	Arthritis Tendinitis Bursitis Rheumatoid arthritis Neuropathic pain

—*Continued next page*

Continued—

Associated symptoms	
Is there swelling:	
• *In the area of the pain?*	In rheumatoid arthritis, the joints are painful and swollen.
• *Around or near it?*	In RSD, the entire region may be swollen. With deep structures of the hip and buttocks, stiffness or immobility may be the only clue to deep tissue swelling.
Is the skin red?	Tendinitis may have erythema (redness) over the affected tendon. Infected structures often have surrounding erythema, as does DVT.
Modifying factors	
Is the joint pain:	
• *Present only with movement?*	Suggests effusion such as in osteoarthritis
• *Present at rest?*	Suggests inflammation, such as rheumatoid arthritis, or neuropathic pain
• *Increased by motion? Activity?*	Suggests abnormalities of the tendons or bursae Typical of overuse syndromes or athletic injuries
Is the pain in your leg (not related to a joint) induced or made worse:	
• *By sneezing? Coughing? Sitting or hyperextension of the back?*	Lumbar nerve root pain
• *Raising the leg up straight?*	Lumbar spine lesion
• *During stretching?*	Inflamed tendons or bursae Sciatica
• *By light touch?*	Neuropathic pain, such as entrapment neuropathy
Does the pain occur:	
• *When climbing stairs or at night?*	Trochanteric bursitis Piriformis syndrome
• *After activity is over?*	Tendinitis Quadriceps or hamstring strain
• *After recent surgical procedure?*	Coccydynia Entrapment neuropathies
Are you unable to bear weight?	Structural disorders of the hip joint such as fracture or aseptic necrosis of the femoral head
Are you unable to walk?	Related to pain rather than restricted motion Quadriceps muscle or hamstring strain
Are you unable to kick a ball?	Strain or inflammation of the muscles or tendons
Is the pain:	
• *Greatest in the morning?*	Rheumatoid arthritis (morning stiffness)
• *Worse with prolonged use of the joint?*	Osteoarthritis
• *Better with use?*	Hip adductor strain

Do you have:	
• *Fever or chills?*	Septic arthritis or bursitis
• *Numbness, tingling, or burning in the leg?*	Neuropathic pain such as entrapment neuropathy Sciatica LFCN syndrome
• *Swelling, redness, or dyspnea?*	DVT with or without pulmonary embolism

DIAGNOSTIC APPROACH (INCLUDING ALGORITHM)

- Characterize the pain including type, onset, and associated complaints.
- Localize the pain (joints, tendons, soft tissues).
- Look for hints that the pain might be referred or neuropathic.
- Consider the functional anatomy of the region, including specific movements that cause, exacerbate, or relieve the pain.
- Identify potential causes, such as occupation, athletics, habits, and other musculoskeletal problems (eg, gait disorder, injury).

See Figure 55–1 for the diagnostic approach to lower extremity pain.

CAVEATS

Although significant morbidity from musculoskeletal disorders of the lower extremity is rare, life- or limb-threatening disease may result from joint or soft tissue infection, DVT and its cardiopulmonary complications, or malignancy.

Neuropathic pain is the great mimicker. Although investigation of the painful structure is necessary, also consider inflamed nerves, nerve roots, pain referred from other structures, or conditions that put the patient at risk for RSD/CRPS.

Descriptions are helpful when considering lower extremity pain, but there is no substitute for pointing to the area in question, performing the movement that causes the pain, or demonstrating the work-related or athletic activity that precipitates the pain.

PROGNOSIS

The vast majority of causes of lower extremity pain resolve spontaneously or with cessation of the inciting activity. Physical therapy helps many patients. Learning the importance of adequate warm-up and stretching limits recurrences. Permanent disability is unusual, although systemic illnesses such as hypercoagulability or inflammatory disorders significantly affect the prognosis.

CASE SCENARIO | Resolution

A 72-year-old woman presents to your clinic complaining of left hip pain. She denies antecedent trauma and localizes the pain to the lateral hip. It radiates down her left lateral thigh but not to her groin. The pain is exacerbated when she lays on it at night. The pain has progressed, prompting her visit today.

ADDITIONAL HISTORY

The pain is located only on her left side. When asked to point with one finger to the point of maximal pain, she localizes it to her upper left lateral thigh. There has been no redness of her skin. She also reports that one of her legs is about 3 inches longer than the other. Several years ago, she had similar pain that went away when she added a lift to the shoe of her shorter leg. She has no history of sickle cell anemia, corticosteroid use, or osteoporosis.

Question: What is the most likely diagnosis?

A. Avascular necrosis of the femoral head
B. Hip fracture
C. Hip osteoarthritis
D. Trochanteric bursitis

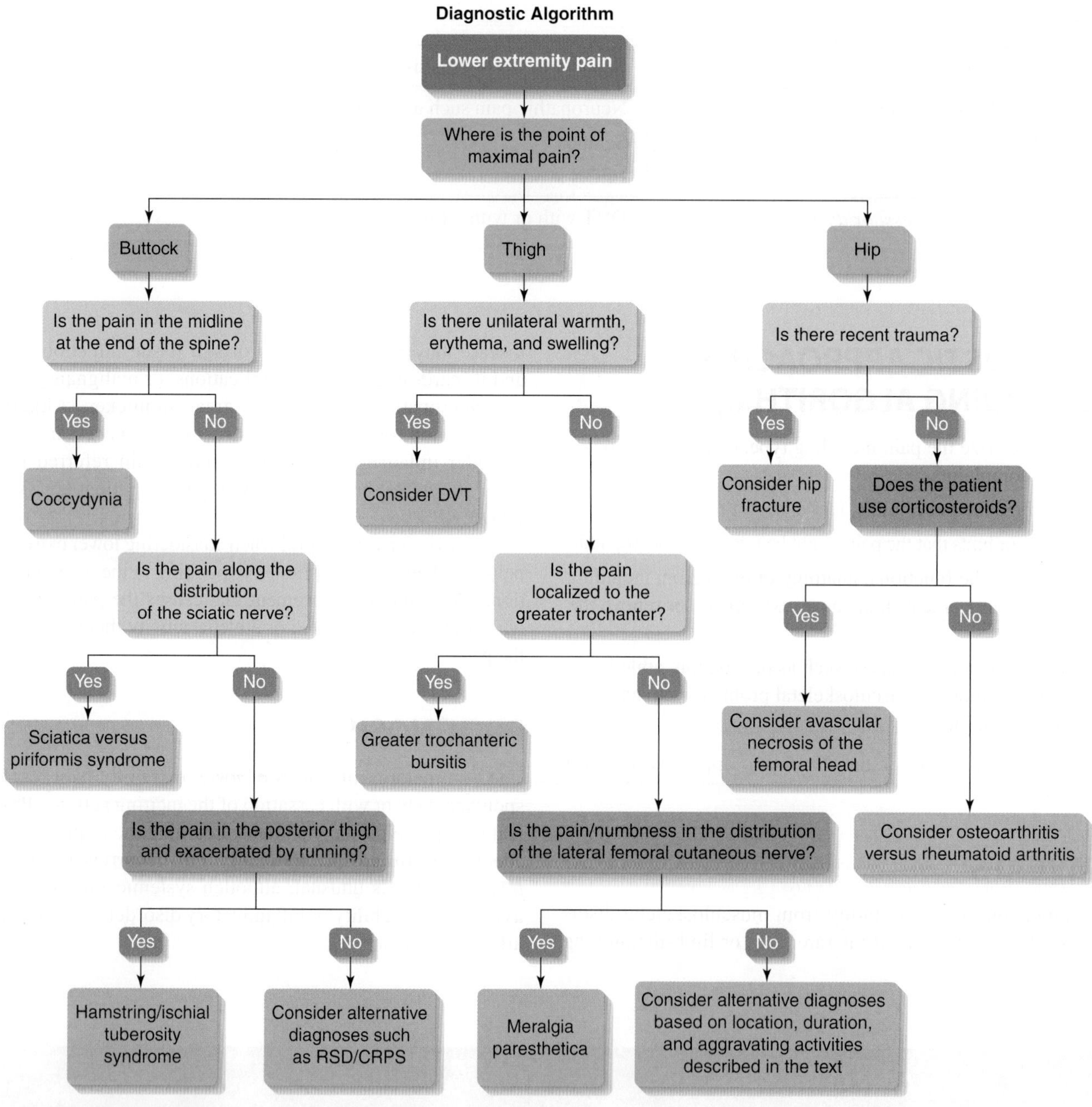

FIGURE 55–1 Diagnostic approach: Lower extremity pain. DVT, deep vein thrombosis; N, no; RSD/CRPS, reflex sympathetic dystrophy/chronic regional pain syndrome; Y, yes.

Test Your Knowledge

1. A 72-year-old man with a history of emphysema presents to your outpatient clinic with left hip pain. The pain radiates to the groin and has been present for greater than a year. His emphysema is poorly controlled, and he has had multiple exacerbations in the past 5 years. An x-ray of the hip shows avascular necrosis of the femoral head.

   Which medication put this patient at increased risk for this condition?

   A. Ibuprofen (a nonsteroidal anti-inflammatory drug [NSAID])
   B. Prednisone (a corticosteroid)
   C. Salmeterol inhaler (a long-acting β-agonist)
   D. Aspirin
   E. Simvastatin (an HMG-CoA reductase inhibitor)

2. A 24-year-old woman presents to your clinic 4 weeks after delivering a healthy, 9 lb, 4 oz baby boy. She reports feeling well except for pain in her lower back, which she describes as an aching sensation in the midline.
   What is the most likely diagnosis?
   A. Sciatica
   B. Piriformis syndrome
   C. Meralgia paresthetica
   D. Reflex sympathetic dystrophy
   E. Coccydynia

3. A 21-year-old man presents to your clinic with pain in his thighs. He describes the pain as a burning sensation localized to the lateral aspect of both thighs. He is on the college wrestling team and frequently lifts weights.
   What is the most likely cause of his pain?
   A. Trochanteric bursitis
   B. Hamstring strain
   C. Quadriceps muscle strain
   D. Meralgia paresthetica
   E. Sciatica

References

1. Maigne JY, Doursounian L, Chatellier G. Causes and mechanisms of common coccydynia: role of body mass index and coccygeal trauma. *Spine.* 2000;25:3072–3079.
2. Hagen KB, Hilde G, Jamtvedt G, Winnem MF. The Cochran review of advice to stay active as a single treatment for low back pain and sciatica. *Spine.* 2002;27:1736–1741.
3. Kujala UM, Orava S, Jarvinen M. Hamstring injuries. Current trends in treatment and prevention. *Sports Med.* 1997;23: 397–404.
4. Browning KH. Hip and pelvis injuries in runners: careful evaluation and tailored management. *Phys Sportsmed.* 2001;29:23–34.
5. Rich B, McKeag D. When sciatica is not disc disease: detecting piriformis syndrome in active patients. *Phys Sports Med.* 1992;20:104–115.
6. Reinders MF, Geertzen JH, Dijkstra PU. Complex regional pain syndrome type I: use of the International Association for the Study of Pain diagnostic criteria defined in 1994. *Clin J Pain.* 2002;18:207–215.
7. Grossman MG, Ducey SA, Nadler SS, Levy AS. Meralgia paresthetica: diagnosis and treatment. *J Am Acad Orthop Surg.* 2001;9:336–344.
8. Ryan JB, Wheeler JH, Hopkinson WJ, et al. Quadriceps contusions. West Point update. *Am J Sports Med.* 1991;19:299–304.
9. Holder-Powell HM, Rutherford OM. Unilateral lower limb injury: its long-term effects on quadriceps, hamstring, and plantar flexor muscle strength. *Arch Phys Med Rehab.* 1999;80: 717–720.
10. Shbeeb MI, Matteson EL. Trochanteric bursitis (greater trochanter pain syndrome). *Mayo Clin Proc.* 1996;71:565–569.
11. Biundo JJJ, Irwin RW, Umpierre E. Sports and other soft tissue injuries, tendinitis, bursitis, and occupation-related syndromes. *Curr Opin Rheumatol.* 2001;13:146–149.
12. Prather H. Pelvis and sacral dysfunction in sports and exercise. *Phys Med Rehab Clin N Am.* 2000;11:805–836.
13. Guerra JJ, Steinberg ME. Distinguishing transient osteoporosis from avascular necrosis of the hip. *J Bone Joint Surg.* 1995;77: 616–624.
14. Gottlieb RH, Widjaja J. Clinical outcomes of untreated symptomatic patients with negative findings on sonography of the thigh for deep vein thrombosis: our experience and a review of the literature. *Am J Roentgenol.* 1999;172:1601–1604.
15. Aysar FM, Sahin M, Arikan BU, et al. The possibility of nervus ilioinguinalis and nervus iliohypogastricus injury in lower abdominal incisions and effects on hernia formation. *J Surg Res.* 2002;107:179–185.
16. Braithwaite RS, Col NF, Wong JB. Estimating hip fracture morbidity, mortality and costs. *J Am Geriatr Soc.* 2003;51:364–370.
17. Sowers M. Epidemiology of risk factors for osteoarthritis: systemic factors. *Curr Opin Rheumatol.* 2001;13:447–451.
18. Rasch EK, Hirsch R, Paulose-Ram R, Hochberg MC. Prevalence of rheumatoid arthritis in persons 60 years of age and older in the United States: effect of different methods of case classification. *Arthritis Rheum.* 2003;48:917–926.

Suggested Reading

Greene WB, ed. *Essentials of Musculoskeletal Care.* 2nd ed. Chicago, IL: American Academy of Orthopaedic Surgeons, American Academy of Pediatrics, 2001.

McCue FC III. *The Injured Athlete.* 2nd ed. Philadelphia, PA: JB Lippincott Co., 1992.

Miller MD, Hart JA, MacKnight JM, eds. *Essential Orthopaedics.* New York, NY: Elsevier, Inc., 2010.

Chapter 56

Knee and Calf Pain

Jane E. O'Rorke, MD, FACP, and Deborah L. Cardell, MD

KNEE PAIN

CASE SCENARIO 1

A 42-year-old man comes to your office for evaluation of a painful right knee. He reports that he awoke 3 days ago with pain and swelling in the affected knee. The previous day, he had been cleaning out a friend's garage.

- **Are there any alarm symptoms or features?**
- **Which questions help the clinician narrow the differential diagnosis?**
- **Does the patient require urgent evaluation by an orthopedic surgeon?**

INTRODUCTION

Knee pain is common, affecting 10% to 15% of adults at some point in their lifetime. Knee pain accounts for 3% to 5% of physician visits, or 33 million new visits per year.[1,2] Precise anatomic location of the initial pain is key to making the diagnosis. A differential diagnosis can be formulated by considering the local anatomic structures. A thorough history and relevant physical examination should establish the etiology of the knee pain in most cases.

KEY TERMS

Buckling	A complete collapse of the knee, often secondary to pain or muscle weakness of the quadriceps.[3]
Effusion	Fluid accumulation in the knee joint causing swelling.
Giving way	Symptom usually associated with ligamentous injuries.[4] Occurs with normal walking but may be most prominent during pivoting movements, such as quick changes in direction. Results from a bony structure sliding on another in an abnormal way.
Intermittent claudication	An aching, crampy, sometimes burning pain in the legs that typically occurs with walking and goes away with rest.
Likelihood ratio (LR)	Incorporates both the sensitivity and specificity of a test (or clinical finding), providing a direct estimate of how much a test result will change the odds of having a disease.
Locking	When the knee becomes stuck, usually in 45 degrees of flexion, and patient is unable to unlock the knee without manipulating it in some fashion.[3]
Negative predictive value	Probability that an individual is not affected with the condition when a negative test result is observed.

—Continued next page

Continued—

Odds ratio (OR)	Ratio of the odds of an event occurring in the exposed group versus the unexposed group.
Positive predictive value	Probability that an individual is affected with the condition when a positive test result (or clinical finding) is observed.
Pseudolocking	Occurs with arthritis, when the adjacent rough articular surfaces stick momentarily as they glide over one another.[3]

ETIOLOGY OF KNEE PAIN

	Possible Causes	Prevalence Among Patients Presenting to Primary Care Setting[1]
Knee pain	Unclassified strains/sprains	42%
	Osteoarthritis	34%
	Meniscal tear	9%
	Collateral ligament	7%
	Cruciate ligament	4%
	Gout	2%
	Fracture	1.2%
	Rheumatoid arthritis	0.5%
	Infectious arthritis	0.3%
	Pseudogout	0.2%
Anatomic location of the pain		
Anterior knee	Patellofemoral syndrome	
	Prepatellar bursitis	
	Patellar fracture	
	Patellar tendinitis	
	Quadriceps femoris strain	
	Osteoarthritis	
Posterior knee	Hamstring strain	
	Bursitis (semimembranous, popliteal, gastrocnemius)	
	Baker cyst	
	Deep venous thrombosis	
	Popliteal aneurysm	
Medial knee	Osteoarthritis	
	Medial meniscal tear	
	Medial collateral ligament sprain	
	Anserine bursitis	
	Hamstring (semimembranous) strain	
	Patellofemoral syndrome	

Lateral knee	Lateral meniscal tear Lateral collateral ligament tear Iliotibial band syndrome Biceps femoris strain Fibular head fracture/dislocation	
Presenting symptoms		
Knee laxity (giving way not buckling)	Anterior cruciate ligament tear Posterior cruciate ligament tear Lateral collateral ligament tear Medial collateral ligament tear	
Knee locking or clicking	Medial meniscal tear Lateral meniscal tear	
Acute swelling (immediately following injury)	Anterior cruciate ligament tear Posterior cruciate ligament tear Patellar fracture Tibiofemoral dislocation	
Delayed swelling (occurs hours after injury)	Medial meniscal tear Lateral meniscal tear	
Swelling without known trauma	Septic knee Acute gout/pseudogout attack Degenerative meniscal tear Gonococcal infection	

GETTING STARTED WITH THE HISTORY

- Start with open-ended questions.
- Be methodical in your history taking.

Questions	Remember
Tell me about the problem with your knee or calf.	Let patients describe symptoms in their own words.
Point with one finger to the area that is bothering you.	Prompt patient for exact details concerning initial episode of pain. If recurrent ask about the very first incident.
*Describe the first time you felt this pain, and what **exactly** you were doing at the time.*	Be persistent about having the patient point with one finger. If entire area hurts, instruct patient to point to the spot where initial pain was felt.
Have you ever had this problem before?	

INTERVIEW FRAMEWORK

- Categorize pain into one of the 4 anatomic areas of the knee: anterior, posterior, medial, or lateral.
- If there was trauma, obtain details about the mechanism of injury.
- Follow standard format for attributes of a symptom.
    - Location: Fundamental to narrowing the differential diagnosis
    - Quality and severity: Can be assessed with pain rating scale or by functional limitations to their daily activities (eg, "What can't you do because of your pain?")

- Timing: Was there an inciting event? Did pain develop quickly over hours or insidiously over weeks/months? Is it intermittent? What is the pain like at different times during the day?
- What aggravates pain (eg, exercise versus rest)?
- What relieves pain (eg, over-the-counter treatments, prescription medications, alternative and complimentary therapies)?
- Associated symptoms (eg, swelling, stiffness, or fever)

IDENTIFYING ALARM SYMPTOMS

Immediate referral to a specialist should be considered for the following symptoms.

Alarm Symptoms	Sensitivity (95% Confidence Interval)	If Present, Consider...
Locking		Meniscal tear
Giving way		Ligamentous injury causing instability of the joint
Neurovascular symptoms		Injury to nerve or damage to blood supply
Severe pain	85% (78%–90%)[5]	Septic joint
Effusion	78% (71%–85%)[5]	
Fever	57% (52%–62%)[5]	

FOCUSED QUESTIONS FOR KNEE PAIN

Close-ended questions are important in evaluating knee pain.

QUESTIONS	OR/LR (95% CONFIDENCE INTERVAL)	THINK ABOUT...
What were you doing when you first felt the pain?		Anatomic structures that may have been affected
Have you had this pain before? If yes, what was the diagnosis?		Recurrent musculoskeletal condition
Did the knee pain have a sudden or acute onset?		Contusions, fractures or physeal injuries, ligamentous injuries, meniscal tears, patellar subluxations or dislocations
Is the knee pain chronic?		Osteoarthritis, tumors, overuse syndromes (bursitis/tendinitis)
Is there locking of the knee in a flexed position?		Meniscal injuries
Age > 40 years?	OR 4.1 (1.7–9.9), LR+ 2.0[6]	
Weight bearing during trauma?	OR 3.4 (1.1–9.9), LR– 0.4 (0.2–0.9)[6]	
Is there clicking when walking?		

If swelling occurred, was it immediate or delayed?		Immediate: ligament injury Delayed: meniscal injury
Was there twisting or rotational trauma of the knee?	OR 5.7 (1.5–21.8)[7]	Ligamentous injuries
Was there trauma by external force?	OR 4.1 (0.8–20.9)[7]	
Does the knee give way?		
Was the knee in full extension?		
Is the pain aggravated by climbing stairs, standing from a seated position, or walking up hill?		Patellofemoral syndrome
Do you have pain at night or at rest?		Night pain may indicate higher severity.
What have you done to treat the pain? *Prescription medications?* *Over-the-counter medications?* *Herbs, salves, or alternative therapies?* *Physical therapy?*		Indicates potential treatment options
Have you played sports in your lifetime? Which ones?		More likely to have osteoarthritis if played sports
Are you a runner or jogger with lateral knee pain?		Consider iliotibial band syndrome
Have you had any past injuries to your knee?		More likely to have osteoarthritis with past injuries
What type of work have you done in your lifetime?		
What activities did you do before the knee pain that you are unable to do now?		Good assessment of how much knee pain is affecting daily life
Ask about sexual history, especially in young patients with no history of trauma and a warm, tender, swollen joint.		Gonococcal arthritis

DIAGNOSTIC APPROACH (INCLUDING ALGORITHM)

The most important step is to exclude septic arthritis because it could be potentially life or limb threatening. The presence of fever; a red, hot, swollen joint; and exquisite pain with decreased range of motion is suggestive but not diagnostic of a septic joint. Besides infection, knee effusion may result from gout or pseudogout, inflammatory arthritis, or meniscal or ligament tears. Physical examination and arthrocentesis are needed to establish the diagnosis.

If the knee is not inflamed, consider the location of pain to help narrow the differential diagnosis. Osteoarthritis often causes the gradual onset of pain that progresses over years; it is aggravated by standing or walking and relieved with rest. Otherwise the following clinical features may be helpful (see diagnostic algorithm in Figure 56–1).

- Anterior knee pain
    - Patellar fracture: history of fall or trauma to the anterior knee
    - Patellofemoral syndrome: pain aggravated by walking up stairs or a hill or rising from a seated position

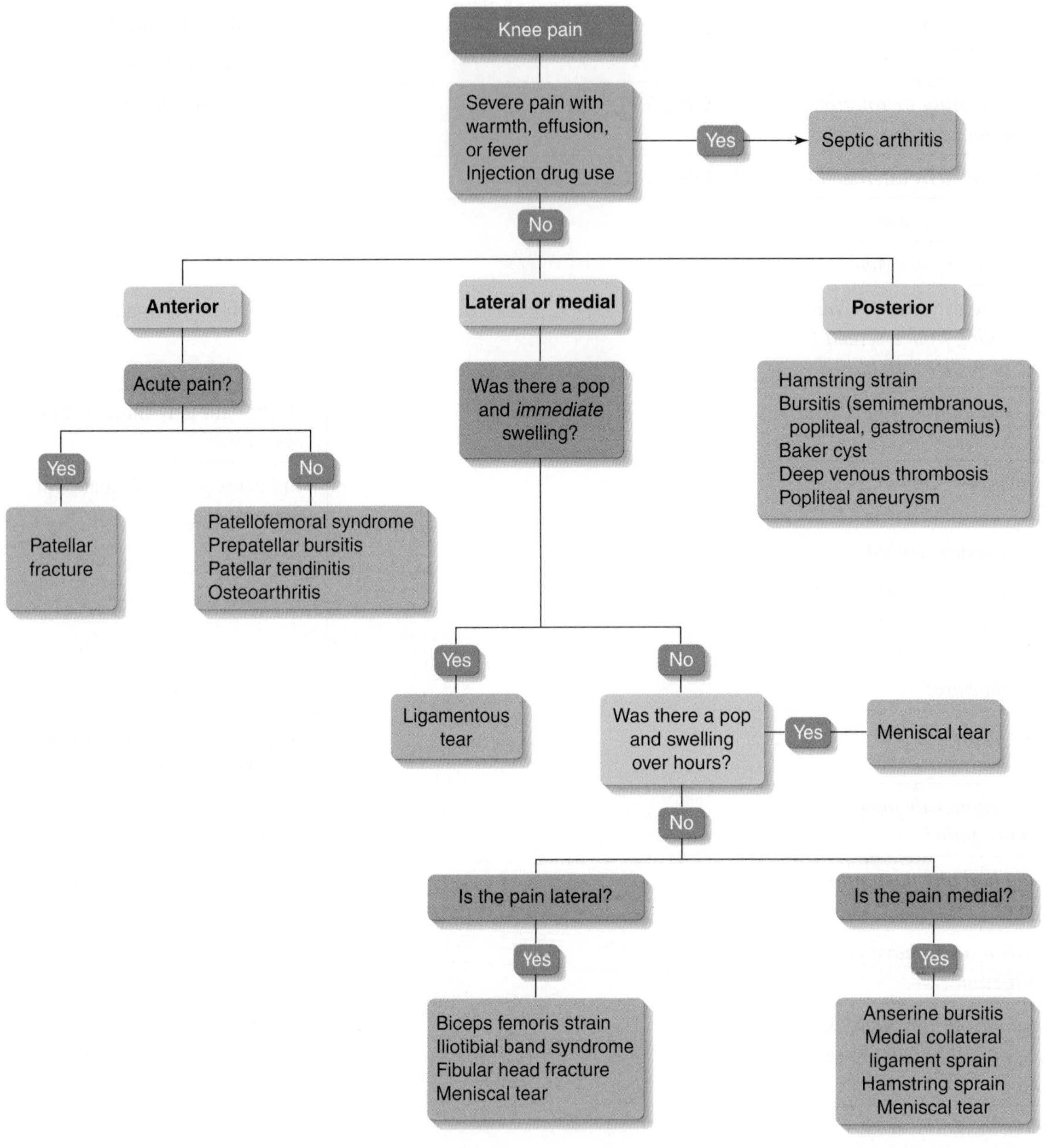

FIGURE 56–1 Diagnostic approach: Knee pain.

   - Prepatellar bursitis: swelling over the patella with history of kneeling, for example, in a bricklayer or mason
   - Patellar tendinitis: pain at the superior or inferior aspect of the patella, aggravated by flexing and extending the knee
- Lateral knee pain
   - Meniscal tear: history of trauma, a popping sound, and swelling of the knee hours after the injury; also consider in patients who have known osteoarthritis and lateral pain with intermittent or persistent swelling
   - Iliotibial band syndrome: occurs most frequently in runners and joggers; tenderness is greatest slightly distal to the lateral joint line
   - Fibular head fracture: history of trauma and pain over the fibular head
- Medial knee pain
   - Meniscal tear: history of trauma, a popping sound, and swelling of the knee hours after the injury; also consider in patients who have known osteoarthritis and lateral pain with intermittent or persistent swelling
   - Anserine bursitis: pain aggravated when the patient lays on his or her side at night with legs together

- Posterior knee pain
  - Baker cyst: fullness or tightness in the posterior knee with decreased flexion
  - Hamstring strain: increased activity level or recently started a new activity
  - Deep venous thrombosis: pain and swelling in the corresponding calf

CAVEATS

- Always ask about the presence of fever, warmth, swelling, and pain, which may herald septic arthritis.
- Osteoarthritis may present as generalized, anterior, lateral, or medial knee pain.
- Even if a patient reports acute knee pain, be sure to ask about previous episodes (indicating more of a chronic intermittent process).
- Get the patient to commit to the location of the pain with one finger.
- When asking about medications used to treat pain, determine the exact dose and frequency. Patients may report that a medication is ineffective when they are not taking a therapeutic dose or allowing sufficient time for it to work.
- Occasionally patients will suffer knee trauma during activities such as dancing but will not recognize it as such. Hence, it is critical to ask exactly what the patient was doing at the time the pain started.
- Always ask about occupational and sports history, past and present.

CASE SCENARIO 1 | Resolution

A 42-year-old man comes to your office for evaluation of a painful right knee. He reports that he awoke 3 days ago with pain and swelling in the affected knee. The previous day, he had been cleaning out a friend's garage.

ADDITIONAL HISTORY

On further questioning, the patient reports redness, warmth, and subjective fevers. He also reports using intravenous heroin 1 week ago.

Question: What diagnosis must be urgently excluded?

A. Gout
B. Ligament tear
C. Meniscal tear
D. Osteoarthritis
E. Septic joint

CALF PAIN

CASE SCENARIO 2

A 45-year-old woman presents to your office with a 3-day history of left calf pain, which is constant and unaffected by activity. She has tried heat and acetaminophen, but neither helps for long.

- **What are the major etiologies of calf pain?**
- **What historical questions help differentiate the various causes?**

INTRODUCTION

There are no studies evaluating the prevalence of various etiologies of calf pain. History taking remains a key element in determining the diagnosis. Deep venous thrombosis (DVT) and intermittent claudication are serious diagnoses that must be considered. The prevalence of intermittent claudication depends on the population studied but ranges from 3% to 10%, sharply increasing in patients age 70 or older. Of patients with claudication, 2% to 4% will require amputation.[3] In patients with DVT, calf pain has a positive likelihood ratio of 1.1 and positive predictive value of 17.[8]

ETIOLOGY OF CALF PAIN

Differential Diagnosis

Calf pain	Intermittent claudication DVT Cellulitis Popliteal artery entrapment syndrome (young individuals without atherosclerotic risk factors) Gastrocnemius or soleus muscle tear or contusion Distal dissection of a Baker cyst Soft tissue sarcoma

IDENTIFYING ALARM SYMPTOMS

Alarm Symptoms	If Present Consider…
Fever, calf swelling, shortness of breath, pleuritic chest pain	DVT, pulmonary embolism
Calf redness, warmth, swelling	Cellulitis, DVT

FOCUSED QUESTIONS FOR CALF PAIN

QUESTIONS	OR (95% CONFIDENCE INTERVAL)	THINK ABOUT...
Does the pain occur with walking? *Is the pain relieved with rest?* *Does the pain reoccur at the same distance every time?* *Is the pain unilateral?* *Do you have pain in the thighs, buttocks, or hips?* *Have you ever had a nonhealing ulcer?*[4]		Intermittent claudication (consider in older individuals)
Wells Criteria		
• *Is the limb paralyzed? (+1 point)*		DVT Apply Wells criteria (score ranges from −2 to 9).
• *Have you been bedridden for > 3 days OR had major surgery in the past 4 weeks? (+1 point)*	OR 1.8 (1.3–2.48)[9]	High risk: ≥ 3 points (53% probability of DVT)
• *Do you have local tenderness in lower limb? (+1 point)*		Moderate risk: 1–2 points (22% probability of DVT)

• *Do you have cancer? (+1 point)* • *Is the entire leg swollen? (+1 point)* • *Do you have calf swelling > 3 cm? (+1 point)* • *Do you have pitting edema? (+1 point)* • *Have you had a previous DVT? (+1 point)* • *Do you have collateral superficial veins? (+1 point)* • *Is another diagnosis more likely? (–2 points)*	OR 2.11 (1.34–3.32)[9]	Low risk: ≤ 0 points (9% probability of DVT)[10]
Is there absence of trauma? *Is there a family history of blood clots?* *Do you take oral contraceptives?* *Do you take anabolic steroids or hormones for body building?*[8]	OR 1.72 (1.18–2.5)[9]	
Did you have swelling behind your knee prior to the calf pain? *Do you have osteoarthritis of the knee?*		Dissecting Baker cyst
Have you had any trauma to the calf? *Do you play sports?* *Were you doing an activity when the pain started?*		Tear or contusion of the gastrocnemius or soleus muscle

DIAGNOSTIC APPROACH (INCLUDING ALGORITHM)

See Figure 56–2 for the diagnostic approach algorithm for calf pain.

PROGNOSIS

Most knee and calf pathology can be diagnosed with a thorough history and physical. If initial diagnosis is correct, treatment can begin immediately. Although musculoskeletal problems often take weeks to months to resolve, many problems will resolve with conservative therapy.

CAVEAT

Always consider DVT in patients with calf pain, especially if unilateral. Wells Criteria (a clinical prediction rule) helps identify patients with low pretest probability of DVT but has limited specificity or ability to establish the diagnosis. Patients in the low-risk category had a negative predictive value for DVT of 96% (range, 87%–100%). It may not perform as well in primary care settings that include more elderly patients and patients with prior DVT or multiple comorbidities. The physical examination is of limited value in identifying patients with DVT. The diagnosis is generally established with Doppler ultrasonography.

CASE SCENARIO 2 | Resolution

A 45-year-old woman presents to your office with a 3-day history of left calf pain, which is constant and unaffected by activity. She has tried heat and acetaminophen, but neither helps for long.

ADDITIONAL HISTORY

The pain started the day after a 24-hour drive from her sister's home. She initially thought her calf was just stiff from driving. She denies any trauma, shortness of breath, swelling, or redness. Her only medication is oral contraceptives.

Question: What is the most likely diagnosis?

A. Deep venous thrombosis
B. Intermittent claudication
C. Muscle strain
D. Ruptured Baker cyst

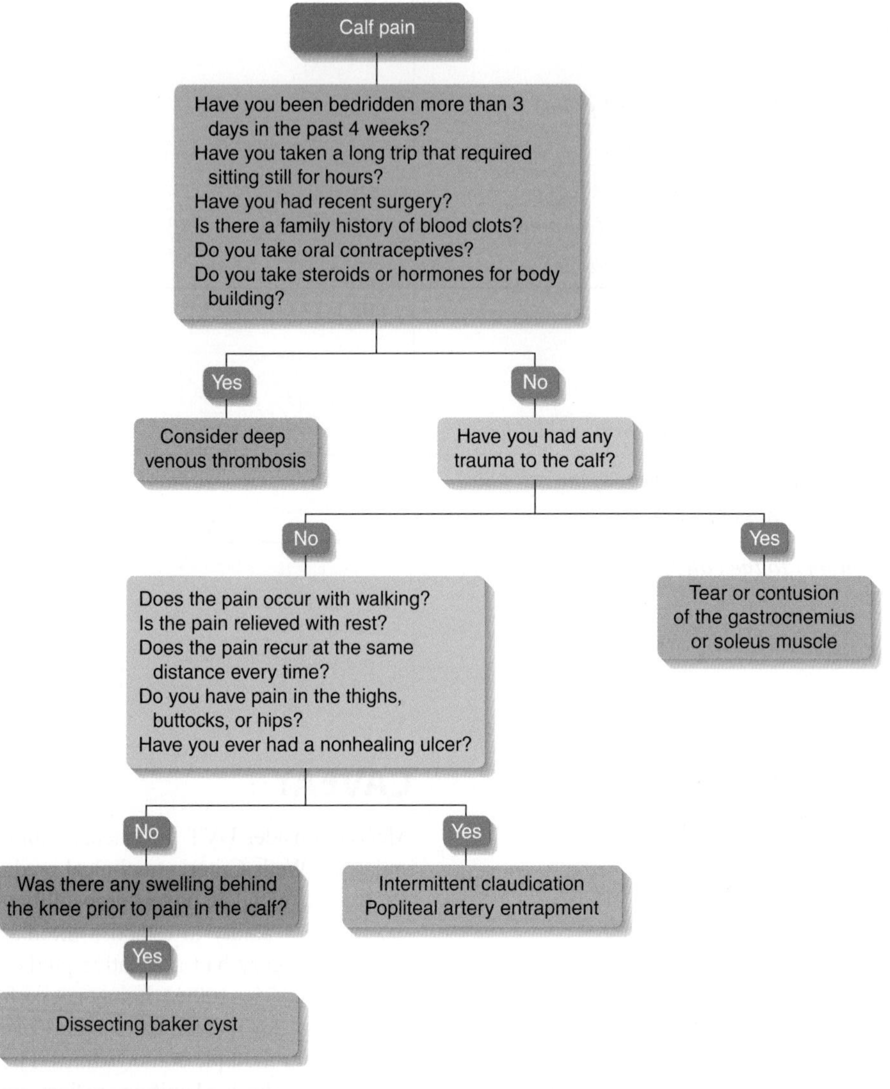

FIGURE 56–2 Diagnostic approach: Calf pain.

Test Your Knowledge

1. A 25-year-old woman presents to an urgent care center with a swollen, painful right knee. The patient was playing soccer and ran into another player, causing her to twist and fall. She reports immediate swelling of her knee.

   What is the most likely diagnosis?

   A. Fracture
   B. Ligamentous tear
   C. Meniscal tear
   D. Septic joint

2. A 65-year-old retired male bricklayer presents with bilateral anterior knee pain that has worsened over the past month. He reports intermittent knee pain for the past 5 years. He denies swelling, warmth, fever, or erythema. There is no history of trauma. The pain worsens with climbing stairs and when standing from a seated position.

   What is the most likely diagnosis?

   A. Ligamentous tear
   B. Patellar fracture
   C. Patellofemoral syndrome
   D. Septic arthritis

3. A 50-year-old woman presents with calf pain and swelling for 1 day. She had a cholecystectomy 3 weeks ago. On examination, she has a swollen left calf with 2+ pitting edema.

   What diagnosis must be urgently excluded?

   A. Baker cyst
   B. Deep venous thrombosis
   C. Muscle strain
   D. Intermittent claudication

References

1. Jackson JL, O'Malley PG, Kroenke K. Evaluation of acute knee pain in primary care. *Ann Intern Med*. 2003;139: 575–588.
2. Solomon DH, Simel D, Bates D, et al. The rational clinical examination. Does this patient have a torn meniscus or ligament of the knee? Value of the physical examination. *JAMA*. 2001;286:1610–1620.
3. Schmieder FA, Comerota AJ. Intermittent claudication: magnitude of the problem, patient evaluation, and therapeutic strategies. *Am J Cardiol*. 2001;87:3D–13D.
4. Fernandez BB Jr. A rational approach to diagnosis and treatment of intermittent claudication. *Am J Med Sci*. 2002;323:244–251.
5. Margaretten ME, Kohlwes J, Moore D, et al. Does this adult patient have septic arthritis? *JAMA*. 2007;297:1478–1488.
6. Wagemakers HPA, Heintjes EM, Boks SS, et al. Diagnostic value of history-taking and physical examination for assessing meniscal tears of the knee in general practice. *Clin J Sport Med*. 2008;18:24–30.
7. Kastelein M, Wagemakers HP, Luijsterburg PA, et al. Assessing medial collateral ligament knee lesions in general practice. *Am J Med*. 2008;121:982–988.
8. Wells PS, Anderson DR, Bormanis J, et al. Value of assessment of pretest probability of deep-vein thrombosis in clinical management. *Lancet*. 1997;350:1795–1798.
9. Oudega R, Moons K, Hoes A. Limited value of patient history and physical examination in diagnosing deep vein thrombosis in primary care. *Fam Pract*. 2005;22:86–91.
10. Goodacre S. In the clinic: deep venous thrombosis. *Ann Intern Med*. 2008;149:ITC3-1.

Suggested Reading

Anderson BC. *Office Orthopedics for Primary Care: Diagnosis and Treatment*. Philadelphia, PA: W.B. Saunders Company, 1999.

Griffin LY. *Essentials of Musculoskeletal Care*. 3rd ed. Rosemont, IL: American Academy of Orthopedic Surgeons, 2005.

Jackson JL. Evaluation of acute knee pain in primary care. *Ann Intern Med*. 2003;139:575–588.

Chapter 57

Foot and Ankle Pain

Deborah L. Cardell, MD, and Jane E. O'Rorke, MD, FACP

CASE SCENARIO

A 63-year-old man comes to clinic with a 2-hour history of ankle pain after stepping off the curb and twisting his ankle.

- **What other aspects of the history will be helpful in determining the etiology of his ankle pain?**

INTRODUCTION

Ankle pain accounts for 20% of musculoskeletal complaints in outpatients.[1] Etiologies of foot and ankle pain include trauma, inflammatory arthritis, sprains, shoe problems, and local manifestations of systemic diseases. The history is critical for determining which diagnoses to consider.

Foot problems are rare among populations that do not wear shoes. Females are 9 times more likely than men to have foot problems. Chronic foot pain (lasting > 2 weeks) is more common than acute foot pain (lasting < 2 weeks).[2]

Between 5 and 10 million ankle injuries occur in the United States each year. Of these injuries, 85% are sprains. Adult age 21 to 30 years old are at greatest risk.

KEY TERMS

Ankle	Joint created by the calcaneus, talus, tibia, and fibula.
Arthritis	Inflammation of the joint characterized by swelling, warmth, redness, pain, and restriction of motion.
Bunion	Bony prominence and abnormal angle of the great toe and first metatarsophalangeal (MTP) joint.
Callus	A hard thick area of skin occurring in parts of the body subject to pressure or friction.[5]
Corn	An area of hard or thickened skin on or between the toes.[5]
Deltoid ligament	A triangular-shaped ligament found on the medial side of the ankle, connecting the tibia to the navicular, calcaneus, and talus.
Eversion	Turning outward of the ankle; the plantar aspect of the foot is directed medially.
Forefoot	Includes toes and the distal aspect of metatarsals.
Hindfoot	Includes the entire heel.
Inversion	Turning inward of the ankle; the plantar aspect of the foot is directed laterally.
Lateral malleolus	Joint created by fibula and talus.
Medial malleolus	Joint created by tibia and talus.
Midfoot	Area between distal metatarsals and beginning of the calcaneus.
Pes cavus	High arched foot.

—Continued next page

Continued—

Pes planus	Flat foot.
Podagra	Gout affecting the first MTP.
Pronation	The act of turning the foot outward so that the lateral margin of the foot is elevated.
Sprain	Injury to a ligament caused by sudden stretching.[5]
Supination	The act of turning the foot inward so that the medial margin is elevated.[5]
Tarsal tunnel	The tunnel formed by the flexor retinaculum.

ETIOLOGY

Foot Pain

In an Italian study of 459 individuals, 21.8% had foot pain with standing, and 9.6% had pain at rest. The most common physical findings included calluses/corns (64.8%), hypertrophic nails (29.6%), hallux deformities (21.2%), and absent arterial pulses (15.9%).[3] The Women's Health and Aging Study reported that 32% of disabled women had moderate to severe foot pain; obesity and osteoarthritis of the hands and feet were more common in these women.[4] Ultimately, determining the etiology of foot pain depends on the location and duration of pain.

Ankle Pain

There are no studies addressing the etiology of ankle pain. Most ankle pain results from injury to the lateral ligaments of the ankle. The location of pain is essential to determining the etiology (Figure 57–1).

Differential Diagnosis (By Location of Pain)

Ankle pain	
Lateral ankle pain	Anterior talofibular ligament (ATFL) sprain is most common; 85% of sprains involve the lateral ligaments.[6] Distal fibular fracture Chronic ankle instability Peroneal tendinitis
Medial ankle pain	Deltoid ligament sprain; 15% of sprains are caused by medial and syndesmosis sprains[6] Posterior tibial tendinitis Tarsal tunnel syndrome Distal tibial fracture
Posterior ankle pain	Achilles tendinitis, Haglund's deformity Achilles tendon rupture Retrocalcaneal bursitis Pre-Achilles bursitis
Chronic ankle pain	Arthritis: rheumatoid arthritis (RA), gout, pseudogout, reactive arthritis

—Continued next page

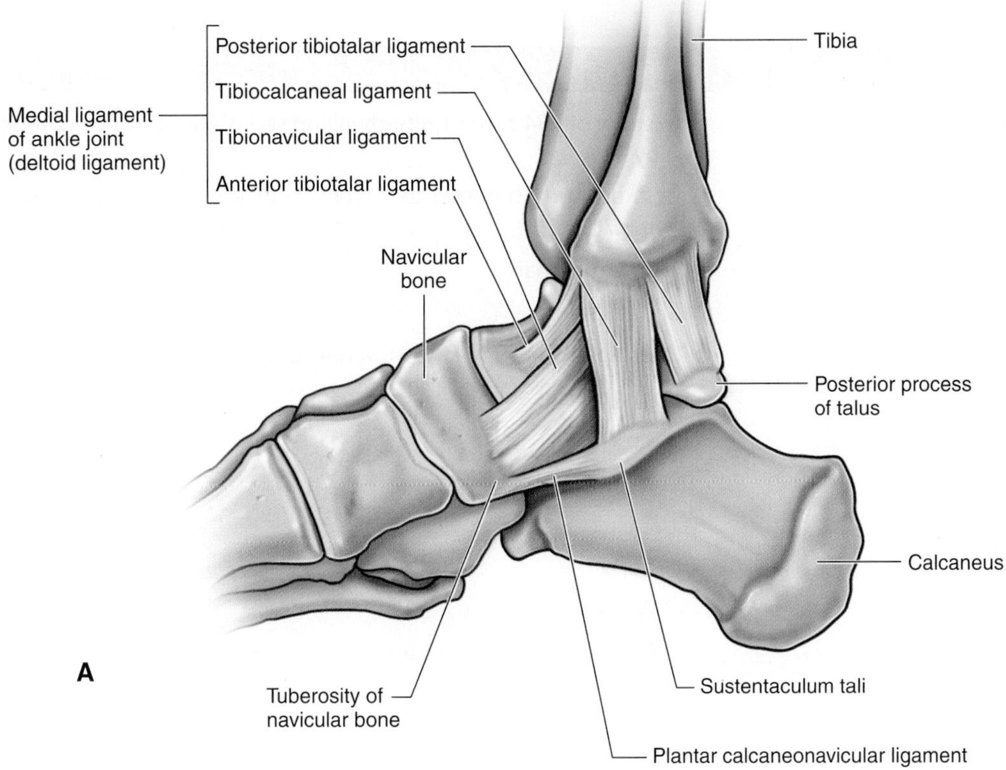

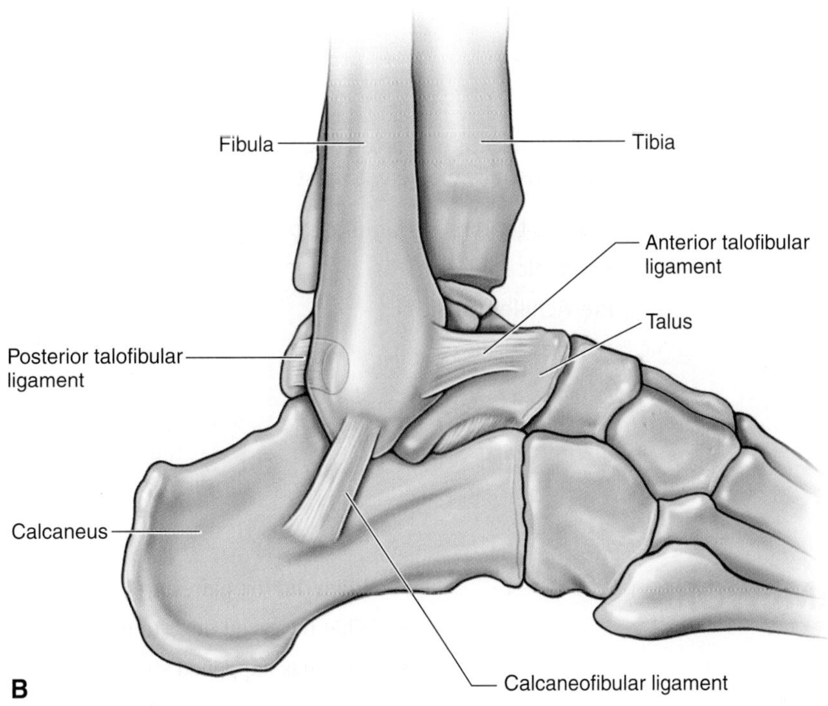

FIGURE 57–1 **(A)** Medial and **(B)** lateral views of the right ankle joint.

Continued—

Foot pain	*Affects 39.5% of adults over age 50[7]*
Forefoot pain	In study of 784 community-dwelling seniors, bunions were reported by 37.4%.[8] In same study, hammer toes were reported in 34.5% and claw toes in 8.7%.[8] Ingrown toenails Metatarsalgia Interdigital neuromas: Morton neuroma Hallux rigidus Sesamoiditis Bunionette Callus Corn Warts Metatarsal stress fracture
Midfoot pain	Osteoarthritis Midfoot plantar fasciitis Plantar fibromas Tarsal tunnel syndrome Pes planus Pes cavus
Hindfoot pain	
Pain at plantar anterior heel or arch	Plantar fasciitis (reported in 6.9% of community-dwelling seniors[8]); pain usually worse with first step in the morning
Posterior heel pain	Achilles tendinitis, Haglund's deformity Retrocalcaneal bursitis Pre-Achilles bursitis Achilles rupture
Plantar heel	Calcaneal fracture
Plantar surface	Plantar warts

INTERVIEW FRAMEWORK

Start with-open ended questions.

- Can you tell me about your pain?
- How did the injury occur?
- When did the pain start?
- What have you done to make it feel better?
- What has happened since it began?

Open-Ended Questions	Tips for Effective Interviewing
Tell me about the problem with your foot or ankle.	Let patients describe the problem in their own words.
Point with one finger to the area that is bothering you the most. Point to where you first felt the pain.	Push patients for exact details concerning initial episode of pain. If recurrent, ask about the first episode.
Describe the first time you felt this pain. What exactly were you doing?	Be firm when asking patients to point with one finger. If entire area hurts, have them point to the spot where initial pain was felt.
Have you ever had this pain before? If so, how was it treated?	

IDENTIFYING ALARM SYMPTOMS

- Patients who have had a joint replacement or have joint hardware are at increased risk of a septic joint (especially if constitutional symptoms are present).

Alarm Symptoms	Serious Causes	Benign Causes
Fever, ulceration, or skin redness (warmth)	Cellulitis Septic arthritis	
History of trauma with inability to bear weight	Fracture	Bone contusion Sprain
Pain on weight bearing, swelling after a recent increase in activity	Stress fracture	Plantar fasciitis
Persistent rolling in or out of the foot	Ligamentous instability Posterior tibial dysfunction	Weakness of the muscles supporting the ankle
Pain on the medial aspect of the ankle anterior to the medial malleolus	Deltoid ligament sprain	Trauma without ankle instability
Pain in the lower anterior portion of the leg just above the ankle	High ankle (syndesmotic) sprain	Strain without ankle instability
Inability to walk 4 steps immediately after injury or during initial evaluation	Ankle fracture	Simple sprain
Numbness, weakness in the foot	Fracture with compromise of a nerve	
Feeling of being shot or kicked in the back of the ankle, sometimes with an audible pop	Achilles tendon rupture	Contusion of the Achilles tendon

FOCUSED QUESTIONS

- Follow format for attributes of a symptom.
  - Where does it hurt? (Determining location helps narrow the differential diagnosis.)
  - What does the pain feel like (ie, burning, sharp)?
  - How severe is the pain? Can you rate the pain on a scale of 0 to 10? What is the pain like at different times during the day or with different activities?
  - Did the pain develop quickly over hours or insidiously (over weeks or months)? Is it intermittent or constant?
  - What aggravates the pain?
  - What relieves the pain (eg, over-the-counter medications, prescription medications, alternative and complementary medicines or therapies, positions)?
  - Do you have any associated symptoms such as swelling, stiffness, or fever?
- Occupational and sports history may give a clue to the etiology.
  - What type of work do you do now? What work have you done in the past?
  - What sports do you play? What have you played in the past?
- Functional limitations are important in assessing severity of pain.
  - What activities can you not do now that you could do before developing the pain?
  - Are there any activities you have stopped due to the pain?
  - Are you able to do your activities of daily living, such as dressing, bathing, and shopping?

QUESTIONS	THINK ABOUT...
Foot	
Are you having problems wearing your shoes?	Foot deformities, including ganglion cysts and plantar fibromas
Do your shoes rub on your big toe?	Bunions
Is there rubbing on any other toes?	Adventitial bursitis of the first MTP joint Hammer toes, corns
Does the weight of a sheet cause pain in your toe?	Gout
Are any of your toes numb?	Morton neuroma, diabetic neuropathy
Is there pain between your toes?	Corn
Do tight shoes make your toes tingle?	Tarsal tunnel
Do you have diabetes mellitus?	Diabetic foot Charcot foot
Do you have pain at night?	Diabetic foot Charcot foot
Do you have burning?	Diabetic foot Charcot foot
Do you have tingling?	Diabetic foot Charcot foot
Do you have progressive deformity?	Diabetic foot Charcot foot
Is the pain in your heel at its worst when you first step on it?	Plantar fasciitis
Does the pain improve with non–weight bearing?	Fracture
Do you have tingling and burning along the bottom of your foot?	Tarsal tunnel syndrome

Ankle	
Was there any twisting or rotation of the ankle? Did you land on the side of your foot?	Ankle sprain Fracture
Do have any lumps on the back of your heel?	Pre-Achilles bursitis
Does the back of your ankle hurt when climbing stairs?	Retrocalcaneal bursitis
Is there swelling around the back of your ankle? Are your shoes rubbing the inside of your ankle?	Posterior tibialis tenosynovitis
Have you played sports in your lifetime? Any history of dance?	Ankle instability Osteoarthritis
Have you had any past injuries to your ankle?	Chronic ankle instability, arthritis

DIAGNOSTIC APPROACH (INCLUDING ALGORITHMS)

The diagnostic approach algorithms for foot pain and ankle pain are shown in Figures 57–2 and 57–3, respectively.

CAVEATS

- Even if a patient reports acute pain, ask about previous episodes because they may indicate a more chronic intermittent process.
- Encourage the patient to commit to the location of pain with one finger.
- When asking about medications used to treat the pain, determine the exact dose and frequency. Patients may report that a medication is not effective when they were not taking a therapeutic dose or not allowing sufficient time for it to work.
- Patients will occasionally have foot or ankle trauma but not recognize it as such, for instance with dancing. Therefore, determine exactly what the patient was doing at the time the pain started.
- Remember to perform a thorough occupational and sports history.
- Ankle arthritis may cause pain in any part of the ankle.
- Posterior heel bursitis can cause either ankle or heel pain.

PROGNOSIS

Most foot and ankle disorders can be diagnosed with a thorough history and physical examination. Although musculoskeletal problems often take weeks to months to resolve, many will improve with conservative therapy.

CASE SCENARIO | Resolution

A 63-year-old man comes to clinic with a 2-hour history of ankle pain after stepping off the curb and twisting his ankle. What other aspects of the history will be helpful in determining the etiology of his ankle pain?

ADDITIONAL HISTORY

As he stepped off of the curb, the patient recalls inverting the ankle but denies hearing a pop. After sitting for 5 minutes, he was able to walk with a limp. He has never previously injured his ankle. He works as a salesman and has never played sports. The pain is worse on the lateral surface of his ankle. It is worse when he walks and better when he sits down.

Question: What is the most likely diagnosis?

A. Deltoid ligament sprain
B. Lateral ligament sprain
C. Plantar fasciitis
D. Bunion

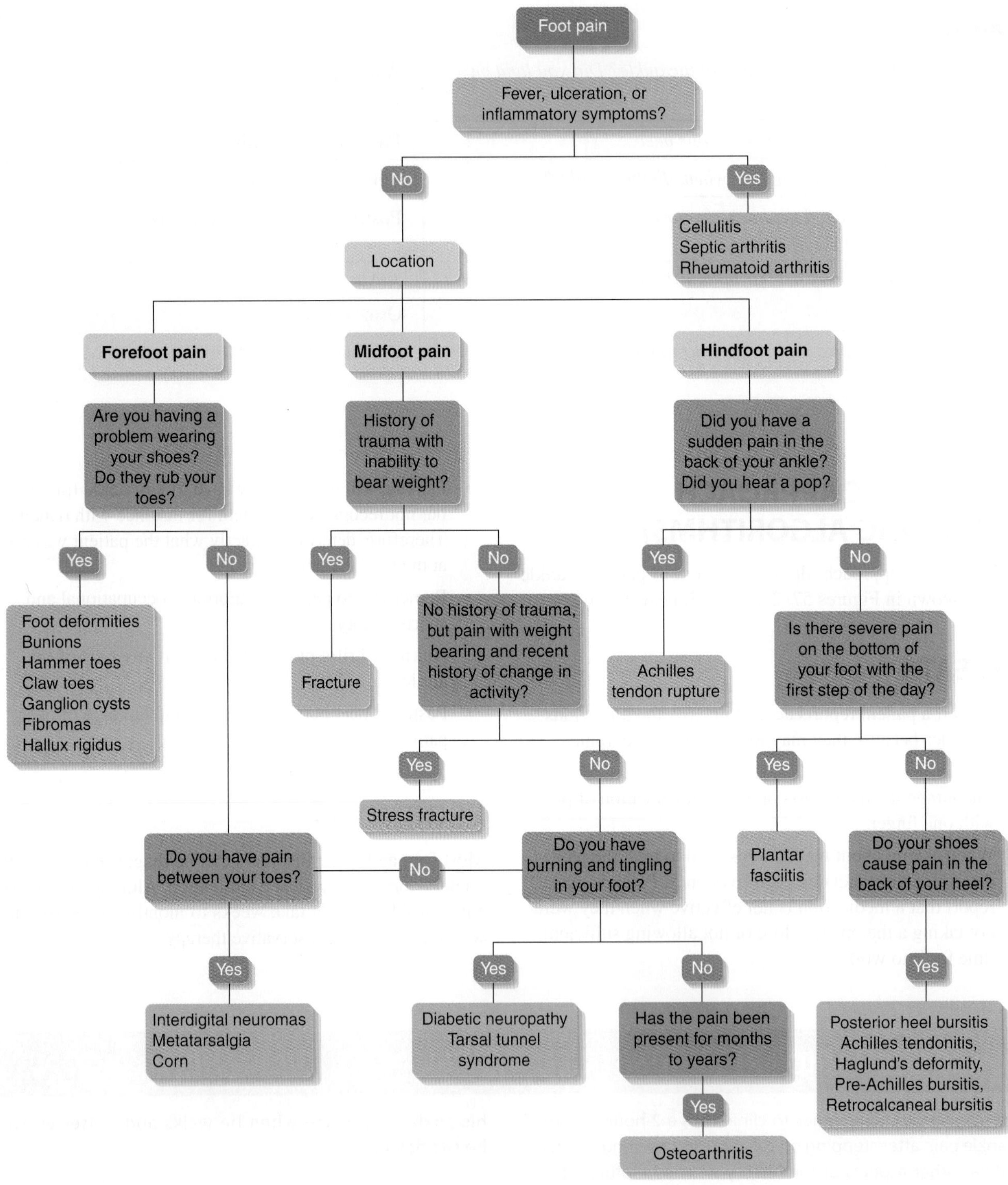

FIGURE 57–2 Diagnostic approach: Foot pain.

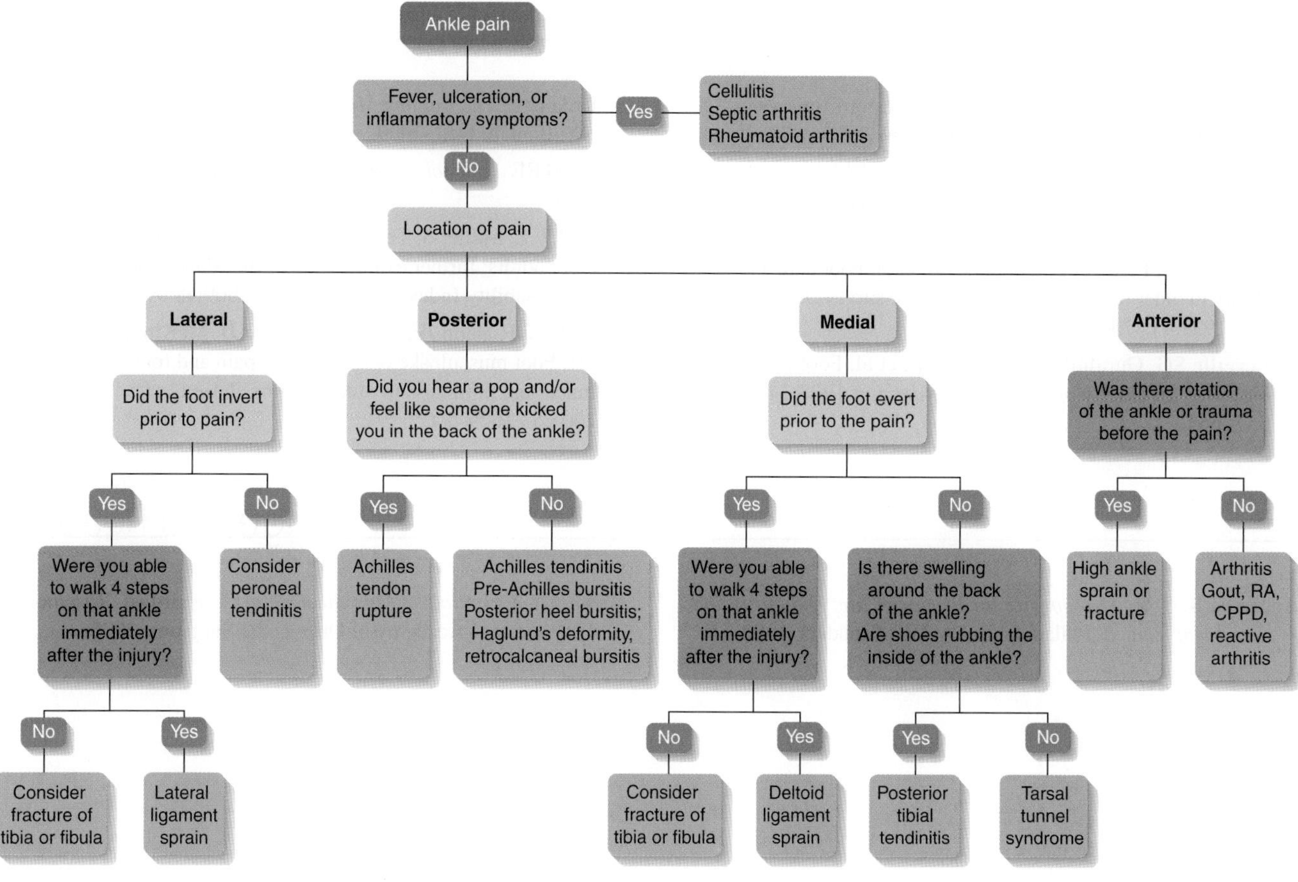

FIGURE 57–3 Diagnostic approach: Ankle pain. CPPD, calcium pyrophosphate deposition disease; RA, rheumatoid arthritis.

Test Your Knowledge

1. A 69-year-old woman comes to see you for worsening ankle pain. She underwent an open reduction, internal fixation with hardware insertion for a right ankle fracture 3 weeks earlier and reports the ankle has become increasingly red, warm, and swollen. This morning, she developed a temperature of 102°F.
   What is the most important diagnosis that must be considered?
   A. Ligamentous strain
   B. Osteoarthritis
   C. Plantar fasciitis
   D. Septic arthritis

2. A 32-year-old man comes to the office complaining of heel pain. He does not recall injuring himself or stepping on anything. The pain is greatest in the morning when he first gets out of bed and is most intense at the medial plantar edge of his heel. He is not an athlete.
   What is the most likely diagnosis?
   A. Bunion
   B. Calcaneal fracture
   C. Callus
   D. Plantar fasciitis

3. A 45-year-old man presents with 2 days of intense pain in his first metatarsophalangeal (MTP) joint. The pain began suddenly, without any previous trauma. He has never played sports. His toe feels hot and very tender to touch. He mentions that he cannot even sleep with the sheets on his foot.
   What is the most likely diagnosis?
   A. Bunion
   B. Gout
   C. Osteoarthritis
   D. Plantar warts

References

1. Watters DAK, Brooks S, Elton RA, et al. Sports injuries in an accident and emergency department. *Arch Emerg Med.* 1984;2:105–111.
2. Balint GP. Foot and ankle disorders. *Best Pract Res Clin Rheumatol.* 2003:87–111.
3. Benvenuti F, Ferrucci L, Guralnik JM, et al. Foot pain and disability in older persons: an epidemiologic survey. *J Am Geriatr Soc.* 1995;43:479–484.
4. Leveille SG, Guralnik JM, Ferrucci L, et al. Foot pain and disability in older women. *Am J Epidemiol.* 1998;148:657–665.
5. Urdang L. *The Bantam Medical Dictionary*. 6th ed. New York, NY: Bantam Dell, 2009.
6. Rakel RE. *Textbook of Family Medicine*. 7th ed. Philadelphia, PA: 2007.
7. Roddy E, Muller S, Thomas E. Defining disability foot pain in older adults: further examination of the Manchester Foot Pain and Disability Index. *Rheumatology*. 2009;48:992–996.
8. Badlissi F, Dunn JE, Link CL, Keysor JJ, McKinlay JB, Felson DT. Foot musculoskeletal disorders, pain and foot-related functional limitation in older persons. *J Am Geriatr Soc.* 2005;53:1029–1033.

Suggested Reading

Anderson B. *Office Orthopedics for Primary Care: Diagnosis and Treatment*. 2nd ed. Philadelphia, PA: WB Saunders, 1999.

Griffin LY. *Essentials of Musculoskeletal Care*. 3rd ed. Rosemont, IL: American Academy of Orthopedic Surgeons, 2005.

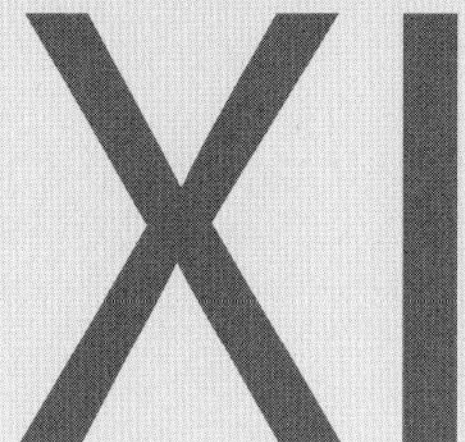

XI NEUROLOGY

Chapter 58

Confusion

Daniel Press, MD, and Michael Ronthal, MD

CASE SCENARIO

A 70-year-old man lives with his daughter. She is awakened one night and finds him wandering in the kitchen with the pots in disarray. He cannot explain clearly what he is doing, and she is worried because this is a dramatic change for him. She takes him to see you for immediate evaluation.

- **What additional questions can you ask to determine the cause of his change in mental status?**
- **What are the possible causes for the quick onset of confusion?**
- **What life-threatening conditions need to be considered immediately?**
- **How can you use the patient history to determine whether this is occurring in the setting of previously normal cognitive function versus underlying cognitive impairment?**

INTRODUCTION

Confusion is an impairment in attention and is characterized by an inability to maintain a coherent stream of thought or action. An "acute confusional state" is a prolonged period of confusion and is synonymous with "delirium." An acute confusional state is usually of abrupt onset, and the mental status fluctuates from alert and hypervigilant to obtunded. An altered level of consciousness is common and can be the predecessor of stupor and coma if the underlying cause is not found and reversed. Confusion presents a unique challenge in acquiring a direct patient history because the patient is inattentive and distractible. In a confusional state, the organ system that is required to report on symptoms (the central nervous system [CNS]) is itself dysfunctional. For that reason, most of the historical information must be acquired from caregivers and family members. Although this poses an extra level of challenge in acquiring accurate historical information, the history is often crucial in determining the correct diagnosis.

Dementia is a chronic, progressive loss of cognitive function that impairs day-to-day abilities and predisposes to confusion if the brain is challenged with even a relatively minor toxic or metabolic disturbance. A major diagnostic challenge is to determine whether the altered mental status is due solely to an acute condition or whether an underlying dementia is acting as a predisposing factor.[1] The diagnosis of delirium is missed in up to 40% to 60%[2] of those affected and is a sign of a worse prognosis with higher hospital readmission rates and 30-day mortality, especially if untreated. Confusion may be seen in up to 20% of elderly patients admitted to hospital, and of those admitted not confused, 25% to 50% will develop an episode of confusion during the admission. Regardless of cause, delirium confers a worse prognosis with higher hospital readmission rates and 30-day mortality, especially if untreated.[3] The causes of delirium differ greatly depending on the setting (ie, hospital versus nonhospital setting).

KEY TERMS

Delirium/acute confusional state/ diffuse encephalopathy	Synonymous terms for an acute impairment in attention or disorganized thinking, with a fluctuating course and altered level of consciousness.
Dementia	Chronic progressive degenerative condition affecting memory, behavior, and cognition.

—Continued next page

Continued—	
Attention	The ability to focus on specific stimuli and change from one stimulus to another when salient.
Alertness	The level of arousal or responsiveness to external cues.
Coherence	The ability to maintain selective attention over time.
Asterixis	Failure to maintain continuous voluntary tone in the limbs resulting in very brief loss of strength.
Meningismus	Neck stiffness and pain on neck flexion and extension, a sign of meningitis.

ETIOLOGY

The causes of confusion differ depending on whether it develops in people residing in the community or in those already hospitalized for a medical illness. Confusion in hospitalized patients generally occurs in those with predisposing risk factors.[4] Although a severe insult can cause confusion even in patients at low vulnerability, only a relatively mild insult can trigger it in patients with multiple risk factors (see Differential Diagnosis box). The list of potential causes of confusion in the community can be divided into 3 categories: (1) primary insults to the CNS (such as seizures, stroke, or meningitis), (2) systemic metabolic conditions impairing CNS function (organ failure) resulting in the production of endogenous toxins, and (3) exogenous toxins such as systemic infections, medications, or drugs.

Risk Factors for Confusion in Hospitalized Patients (Inouye and Charpentier, 1996)

Risk Factor	Relative Risk
Use of physical restraints	4.4 (2.5-7.9)
Malnutrition	4.0 (2.2-7.4)
>3 Medications added	2.9 (1.6-5.4)
Use of bladder catheter	2.4 (1.2-4.7)
Any iatrogenic event	1.9 (1.1-3.2)

Differential Diagnosis[a]

	Prevalence[b]
Primary CNS causes	***35%***
Meningitis/encephalitis	
Stroke (primarily right hemisphere, either frontal, parietal, or occipital lobes)	
Seizures (postictal state or partial seizures)	
Head trauma	
Secondary CNS causes	***60%***
Infections, especially urinary tract infection (UTI), pneumonia, or sepsis	5%
Hypoxia	25%
Hypoperfusion (eg, congestive heart failure, shock)	5%
Hypoglycemia	5%
Renal failure	5%
Hepatic failure	
Toxins (carbon monoxide, heavy metals)	

Medications	5%
Alcohol (intoxication or withdrawal)	3%
Narcotic analgesics	
Opiates	
Amphetamines	
Anticholinergic drugs (especially diphenhydramine)	
Drug withdrawal syndromes	

[a]Causes of delirium among elderly patients presenting to emergency department.[2]
[b]Prevalence is unknown when not indicated.

GETTING STARTED WITH THE HISTORY

- The patient is unlikely to be able to convey much information, but one should ask focused questions; inquire about headache, recent drug use, and fevers.
- Make every effort to contact a caregiver if none is present with the patient. The task may require some detective work, but it is crucial.
- Always determine the patient's current medications and whether any have changed. This may require calls to the patient's pharmacy or requests to have the family bring in all the medication bottles.
- In young patients, consider both the acute effects of drugs of abuse and withdrawal states.

INTERVIEW FRAMEWORK

The goal is to determine both the acute cause of the confusion and the presence of any baseline risk factors (such as dementia or malnutrition).

- Inquire about timing of the episode.
    - Previous episodes
    - Suddenness of onset
    - Any baseline cognitive impairment
    - Any history of seizures
- Inquire about associated symptoms.
    - Fever
    - Shortness of breath
    - Headache
    - Abnormal motor activity
- Inquire about drug usage.
    - Any recent change in drug regimen
    - Use of drugs of abuse or pain medications
    - Recent drug withdrawal

IDENTIFYING ALARM SYMPTOMS

Delirium usually reflects serious CNS dysfunction, especially if the onset has been acute. Delirium is a common presentation of life-threatening conditions, including subarachnoid hemorrhage, meningitis, and increased intracranial pressure due to a mass lesion. A number of investigations are often necessary to determine the cause; certain symptoms will suggest which tests should be done first.

Serious Diagnoses

Alarm Symptoms	Serious Causes	Benign Causes
Fever or hypothermia	Meningitis Sepsis	UTI Upper respiratory tract infection (URI)
Abnormal motor activity or history of epilepsy	Seizures (status epilepticus) or postictal state	Myoclonus or asterixis from metabolic disturbance
Headache	Stroke Meningitis Mass lesion/trauma	Migraine and confusion due to excessive pain medication
Shortness of breath	Hypoxia (congestive heart failure, pneumonia)	URI
Diaphoresis, tremors	Hypoglycemia	Fever
Neglect (inattention to one side of space) or visual field loss	Stroke	Glaucoma Macular degeneration
Ataxia, nystagmus	Wernicke encephalopathy	Alcohol or drug intoxication

FOCUSED QUESTIONS

After hearing the story in the words of the patient and caregiver and considering possible alarm symptoms, the following questions help to narrow down the diagnostic possibilities.

QUESTIONS*	THINK ABOUT...
Do you have:	
• *History of seizures?*	Postictal state
	Nonconvulsive status epilepticus
• *Pain on urination or recent urinary catheter?*	UTI
	Urosepsis
• *Shortness of breath?*	Congestive heart failure
	Pneumonia
	Pulmonary embolism in postoperative patient
• *History of insulin-requiring diabetes?*	Hypoglycemia
• *History of liver problems?*	Hepatic encephalopathy
• *Headache?*	Meningitis
	Stroke
	Subarachnoid or subdural hemorrhage
Have you recently used sleep medications?	Anticholinergic or sedative toxicity
Have you fallen recently?	Unwitnessed head trauma
Have you experienced memory problems previously?	Underlying dementia
Quality	
Is the confusion primarily a memory problem?	Dementia
Does the patient have poor attention, especially with fluctuations?	Delirium
Time course	
Is the onset:	
• *Sudden (over seconds)?*	Seizure
	Stroke
	Subarachnoid hemorrhage
• *Over minutes to hours?*	Drug-induced
	Hypoxia
	Hypoglycemia
• *Over hours to days?*	Infection
	Renal failure
	Hepatic failure
• *Gradual progression over months?*	Dementia

Associated symptoms	
Do you have:	
• *Altered level of consciousness?*	Delirium of any cause
• *Hypervigilance?*	Drug or alcohol withdrawal
	Wernicke encephalopathy
• *Shortness of breath?*	Congestive heart failure
	Myocardial infarction
	Pulmonary embolism
• *Headache?*	Subarachnoid hemorrhage
	Mass lesion
	Meningitis
• *Blurred vision? (monocular)*	Cavernous sinus disease
	Pituitary apoplexy
• *Blurred vision? (binocular)*	Parietal or occipital lobe stroke or mass lesion
	Hypertensive encephalopathy
• *Stiff neck?*	Meningitis (bacterial, viral, neoplastic, or aseptic)
• *Vertigo?*	Cerebellar or brainstem lesion
• *Jaundice?*	Hepatic encephalopathy
• *Dysuria or anuria?*	UTI
	Pyelonephritis
	Uremic encephalopathy
Modifying factors	
Are symptoms worse at nighttime?	"Sundowning" (may be due to delirium or underlying dementia)
Is there rapid improvement over seconds?	Postsyncope (see Chapter 29)
Is there improvement over minutes to hours?	Postictal state
Are symptoms worse when standing?	Hypoperfusion
Is there a history of seizures?	Nonconvulsive status epilepticus

[*]Ask both patient and caregiver.

DIAGNOSTIC APPROACH (INCLUDING ALGORITHM)

The diagnostic approach to confusion depends on 3 factors:

- Temporal course
- Presence of focal neurologic symptoms
- Age of the patient

An acute onset over hours to days suggests delirium, whereas a gradual onset of cognitive dysfunction over months suggests underlying dementia. If the onset is acute, rapidly search for an underlying reversible cause that may be life threatening without treatment. Focal symptoms (visual changes, headache, focal weakness, or numbness) suggest a primary CNS process. The central causes include CNS infections (meningitis, abscess), strokes (ischemic or hemorrhagic), mass lesions (tumors), or seizures (with postictal state). If delirium develops without focal signs or symptoms, the patient's age may help determine the likely cause.

In younger patients without a focal CNS cause, consider drug use or withdrawal, unwitnessed head trauma, and unwitnessed seizures. When delirium develops in the elderly, likely causes include systemic infections (UTI, pneumonia), drugs (especially opiates and anticholinergic medications), hypoxia, hypoperfusion, and metabolic disturbances (renal failure, hepatic failure). In hospitalized patients, questions should focus both on the cause of the delirium and predisposing risk factors (see Focused Questions).

A number of concomitant medical conditions bring up special concerns.

- **Epilepsy:** Confusion is most often due to a postictal state, but a sudden worsening in confusion or fluctuating course suggests ongoing seizures or nonconvulsive status epilepticus.
- **Diabetes:** Both hypoglycemia and hyperglycemia (with either acidosis or a hyperosmolar state) can lead to confusion. In patients with diabetes, confusion can also develop from either cerebral ischemia (stroke) or coronary ischemia (myocardial infarction).
- **Hepatic cirrhosis:** Confusion can be a sign of worsening cirrhosis but may also herald upper gastrointestinal bleeding from varices (causing cerebral hypoperfusion or hepatic encephalopathy). Drug-induced delirium is also more common in patients with cirrhosis due to impaired hepatic metabolism.
- **Parkinson's disease:** In addition to the usual causes in the elderly, anticholinergic drugs and dopamine agonists can cause confusion.

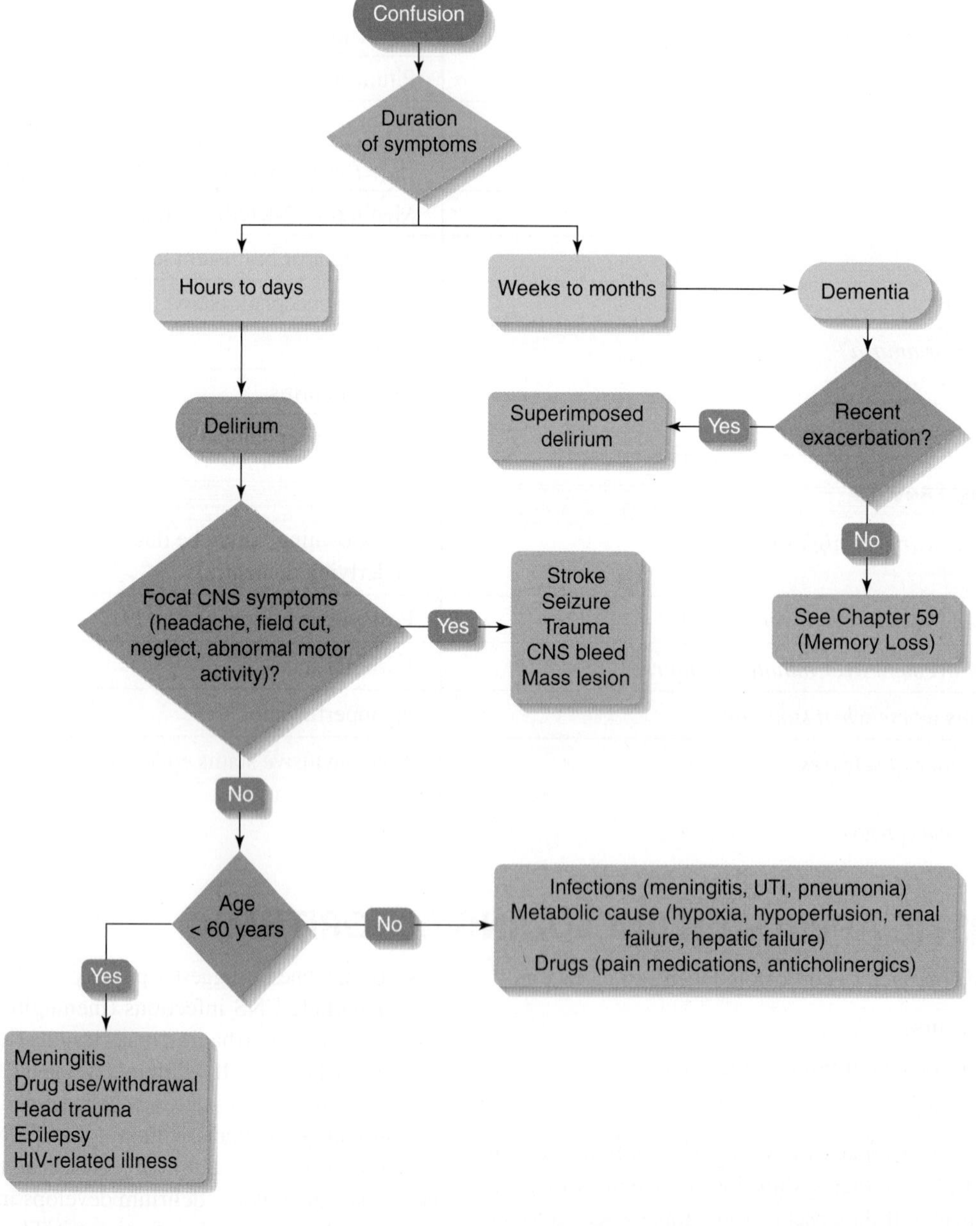

FIGURE 58–1 Diagnostic approach: Confusion. CNS, central nervous system; HIV, human immunodeficiency virus; UTI, urinary tract infection.

- **Cancer:** Cancer may cause confusion via direct cerebral mechanisms (metastases, carcinomatous meningitis), indirect mechanisms (drug effects, paraneoplastic states), and systemic mechanisms (hypercalcemia, hyponatremia, hepatic encephalopathy due to liver metastases, uremic encephalopathy due to obstructive uropathy).
- **Human immunodeficiency virus (HIV)/acquired immunodeficiency syndrome (AIDS):** HIV can predispose to confusion through CNS infections (toxoplasmosis, cryptococcal meningitis, progressive multifocal leukoencephalopathy) as well as directly (HIV dementia). Complicated treatment regimens with large numbers of medications can also predispose to confusion.
- **Postoperative patients:** If confusion is present immediately upon awakening from surgery, consider an intraoperative event (eg, global hypoxia/hypoperfusion or a focal stroke). In days 1 to 3 after surgery, consider hypoxia (from pneumonia or a pulmonary embolism) and drug withdrawal in addition to other causes of confusion in hospitalized patients.

Figure 58–1 shows the diagnostic approach algorithm for confusion.

CAVEATS

- The confused patient's ability to communicate and provide useful history can fluctuate markedly. Be sure to obtain ancillary information from other caregivers, and when in doubt, evaluate the patient at different times.
- Do not assume that confusion has been longstanding in a patient who appears "demented." Err on the side of assuming there is a treatable delirium present, even in patients with chronic cognitive deficits.
- Delirium and dementia often coexist. Determining whether an underlying dementia is present is challenging in the setting of a delirium. Appropriate testing and interventions should be planned after the causes of the confusion have been treated.

PROGNOSIS

Some symptoms of delirium can persist for 6 months or longer in up to 80% of patients.[5] Those persons in whom delirium develops during a hospital stay are much more likely to require long-term institutional care; 43% reside in an institution at 6 months. The 1-month mortality for hospitalized patients with delirium is approximately 14% and is significantly higher than controls even when accounting for comorbid conditions.[6] Mortality for those with delirium is 39% at 1 year, roughly twice the likelihood compared with age-matched controls.[4] Although delirium is frequently completely reversible, it is often the harbinger of more serious and chronic cognitive deficits. In those with an underlying dementia, delirium heralds a more rapidly progressive course.

CASE SCENARIO | Resolution

A 70-year-old man lives with his daughter. She is awakened one night and finds him wandering in the kitchen with the pots in disarray. He cannot explain clearly what he is doing, and she is worried because this is a dramatic change for him. She takes him to see you for immediate evaluation.

ADDITIONAL HISTORY

On focused questioning, the daughter reports that the patient has fallen occasionally over the last few weeks. He has been more confused over the last few days and has had a few episodes of urinary incontinence. Although he has had some memory problems for a year or 2, he has been unable to dress himself or to tend to hygiene only in the last few days. He has also had some headaches over the last few days. He has not had any fever or any change in medications.

Question: What is the most likely diagnosis?

A. Meningitis
B. Subdural hematoma from trauma
C. Unwitnessed seizure with postictal confusion
D. Stroke

Test Your Knowledge

1. An 80-year-old man is brought to see you for the sudden onset of confusion earlier today. On questioning, the caregiver mentions that he has had some memory symptoms for a number of months but that "this is different." He has had some difficulty sleeping, and the caregiver thinks he might have taken medication for this. The caregiver has not noticed any weakness or jerking movements but is unsure as to whether he has had a fever.

   Which of the following features, if present, would be an alarm symptom in him?

   A. Disorientation to the location or time
   B. Having word-finding trouble and making up new words
   C. Having pain with neck movement
   D. Having periodic jerking movements in the arms and legs

2. A 25-year-old woman is found wandering in the street, confused and unable to answer questions. Her roommate reports that for the last 2 or 3 days, she has become progressively more confused. She has had some fever and has had 2 or 3 episodes where she seemed to "blank out" for about a minute.

   Which of the following symptoms would be most concerning for meningitis or encephalitis?

   A. Blurred vision
   B. Fever
   C. Neglect of the left side of space
   D. A history of seizures

References

1. Rahkonen TR, Luukkainen-Markkula R, Paanila S, et al. Delirium episode as a sign of undetected dementia among community dwelling elderly subjects: a 2 year follow up study. *J Neurol Neurosurg Psychiatry.* 2000;69:519–521.
2. Lewis LM, Miller D, Morley JE, et al. Unrecognized delirium in ED geriatric patients. *Am J Emerg Med.* 1995;13:142–145.
3. Francis J, Kapoor WN. Prognosis after hospital discharge of older medical patients with delirium. *J Am Geriatr Soc.* 1992;40:601–606.
4. Inouye SK, Charpentier PA. Precipitating factors for delirium in hospitalized elderly persons. Predictive model and interrelationship with baseline vulnerability. *JAMA.* 1996;275:852–857.
5. Francis J, Martin D, Kapoor WN. A prospective study of delirium in hospitalized elderly. *JAMA.* 1990;263:1097–1101.
6. Cole MG, Primeau FJ. Prognosis of delirium in elderly hospital patients. *CMAJ.* 1993;149:41–46.

Suggested Reading

Amador LF, Goodwin JS. Postoperative delirium in the older patient. *J Am Coll Surg.* 2005;200:767–773.

Brown TM, Boyle MF. Delirium. *BMJ.* 2002;325:644–647.

Edlund A, Lundstrom M, Karlsson S, et al. Delirium in older patients admitted to general internal medicine. *J Geriatr Psychiatry Neurol.* 2006;19:83–90.

Francis J, Young GB. Diagnosis of delirium and confusional states. 2010. UpToDate. B. Rose. Wellesley, MA. Available at: http://www.uptodate.com. Accessed November 5, 2011.

Holroyd-Leduc JM, Khandwala F, Sink KM. How can delirium best be prevented and managed in older patients in the hospital? *CMAJ.* 2010;182:465–470.

Inouye SK. Delirium in older persons. *N Engl J Med.* 2006;354:1157–1165.

Young J, Murthy L, Westby M, et al. Diagnosis, prevention, and management of delirium: summary of NICE guidance. *BMJ.* 2010;341:c3704.

Chapter 59

Memory Loss

Calvin H. Hirsch, MD

CASE SCENARIO

A 74-year-old retired auto mechanic presents to clinic with his wife and daughter, who are concerned about his behavior. The patient has become more irritable and spends most of his days watching television instead of going out to his shop to tinker with old lawnmowers, which he used to fix and sell. He has also begun accusing his wife and daughter of stealing or hiding his wallet and keys, which his wife eventually finds somewhere in the house. He still drives the car downtown, but the wife admits not liking to drive with him because he gets angry when she tells him he has taken a wrong turn. When you ask about the patient's memory, his daughter states that it still seems "good, because he can remember events from a long time ago as if they were yesterday." The patient agrees: "I think I remember as well as you'd expect for a person my age."

- **What additional questions should you ask to better understand the patient's behavioral changes?**
- **What additional medical, social, and family history would be important to obtain?**
- **Does the report of good long-term memory preclude the diagnosis of dementia?**
- **What is the relationship between mood change and memory loss?**

INTRODUCTION

Although recall and the speed of cognitive processing decline slightly with normal aging,[1] substantial memory loss is abnormal and reflects underlying pathology. While memory loss characteristically is the most prominent feature of early dementia, impairment in other domains of cognitive function, personality changes, or behavioral disturbances may be the earliest symptoms noted by observers. The prevalence of dementia roughly doubles every 5 years after the age of 60, rising from 1% at age 60 to 25% to 30% at age 85.[2] Nearly two-thirds of patients age 75 and older with dementia will have Alzheimer's disease.

KEY TERMS

Term	Synonyms	Definition
Dementia	Obsolete: senility, organic brain syndrome	A decline from a previous state of mental functioning that interferes with social or occupational activities. Dementia involves memory plus at least one of the following: (1) aphasia (language impairment); (2) impairment in executive function (eg, organizing, abstracting, judgment); (3) apraxia (impaired ability to carry out familiar motor tasks despite intact motor function); and (4) agnosia (inability to identify familiar objects or substances despite intact sensation, such as failure to recognize the smell of coffee grounds).
Mild cognitive impairment (MCI)	Cognitive impairment—no dementia	A decline from a previous state of mental functioning that causes no or minimal interference with daily activities. MCI is considered a transitional state between normal, age-associated memory impairment and dementia. Multiple definitions exist. It is most commonly classified as amnestic (subjective or objective evidence of memory impairment) or nonamnestic (memory sparing). Amnestic and nonamnestic MCI are further subclassified as involving single or multiple cognitive domains.[3]

—Continued next page

Continued—		
Delirium	Acute confusional state	A state of global cognitive impairment with an acute onset, fluctuating course, short-term memory dysfunction, inattention, and disorganized thinking or altered level of consciousness. Psychosis is common.

ETIOLOGY

The accuracy and reliability of the diagnostic criteria for dementia vary, depending on the type of dementia. For Alzheimer's disease, the National Institute of Neurologic and Communicative Disorders and Stroke/Alzheimer's Disease and Related Disorders Association (NINCDS/ADRDA) criteria[4] enable expert clinicians to make an accurate diagnosis about 85% of the time. The several commonly used criteria for vascular dementia show accuracy in the range of 60% to 70%.

Major Causes of Memory Loss

Type	Prevalence in Persons Over Age 65[a,b]	Relative Distribution[b]	Definition
MCI	2%–9% (> age 75)		See Key Terms box. Depending on the definition used, between 5% and 16% per year will progress to dementia.[5]
Alzheimer's disease	4.4%	45%–54%	Dementia that has an insidious onset and progresses steadily in the absence of focal neurologic signs or other identifiable causes. Autopsy reveals characteristic cortical degeneration with amyloid plaques and neurofibrillary tangles.
Vascular dementia	1.6%	12%–24%	Dementia temporally related to a stroke or due to chronic cerebral ischemia. Classically, the dementia progresses in a stepwise manner, but it may be steadily progressive. It may be difficult to distinguish from Alzheimer's disease. In the early stages, subcortical signs (eg, depression, subtle gait disturbances) and language difficulties often outweigh memory impairment, in contrast to early Alzheimer's disease, in which memory loss typically predominates.
Mixed dementia		22%–28%	The coexistence of Alzheimer's disease and vascular dementia.

Parkinson's disease	1%	NA	Dementia occurs in about 30% of Parkinson's disease patients as a late manifestation of the disease. Two very rare extrapyramidal disorders, corticobasal degeneration (CBD) and progressive supranuclear palsy (PSP), cause parkinsonism together with other neurologic abnormalities. Dementia occurs very early in CBD and in the middle stages of PSP.
Diffuse Lewy body disease (DLBD)	NA	5%	The **early** coexistence of dementia and Parkinson's disease. Unlike Parkinson's disease, the dementia of DLBD either precedes or occurs within 12 months of the onset of extrapyramidal symptoms. The cognitive impairment often fluctuates, and psychiatric symptoms (commonly visual hallucinations) occur early in the course of the illness.
Frontotemporal dementia	NA	4%	A progressive dementia in which personality changes (eg, apathy, self-neglect, perseveration, hyperorality) and speech impairment typically exceed memory loss during the early stages.[6]

NA, not applicable.

[a]In persons over age 60, unless otherwise specified.

[b]Prevalence or distribution is not available when not indicated.

GETTING STARTED WITH THE HISTORY

Screening

Clinicians often fail to detect early dementia, in part because patients commonly deny having memory or other cognitive deficits and in part because well-preserved social skills may conceal these deficits. In the absence of a complaint of memory loss, it is reasonable to screen patients for cognitive impairment approximately every 3 years from age 75 to 81, and then every other year thereafter. The most widely used screening instrument is the Folstein Mini-Mental State Examination (MMSE).[7] However, the MMSE does not cover executive function (reasoning, judgment, organization, and planning) and is insensitive to very early impairment. A time-efficient alternative to the MMSE, but possessing comparable sensitivity and specificity, is the Mini-Cog.[8] It consists of recall of 3 unrelated objects (eg, baseball, penny, chair) at 3 minutes and the drawing of a clock, involving inserting all the numbers and setting the hands to the requested time (Figure 59–1). Clock drawing tests both visuospatial skills and aspects of executive function. Cognitive impairment is suggested if the patient fails to recall 2 of the 3 items or draws an abnormal clock. The Montreal Cognitive Assessment (MoCA),[9] available free on the Internet,[10] tests executive function and has a more extensive memory battery than the MMSE, making it more suitable as a screen for MCI and early dementia, especially when paired with history from a family member or knowledgeable informant. An instrument like the Informant Questionnaire for Cognitive Decline in the Elderly (IQCODE)[11] gathers this information systematically, and can improve diagnostic sensitivity for dementia.

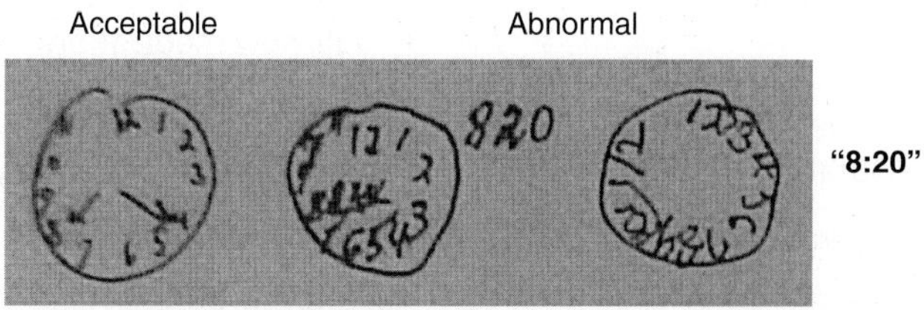

FIGURE 59–1 Clock drawing test showing acceptable and abnormal results.

Questions[a]	Remember
Do you sometimes have trouble remembering things, or finding the right word?	If an informant is present, discretely interview the informant separately from the patient.
Has there been a change in your ability to accomplish familiar tasks?	If a patient is suspicious or resentful of discussions behind his/her back, asking the nurse to obtain additional vital signs before the physical examination provides an excuse for you and the informant to leave the room.
Can you give some recent examples?	Some patients and family members assume that memory loss is part of normal aging and so discount its importance.

[a]*Consider asking these questions when there is a positive screen or a complaint of memory (or other type of cognitive) impairment.*

INTERVIEW FRAMEWORK

A challenge in assessing memory loss is that other psychiatric and neurologic complaints may overshadow cognitive symptoms, which may go undetected unless specifically inquired about through directed questioning. For example, a family member might complain that, over the course of months, the patient has become more irritable and reluctant to leave the house. Such symptoms could be a sign of late-life depression (a risk factor for Alzheimer's disease) or could represent depressive symptoms that accompany Alzheimer's disease up to 50% of the time. A patient who reports frequent falls, a hand tremor, and occasional visual hallucinations could have early Lewy body dementia.

The history should include the following information.

Feature	Specific Information
Onset	Abrupt (onset can be dated to within days or weeks); if abrupt, associated events (eg, fall, new medication) Insidious (exact onset impossible to pinpoint)
Duration	Days, weeks, months, or years
Overall course	Stable (no progression) Steadily progressive Stepwise decline (sudden worsening, period of stability, then sudden worsening)
Daily changes	Amount of fluctuation during the day and from 1 day to the next
Characteristics	Specific examples of memory problems
Associated cognitive problems	Language: word finding, fluency, naming Executive function: judgment, reasoning, planning, organization
Associated functional problems	Loss of ability to perform high-level intellectual tasks (recreational, occupational) Loss of ability to manage higher domains of functioning, such as driving, finances, shopping, meal preparation, housework Loss of ability to perform basic self-care, such as maintaining continence, hygiene, and appearance
Associated neurologic symptoms	Headache Focal neurologic symptoms Gait disorder

Concurrent medical conditions	Untreated or undertreated medical conditions, such as hyper- and hypothyroidism, vitamin B_{12} deficiency, chronic ethanol abuse, human immunodeficiency virus (HIV) infection
Prescribed and over-the-counter medications	Medications that can cause confusion, such as narcotics, benzodiazepines, tranquilizers, and anticholinergic medications (eg, antihistamines)
Associated psychiatric symptoms	Personality changes Mood changes Behavioral problems Aggression Agitation Psychosis Paranoia

IDENTIFYING ALARM SYMPTOMS

Alarm symptoms can be classified into 2 types: (1) those reflecting the seriousness of the underlying cause of memory loss, and (2) those reflecting serious complications. Many autoimmune, infectious, and cancer-associated dementias can be treated successfully, but if their underlying cause is missed, they may lead to irreversible neurologic damage or death.

Alarm Symptoms	If Present, Consider...
Abrupt onset	Delirium, stroke-related vascular dementia, subdural hematoma
Dementia associated with urinary incontinence and wide-based gait	Normal-pressure hydrocephalus
Rapid progression over weeks to months	**Common:** subdural hematoma, brain tumor **Uncommon:** rapidly progressive vascular dementia, frontotemporal dementia, or Alzheimer's disease; autoimmune systemic lupus erythematosus **Rare:** autoimmune and nonautoimmune paraneoplastic (cancer-associated) dementia (eg, limbic encephalitis) Autoimmune antibody-mediated dementia: anti–voltage-gated potassium channel encephalopathy (VGPCE), Hashimoto encephalopathy (HE), anti–glutamic acid decarboxylase antibody syndrome (GADAS), gluten-sensitivity dementia, Sjögren encephalopathy Autoimmune–no antibodies: sarcoidosis, Behçet syndrome, primary angiitis of the central nervous system (CNS) Infectious: subacute spongiform encephalopathy, Whipple disease (Tropheryma whipplei)
Dementia associated with depressed level of consciousness	Delirium, chronic drug toxicity (eg, benzodiazepines), HIV with opportunistic CNS infection
Disruptive behavior (agitation, aggressive or threatening behavior, purposeless behavior, wandering, inverted sleep-wake cycle, resistance to care)	Common in the middle to late stages of dementias. Assess caregiver well-being. *—Continued next page*

Continued—	
Psychosis, paranoia	Common in middle to late dementia. If visual hallucinations experienced early on, consider DLBD.
Inappropriate, involuntary movements of face or body	Extrapyramidal side effects of neuroleptic medication, Huntington's chorea, CBD
Difficulty with gait, stiffness, postural instability	Acquired immunodeficiency syndrome (AIDS) dementia complex, subacute spongiform encephalopathy, Parkinson's disease with dementia, DLBD, CBD, PSP, vascular dementia, side effects of neuroleptic medication, late Alzheimer's disease
Seizures	Mid to late stages of Alzheimer's disease, Korsakoff syndrome with alcohol withdrawal, brain tumor, delirium from repeated seizures, autoimmune dementia (antibody-mediated or CNS vasculitis), vascular (poststroke) dementia
Signs or suspicion of abuse of patient by caregiver or abuse of caregiver by patient	If present or strongly suspected, contact Adult Protective Services. Risk of reciprocal abuse is highest when demented patient is physically aggressive and when premorbid relationship between patient and caregiver was poor.
Caregiver acts angry, short-tempered, depressed, or anxious; complains of not being able to cope	Assess for caregiver stress, need for counseling, institutionalization of patient

Serious Diagnoses

All dementias affect daily functioning and therefore are serious; most degenerative (progressive) dementias are irreversible. However, treatment of underlying conditions may halt the progression or even lead to partial or complete reversal of dementia. Some causes of memory loss or dementia can be life threatening or produce substantial morbidity if not recognized. Although there is no known treatment for subacute spongiform encephalopathy, its potential for human-to-human transmission through organ transplantation or blood inoculation renders it a public health hazard if undiagnosed.[12]

Serious Diagnoses	Suggestive History	Differential Diagnosis
Chronic subdural hematoma	Dementia of acute or subacute origin. May or may not progress. History of falling or known fall risk. Recent head trauma. Focal neurologic symptoms may or may not be present.	Vascular dementia, "chronic" delirium (ie, lasting > 2 weeks)
Delirium	Short-term memory loss only part of syndrome. Cardinal symptoms include acute onset with fluctuating course during the day, inattention, and disorganized thinking and/or altered level of consciousness (hyperalert, agitated versus somnolent, passive).	Ethanol or benzodiazepine withdrawal
AIDS dementia complex	An infrequent (< 2%) initial presentation of AIDS with features of a subcortical dementia. Early on, there is psychomotor slowing and apathy, with later development of bradykinesia, altered posture, and parkinsonian gait disturbance. Consider in a patient with HIV risk factors or who is HIV positive.	Frontotemporal dementia, neurosyphilis, brain tumor, subacute spongiform encephalopathy, DLBD (in older patient)

Subacute spongiform encephalopathy (SSE)	The generic name given to prion-associated encephalopathies like Creutzfeldt-Jakob disease. Rapidly progressive. SSE should be considered when memory loss occurs at a younger age. Early stages dominated by psychiatric symptoms (dysphoria, withdrawal, irritability, apathy), with memory loss prominent in the middle stages.[13]	Depression, frontotemporal dementia, neurosyphilis, AIDS dementia complex, Whipple disease, vascular dementia, early-onset Alzheimer's disease (genetic; family history usually positive), autoimmune dementia
Late neurosyphilis	Memory loss often accompanied by delusions, paranoia, and emotional lability. Signs of tabes dorsalis may be present (paresthesias, impaired proprioception, wide-based gait).[14]	AIDS dementia complex, SSE, Alzheimer's disease
Systemic autoimmune disorders (eg, systemic lupus erythematosus, sarcoidosis, Behçet syndrome)	Cognitive decline usually occurs in association with more common features of the autoimmune disorder. Rarely, cognitive changes may be the presenting symptom. Patients tend to be younger, and the cognitive changes usually have a subacute onset with a waxing and waning course.	Frontotemporal dementia, neurosyphilis, AIDS dementia complex, SSE, Whipple disease, vascular dementia, early-onset Alzheimer's disease, other autoimmune dementias
Autoimmune disorders with antineuronal antibodies (eg, paraneoplastic dementia, Hashimoto encephalopathy, VGPCE, GADAS)	Rapid cognitive decline with reports by the informant of poor judgment or decision making, personality changes, and/or memory loss. Other neurologic complaints may be prominent (eg, focal shaking [myoclonus], seizures, ataxia).	SSE, frontotemporal dementia, neurosyphilis, AIDS dementia complex, Whipple disease, vascular dementia, Alzheimer's disease, systemic autoimmune disorders
Whipple disease	Rapidly progressive cognitive decline associated with a history of unintentional weight loss and diarrhea (due to malabsorption). Rarely, dementia occurs without the classic gastrointestinal symptoms. Cognitive changes are often accompanied by neurologic complaints such as tremor or ataxia.	SSE, paraneoplastic dementia, neurosyphilis, AIDS dementia complex, vascular dementia, Alzheimer's disease, autoimmune dementia
Brain tumor	Complaints of memory loss usually associated with psychomotor retardation or apathy. Patient or family may also report headaches, altered level of consciousness, or focal neurologic changes.	Depression, frontotemporal dementia
Korsakoff syndrome	Memory loss due to thiamine deficiency. Usually, history of alcohol abuse. Patient typically unaware of deficit and confabulates.	MCI, early Alzheimer's disease, vitamin B_{12} deficiency
Vitamin B_{12} deficiency	Symptoms of memory loss or mild dementia. Complaints of ataxia and decreased lower extremity sensation (dorsal column disease) should increase suspicion. (Note: Neuropsychiatric symptoms may precede anemia.)	Early Alzheimer's disease, MCI, Korsakoff syndrome
Normal-pressure hydrocephalus	Dementia associated with urinary incontinence and wide-based gait. Low likelihood if complete triad not present.[15]	Vitamin B_{12} deficiency, late neurosyphilis
		—Continued next page

Continued—		
Hyperthyroidism	A rare but reversible cause of dementia in older persons. Because older individuals may not display the typical symptoms of hyperthyroidism (so-called "apathetic hyperthyroidism"), it should be ruled out in most cases of dementia.	Alzheimer's disease, vitamin B_{12} deficiency
Hypothyroidism	Hypothyroidism has been associated with dementia, but the incidence of complete reversibility with treatment is low.	Alzheimer's disease, apathetic hyperthyroidism, AIDS dementia complex, vitamin B_{12} deficiency, depression
Pseudodementia	Defined as dementia-like symptoms due to depression. Variable onset, usually traceable to within weeks. Both subjective and objective evidence of memory loss. Depressed mood and affect, apathy, and weight loss support this diagnosis. Patient may have variable somatic complaints. (Note: Depression occurs in up to 50% of Alzheimer's disease patients.)	Alzheimer's disease, MCI, frontotemporal dementia, hypothyroidism, AIDS dementia complex

FOCUSED QUESTIONS

Use focused questions to determine the presence of associated and alarm symptoms. Questions about the order in which symptoms developed can help narrow the differential diagnosis. Screening tools like the MMSE can only partially determine the severity of dementia; systematic questioning about the impact of the memory loss or dementia on daily activities should comprise part of the evaluation.

QUESTIONS	THINK ABOUT...
What sort of activities or hobbies did you do 6 months ago? Have you had trouble or stopped doing any of these in recent months? Why?	Impairment of daily activities due to difficulties with memory or executive function suggests dementia rather than MCI or benign age-related changes. Depression also should be considered.
In the last few months, have you lost your way while driving to a familiar destination?	Loss of visuospatial functioning suggests dementia.
Which came first, memory problems or stiffness and a shuffling gait?	If memory problems came first, think about Lewy body dementia or vascular dementia. If memory problems began more than a year after parkinsonian symptoms, consider Parkinson's disease with dementia.
(To the caregiver) What time of day does (specific disruptive behavior) occur or get worse? Are there any precipitating factors? What happens when the behavior occurs? How troublesome is this behavior to you? What do you do when it happens?	Think about ways to prevent disruptive behaviors and ways the caregiver can manage them without medications. If unsuccessful, consider a trial of a major tranquilizer.

ADDITIONAL AREAS OF FOCUS		THINK ABOUT...
Quality	Involves only memory loss.	• MCI • Early dementia (impairment in other cognitive domains unrecognized) • Korsakoff syndrome • Depression/pseudodementia
	Predominantly memory loss, but other cognitive domains affected	• Dementia, not otherwise specified
	Language affected more than memory	• Subcortical dementia
	Age of onset under 65	• Early-onset Alzheimer's disease • Frontotemporal dementia • SSE • AIDS dementia complex • Autoimmune and paraneoplastic dementias • Brain tumor
Time course	Acute onset	
	• Fluctuating course throughout day	• Delirium
	• Minimal diurnal variation or slow progression over days	• Subdural hematoma
	• Minimal diurnal variation, stable over weeks to months or stepwise progression	• Stroke (vascular dementia)
	Subacute onset	
	• Rapidly progressive over weeks to months with or without spontaneous remissions	• Autoimmune dementia • Paraneoplastic dementia
	Insidious onset	
	• Moderate diurnal variation early in course; slow, steady progression over months	• DLBD
	• Minimal diurnal variation; slow, steady progression over months	• Alzheimer's disease • Vascular dementia • Frontotemporal dementia • SSE (relatively more rapid) • AIDS dementia complex (relatively more rapid) • Whipple disease
	• Stepwise progression over months	• Vascular dementia

—Continued next page

Continued—

Associated symptoms	Apathy	• Depression/pseudodementia • Frontotemporal dementia • AIDS dementia complex • SSE • Hypothyroidism
	Depression	• Depression/pseudodementia • Subcortical (vascular) dementia • Alzheimer's disease
	Hallucinations	
	• In early stages of dementia	• DLBD
	• In middle to late stages	• Any progressive dementia
	Disruptive behavior (agitation, aggression, wandering, disrupted sleep-wake cycle, etc)	• Any moderate to advanced dementia
	Extrapyramidal signs and symptoms (gait disturbance, stooped posture, decreased spontaneous movement)	• Late Alzheimer's disease • DLBD • Dementia associated with Parkinson's disease • CBD • PSP • Late SSE • Vascular dementia
	Slow, wide-based, unsteady gait	• Normal-pressure hydrocephalus • Subcortical (vascular) dementia • CBD
	Incontinence	• Any advanced dementia
	• with wide-based gait	• Normal-pressure hydrocephalus
Modifying factors	Acute illness	• Superimposed delirium exacerbating memory loss or dementia
	Chronic metabolic disorder • Hypothyroidism • Hyperthyroidism • Vitamin B_{12} deficiency	• May cause or exacerbate memory loss or dementia
	Medications (major and minor tranquilizers, centrally acting antihypertensives [eg, clonidine], narcotics, anticonvulsants, nonsteroidal anti-inflammatory drugs, anticholinergic medications, others)	• May cause or exacerbate memory loss or dementia

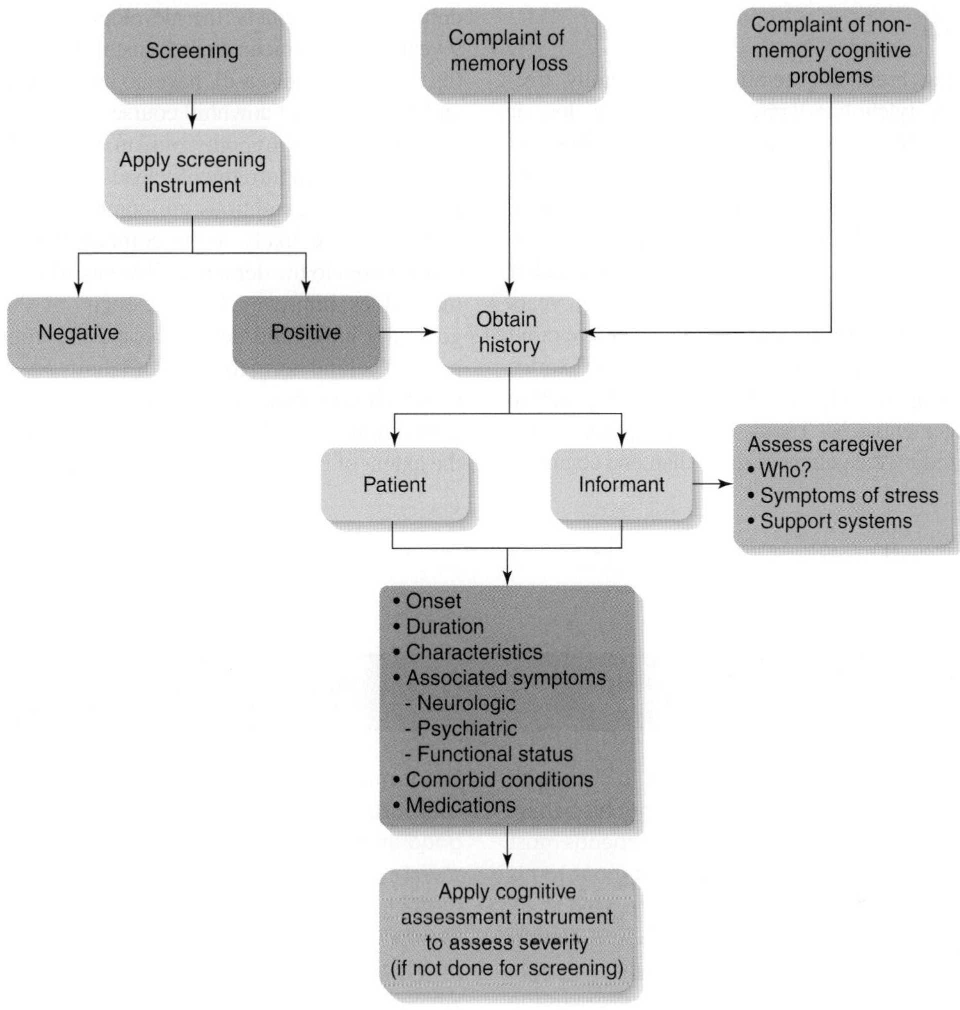

FIGURE 59–2 Diagnostic approach: Memory loss.

DIAGNOSTIC APPROACH (INCLUDING ALGORITHM)

See Figure 59–2 for the diagnostic approach algorithm for memory loss.

CAVEATS

- Do not assume that every older patient with dementia has Alzheimer's disease. The diagnosis of dementia should follow a rigorous systematic process including a careful physical examination (with attention to neurologic findings) and, if indicated, blood tests, cranial imaging, and (infrequently) lumbar puncture and electroencephalogram.[1]
- The distinction between "benign" age-associated memory impairment (subjective but without objective memory loss) and MCI (subjective plus objective memory or other cognitive loss) may be difficult without neuropsychological testing. An affective disorder (depression) should be considered in either case.
- There is no such thing as "acute" Alzheimer's disease. A diagnosis of dementia cannot be made in the acutely ill patient, in whom delirium may cloud the picture.
- Given the prevalence of polypharmacy among older patients, the potential for adverse CNS effects, including chronic confusion due to medications mimicking dementia, is substantial.
- Because demented individuals residing in the community cannot survive without the close involvement of a caregiver, caregiver stress must also be monitored as part of overall patient management.

[1]A detailed description of pertinent neurological findings and diagnostic studies is beyond the scope of this textbook.

PROGNOSIS

Dementias involving brain degeneration are generally irreversible, although acetylcholinesterase inhibitors may slow or delay progression slightly in Alzheimer's disease, DLBD, and (to a lesser extent) vascular and mixed dementia. Memantine has been shown to slow the progression of moderate to severe Alzheimer's disease and early vascular dementia. The prognosis for Alzheimer's disease varies according to the stage at which it was diagnosed, with a mean survival of approximately 8 years from diagnosis. Vascular dementia tends to follow a more rapid course than Alzheimer's disease. The prognosis for MCI varies by type. MCI involving memory only has the lowest 9-year rate of conversion to dementia. MCI with objective performance deficits unrecognized by the patient in more than one cognitive domain best predicts the development of dementia within 9 years. SSEs, which can be transmitted from animal to human (eg, "mad cow" disease), have no currently available treatment and follow a rapid downhill course measured in months.

Treatment of hypothyroidism, vitamin B_{12} deficiency, and hyperthyroidism infrequently leads to cognitive improvement. Because these conditions are common among older persons, they are more likely to be coincidental comorbidities than contributors to the dementia. Patients whose cognitive impairment does improve after treatment of the endocrinopathy generally have mild dementia, and the improvement can lag months behind normalization of laboratory values. The degree to which cognitive deficits can be reversed by treatment of autoimmune disorders causing dementia varies depending on the extent of brain damage caused by the autoimmune process.

CASE SCENARIO | Resolution

A 74-year-old retired auto mechanic presents to clinic with his wife and daughter, who are concerned about his behavior. The patient has become more irritable and spends most of his days watching television instead of going out to his shop to tinker with old lawnmowers, which he used to fix and sell. He has also begun accusing his wife and daughter of stealing or hiding his wallet and keys, which his wife eventually finds somewhere in the house. He still drives the car downtown, but the wife admits not liking to drive with him because he gets angry when she tells him he has taken a wrong turn. When you ask about the patient's memory, his daughter states that it still seems "good, because he can remember events from a long time ago as if they were yesterday." The patient agrees: "I think I remember as well as you'd expect for a person my age."

ADDITIONAL HISTORY

The patient's wife reports that he began to lose interest in lawnmower repair perhaps 6 to 12 months earlier. She remembers him stating that the motors had gotten too complicated in recent years. He first got lost while driving 18 months ago, when she told him to pick up the dry cleaning at a new strip mall. In recent months, he has gotten lost twice on the way to his regular barbershop. She states, "He is not much of a talker," and she has always paid the bills "because, with a sixth-grade education, he never was very good at math." His 80-year-old older brother has had "real memory problems" since his bypass operation, and his mother, who died from a stroke, became forgetful a year or 2 before she died. The patient has a past medical history of hypertension, prostatic hyperplasia, and insomnia, for which he takes over-the-counter sleeping aids.

Question: Which of the following statements is true?

A. The family history of dementia strongly supports a diagnosis of probable Alzheimer's disease.
B. Depression is unlikely to be a cause of the patient's irritability.
C. This patient does not meet the criteria for dementia because of his ability to recall distant events.
D. The patient's paranoia (believing his family is stealing his wallet and keys) is consistent with a diagnosis of Alzheimer's disease.
E. Nonprescription sleeping pills are unlikely to contribute to cognitive impairment.

Test Your Knowledge

1. A 51-year-old previously healthy former high school biology teacher comes to the clinic with his wife, who wants you to evaluate him for depression. Over the last year, he has become increasingly slovenly in his appearance, wearing the same clothes for days and not regularly shaving or brushing his teeth. For the last few months, he has preferred sitting around the house watching television. He readily admits drinking 1 to 2 beers per day while watching television. He acknowledges a substantial weight gain in the past year, which he attributes to his dislike of exercise and love of snack food. He was fired from his job 11 months earlier for making a comment about a female student's physical attributes and asking her out on a date. Previously a very polite man, he now regularly punctuates his sentences with the "f-word." When not watching television, he surfs the Internet and has racked up thousands of dollars in Internet purchases. On mental status testing, he scores 29 out of 30 on the Mini-Mental State Examination.

   What is the most likely diagnosis?

   A. The early stage of early-onset Alzheimer's disease
   B. Depression following dismissal from his teaching post
   C. Frontotemporal dementia
   D. Alcohol-related dementia
   E. Creutzfeldt-Jakob disease

2. Mr. M. is a 78-year-old retired superior court judge who is brought to your office by his son for evaluation of worsening falls. His last fall resulted in a large scalp laceration and small subdural hematoma, which did not require evacuation. Nine months earlier, the patient was given a diagnosis of Alzheimer's disease and prescribed a cholinesterase inhibitor for memory difficulties. The son says that on some days his father is as "sharp as a tack," whereas on other days, he asks the same question over and over and cannot remember the answer. Until the age of 76, his father was an avid outdoorsman, but in the past year, his posture has become stooped and he has developed a short-stepped, shuffling gait. Three months ago, the patient went to his primary doctor because of vivid hallucinations of his deceased wife and was prescribed risperidone, an atypical antipsychotic. The son states that, although the hallucinations disappeared, his father has become so stiff that he now resembles a mannequin, requires a front-wheel walker for support, and tends to fall backward when he first stands up.

   What is the most likely diagnosis?

   A. Alzheimer's disease
   B. Parkinson's disease with dementia
   C. Dementia due to traumatic brain injury
   D. Lewy body dementia
   E. Vascular dementia

3. A 76-year-old woman is brought in because of progressive difficulty walking and worsening short-term memory over the past 6 months. She was diagnosed with mild dementia 1 year earlier based on reports by her husband and daughter that she seemed noticeably slower mentally and was having difficulty following recipes, although previously a good cook. Her past medical history includes obesity (body mass index = 31 kg/m^2), diabetes mellitus, hyperlipidemia, and hypertension, all of which are well controlled on medications. Her husband describes her walking as slow, wide-based, and unsteady. In the last month, she started wearing diapers because of difficulty getting to the bathroom in time.

   Which of the following statements is true?

   A. The triad of broad-based gait, urinary incontinence, and dementia is consistent with normal-pressure hydrocephalus.
   B. Lewy body dementia is excluded because she does not have hallucinations.
   C. The patient's dementia can be attributed to chronic hypoxemia from undiagnosed obstructive sleep apnea associated with obesity.
   D. The features and progression of her dementia are most consistent with a diagnosis of Alzheimer's disease.
   E. Vascular dementia is unlikely because her diabetes and hypertension are well controlled.

References

1. Christensen H. What cognitive changes can be expected with normal ageing? *Aust N Z J Psychiatry.* 2001;35:768–775.
2. Ferri CP, Prince M, Brayne C, et al. Global prevalence of dementia: a Delphi consensus study. *Lancet.* 2005;366:2112–2117.
3. Winblad B, Palmer K, Kivipelto M, et al. Mild cognitive impairment—beyond controversies, towards a consensus: report of the International Working Group on Mild Cognitive Impairment. *J Intern Med.* 2004;256:240–246.
4. McKhann G, Drachman D, Folstein M, Katzman R, Price D, Stadlan EM. Clinical diagnosis of Alzheimer's disease: report of the NINCDS-ADRDA Work Group under the auspices of Department of Health and Human Services Task Force on Alzheimer's Disease. *Neurology.* 1984;34:939–944.
5. Gauthier S, Reisberg B, Zaudig M, et al. Mild cognitive impairment. *Lancet.* 2006;367:1262–1270.
6. Kertesz A. Clinical features and diagnosis of frontotemporal dementia. *Front Neurol Neurosci.* 2009;24:140–148.
7. Folstein MF, Folstein SE, McHugh PR. "Mini-mental state": a practical method for grading the cognitive state of patients for the clinician. *J Psychiatr Res.* 1975;12:189–198.
8. Borson S, Scanlan J, Brush M, Vitaliano P, Dokmak A. The Mini-Cog: a cognitive 'vital signs' measure for dementia screening in multi-lingual elderly. *Int J Geriatr Psychiatry.* 2000;15:1021–1027.

9. Nasreddine ZS, Phillips NA, Bedirian V, et al. The Montreal Cognitive Assessment, MoCA: a brief screening tool for mild cognitive impairment. *J Am Geriatr Soc.* 2005;53:695–699.

10. Welcome to the Montreal Cognitive Assessment. Available at: http://www.mocatest.org/. Accessed March 3, 2010.

11. Jorm AF. A short form of the Informant Questionnaire on Cognitive Decline in the Elderly (IQCODE): development and cross-validation. *Psychol Med.* 1994;24:145–153.

12. Glatzel M, Stoeck K, Seeger H, Luhrs T, Aguzzi A. Human prion diseases: molecular and clinical aspects. *Arch Neurol.* 2005;62:545–552.

13. Spencer MD, Knight RS, Will RG. First hundred cases of variant Creutzfeldt-Jakob disease: retrospective case note review of early psychiatric and neurological features. *BMJ.* 2002;324:1479–1482.

14. Cintron R, Pachner AR. Spirochetal diseases of the nervous system. *Curr Opin Neurol.* 1994;7:217–222.

15. Dippel DW, Habbema JD. Probabilistic diagnosis of normal pressure hydrocephalus and other treatable cerebral lesions in dementia. *J Neurol Sci.* 1993;119:123–133.

Suggested Reading

Caserta MT, Bannon Y, Fernandez F, Giunta B, Schoenberg MR, Tan J. Normal brain aging clinical, immunological, neuropsychological, and neuroimaging features. *Int Rev Neurobiol.* 2009;84:1–19.

Chertkow H, Massoud F, Nasreddine Z, et al. Diagnosis and treatment of dementia: 3. Mild cognitive impairment and cognitive impairment without dementia. *CMAJ.* 2008;178:1273–1285.

Croes EA, van Duijn CM. Variant Creutzfeldt-Jakob disease. *Eur J Epidemiol.* 2003;18:473–477.

Geschwind MD, Shu H, Haman A, Sejvar JJ, Miller BL. Rapidly progressive dementia. *Ann Neurol.* 2008;64:97–108.

Hanson JC, Lippa CF. Lewy body dementia. *Int Rev Neurobiol.* 2009;84:215–228.

Kertesz A. Clinical features and diagnosis of frontotemporal dementia. *Front Neurol Neurosci.* 2009;24:140–148.

Langa KM, Foster NL, Larson EB. Mixed dementia: emerging concepts and therapeutic implications. *JAMA.* 2004;292:2901–2908.

Querfurth HW, LaFerla FM. Alzheimer's disease. *N Engl J Med.* 2010;362:329–344.

Ritchie K, Lovestone S. The dementias. *Lancet.* 2002;360:1759–1766.

Schneck MJ. Vascular dementia. *Top Stroke Rehabil.* 2008;15:22–26.

Chapter 60

Diplopia

Jason J. S. Barton, MD, PhD, FRCPC

CASE SCENARIO

A 40-year-old woman presents with sudden diplopia and bad headache while at work. She notes that the left image is higher than the right one and that the images get further apart when she looks up, down, or to the left. On examination, she has an exotropia and left hypotropia when looking straight ahead, and there is reduced adduction, depression, and elevation of the right eye.

- **What additional signs should you look for?**
- **What nerve, muscle, or structure has been affected?**
- **What is your chief worry in a case like this, and how would you investigate it?**

INTRODUCTION

Diplopia is the experience of seeing more than a single image. In the majority of cases, it is due to the fact that the 2 eyes are not pointing at the same location in space (ocular misalignment). Thus, images of an object fall on different locations of the retinae of the 2 eyes, giving rise to the impression of 2 objects rather than 1.

KEY TERMS

Diplopia	Seeing a duplicate copy of an image, colloquially referred to as "double vision."
Monocular diplopia	Diplopia with only one eye viewing.
Binocular diplopia	Diplopia present only when both eyes are open.
Polyopia	Seeing multiple copies of an image.
Abduction	Moving the eye away from the nose.
Adduction	Moving the eye toward the nose.
Elevation	Moving the eye up.
Depression	Moving the eye down.
Comitant	Diplopia that does not vary with gaze direction.
Esotropia	Crossed eyes; eyes pointing medially with respect to each other.
Exotropia	Eyes that are pointing laterally with respect to each other.
Hypertropia	One eye elevated with respect to the other.
Phoria	A tendency for the eyes to be misaligned when one eye is covered; with both eyes open, the subject's ocular motor control system can use vision to align the eyes so that there is no diplopia.
Microvascular palsy	Palsies attributed to small-vessel ischemia, often related to hypertension or diabetes.

ETIOLOGY

Binocular diplopia stems from dysfunction of a broad range of motor structures, ranging from muscle, neuromuscular junction, nerves in their course within and outside the brainstem, and prenuclear brainstem control problems. This anatomic division is a useful approach to evaluation and differential diagnosis.

Differential Diagnosis

Site of Pathology	Diagnosis
Ocular myopathy	Graves ophthalmopathy[1] (Figure 60–1) Orbital myositis Muscle entrapment (Figure 60–2)
Neuromuscular junction	Myasthenia gravis[2] Botulism
Cranial neuropathy (III, IV, VI)[3–5] (Figures 60–3 and 60–4)	Microvascular disease (diabetes) Tumor Infection Inflammation Cerebral aneurysm
Supranuclear (brainstem) disorders[6]	Stroke Tumor Demyelination Infection

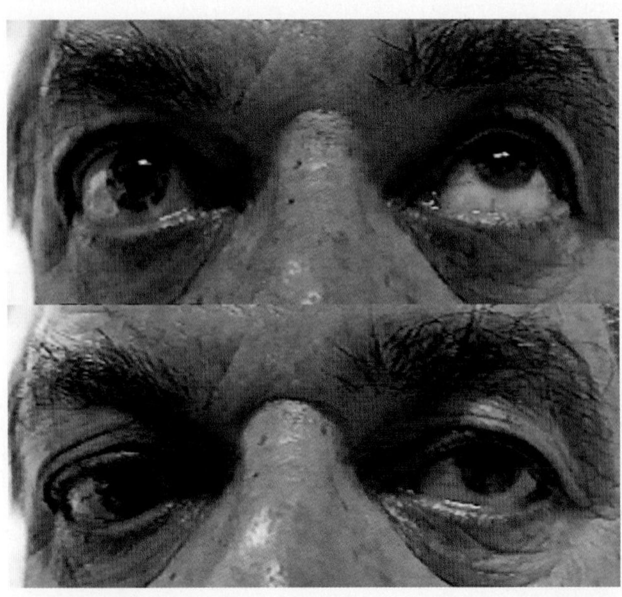

FIGURE 60–1 Graves ophthalmopathy. Note that in straight-ahead gaze (*bottom image*) the eye is slightly lower and is proptotic. In upward gaze (right *top image*), the right eye cannot elevate. The patient has vertical diplopia worse in up gaze. (Image reprinted with permission from www.neuroophthalmology.ca.)

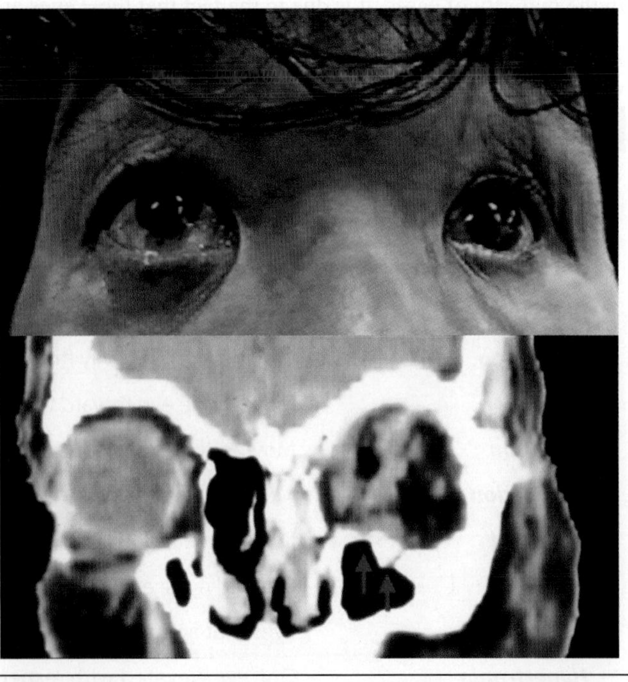

FIGURE 60–2 Orbital blowout fracture. This woman fell down the stairs, and now the left eye cannot look upward. The coronal computed tomography scan shows air in the left orbit, indicating an orbital wall fracture allowing air to enter the orbit, and arrows indicate the disruption of the bony orbital floor that is entrapping the inferior rectus and not allowing the eye to look up. (Image reprinted with permission from www.neuroophthalmology.ca.)

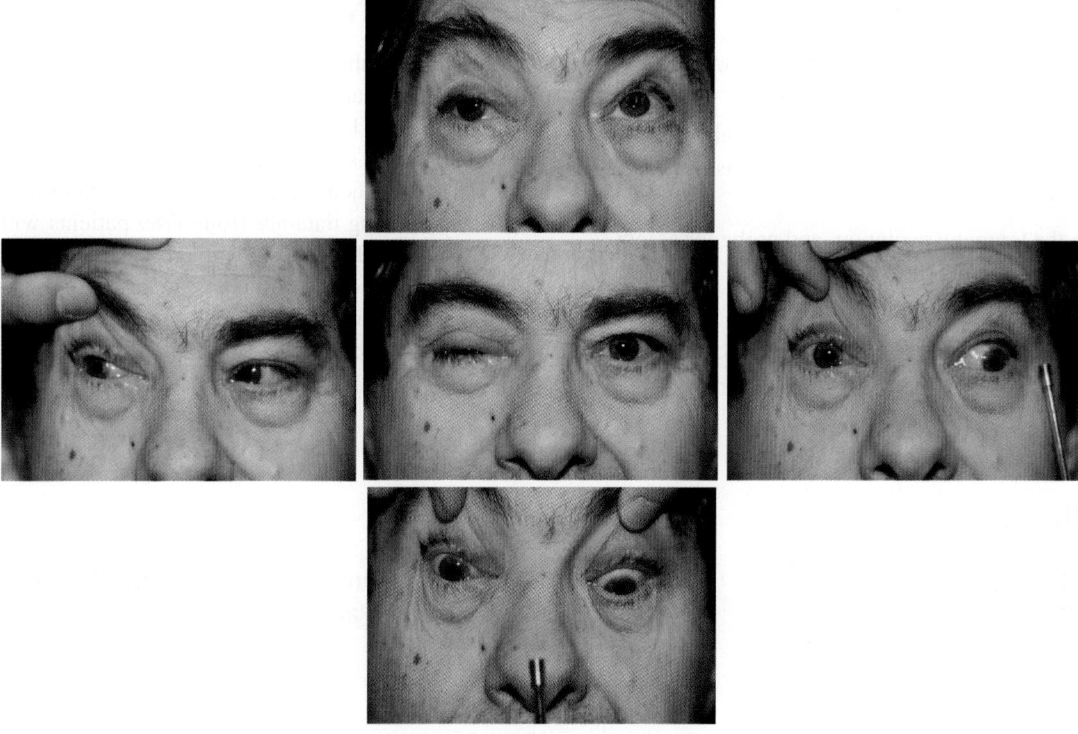

FIGURE 60–3 Complete right III nerve palsy, with pupil sparing. Note the complete ptosis and the failure to adduct, elevate, or depress the right eye. Abduction is normal. (Image reprinted with permission from www.neuroophthalmology.ca.)

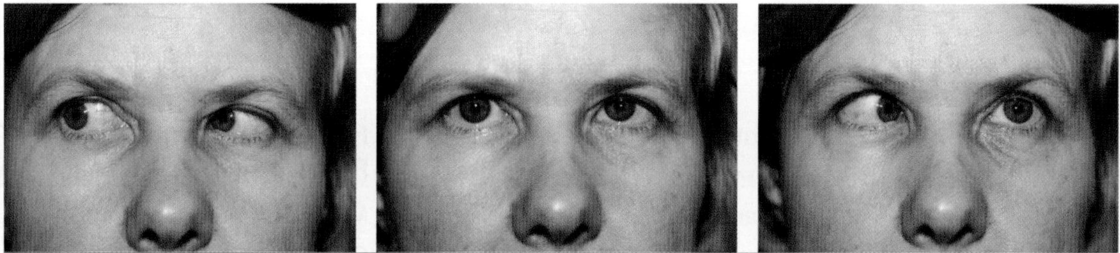

FIGURE 60–4 Complete left VI nerve palsy. Abduction is absent, but all other eye movements are spared (vertical range not shown). (Image reprinted with permission from www.neuroophthalmology.ca.)

GETTING STARTED WITH THE HISTORY

Questions	Remember
Does double vision disappear when one eye is closed?	If diplopia persists with one eye closed, the cause is a simple refractive problem, not an ocular motor one.
Does it hurt?	Pain should raise considerations of more ominous pathology, even though it can occur with benign microvascular palsies.
How long have you had double vision? Is it getting worse?	Progression is an ominous feature, suggesting a mass lesion.

INTERVIEW FRAMEWORK

- Determine whether the problem is due to a refractive problem or ocular misalignment.
- For ocular misalignment, determine the pattern of diplopia in order to isolate which eye movement is weak and in which eye.
- Determine the temporal evolution, and probe for associated symptoms of ominous pathology.
- Identify risk factors from prior history, especially diabetes or symptoms compatible with vasculitis.

IDENTIFYING ALARM SYMPTOMS

Diplopia can be the sign of ominous, even life-threatening pathology. Fortunately, this is unusual. Most often, serious problems reflect a lesion of the peripheral nerve or brainstem. The likelihood of serious causes varies depending on which nerve is involved, hence the importance of anatomic diagnosis first. The following data are from 4789 patients with cranial nerve palsies (III, IV, and VI) who presented either to a hospital or an ophthalmology clinic.[3–5] The distribution also differs by age; pediatric patients have less microvascular palsies and more mass lesions.[7]

Serious Diagnoses

Diagnosis	Prevalence Among Patients With Cranial Nerve Palsies[a]
Cerebral aneurysm	6%
Brain tumor	13%
Cavernous sinus mass lesion	
Increased intracranial pressure	
Infection	

[a]Empty cells indicate that prevalence is not known.

Alarm Symptoms	If Present, Consider Serious Causes...	However, Benign Causes for This Feature Include...
Eye pain or headache	Cerebral aneurysm Cavernous sinus mass Increased intracranial pressure Meningitis	Microvascular palsy Orbital inflammation Unrelated migraine
Facial numbness	Cavernous sinus mass	
Facial weakness Limb weakness Limb numbness Imbalance Drowsiness	Brainstem lesion Meningitis	

FOCUSED QUESTIONS

QUESTIONS	THINK ABOUT...
Is double vision still present when you close one eye?	Refractive cause, that is, cataract, keratoconus
Does double vision vary through the day?	Myasthenia gravis
Can you make vision single with concentration?	Congenital eso- or exophoria, a latent tendency to ocular deviation that can emerge in later life with diplopia, with no dire significance
Quality	
Is it vertical?	III nerve palsy (see Figure 60–3), IV nerve palsy, Graves ophthalmopathy (see Figure 60–1),[1] skew deviation[6]
Is it horizontal?	VI nerve palsy (Figure 60–4), internuclear ophthalmoplegia, Graves ophthalmopathy, convergence insufficiency
Does it change with which way you look?	Nerve or muscle palsy
Time course	
Is the distance between the images about the same as when you first noticed diplopia?	Microvascular palsies Skew deviation from strokes Decompensation of congenital strabismus
Is it increasing over time?	Tumor, meningeal infection, aneurysmal compression
Does it vary from day to day?	Myasthenia gravis
Associated symptoms	
Do you have eye, head, or facial pain?	Infection, tumor, or aneurysm, if pain is prolonged; microvascular palsies can hurt, but generally for less than a week
Has your eye changed in appearance?	Proptosis in Graves ophthalmopathy, or other orbital mass
Has your speech or swallowing changed?	Bulbar symptoms in myasthenia gravis, brainstem strokes, Miller Fisher syndrome
Do you have numbness anywhere in your face?	Cavernous sinus lesion (likely a mass) or brainstem lesion
Do you have weakness or numbness of one side of your body?	Brainstem lesion
Is your balance affected?	Brainstem or cerebellar lesion
Modifying symptoms	
Does the double vision increase with certain visual activities like driving or reading?	Myasthenia gravis

DIAGNOSTIC APPROACH (INCLUDING ALGORITHMS)

See diplopia algorithm (Figure 60–5; see also Figure 60–7) for an overview of the diagnostic approach. First, determine whether diplopia is monocular or binocular: Does each eye alone see single?

Monocular Diplopia

If one eye sees double while the other is covered, this is a refractive problem. Among elderly patients, this is most commonly a cataract. More serious corneal problems like keratoconus can also do this. Transient monocular diplopia is not uncommon and probably reflects a problem with the corneal surface such as dry eyes; often there is little to find.

Binocular Diplopia

If diplopia only occurs with both eyes open, the problem is a misalignment between the two eyes. Next, one must determine whether the diplopia is horizontal or vertical.

Horizontal Diplopia

- **Which eye sees the right-most image?** Because of the optics, the eye that sees the right-most image is pointing left of the other eye. For example, if the left eye sees the right image, it is pointing left of where the right eye is looking. Hence the eyes are diverged, or exotropic, usually indicating a weakness of adduction. If the left eye sees the left image, the eyes are crossed, or esotropic, from abduction weakness (Figure 60–6). This does not yet establish which eye is the weak eye. It just tells the relative position of the 2 eyes.
- **Is diplopia worse (separation between the images increases) in left or right gaze? Is diplopia worse for near vision or far vision?** Diplopia worsens when you make the weak nerve or muscle work. For example, if diplopia gets worse in left gaze, this implies a problem with either abducting the left eye or adducting the right eye. If diplopia is worse looking close, one or both of the adducting muscles (ie, the medial recti) is the problem (because we cross our eyes to look close). If it is worse

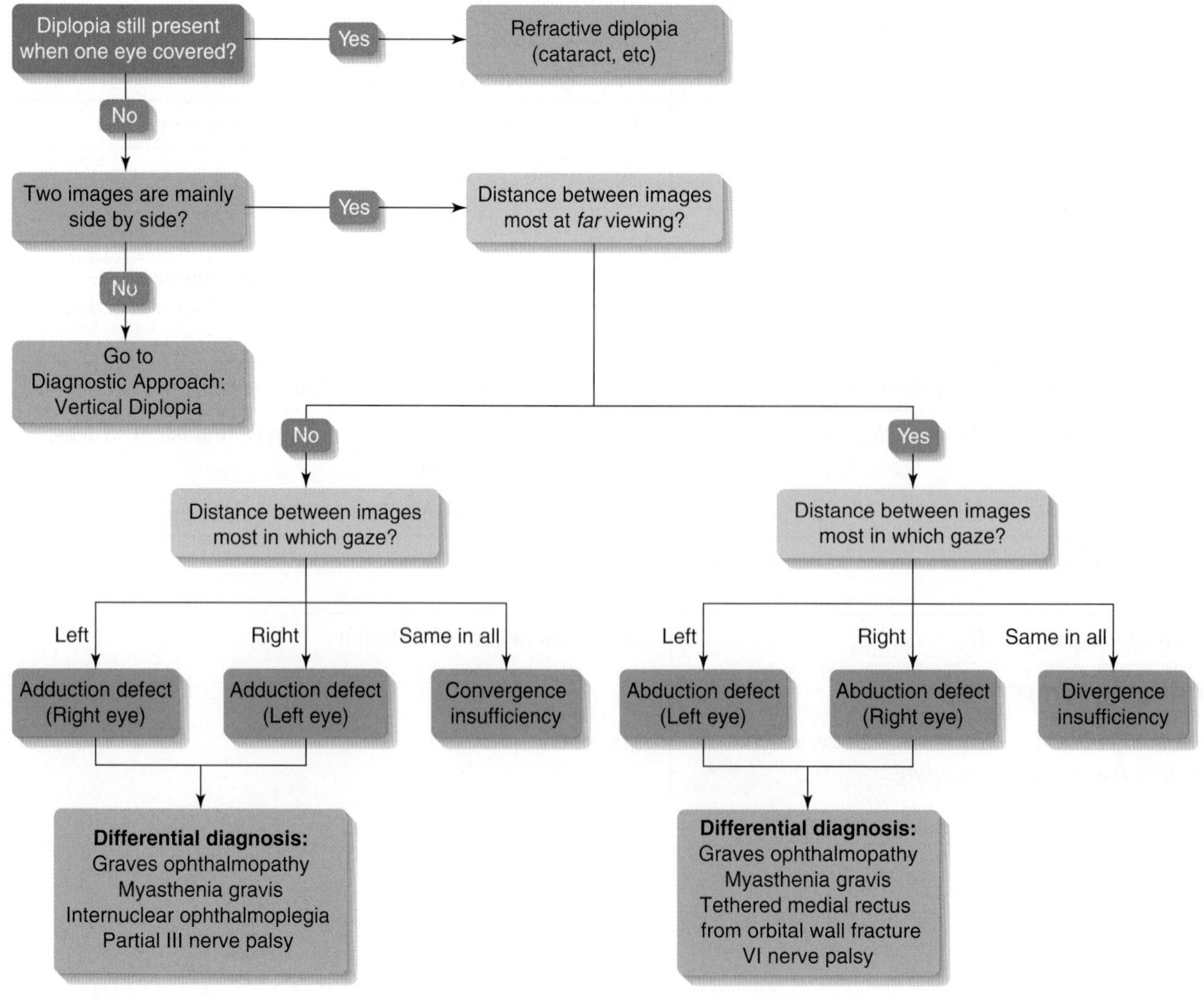

FIGURE 60–5 Diagnostic approach: Diplopia.

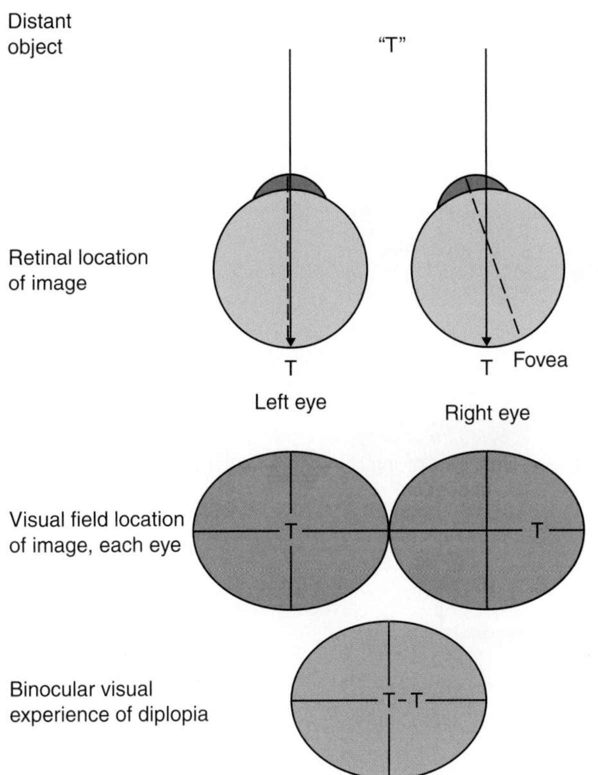

FIGURE 60–6 Image pattern in esotropia. The position of the eyes in a patient with a right VI nerve palsy is shown, as the patient fixates the letter "T" in the distance. Because the right eye is deviated toward the nose, the image of the "T" in this eye falls to the left of the fovea, whereas in the good left eye, the "T" is projected onto the fovea. Because of the inversion of images projected onto the retina, a retinal image left of the fovea is perceived as right of center (see "Visual field location of image"). Thus the "T" seen by the right eye is right of the "T" seen by the left eye. This is an "uncrossed diplopia," meaning that the right eye sees the right image.

at far, abduction is the problem (ie, the lateral recti). Here are 2 examples. First, a left VI nerve palsy, which causes weakness of the lateral rectus that abducts the left eye, will cause a horizontal diplopia worse at far and in left gaze. Second, a convergence insufficiency, in which there is a brainstem problem with getting both medial recti to adduct fully when looking up close, will cause a horizontal diplopia worse at near, but because both sides are involved, it does not vary with looking right or left.

Vertical Diplopia

The 3 questions for vertical diplopia are similar to the 3 questions for horizontal diplopia (Figure 60–7).

- **Which eye sees the lower image?** The higher eye sees the lower image. Diplopia may be due to weakness of the depressor muscles (inferior rectus or superior oblique) of the higher eye or the elevator muscles (superior rectus or inferior oblique) of the lower eye.
- **Is the diplopia worse in left gaze or right gaze?**
- **Is the diplopia worse in up gaze or down gaze?**

The 3 questions above can isolate a weakness of any single oblique or vertical rectus muscle. However, in practical terms, the main differential of vertical diplopia is between 5 items (see vertical diplopia algorithm, Figure 60–7):

1. Graves ophthalmopathy[1]: Look for associated signs of proptosis, conjunctival injection, and lid lag or retraction. Patients may have other signs of hyperthyroidism or hypothyroidism, but euthyroid Graves is not uncommon.
2. Myasthenia gravis[2]: This disorder can mimic any palsy. The hallmark is variability, with diplopia changing throughout the day, sometimes being worse with visually demanding tasks like driving or reading and sometimes with different findings by different examiners or between different visits. A subtle ptosis may also be a good clue.
3. IV nerve palsy: The 3 questions will show that the eye with a IV nerve palsy is higher, and this separation is worse when looking in the direction of the lower (normal) eye or when looking down. Also, IV nerve palsies are usually worse when tilting the head toward the side of the palsy. All of this can also be remembered as the right-left-right (or left-right-left) rule (eg, a right IV nerve palsy has a right hypertropia, worse in left gaze and on right head tilt).
4. III nerve palsy: This involves various combinations of weakness of adduction, elevation, and depression, as well as ptosis and/or a larger pupil in the affected eye (see Figure 60–3)
5. Skew deviation[6]: This results from disruption of brainstem vestibular pathways. Signs of the other 4 conditions should be sought and excluded. A neurologic examination may reveal associated damage to sensory or motor tracts to the limbs as they pass through the brainstem, other cranial neuropathies, a Horner syndrome, or cerebellar signs.

CAVEATS AND PEARLS

- Although binocular diplopia is most often due to a weakness of a muscle or nerve, less frequently it is due to restriction. That is, an eye fails to move because the muscle that moves it in the other direction is tethered and unable to stretch. The 2 main causes of this are muscle inflammation (eg, Graves ophthalmopathy) and orbital wall or floor fractures from facial trauma, which usually should be evident from the history. Suspect these entities if there is proptosis, conjunctival redness, a history of thyroid disease, or recent facial trauma.
- If you suspect myasthenia, ask about generalized symptoms of limb weakness, dyspnea, or dysphagia. These patients may be at risk of respiratory failure or aspiration.

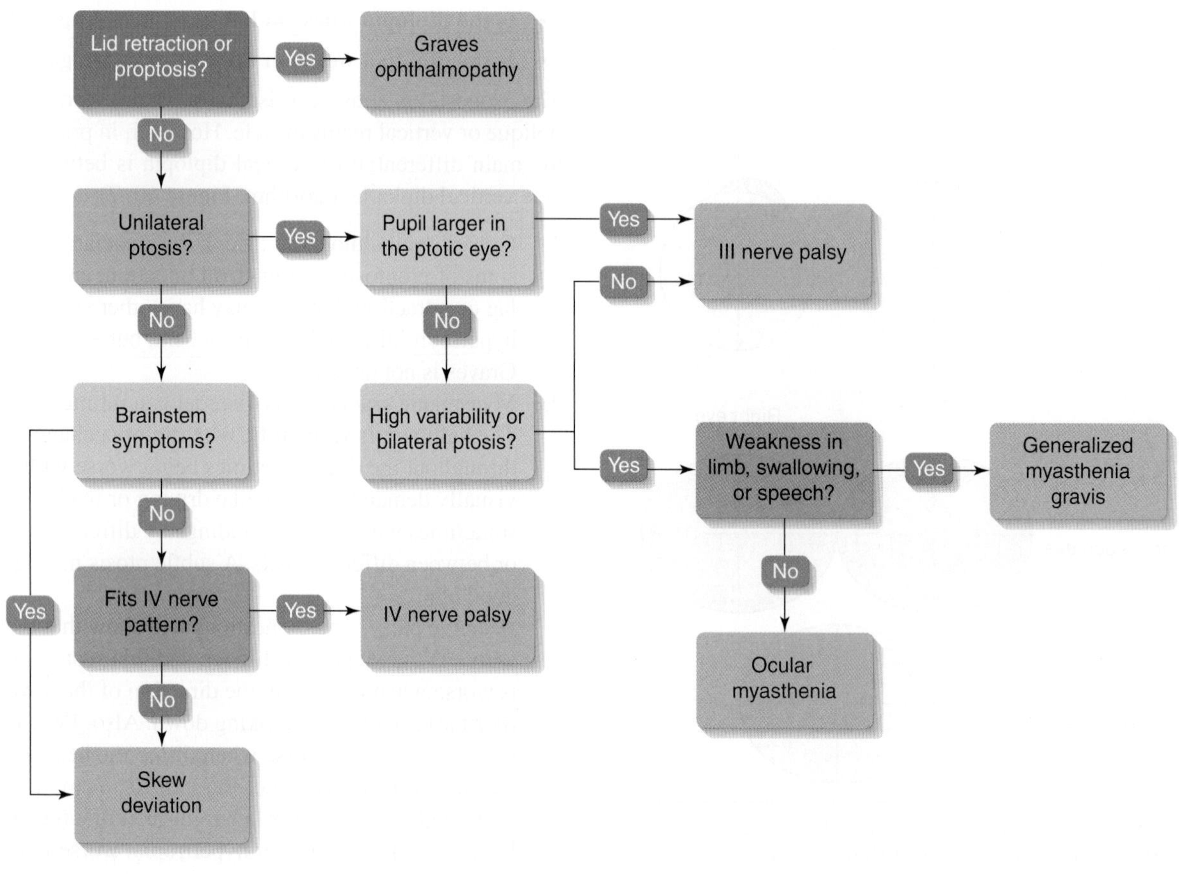

FIGURE 60–7 Diagnostic approach: Vertical diplopia.

- If painful diplopia is present, always obtain neuroimaging to screen for the possibility of a parasellar mass, infection, or cerebral aneurysm.
- If a patient has mild ocular motor weakness that causes diplopia only in one or a few directions of gaze, he or she may say that the diplopia is intermittent. However, if the diplopia is always present when looking in that direction, the problem is not really intermittent but persistent.
- The history of onset is not useful in trying to determine whether the problem is an acute or chronically progressive one. Diplopia is either there or it is not. What is more useful is to determine whether the *distance* between the 2 images has been gradually increasing with time. Another gauge of progression is that, if diplopia is present only when looking in a certain direction, the patient does not have to look as far over to that side before starting to seeing double. Similarly, a patient with a progressive VI nerve palsy may note that initially he or she had to look far into the distance to appreciate the doubling, but now it is apparent for objects that are a lot closer.
- The "Pupil Rule": Cranial nerve III innervates the lid, the pupil constrictor, and all extraocular muscles except the lateral rectus and superior oblique, If a patient has a complete III nerve palsy except for completely normal pupil function (ie, same size as other pupil in both light and dark), as in Figure 60–3, then this is very unlikely to be due to a cerebral aneurysm pressing on the III nerve.[8] This is because the location of the pupil fibers in the III nerve makes them prone to compression by an adjacent aneurysm.

PROGNOSIS

This depends on the cause of diplopia. Patients with ocular myopathy generally have a very slowly progressive diplopia. This is particularly true of Graves ophthalmopathy. Occasionally this disease leads to more rapid orbital mass effect with risk of corneal exposure and compressive optic neuropathy. Paradoxically, the latter may be more likely in those with less impressive proptosis. Monitoring with regular visual field examinations is a good idea.

A diagnosis of ocular myasthenia is important, because 50% of these patients will progress to generalized myasthenia (80% of these doing so within 2 years of diagnosis).[9] As such, one must follow these patients carefully, particularly regarding their risk of respiratory failure or aspiration.

Cranial neuropathies are most often microvascular, and most patients recover spontaneously within 12 to 14 weeks. Aneurysms are less common, but one must promptly identify and treat aneurysms because of a high risk of subarachnoid hemorrhage and death.

Infections are usually from meningitis and require specific treatment. Neoplastic palsies are usually due to benign tumors in the region of the cavernous sinus and thus progress slowly. Carcinomatous or lymphomatous involvement is rare but usually implies meningeal or bony disease with poor survival, regardless of intervention.

Brainstem causes of double vision are most frequently strokes and carry the long-term prognostic characteristics of cerebrovascular disease. Diplopia from a limited stroke that causes few other symptoms can do well, with frequent recovery over weeks, but may persist. Management must really focus on long-term stroke risk management.

CASE SCENARIO | Resolution

A 40-year-old woman presents with sudden diplopia and bad headache while at work. She notes that the left image is higher than the right one and that the images get further apart when she looks up, down, or to the left. On examination, she has an exotropia and left hypotropia when looking straight ahead, and there is reduced adduction, depression, and elevation of the right eye.

ADDITIONAL HISTORY

An ocular motor examination is not complete without examining the lid and the pupil. In this case, there is also a mild right ptosis and anisocoria that is greater in bright light, with the right pupil being the larger one.

The patient has limited function of the medial rectus, superior rectus, and inferior rectus, as well as the levator palpebrae superioris and pupil constrictor muscle. This strongly suggests a right III nerve palsy.

Question: What is the most likely diagnosis?

A. Microvascular III nerve palsy from incipient diabetes
B. Ocular myasthenia
C. Compressive III nerve palsy from an aneurysm
D. Compressive III nerve palsy from pituitary apoplexy
E. Ophthalmoplegic migraine

Test Your Knowledge

1. A 45-year-old man has noted horizontal double vision when driving, starting about 15 minutes after he gets in the car, for about a month. It seems to be getting more frequent. He never has double vision when reading. He has no other complaints. When seen, he also appears to have a slight ptosis on the left.

   Which of the following would be useful signs to evaluate? (You may select more than one answer.)

   A. Anisocoria
   B. Increase in ptosis after prolonged up gaze
   C. Weakness of eyelid closure
   D. Dysarthric speech
   E. Effect of head tilt on his double vision

2. A 39-year-old woman awoke 6 weeks ago with horizontal diplopia that was worse looking to the left. She was seen in the emergency department when it started and had a normal noncontrast computed tomography scan of her head. She was told it was a small stroke of her VI nerve and that it would improve in a few months.

   Which of the following would you consider alarming? (You may select more than one answer.)

   A. Double vision is still present when one eye is covered.
   B. The 2 images are slowly getting further apart.
   C. She has new facial pain and numbness of her cheek.
   D. She has long-standing migraines with scalp tenderness.
   E. She has diabetes.

3. A 30-year-old man with a prior history of hyperthyroidism presents now with a few months of double vision.

   Which sign would be *inconsistent* with Graves ophthalmopathy?

   A. Ptosis
   B. Horizontal diplopia worse in far gaze
   C. Vertical diplopia worse in up gaze
   D. Proptosis
   E. Conjunctival injection

References

1. Bartley G, Gorman C. Diagnostic criteria for Graves' ophthalmopathy. *Am J Ophthalmol.* 1995;119:792–795.
2. Barton JJS, Fouladvand M. Ocular aspects of myasthenia gravis. *Semin Neurol.* 2000;20:7–20.
3. Berlit P. Isolated and combined pareses of cranial nerves III, IV and VI. A retrospective review of 412 patients. *J Neurol Sci.* 1991;103:10–15.
4. Green W, Hackett E, Schlezinger N. Neuro-ophthalmologic evaluation of oculomotor nerve paralysis. *Arch Ophthalmol.* 1964;72:154–167.
5. Richards BW, Jones FR, Younge BR. Causes and prognosis in 4278 cases of paralysis of the oculomotor, trochlear, and abducens cranial nerves. *Am J Ophthalmol.* 1992;113:489–496.
6. Keane J. Ocular skew deviation. Analysis of 100 cases. *Arch Neurol.* 1975;32:185–190
7. Kodsi SR, Younge BR. Acquired oculomotor, trochlear and abducent cranial nerve palsies in pediatric patients. *Am J Ophthalmol.* 1992;114:568–574.
8. Nadeau S, Trobe J. Pupil sparing in oculomotor palsy: a brief review. *Ann Neurol.* 1983;13:143–148.
9. Bever CJ, Aquino A, Penn A, Lovelace RE, Rowland LP. Prognosis of ocular myasthenia. *Ann Neurol.* 1983;14:516–519.

Suggested Reading

Acierno M. Vertical diplopia. *Semin Neurol.* 2000;20:21–30.

Barton JJS. Infranuclear and nuclear ocular motor palsies. In: Rosen ES, Eustace P, Thompson HS, Cumming WJK, eds. *Neuro-ophthalmology*. London, UK: Mosby, 1998:15.1–15.13.

Barton JJS. Neuroophthalmology III: eye movements. In: Joynt R, Griggs R, eds. *Baker's Clinical Neurology*. CD-ROM. Philadelphia, PA: Lippincott-Williams & Wilkins, 2002.

Leigh RJ, Zee DS. The diagnosis of peripheral ocular motor palsies and strabismus. In: *The Neurology of Eye Movements*. 3rd ed. Oxford, UK: Oxford University Press, 1999:321–404.

Chapter 61

Gait Abnormalities

Jeff Wiese, MD, and Michelle Guidry, MD

CASE SCENARIO

A 34-year-old man comes to your office because he is "having a hard time walking." Two weeks ago, he noticed "weakness" in his right leg that has changed the way he walks.

- **What additional questions would you ask to characterize his gait abnormality?**
- **What are the 5 physiologic components essential to normal ambulation?**
- **Can a definitive cause of his gait abnormality be determined by historical information alone?**
- **What historical questions will be useful in determining the appropriate evaluation of his gait abnormality?**

INTRODUCTION

Ambulation (gait) is an exercise in controlled falling. The upright body falls forward and the outstretched foot and leg must prevent the body from falling by supporting the body's weight and rotating the weight over the limb. Gait abnormalities result from 1 of 5 disorders:

1. Inadequate muscle strength to flex the hip (to raise the knee), flex the knee (to lift the foot), or dorsiflex the ankle (to keep the foot from dragging on the ground).
2. Inadequate sensation in the foot (or excess sensation with neuropathies) to tell the brain when the foot has planted and is ready for the body to rotate over the limb.
3. Inadequate muscle strength in the leg to maintain extension of the leg (knee) to support the body's weight.
4. Inability to relax the muscles of the leg as the body moves over the extended leg and transfers weight to the opposite leg (in preparation for extending the leg for the next step).
5. Disorders of the cerebellum, which normally receives sensory input and coordinates muscle contraction (the stepping limb) and relaxation (the opposite limb).

KEY TERMS

Ataxia	Unbalanced or uncoordinated ambulation.
Cerebellar ataxia	Ataxia due to impaired cerebellar function.
Normal-pressure hydrocephalus	A triad of dementia, ataxia, and urinary incontinence that results from obstruction of the arachnoid granulations that drain cerebrospinal fluid. The fluid accumulation compresses the brain, causing the symptoms.
Peripheral neuropathy	Abnormal sensory or motor nerve function leading to weakness, altered sensory perception, or both.
Sensory ataxia	Ataxia due to impaired proprioceptive or sensory feedback from the lower extremities.
Spastic paraplegia	Tonic muscular contraction leading to an inability to relax the muscles. The increased tone is due to damage of the inhibitory neurons in the spinal cord or brain.

ETIOLOGY

Gait disorders result from disease of muscles, nerves, bones and joints, or the cerebellum.

GETTING STARTED WITH THE HISTORY

- Review the patient's past medical history. Most gait abnormalities are due to chronic or congenital diseases.
- Assess the time course of the symptoms. Acute changes in gait suggest an injury or stroke. A gradual, protracted onset suggests a systemic disease, peripheral neuropathy, or cerebellar disease of any type.
- Avoid leading questions. It may be necessary to follow-up with a close-ended questions directed at the most likely disorder.

INTERVIEW FRAMEWORK

- Assess for alarm symptoms.
- Ask about conditions that make the gait abnormality worse (ie, walking in darkness or walking upstairs).
- Ask about weakness involving other parts of the body (ie, the arms, neck).
- Ask about sensory abnormalities involving other parts of the body.
- Ask about alcohol and drug use.
- Take a thorough dietary history.
- Determine the temporal pattern and duration of symptoms, accompanying symptoms, and precipitating factors.

IDENTIFYING ALARM SYMPTOMS

Outside of spinal cord impingement and stroke, gait abnormalities are rarely a life-threatening condition. For all cases of gait abnormalities, a sudden onset of the abnormality is alarming; the less serious etiologies, such as degenerative joint disease, are insidious in onset. Chronic neurologic degenerative diseases, such as parkinsonism and cerebellar degeneration, are also insidious.

Alarm Symptoms	Consider
Use of injection drugs Recent bacterial infection Fever	Spinal cord impingement from an epidural or spinal abscess
History of cancer Incontinence Numbness in your buttocks and groin area (saddle anesthesia)	Spinal cord impingement from a metastatic malignancy
Atrial fibrillation Hypertension History of stroke Lost vision Arm weakness	Stroke
Incontinence Decline in thinking ability (ask family members)	Normal-pressure hydrocephalus
Chest pain Hypertension	Aortic dissection causing spinal cord ischemia

Serious Diagnoses

- Spinal cord impingement by tumor or infection
- Stroke
- Normal-pressure hydrocephalus
- Aortic dissection causing spinal cord ischemia

FOCUSED QUESTIONS

Causes of Muscle Weakness

See Chapter 13 (Muscle Weakness) for causes of muscle weakness. It is important to distinguish whether the weakness is isolated to one muscle (traumatic injury, radiculopathy), one limb (stroke), or both limbs (systemic disease or spinal cord disease).

QUESTIONS	THINK ABOUT...
When you walk, do you waddle like a duck? *Are other parts of your body weak?*	**Gluteal or quadriceps weakness:** To begin walking, the body must lift the leg to keep it from dragging on the ground. To do this, the hip must be raised by contraction of the gluteal (buttocks) and quadriceps muscles. If either is weak, the patient swings the leg laterally to keep it from dragging, creating a gait that resembles the waddle of a duck.
When you walk, do you feel as if you are walking up steps?	**Damage to the peroneal nerve:** Weakness of dorsiflexion due to peroneal nerve damage prevents the patient from lifting the toes as he or she moves forward. The patient will compensate by lifting the knee higher than normal to lift the foot so that the toes clear the ground. This has the appearance of the patient walking up steps.
Have you had recent surgery? Have you had trauma to the lower extremity?	**Damage to the peroneal nerve:** Occurs commonly following trauma to the lower extremity or surgery during which the patient's leg has become pinned against the bed rail, paralyzing the peroneal nerve.
Are you unable to stand prior to initiating gait?	**Systemic weakness** (see Chapter 13)

Sensory Abnormalities

QUESTIONS	THINK ABOUT...
Do you slap your feet down as you walk? *Do you walk with a wider stance than normal?* *Describe your diet. Are you a strict (vegan) vegetarian? (vitamin B_{12} deficiency)* *Have you had unprotected sex or a history of sexually transmitted diseases? (Syphilis)* *Do you have a history of diabetes?* *Do you consume excessive amounts of alcohol?*	**Sensory abnormality:** Normal gait requires adequate position sense, which is accomplished by proprioceptive input from the leg muscles. Disease of the dorsal columns (eg, vitamin B_{12} deficiency, syphilis, diabetes mellitus) impairs proprioception, causing the patient to fall. To increase stability, the patient widens the distance between the legs while walking. The patient may also slap the feet down to increase sensory input.
Is your gait worse with the eyes closed?	**Dorsal column disease:** Visual input compensates for lack of proprioceptive sensory input.
Is your gait equally bad with eyes open or closed?	**Cerebellar dysfunction**
Do your feet hurt or burn as you walk?	**Hyperesthetic gait (due to a sensory neuropathy):** With hyperesthesia, the patient walks as if on hot coals (antalgic gait); similar to walking on a foot after it has fallen asleep (pins and needles).

Inability to Relax Muscles

All causes of spastic paraparesis are due to upper motor neuron disease (from the cerebral cortex to the anterior horn).

QUESTIONS	THINK ABOUT...
Do you have trouble getting yourself going forward when you try to walk? (Festination) *Do you have trouble stopping yourself once you begin walking? (Propulsion)* *Do you walk in small steps?*	**Parkinsonism:** Motor output to legs is chronically hyperstimulated. The muscles are tonically contracted, making it difficult to relax and allow the leg to be lifted as the patient tries to extend it forward during gait. To compensate, the patient takes small, short steps like a wind-up robot (march à petite pas).
Were there any complications associated with your birth? *Do you have a history of multiple sclerosis?*	**Spastic paraplegia:** The legs are locked in spastic contraction. The patient takes short steps with toes never leaving the floor. The knees cross and rub against each other as the patient moves forward, like the blades of a scissors (scissors gait). The most common causes of this gait are cerebral palsy and multiple sclerosis.
Have you experienced a decline in the sharpness of your thinking ability? *Have you had difficulty holding your urine?* *When you walk, do you feel like your feet are magnetically "stuck" to the floor?*	**Normal-pressure hydrocephalus:** A disease of older patients characterized by dementia, urinary incontinence, and apraxia. The characteristic gait is sometimes called an apraxic gait.

Cerebellar Disorders

QUESTIONS	THINK ABOUT...
Have you noticed difficulty keeping your balance? *Do you consume alcohol on a regular basis?* *Do you have a history of lung cancer?*	Cerebellar disease: The midline cerebellum (vermis) processes proprioceptive input from the legs and adjusts motor input to the legs accordingly. When damaged or impaired (by alcohol), the patient cannot make fine motor adjustments to keep moving forward, resulting in truncal imbalance.
When you walk, do you stumble from side to side as you try to move forward?	Acute intoxication, especially from alcohol
When you walk, do you consistently deviate or "fall" toward one side?	Unilateral cerebellar disease (eg, tumor, abscess, hematoma)

DIAGNOSTIC APPROACH (INCLUDING ALGORITHM)

See Figure 61–1 for the diagnostic approach algorithm for gait abnormalities.

CAVEATS

- The observed pattern of gait abnormalities can be a helpful clue to the etiology.
- The gait of the malingering patient is characterized by wide swings from left to right, hitting the walls of the hall as the patient moves forward.
- The malingering patient will lurch from the hips (maintaining enough control to avoid falling until he means to), whereas the patient with cerebellar disease will lurch from the knees.
- Unless intoxicated, patients with cerebellar damage will consistently deviate to one side of the hall (the side of the lesion).

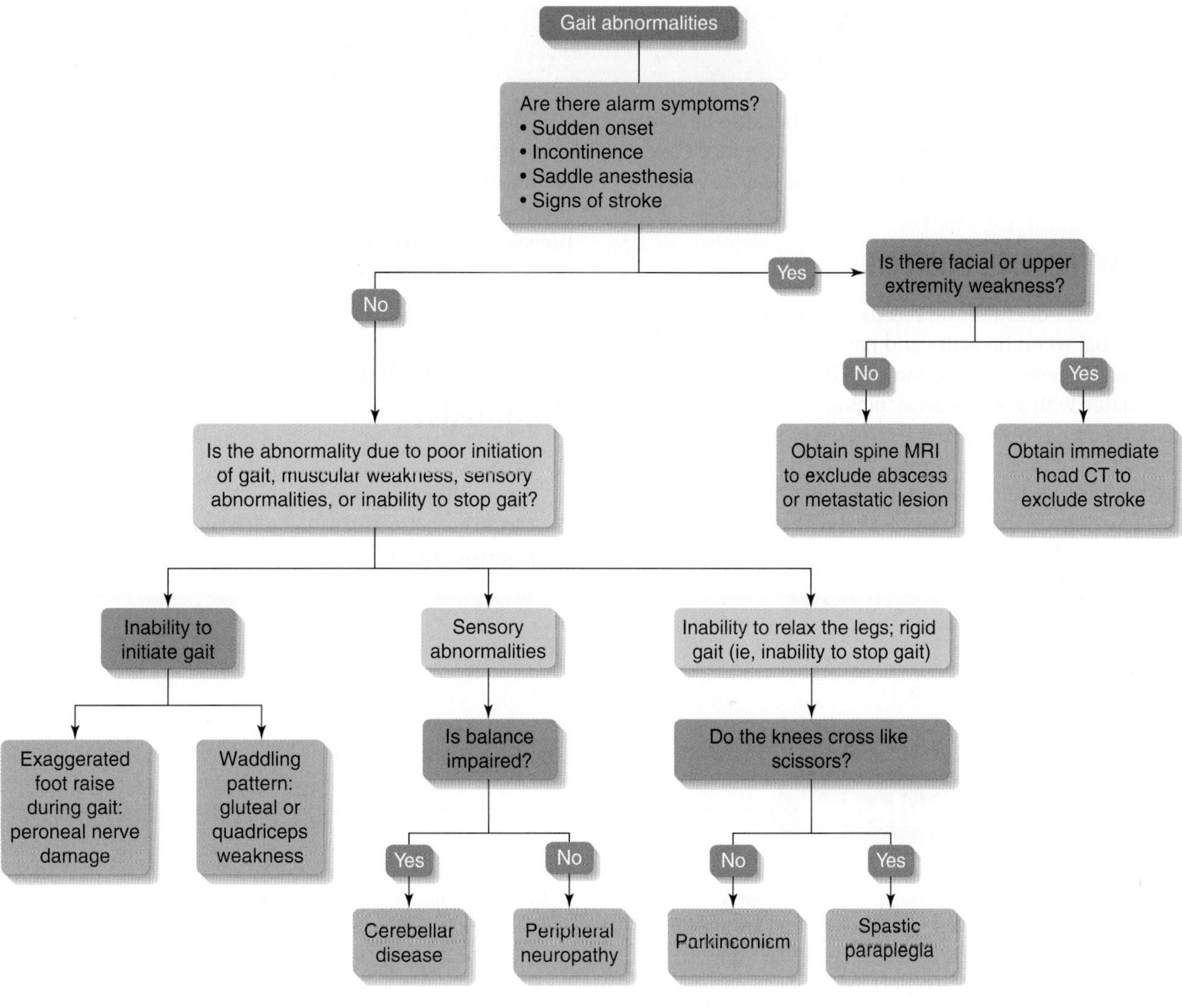

FIGURE 61–1 Diagnostic approach: Gait abnormalities. CT, computed tomography; MRI, magnetic resonance imaging.

- Do not assume that the cerebellum is healthy because the patient can successfully perform finger-to-nose and heel-shin testing, which tests only the appendicular or lateral cerebellar hemispheres. All patients should have their ambulation observed if cerebellar disease is suspected; this tests the vermicular or midline cerebellum.

PROGNOSIS

The prognosis of gait abnormalities depends on the underlying disease.

CASE SCENARIO | Resolution

A 34-year-old man comes to your office because he is "having a hard time walking." Two weeks ago, he noticed "weakness" in his right leg that has changed the way he walks.

ADDITIONAL HISTORY

The patient notes that he has to raise his right leg higher than usual when he walks and has to "throw his right foot forward" in order to keep moving. The gait abnormality is associated with a sensation of "pins and needles" in his right foot. He denies trauma to the right leg or similar symptoms in the past, although 2 months ago he began having trouble "picking up things" with his left hand. This weakness has improved but is still present. He reports no problems with balance.

His past medical history includes advanced human immunodeficiency virus (HIV) infection, for which he is taking highly active antiretroviral medications, as well as prophylactic antimicrobial therapy. He has had no opportunistic infections or complications of HIV infection. He does not drink or smoke tobacco and denies environmental exposures.

Question: What is the most likely diagnosis?

A. Stroke
B. Cerebellar degeneration
C. Mononeuritis multiplex with peroneal nerve palsy
D. Parkinsonism

Test Your Knowledge

1. A 62-year-old woman is brought to the emergency department. Two days ago, she noted the sudden inability to get out of bed due to "weakness in my legs." She subsequently called her daughter, who brought the patient to the hospital. The patient notes no previous episodes of weakness. The weakness is localized to both legs and is associated with urinary incontinence and back pain. She has a history of moderate alcohol use and a 30 pack-year history of smoking. She has no prior medical history, although she has not seen a doctor in several years. She takes no medications.
   Which of the following is the most appropriate next diagnostic step?
   A. Computed tomography (CT) of the head
   B. Magnetic resonance imaging (MRI) of the spine
   C. Nerve conduction studies
   D. Lumbar puncture for oligoclonal bands

2. A 54-year-old man presents with a 3-month history of gait abnormalities characterized as "unsteadiness when I walk." He notes that the abnormality is persistent but worse at night, resulting in several falls upon ambulating to the bathroom. He also reports associated numbness in his feet but no leg weakness. He has hypertension and a 10 pack-year tobacco history. He has consumed a 6-pack of beer each day for many years.
   What is the most likely cause of his gait abnormality?
   A. Stroke
   B. Early-onset Parkinson's disease
   C. Cerebellar degeneration
   D. Multiple sclerosis
   E. Peripheral neuropathy

3. A 72-year-old man presents for evaluation of "inability to walk the way that he used to." Although the patient has no complaints, his daughter describes his gate as slower than normal. She says he has a hard time getting started when they walk together, and even when he gets going, he walks with "little steps." He reports no other symptoms, although his daughter is concerned about several recent "choking fits" following meals.
   What is the most likely diagnosis?
   A. Parkinson's disease
   B. Spastic paraplegia
   C. Wilson's disease
   D. Stroke
   E. Huntington's disease

Suggested Reading

Jackson GR, Owsley C. Visual dysfunction, neurodegenerative diseases, and aging. *Neurol Clin*. 2003;21:709–728.

Mayer M. Neurophysiological and kinesiological aspects of spastic gait: the need for a functional approach. *Funct Neurol*. 2002;17:11–17.

Mayeux R. Epidemiology of neurodegeneration. *Annu Rev Neurosci*. 2003;26:81–104.

Nielsen JB, Sinkjaer T. Afferent feedback in the control of human gait. *J Electromyogr Kinesiol*. 2002;12:213–217.

Patrick JH. Case for gait analysis as part of the management of incomplete spinal cord injury. *Spinal Cord*. 2003;41:479–482.

Rietman JS, Postema K, Geertzen JH. Gait analysis in prosthetics: opinions, ideas and conclusions. *Prosthet Orthot Int*. 2002;26:50–57.

Rodda J, Graham HK. Classification of gait patterns in spastic hemiplegia and spastic diplegia: a basis for a management algorithm. *Eur J Neurol*. 2001;8(Suppl 5):98–108.

Wilder RP, Wind TC, Jones EV, Crider BE, Edlich RF. Functional electrical stimulation for a dropped foot. *J Long Term Eff Med Implants*. 2002;12:149–159.

Chapter 62

Tremor

Laurie Gordon, MD, and Daniel Tarsy, MD

CASE SCENARIO

A 45-year-old man comes to your office for evaluation of tremor. He started to notice the tremor recently, when he began building model airplanes with his son and had difficulty doing the fine motor tasks required for this hobby. His son has been making jokes about the shaking to his mother, who was concerned about this new tremor and scheduled an appointment for her husband to see you.

- **What additional questions should you ask to gather more details regarding his tremor?**
- **How do you classify tremors?**
- **What warning symptoms can help you determine if this is indicative of a concerning disease or something more benign?**
- **How do you determine the cause of his tremor through the history?**

INTRODUCTION

Tremor is the most common movement disorder of adult life.[1] In most cases, it is secondary to either essential tremor or Parkinson's disease. Patients often seek medical attention due to concern about possible Parkinson's disease or another serious illness. The most common etiology is essential tremor, although there are many other causes of tremor in adults.

Although the physical examination is important in the evaluation of tremor, the history alone can provide the necessary clues to a correct diagnosis. The initial approach is to first determine whether it occurs primarily with rest, holding a posture, or action. This will narrow the differential diagnosis and allow for a more directed history. Although a few alarm symptoms indicate the need for urgent assessment of tremor, the evaluation usually occurs in the outpatient setting.

KEY TERMS

Tremor	A rhythmic oscillation of antagonist groups of muscles, in either an alternating or synchronous fashion.
Action tremor	An oscillation that occurs or increases during voluntary movement, generally of midrange frequency (6–8 Hz). Also called kinetic tremor.
Postural tremor	An oscillation that occurs while maintaining a fixed posture against gravity or during other fixed postures (clenched fist, standing), generally at a higher frequency (8–14 Hz).
Rest tremor	An oscillation that occurs with the affected body part at rest, during no action (voluntary contraction of muscles) and without resisting gravity, generally at a lower frequency (3–6 Hz).
Intention tremor	A type of action tremor in which an oscillation occurs orthogonal to the direction of movement and increases in amplitude as the target is approached. Usually denotes disease of the cerebellum and/or its connections.
Physiologic tremor	Irregular oscillations of 8–10 Hz occurring during maintenance of a posture, which usually disappear when the eyes are closed or a gravity load is placed on the muscles. By definition, mild physiologic tremor may be a normal finding and is common in the general population.

—Continued next page

Continued—

Enhanced physiologic tremor	Physiologic tremor is increased in amplitude due to fatigue, sleep deprivation, treatment with certain drugs, some endocrine disorders, caffeine use, or stress.
Essential tremor	Isolated postural or action tremor involving the hands and sometimes the head and voice without other neurologic findings. Genetically determined with a positive family history ("familial tremor") in approximately 50% of cases.
Parkinsonian tremor	Rest tremor that usually has a very regular "pill-rolling" quality and is frequently, but not always, associated with other symptoms of Parkinson's disease (stiffness, slowness, gait changes).
Task-specific tremor	A tremor elicited by a specific task, such as speaking or writing.

ETIOLOGY (INCLUDING PREVALENCE OF VARIOUS CAUSES)

Although many tremors are actually physiologic or enhanced physiologic tremors, pathologic tremors due to neurologic disorders are most commonly secondary to essential tremor (if postural or kinetic) or Parkinson's disease (if a rest tremor). It is important to determine whether tremor is the primary condition or secondary to another neurologic cause, such as toxic, metabolic, structural, or vascular abnormalities.

Differential Diagnosis

	Prevalence[a]
Primary tremors	
Essential tremor	0.4%–0.9%[1,b]
Parkinson's disease	0.01%–0.4%[2,c]
Parkinsonian syndromes	
• Multiple system atrophy (MSA)	0.002%–0.007%[3]
• Progressive supranuclear palsy (PSP)	0.0003%–0.008%[3,4]
Wilson's disease	0.002%–0.003%[5–7]
Dystonic tremor	
Psychogenic tremor	
Cerebellar dysfunction	
Midbrain tremor (rubral)	
Secondary tremors	
Medications (see following box)	
Fatigue, anxiety, fear	

[a]In the general population; prevalence data are unavailable when not indicated.

[b]Increasing with age; prevalence 4.6%–6.3% for age ≥ 65 years.[1]

[c]Increasing with age; prevalence 1.6% for age ≥ 65 years.[8]

Medications That May Cause Tremor

Adrenergic Agents	Miscellaneous
Amphetamines	Lithium
Bronchodilators	Corticosteroids
β-Adrenergic agonists	Antipsychotic drugs
Peripheral vasoconstrictors	Caffeine
Tricyclic antidepressants	Cyclosporine
Serotonin reuptake inhibitors	Valproic acid
	Amiodarone
	Levothyroxine

GETTING STARTED WITH THE HISTORY

As with any chief complaint, encourage the patient to tell the history as much as possible in his or her own words. Try to prevent the patient from simply showing you the tremor.

Questions	Remember
What brings you into the office? *What made you decide to come in at this time?* *What concerns you about the tremor?* *Tell me more about the tremor.*	Establishes tremor as the complaint and delineates activities affected, progression and acuity, and the patient's concerns and goals for the visit, while encouraging the patient to tell his or her own story.

INTERVIEW FRAMEWORK

There are 3 main goals in eliciting a tremor history: identifying alarm symptoms, determining tremor type (resting, postural, or action), and recognizing associated symptoms that will help establish a diagnosis.

Inquire about the following tremor characteristics:

- Onset
- Progression
- Quality (rest, postural, action)
- Location
- Effect on daily function
- Associated symptoms
- Aggravating and alleviating factors

IDENTIFYING ALARM SYMPTOMS

Tremor is rarely an emergency, but the following features suggest that a serious diagnosis should be considered and indicate urgent evaluation:

1. Recent, sudden onset (within hours to days)
2. Rapid progression (over hours to days)
3. Exposure to new medications, controlled substances, intoxicants, or toxins
4. Associated with sudden alteration in mental status
5. Underlying disease (such as cancer or immunodeficiency), particularly in association with any of the above

Alarm Symptoms[a]	Serious Causes	Benign Causes
R, P, A with altered mental status, seizures, cardiac problems	Intoxication or toxic exposure Iatrogenic (lithium, corticosteroids) Metabolic derangement (hypoglycemia, hyponatremia, hyperthyroidism, hypocalcemia)	Enhanced physiologic tremor Psychogenic Medication-related (eg, β-agonists, levothyroxine, valproic acid)
R, P, A with new-onset hemiparesis, sensory loss, diplopia, or dysarthria	Structural central nervous system (CNS) lesion (stroke, tumor, abscess)	Enhanced physiologic tremor Peripheral neuropathy Psychogenic
P, A with anxiety, emotional lability, pain	Alcohol or drug withdrawal	Enhanced physiologic tremor Essential tremor Anxiety Stress

A, action; P, postural; R, resting.

[a]Tremor type with associated symptoms.

All serious diagnoses do not require emergency evaluation, for example, Parkinson's disease, PSP, MSA, Wilson's disease, or normal-pressure hydrocephalus. However, the latter 2 diagnoses are essential to consider because they are potentially reversible.

FOCUSED QUESTIONS

Although the patient can provide much of the history on his or her own, focused questions will help to clarify the features of the tremor, as well as to more precisely identify the diagnosis.

QUESTIONS	THINK ABOUT...
Chief complaint	
What brings you to the office today?	Goals of evaluation may be different with different patients; some just want reassurance that they do not have a serious condition, others would like a diagnosis, others have dysfunction from their tremor and seek treatment, and in some cases, the tremor has suddenly worsened.
Onset	
When and how did the tremor start? How was it first noticed?	Often people seek medical help because a spouse or coworker has noticed an abnormal movement.
• *It started suddenly.*	Consider acute-onset tremor and ask about alarm symptoms as above. Stroke, structural lesion, intoxication, psychogenic tremor
• *It just started (hours to days).*	Consider acute-onset tremor and ask about alarm symptoms as listed above. Stroke, structural lesion, intoxication, toxic exposure, metabolic derangement, psychogenic tremor

• *It began shortly after I started a new medication.*	May be medication related, due to enhanced physiologic tremor, metabolic derangement
• *I first noticed it several years ago.*	Enhanced physiologic tremor, essential tremor, Parkinson's disease/parkinsonism, peripheral neuropathy
• *I've had it for as long as I can remember.*	Enhanced physiologic tremor, essential tremor
• *It began just after a stressful time/event.*	Psychogenic tremor
Progression	
How has the tremor changed over time?	Many tremors are progressive over time.
• *It has gradually gotten worse.*	Essential tremor, Parkinson's disease/parkinsonism, Wilson's disease, task-specific tremor
• *It has not changed at all.*	Enhanced physiologic tremor, dystonic tremor, task-specific tremor
• *It involves other body parts.*	Essential tremor, Parkinson's disease/parkinsonism
• *It was unilateral and now is bilateral.*	Parkinson's disease (most commonly begins as a unilateral tremor)
Quality	
When do you notice the tremor? When you are completely at rest (lying down before sleep), when you are holding a posture, or with action?	First allow the patient to tell you when the tremor is visible. You may need to prompt the patient with further questions to clarify.
• *At rest (sitting in a chair, watching television, lying down to sleep)*	Parkinson's disease, parkinsonism (MSA, PSP, neuroleptic use)
• *With posture (holding something or maintaining a pose)*	Essential tremor, Parkinson's disease/parkinsonism, enhanced physiologic tremor, metabolic derangements, toxic exposure, intoxication, structural lesions, peripheral neuropathy
• *With action (drinking, eating, writing, putting on makeup, getting dressed).*	Essential tremor, dystonic tremor, central lesion such as stroke, multiple sclerosis, or mass (cerebellar pathways)
• *With action when reaching the target*	Cerebellum or its connections
• *With only one specific action*	Task-specific tremor
• *With walking only*	Parkinson's disease/parkinsonism, orthostatic tremor (if in the legs only)
Location	
Where is the tremor? Is it unilateral or bilateral? Is it in your arms, legs, head, face, jaw, or voice?	The patient may specify the location that causes the most concern or dysfunction (ie, the dominant hand) and may need prompting to mention additional tremor locations.
• *Unilateral or asymmetric*	Parkinson's disease, dystonic tremor, structural, multiple sclerosis, peripheral neuropathy, psychogenic
• *Bilateral and symmetric*	Essential tremor, enhanced physiologic tremor, parkinsonism (MSA, PSP, neuroleptic use)
• *The hand(s)/arm(s)*	Most tremors primarily affect the upper extremities.

—Continued next page

Continued—	
• *The legs only*	Orthostatic tremor
• *The jaw or face*	Parkinson's disease/parkinsonism
• *The head*	Essential tremor, dystonic tremor
• *The voice*	Essential tremor
Functional impact	
How has the tremor affected you?	
• *It is embarrassing.*	Most frequent complaint with a rest tremor because it does not impact actions
• *I have difficulty reading the newspaper.*	Seen with both postural and rest tremors
• *I spill my food and drink.*	Essential tremor, cerebellar dysfunction
• *My handwriting is illegible.*	Essential tremor, cerebellar dysfunction, CNS lesion, task-specific tremor, dystonic tremor
• *I feel uncomfortable standing.*	Orthostatic tremor
Associated symptoms	
Do you have any other problems with movement?	
• *Stiffness (difficulty getting up from a chair, car, or rolling over in bed)*	Parkinson's disease/parkinsonism (rigidity)
• *Slowness of movement (walking, eating, writing)*	Parkinson's disease/parkinsonism (bradykinesia)
• *Brushing teeth, cutting food, tying shoes, doing buttons, tying a tie, washing hair*	Parkinson's disease/parkinsonism (bradykinesia)
• *Weakness of an arm or leg*	Structural lesion
• *Incoordination*	Parkinson's disease/parkinsonism (bradykinesia), essential tremor, cerebellar dysfunction, intoxication
Do you have any problems walking or recent falls?	
• *Lack of arm swing when walking*	Parkinson's disease/parkinsonism
• *Dragging of a leg*	Parkinson's disease/parkinsonism (bradykinesia), a brain or spinal cord lesion causing weakness
• *Imbalance or falls*	Parkinson's disease/parkinsonism (gait instability), CNS lesion (weakness), cerebellar dysfunction (ataxia)
• *Difficulty getting started or shuffling gait*	Parkinson's disease/parkinsonism
Do you have any problems with urinary incontinence, light-headedness when you stand, sexual dysfunction, changes in bowel or bladder habits, uncontrolled sweating for no specific reason, or difficulty swallowing?	Suggests autonomic dysfunction as occurs in MSA. Urinary incontinence can also be seen in normal-pressure hydrocephalus and with cognitive changes.
Have you had a change in your thinking?	
• *Confusion*	CNS lesions, intoxication
• *Hallucinations*	Parkinsonism (Lewy body dementia)
• *Mild cognitive changes (difficulty with finances, for example)*	Parkinson's disease/parkinsonism, toxic exposure, CNS lesions

Relevant medical history	
Do you have any medical problems, and if so, what medications do you take? *Do you smoke?* *Do you drink a lot of coffee, tea, or soda?*	Many medications and drugs (see Medications That May Cause Tremor box) have adrenergic effects that can cause postural tremors, especially theophylline, β-agonist inhalers, and caffeine.
Have you ever taken medication for hallucinations, psychotic episodes, depression, or mood swings?	Neuroleptic medications (eg, haloperidol, chlorpromazine) may cause any type of tremor: resting, postural, or action.
Have you ever taken metoclopramide for nausea, poor gastric motility, or reflux?	Metoclopramide acts in the same way as the neuroleptic medications mentioned above.
Modifying symptoms	
Does stress, anxiety, or fatigue worsen the tremor?	May occur in all tremor types
Does alcohol improve the tremor?	Essential tremor (about 65%–70% of patients report this)
Additional information	
Does anyone in your family have tremor?	Essential tremor, familial Parkinson's disease, Wilson's disease
Have you been exposed to pesticides (organophosphates), heavy metals (mercury, lead), or other chemicals (manganese, arsenic, carbon monoxide, cyanide, alcohol)?	Toxic exposure

DIAGNOSTIC APPROACH (INCLUDING ALGORITHM)

First, establish acuteness of the onset of tremor. If the tremor had an acute onset or rapid progression, ask about alarm symptoms. Next, establish tremor type (resting, postural, or action). Ask questions to determine whether this is a primary tremor from a neurologic cause (such as from essential tremor or parkinsonism) or whether it could be a secondary tremor from a medical rather than neurologic condition (medication, intoxication, metabolic derangement). Once this is determined, ask more focused questions to narrow the differential diagnosis. See Figure 62–1 for the diagnostic approach algorithm for tremor.

CAVEATS

- The patient will describe his or her tremor in functional terms. The interviewer should break down activities step by step to understand if the tremor occurs at rest, while holding a posture, or during activity.
- Many patients and families have access to a variety of information, especially from the Internet. If the patient describes the tremor as "resting" or "postural," do not be misled. For diagnostic purposes, do not assume the informant is using those terms correctly.
- A rest tremor may re-emerge after several seconds with posture and action, and a severe postural or action tremor may overflow into the resting state. Identify the circumstances when the tremor is most prominent in order to classify it as rest, postural, or action.
- The patient may not want or need treatment so much as the comfort or reassurance of a specific diagnosis and often, specifically, to rule out parkinsonism.
- Stress, common stimulants (eg, caffeine, nicotine), and fatigue commonly cause tremor. Ask about coffee consumption, sleep habits, and stressors if the patient describes an enhanced physiologic tremor. Anything that increases adrenergic effect (eg, fatigue, stress, caffeine, and certain medications) can lead to enhanced physiologic tremor. Similarly, fatigue, stress, and anxiety can worsen any type of tremor.
- Although alcohol and benzodiazepines frequently dampen essential tremor by reducing anxiety, they can reduce other tremor types if they are exacerbated by anxiety.
- Clinicians may not easily distinguish Parkinson's disease from related atypical parkinsonian syndromes (such as MSA and PSP) except at postmortem examination; differentiation often only takes place over time.
- A patient with essential tremor may report a unilateral onset because the dominant hand used for skilled activities was affected.

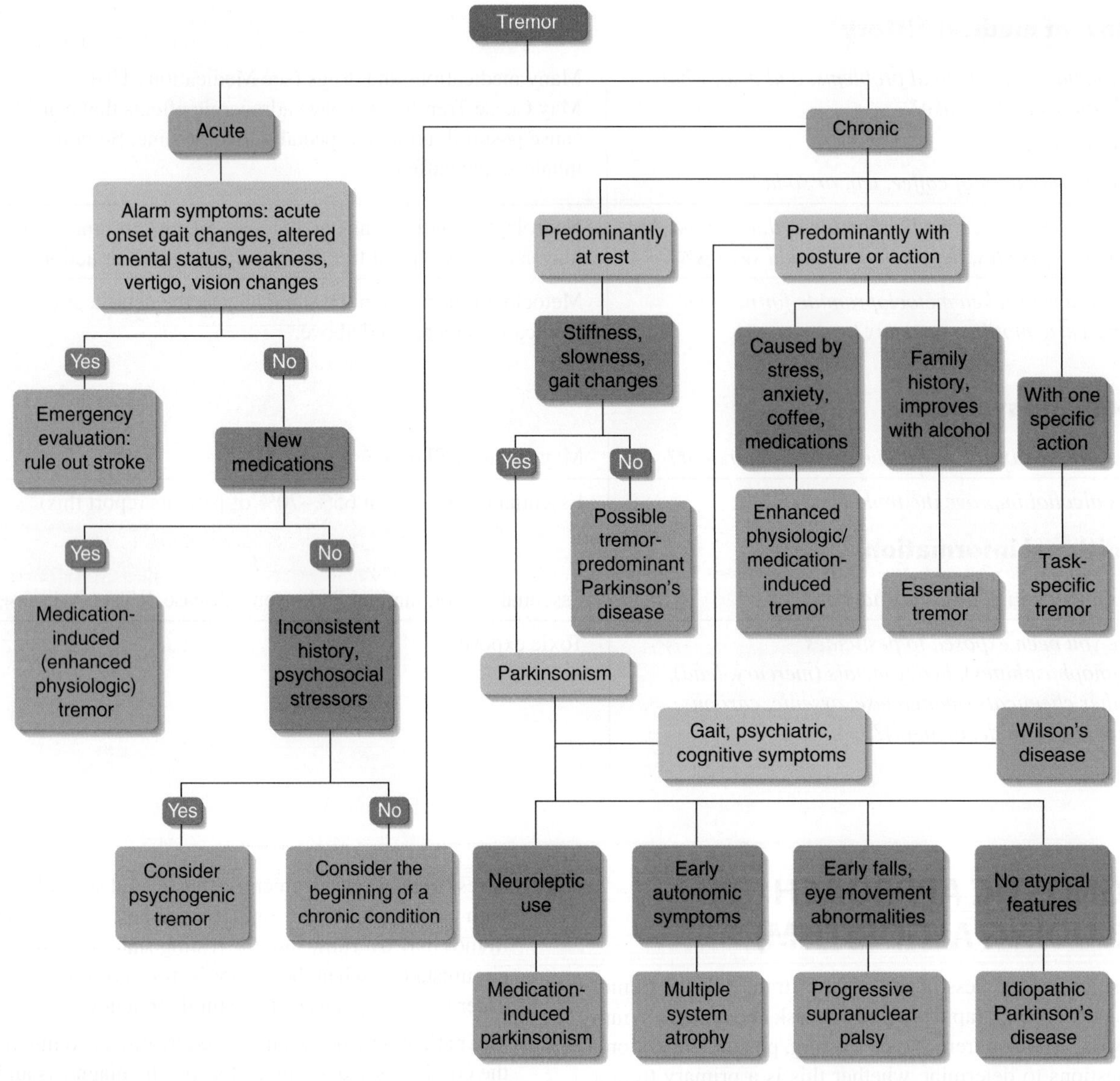

FIGURE 62–1 Diagnostic approach: Tremor.

- Other involuntary movements that may be confused with tremor include:
  - **Myoclonus:** Isolated or serial, high-velocity muscle contractions. Myoclonic jerks are a descriptive term and not a specific diagnosis.
  - **Asterixis:** Sudden, transient, repetitive loss of muscle tone when holding a posture. This is sometimes called "negative myoclonus" and is usually associated with irregular tremor. Asterixis is usually due to decompensated liver disease or other metabolic derangements.
  - **Dystonia:** Fixed spasm of a muscle or group of muscles causing abnormal posturing, which may be associated with an irregular tremor if antagonist muscles are synchronously contracted.
  - **Tic:** Isolated, generally arrhythmic, focal muscle contractions. Usually associated with a premonitory urge and temporary subjective relief.
  - **Athetosis:** An arrhythmic, twisting movement of a limb or limbs.
  - **Chorea:** Another hyperkinetic, involuntary movement causing arrhythmic jerks that are nonpatterned, with unpredictable timing and distribution, more rapid than athetosis. These movements are often incorporated by the patient into what look like voluntary movements.
- History alone may not be able to distinguish between tremor, myoclonus, asterixis, chorea, and other movement disorders. Often this distinction requires physical examination, laboratory findings, and electrophysiologic studies.

PROGNOSIS

Acute tremor usually results from more serious pathology, which ultimately determines prognosis. In primary tremors, prognosis varies, although most tend to progress. Essential tremor, although sometimes called "benign" tremor, can be progressive and debilitating; however, it is not typically associated with the disability of Parkinson's disease and other parkinsonian syndromes. Parkinson's disease has a mean age of onset ranging from 55 to 65 years. PSP and MSA progress more quickly and result in a shorter life expectancy.[3,9] At this time, there are no abortive or regenerative therapies for Parkinson's disease to halt or reverse disease progression. Wilson's disease has a poor prognosis if left untreated but is potentially reversible, so clinicians should consider this diagnosis in any patient with unexplained tremor. Psychogenic tremor has a low rate of remission but a higher reported rate of improvement.[10] The prognosis of secondary tremor from non-neurologic causes depends on the ability to treat the underlying cause but is likely to be good.

CASE SCENARIO | Resolution

A 45-year-old man comes to your office for evaluation of tremor. He started to notice the tremor recently, when he began building model airplanes with his son and had difficulty doing the fine motor tasks required for this hobby. His son has been making jokes about the shaking to his mother, who was concerned about this new tremor and scheduled an appointment for her husband to see you.

ADDITIONAL HISTORY

This tremor is just in his hands and is present in both hands equally. It never occurs when his hands are resting in his lap or when lying in bed before he goes to sleep. He occasionally notices a tremor when doing other things, such as pouring from a full gallon of milk. He had a slight tremor several years ago when building models for the first time, but it was not bothersome to him then. He has one cup of coffee daily, but this has not changed over the last 20 years. He drinks alcohol occasionally but has not noticed an ameliorating effect on his tremor. He has not had any stiffness, slowness, or changes in his gait. He does not have any psychiatric history and denies any problems with his mood now. He is otherwise healthy and does not take any medications. He remembers that his mother had a tremor when she was in her seventies.

Question: What is the most likely diagnosis?

A. Parkinson's disease
B. Enhanced physiologic tremor
C. Essential tremor
D. Task-specific tremor

Test Your Knowledge

1. A 52-year-old right-handed woman comes to see you for evaluation of tremor. It occurs at rest and not with action. It is only in her left hand and so does not affect her function. It has appeared gradually over the last year. She does not have any other symptoms at this time.

   Which of these features is most suggestive of Parkinson's disease rather than essential tremor?

   A. Age
   B. Gradual onset
   C. Presence at rest
   D. Lack of impact on function
   E. Absence of other symptoms

2. A 74-year-old man comes to the emergency room with right hand shaking. It began suddenly this morning and is only present with use. He has also developed difficulty walking; his wife says he is walking like he is drunk. He is also slurring his speech.

   Which of the following is *not* an alarm symptom that should prompt concern for a serious cause of tremor?

   A. Acute onset
   B. Presentation in the emergency room for evaluation
   C. Difficulty walking
   D. Presence only with use
   E. Associated neurologic symptoms

3. A 25-year-old woman presents for evaluation of a resting tremor. The tremor has been present for about 6 months. Her medical history is otherwise remarkable for psychiatric illness for which she has been hospitalized twice. She was started on a new medication prior to the onset of tremor.

   Which of the following medications is most likely to cause a resting tremor?

   A. Haloperidol
   B. Lithium
   C. Valproic acid
   D. Sertraline
   E. Clonazepam

References

1. Louis ED, Ferreira JJ. How common is the most common adult movement disorder? *Mov Disord.* 2010;25:534–541.
2. Louis ED. Clinical practice. Essential tremor. *N Engl J Med.* 2001;345:887–891.
3. Schrag A, Ben-Schlomo Y, Quinn NP. Prevalence of progressive supranuclear palsy and multiple system atrophy: a cross-sectional study. *Lancet.* 1999;354:1771–1775.
4. Nath U, Ben-Shlomo Y, Thomson RG, et al. The prevalence of progressive supranuclear palsy (Steele-Richardson-Olszewski syndrome) in the UK. *Brain.* 2001;124:1438–1449.
5. Pfeiffer RF. Wilson's disease. *Semin Neurol.* 2007;27: 123–132.
6. Reilly M, Daly L, Hutchinson M. An epidemiological study of Wilson's disease in the Republic of Ireland. *J Neurol Neurosurg Psychiatry*. 1993;56:298–300.
7. Fahn S, Jankovic J. *Principles and Practice of Movement Disorders*. Philadelphia, PA: Churchill Livingstone Elsevier, 2007.
8. Willis AW, Evanoff BA, Lian M, et al. Geographic and ethnic variation in Parkinson's disease: a population-based study of US Medicare beneficiaries. *Neuroepidemiology.* 2010;34:143–151.
9. Kollensperger M, Geser F, Seppi K, et al. Red flags for multiple system atrophy. *Mov Disord.* 2008;23:1093–1099.
10. Gupta A, Lang AE. Psychogenic movement disorders. *Curr Opin Neurol*. 2009;22:430–436.

Suggested Reading

Fahn S, Jankovic J. *Principles and Practice of Movement Disorders*. Philadelphia, PA: Churchill Livingstone Elsevier, 2007.

Leffler JB, ed. Essential tremor. Movement disorders. Virtual University. 2008. Available at: http://www.mdvu.org/library/disease/et/. Accessed March 3, 2010.

Robinson R. Parkinson's disease. Movement disorders. Virtual University. 2008. Available at: http://www.mdvu.org/library/disease/pd/. Accessed March 3, 2010.

Tarsy D. Movement disorders. In: Samuels M, Feske SK, eds. *Office Practice of Neurology*. Philadelphia, PA: Churchill Livingston, 2003.

Tarsy D. Overview of tremor. 2009. Available at: http://www.utdol.com. Accessed March 3, 2010.

SECTION

XII PSYCHIATRY

Chapter 63

Anxiety

Michael H. Zaroukian, MD, PhD, FACP, FHIMSS, and Veera Pavan Kotaru, MD

CASE SCENARIO

A 36-year-old woman comes to your office accompanied by her husband to discuss her "nervousness." She says she is nervous and worried almost all of the time. She also feels tired and does not sleep well at night.

- **What additional questions should you ask to learn more about her anxiety?**
- **How would you classify her anxiety problem?**
- **What are the possible causes of her anxiety?**
- **How can you establish a presumptive diagnosis by asking open-ended questions followed by more focused history taking?**
- **How can you use the patient's history to distinguish between anxiety as a normal phenomenon and other types of anxiety that are disabling?**

INTRODUCTION

Anxiety can be a normal and adaptive short-term, fear-based response to perceived threats of physical or psychological harm. An anxiety disorder exists when recurrent or persistent episodes of anxiety are so intense, frequent, or situationally inappropriate that they cause significant distress or impair normal functioning, activities, or relationships. Anxiety disorders are common but are underrecognized both by patients and providers.

Diagnosing anxiety disorders depends heavily on history taking, because physical examination and laboratory testing add little to the evaluation. An important starting point is to keep anxiety disorders in mind, particularly in patients who have a history of unexplained medical symptoms, high utilization of healthcare resources, major life stresses, prior physical or psychological trauma, depression or substance abuse, or disruptions in social or occupational functioning. Once recognized, anxiety disorders can be classified into one of the major categories listed below.

KEY TERMS[1]

Anxiety	Apprehension, uneasiness, or fear in response to a real or perceived threat.
Anxiety disorder	Excessive anxiety and worry, recurring more days than not for at least 6 months.
Generalized anxiety disorder (GAD)	Excessive anxiety, recurring more days than not for at least 6 months, associated with various objects, circumstances, or events.
Phobia	Persistent, irrational, intense anxiety and worry in response to specific external objects, activities, or situations.
Agoraphobia	Anxiety about being confined without easy egress or escape, causing avoidance or endurance with marked distress.
Social phobia	Marked and persistent fear of social activities or performances involving possible scrutiny or evaluation by others, resulting in avoidance or endurance with intense anxiety or stress. Recognized as excessive or unreasonable.

—Continued next page

Continued—

Specific phobia	Marked and persistent fear precipitated immediately and consistently by the presence or anticipation of a specific object or situation, resulting in avoidance or endurance with intense anxiety or stress. Recognized as excessive or unreasonable.
Panic attacks	Rapidly peaking (10 minutes), intense fear or alarm and at least 4 of the following 13 symptoms: abnormal heartbeat, chest discomfort, sweating, shakiness, dyspnea or choking, smothering sensation, abdominal symptoms, dizziness or faintness, sense of unreality, fear of going crazy or losing control, fear of dying, numbness or tingling, or hot flashes or chills.
Panic disorder	Recurrent, unexpected panic attacks, followed by at least 1 month of persistent concern about additional attacks, worry about implications or consequences, or a significant change in behavior in relation to the attacks.
Posttraumatic stress disorder (PTSD)	Persistent re-experience of a traumatic event involving the threat of death or serious injury to self or others, resulting in intense fear, helplessness, or horror. The symptoms should persist for at least 1 month following the traumatic event. If the duration of the symptoms is < 1 month, it is called acute stress disorder.
Obsessive-compulsive disorder (OCD)	Recurrent, persistent, and intrusive thoughts, impulses, or images causing marked anxiety and distress, with an irresistible need to perform repetitive, time-consuming behaviors.
Anxiety due to drugs, medications, and medical illness	Anxiety primarily resulting from the effects of drugs (cocaine, amphetamines, caffeine), drug withdrawal (alcohol, narcotics, sedatives, nicotine, caffeine), medications (decongestants, β-agonists, fluoxetine), or medical conditions (see Alarm Symptoms).

ETIOLOGY

Environmental factors play a more important role in the anxiety disorders than specific genetic abnormalities, although some recent research suggests that genetic factors may make some individuals more vulnerable to developing conditions like PTSD. Studies have identified various alterations in neurotransmitters, regional brain activity, and hypothalamic-pituitary axis function, but no unifying theory has emerged. Among environmental factors, childhood adversity, traumatic experiences, and major stress are associated with anxiety disorders in adulthood.[2]

Differential Diagnosis

	Lifetime Prevalence in US Adults[a]	Women:Men[b]
GAD	3%–5%[3]	3:1
Panic attacks	7.3%[3]	
Panic disorder	2%–5%[3]	3:1
PTSD	9%–12%[4]	2:1
Anxiety due to drugs, medications, and medical illness		
OCD	2%–3%[5]	1:1
Agoraphobia	3.5%–7%[3]	4:1
Social phobia	13.3%[3]	1:1
Specific phobias	15.7%[3]	2:1

[a]Empty cells indicate that a prevalence estimate is unavailable.

[b]*Diagnostic and Statistical Manual of Mental Disorders,* Fourth Edition, Text-Revision (DSM-IV-TR).

GETTING STARTED WITH THE HISTORY

- Before the visit, review the patient's medical diagnoses, medications, and past, family, social, and occupational histories for relevant clues.
- Conduct the interview in an environment that is quiet, comfortable, private, and calming.
- Remind the patient that you will protect his or her confidentiality.
- Avoid distractions.
- Don't rush the patient's description.
- Use open-ended questioning, empathic listening, validation, and affirmation.
- After you have listened to the patient's story, proceed to focused, nonleading questions.
- Consider the NURS (naming, understanding, respecting, and supporting) framework for handling emotions and relationship building.[6]
- Remember that many patients are not consciously aware of their anxiety or the relationship between anxiety and their symptoms.
- Screen for predisposing or aggravating factors, including comorbid mental disorders, stresses, substance abuse, and past abuse or neglect.
- Use decision-support tools and reminder systems as needed, including questionnaires and interview tools. Some useful online resources include the following.

Resource	Website Address
Anxiety Disorders Association of America	http://www.adaa.org/index.cfm
National Institute of Mental Health	http://www.nimh.nih.gov/anxiety/anxietymenu.cfm
Patient Health Questionnaire	http://www.depression-primarycare.org/clinicians/toolkits/materials/forms/phq9/questionnaire/
Hamilton Anxiety Scale	http://www.anxietyhelp.org/information/hama.html
Mini-International Neuropsychiatric Interview	https://www.medical-outcomes.com/index.php
Liebowitz Social Anxiety Scale	http://www.anxietyhelp.org/information/leibowitz.html
Diagnostic and Statistical Manual of Mental Disorders, Fourth Edition, Text-Revision (DSM-IV-TR)	http://dsm.psychiatryonline.org/book.aspx?bookid=22

Open-Ended Questions	Tips for Effective Interviewing
Tell me about your worries, fears, concerns, and stresses, and how they affect you.	Establish a setting of comfort and trust. Listen actively and empathically.
Can you identify anyone or anything that tends to bring on or worsen your feelings of worry, fear, concern, or stress?	Be supportive and nonjudgmental. Handle emotions effectively (NURS).
When you feel worried, fearful, concerned, or stressed, what helps you feel better?	Avoid distractions and leading questions. Involve family members as appropriate.

INTERVIEW FRAMEWORK

- Assess for alarm symptoms.
- Classify the anxiety disorder (eg, generalized, phobic, obsessive-compulsive, posttraumatic, panic, drugs).
- Identify important comorbidities and risk factors.

IDENTIFYING ALARM SYMPTOMS

Anxiety can be serious or even life threatening when it aggravates a serious underlying medical condition (eg, angina, heart failure, asthma) or when it precipitates a reaction that is maladaptive (substance abuse) or actively self-destructive (suicide).

Serious Diagnoses

Diagnosis	Lifetime Prevalence by Condition[a,b]
Major depression	5%–17%[3]
Alcoholism	14%[3]
Suicide	13.5% (ideation); 3.9% (plan); 4.6% (attempt)
Medical illnesses	Panic disorder is 3 times more likely in patients with hypertension and asthma. PTSD is 3.5 times more likely in patients with arthritis.[7]
Dementia	Alzheimer's disease: 1.7%
Eating disorders	Anorexia nervosa: 0.9% (women); 0.3% (men) Bulimia nervosa: 1.5% (women); 0.5% (men) Binge eating disorder: 3.5% (women); 2.0% (men)
Somatization disorder	
Personality disorders	

[a]Empty cells indicate that a prevalence estimate is unavailable.

[b]National Institute of Mental Health. The numbers count: mental disorders in America. http://www.nimh.nih.gov/health/ publications/ the-numbers-count-mental-disorders-in-america/index.shtml.

Alarm Symptoms	If Present, Consider...
Cognitive impairment	Dementia
Confusion or agitation	Substance abuse or withdrawal, medications, hypoxia, infection, head injury, hypoglycemia
Syncope	Temporal lobe epilepsy, cardiac arrhythmia
Severe or changing headache	Head injury, brain infection, central nervous system tumor or hemorrhage, temporal arteritis
Dyspnea	Panic disorder, asthma, pneumothorax, pulmonary embolism, heart failure, hypoxia
Exertional chest pain	Angina pectoris
Thyroid enlargement	Hyperthyroidism, hypothyroidism
Rash, arthralgia, hematuria	Vasculitis, rheumatoid arthritis, systemic lupus erythematosus
Jaundice	Infectious mononucleosis, viral hepatitis

FOCUSED QUESTIONS

After listening to the patient's worries, fears, concerns, stresses, precipitating factors, and coping responses, proceed to focused questions to determine the specific anxiety disorder.[8] Remember that multiple disorders may be present.

QUESTIONS	THINK ABOUT...
If answered in the affirmative...	
Do you often feel nervous, worried, irritable, restless, or tense?	GAD
In general, are you a nervous person?	
Do you have increased fatigue, difficulty concentrating, or sleeplessness?	
Have you ever had a sudden attack of dread or fright that was brief but intense?	Panic disorder
Did anything seem to trigger it?	
Did you also have chest discomfort, abdominal pain, or breathing problems?	
Do you have worrisome symptoms that health professionals have not been able to explain, leaving you feeling unsatisfied and causing you to repeatedly seek care or change doctors?	
Have you ever been in a dangerous or life-threatening situation where you felt helpless to protect yourself against death or serious injury, or where you witnessed violence against another person?	PTSD
Do you have nightmares or flashbacks about the experience?	
What kinds of things remind you of the past trauma?	
Do you become afraid or nervous in places or situations such as tunnels, bridges, crowds, elevators, planes, buses, or automobiles, or when you are outside alone or home alone?	Agoraphobia
Do you become afraid or nervous in situations where you feel you are being watched or evaluated by others and might embarrass or humiliate yourself, such as public speaking or performing, eating in front of others, using a public restroom, attending parties, playing sports, taking tests, using the phone, standing up for yourself, dating, or asking for help?	Social phobia
Do you have any strong fears about a specific situation or thing that distresses you or limits your activities, such as heights, dark places, insects, snakes, strangers, storms, water, blood, or needles?	Specific phobia
Do you find yourself having unpleasant and uninvited thoughts that you cannot make go away and seem to force themselves into your mind, repeating themselves over and over?	OCD
Are there behaviors or habits that you can't resist the urge to repeat over and over, even though they bother you or others you care about?	
Quality	
Is the anxiety:	
• *Related to many different stresses over time?*	GAD
• *A sense of sudden panic that peaks quickly and is over within minutes?*	Panic attack
	Panic disorder
• *Related to situations in which you would have trouble escaping if trapped?*	Agoraphobia
• *Characterized by a fear of embarrassment and humiliation?*	Social phobia
• *Limited to a specific situation or object?*	Specific phobia

—Continued next page

Continued—

• *A repetitive series of intrusive, irrational thoughts and irresistible urges to do something?*	OCD
• *Characterized by nightmares or flashbacks of traumatic experiences?*	PTSD
Time course	
Describe a typical episode of worry, fear, or anxiety. What triggers it and how long does it usually last?	
• *It comes on in a rush, gets very bad very fast, but goes away fast.*	Panic attack Panic disorder
• *It starts when I have to do something in front of a group, but it goes away soon afterward.*	Social phobia
• *It starts when I have to be in a crowded room far from the door, and goes away when I get out or get close to the door.*	Agoraphobia
• *It comes on when I start climbing a ladder, and doesn't go away until my feet are back on the ground.*	Specific phobia
• *Lots of different things can bring it on, and I'm not sure it ever goes away completely. I'm just a worrier!*	GAD
• *It comes on whenever I get thoughts about being responsible for my family getting hurt, and it doesn't go away until I've checked to make sure the stove is off and the doors are locked, 12 times!*	OCD
• *I seem to get it more if I drink less, and I feel better if I have a beer or take a sleeping pill. It seems to be worse since my thyroid medication was increased.*	Anxiety due to medications, sedative-hypnotic withdrawal, or alcohol withdrawal
• *It happens if I get short of breath after I fall asleep, or if I get chest pain when I walk.*	Anxiety due to medical illness
Associated symptoms	
When your worry, fear, or anxiety is bad, do you notice any other symptoms?	
• *My face turns read, my heart beats fast, and my hands get clammy*	Social phobia Specific phobia
• *I get really fatigued, my muscles tighten up, I forget things, and I can't sleep.*	GAD
• *My head, chest, and stomach hurt; my heart beats fast; I feel faint; and my hands go numb.*	Panic attack Panic disorder
• *I "fly off the handle," ache just about everywhere, or just feel numb all over.*	PTSD
• *I get a bad rash on my hands or bald spots.*	OCD
Modifying symptoms	
Does anything in particular tend to trigger an episode of fear, worry, or distress?	
• *It seems like it can be almost anything, depending on what's going on in my life.*	GAD

• *It happens anytime I have to perform a solo on my instrument at a band concert.*	Social phobia
• *It happens whenever I have to clean out the garage, where there might be a spider.*	Specific phobia
• *I get it every time I'm in a crowded room where I can't see a way to get out easily.*	Agoraphobia
• *I get it whenever the thought of germs pops into my head.*	OCD
• *It happens whenever a car engine backfires suddenly.*	PTSD
• *I had it right after my mother died, and again after my car slid across the highway in a snowstorm and I barely missed getting hit by a cement truck.*	Panic disorder
• *It happens every time my asthma gets bad, and I have to go to the emergency department.*	Anxiety due to medical illness

DIAGNOSTIC APPROACH (INCLUDING ALGORITHM)

The first step in diagnosing anxiety disorders is to determine whether a serious underlying medical condition or a separate primary mental health disorder is causing the patient's anxiety. In addition, anxiety due to drugs should be excluded.

Questioning should then focus on whether anxiety comes on as a sudden attack without warning as is characteristic of panic disorder or is more predictably associated with known triggering objects, events, or circumstances. When anxiety triggers are diverse and persistent, GAD is the likely diagnosis. When they are specific and known, phobias, OCD, or PTSD is likely. There are also standard screening tools available for GAD and panic disorder like the Generalized Anxiety Disorder-7 questionnaire, Shedler Quick PsychoDiagnostics Panel (QPD Panel), and the Anxiety Screening Questionnaire (ASQ-15). See Figure 63–1 for the diagnostic approach algorithm for anxiety.

CAVEATS

- Somatic symptoms of severe anxiety can cause affected people to worry that they have a serious undiagnosed medical illness. Such patients are at risk for potentially harmful tests and treatments as well as distress when a diagnosis that explains their symptoms is not forthcoming. The approach to such patients includes careful assessment for underlying medical conditions and patient education about the relationship between anxiety and somatic symptoms.
- Remember that a patient's beliefs about the causes of their symptoms can significantly affect the diagnosis made by their provider. Patients who "explain away" (normalize) their anxiety-associated symptoms ("I'm tired because I don't have time to exercise") are much less likely to be diagnosed with anxiety than patients who use psychological terms ("I'm emotionally worn out").[9]
- Patients with anxiety are often ashamed or embarrassed or concerned that they will be judged by their provider. Establishing a positive relationship with anxious patients may encourage them to reveal, acknowledge, and undergo treatment for the disorder.

PROGNOSIS

Without treatment, anxiety disorders generally persist and cause significant hardship to patients and their families. Because most patients benefit considerably from therapy, accurate and timely diagnosis helps them get the care needed to enhance their functioning and happiness.

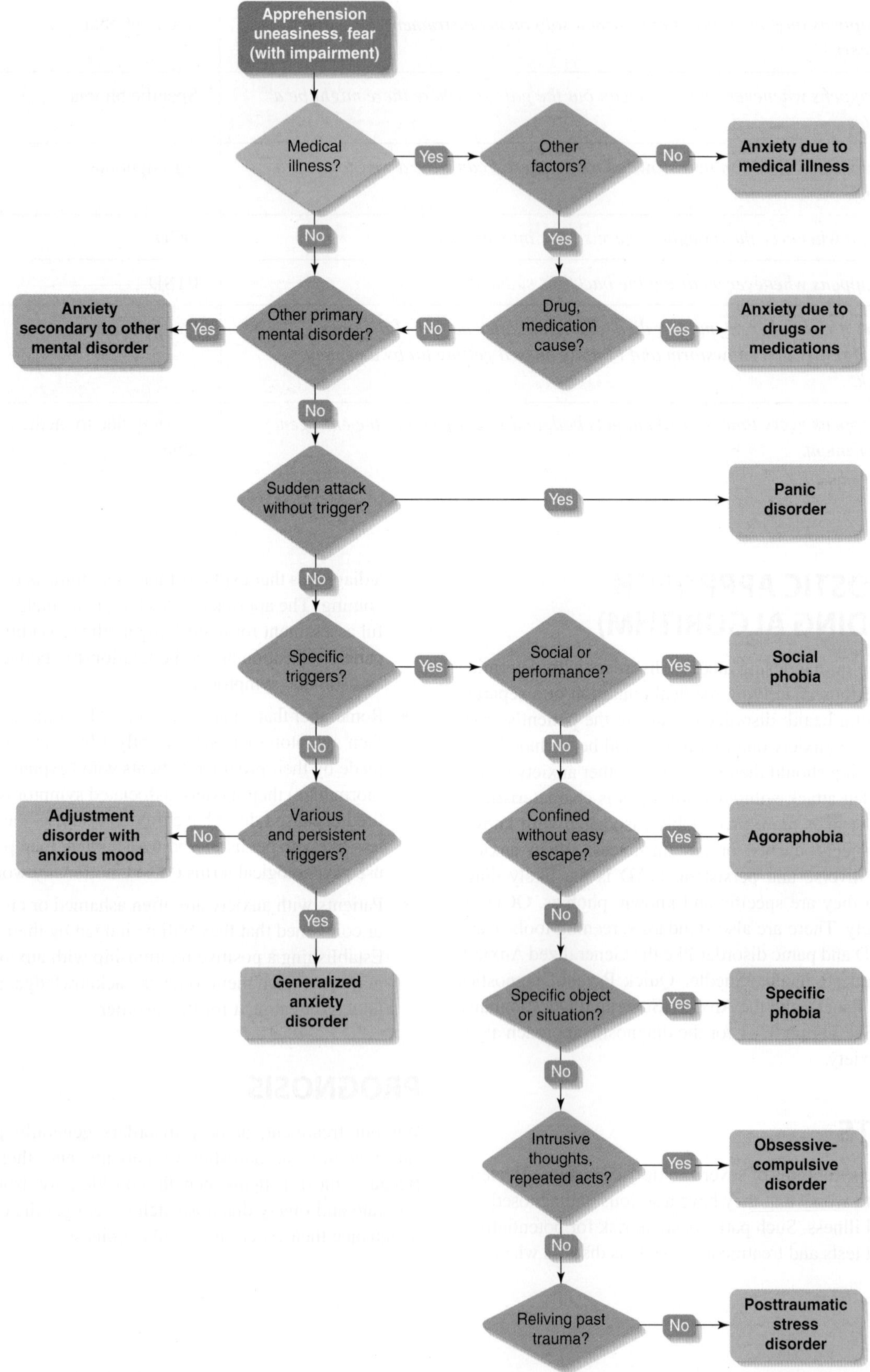

FIGURE 63–1 Diagnostic approach: Anxiety. (Adapted, with permission, from Feldman M. Managing psychiatric disorders in primary care: 2. Anxiety. *Hosp Pract [Minneap]*. 2000;35:77–84.)

GAD	Treated patients generally have a reduction in symptoms but typically relapse if therapy is discontinued.
Agoraphobia	Some untreated patients abuse sedatives and alcohol to allay anxiety. Nearly all agoraphobic patients respond well to therapy.
Social phobia and specific phobia	With treatment, the great majority of patients show at least moderate improvement.
OCD	With the advent of potent serotonin reuptake inhibitors, the great majority of treated patients improve, but few go into remission. Continued therapy is required to prevent relapse.
PTSD	With prompt intervention, most patients with early PTSD respond rapidly and well. Chronic PTSD is more difficult to treat and more likely to be associated with ongoing and variable disability.
Panic disorder	Improvement with residual symptoms and relapses is more common than complete remission.

CASE SCENARIO | Resolution

A 36-year-old woman comes to your office accompanied by her husband to discuss her "nervousness." She says she is nervous and worried almost all of the time. She also feels tired and does not sleep well at night.

ADDITIONAL HISTORY

The patient reports that she has difficulty concentrating even on simple tasks, saying "my mind goes blank." She worries about nearly everything and indicates that her anxiety can be triggered "just like that." She cannot seem to get rid of her concerns, although she understands her anxiety is often more intense than the situation warrants. She has spent much less time with friends, something she used to do a lot. She does not like going out to parties or social events anymore. Her husband indicates that this has been going on for at least 10 months. She denies any known medical problems, prior traumatic life events, or use of alcohol, tobacco, or illicit drugs. Family history is significant for diabetes mellitus and thyroid problems in her mother.

Question: What is the most likely diagnosis?

A. Panic disorder
B. Generalized anxiety disorder
C. Generalized social anxiety
D. Obsessive-compulsive disorder
E. Agoraphobia

Test Your Knowledge

1. Three weeks after a motor vehicle accident, a 32-year-old woman presents to your office with headaches, inability to concentrate, and difficulty sleeping. She witnessed a 6-year-old child die in the accident. The patient reports frequent nightmares since the accident, and her mother reports that the patient has had several emotional outbursts as well. She has avoided driving since the accident and became very nervous even riding in a car to today's visit.

   What is the most likely diagnosis?

   A. Normal grief
   B. Posttraumatic stress disorder (PTSD)
   C. Acute stress disorder
   D. Specific phobia
   E. Panic disorder

2. During a routine office visit, a 24-year-old man reports that he has been thinking of going back to college but is hesitant because he has always found it difficult to go out in public and he hates being the center of attention. He is also afraid that he may look stupid in front of his classmates or teachers. He has been having recurring nightmares in which he trips and falls in front of the whole class. The patient denies any medical problems. He drinks a 12-oz can of beer once a month but does not use tobacco or illicit drugs. He denies any history of traumatic life events or prior abuse.

   What is the most likely diagnosis?

   A. Generalized anxiety disorder (GAD)
   B. Social anxiety disorder (social phobia)
   C. Posttraumatic stress disorder (PTSD)
   D. Agoraphobia
   E. Obsessive-compulsive disorder (OCD)

3. A 29-year-old internal medicine resident comes to the emergency department with palpitations, shortness of breath, and profuse sweating. She is very much convinced that she is having an asthma attack and will die from suffocation. Her symptoms started suddenly while at home, peaked in 10 minutes, and resolved within an hour or so. The patient has had 3 similar episodes in the last 3 weeks. She denies any specific precipitating factor or stressful event and has no history of asthma or any heart problems. She is very concerned about the possibility of future attacks and has stopped exercising for fear of an attack occurring while she is out walking, even though none of her episodes have occurred in association with exercise.

   What is the most likely diagnosis?

   A. Hypochondria
   B. Panic disorder
   C. Acute stress disorder
   D. Specific phobia
   E. Obsessive-compulsive disorder (OCD)

References

1. American Psychiatric Association. *Diagnostic and Statistical Manual of Mental Disorders*. 4th ed. Washington, DC: American Psychiatric Association, 1994.
2. Molnar BE, Buka SL, Kessler RC. Child sexual abuse and subsequent psychopathology: results from the National Comorbidity Survey. *Am J Public Health*. 2001;91:753–760.
3. Kessler RC, McGonagle KA, Zhao S, et al. Lifetime and 12-month prevalence of DSM-III-R psychiatric disorders in the United States. Results from the National Comorbidity Survey. *Arch Gen Psychiatry*. 1994;51:8–19.
4. Breslau N, Davis GC, Andreski P, Peterson E. Traumatic events and posttraumatic stress disorder in an urban population of young adults. *Arch Gen Psychiatry*. 1991;48:216–222.
5. Karno M, Golding JM, Sorenson SB, Burnam MA. The epidemiology of obsessive-compulsive disorder in five US communities. *Arch Gen Psychiatry*. 1988;45:1094–1099.
6. Smith RC. *The Patient's Story: Integrated Patient-Doctor Interviewing*. 1st ed. New York, NY: Little, Brown and Company, 1996.
7. Kessler RC, Ormel J, Demler O, Stang PE. Comorbid mental disorders account for the role impairment of commonly occurring chronic physical disorders: results from the National Comorbidity Survey. *J Occup Environ Med*. 2003;45:1257–1266.
8. Zimmerman M. *Diagnosing DSM-IV Psychiatric Disorders in Primary Care Settings: An Interview Guide for the Nonpsychiatrist Physician*. East Greenwich, RI: Psych Products Press, 1994.
9. Kessler D, Lloyd K, Lewis G, Gray DP. Cross sectional study of symptom attribution and recognition of depression and anxiety in primary care. *BMJ*. 1999;318:436–439.

Suggested Reading

Levinson W, Engel C. Anxiety. In: Feldman M, Christensen J, eds. *Behavioral Medicine in Primary Care: A Practical Guide*. New York, NY: Appleton & Lange, 1997:193–211.

Moses S. Anxiety. In: Moses S, ed. *Family Practice Notebook*. Lino Lakes, MN: Family Practice Notebook, LLC, 2003.

National Institute of Mental Health, National Institutes of Health, U.S. Department of Health and Human Services. The numbers count: mental disorders in America. Available at: http://www.nimh.nih.gov/health/publications/the-numbers-count-mental-disorders-in-america/index.shtml. Accessed March 26, 2010.

Chapter 64

Depressed Mood

John W. Williams, Jr., MD, MHSc, and Jason A. Nieuwsma, PhD

CASE SCENARIO

A 58-year-old woman comes to you complaining of difficulty sleeping. She reports that her sleep problems began about 2 months ago, and since that time, she has felt "drained, weak, and not like my usual self." Over the past 2 months, she also acknowledges having gained 12 lbs. The patient appears visibly lethargic to you, as evidenced by her slumped posture, sluggish movement, delayed replies to your questions, and difficulty sustaining attention.

- **Based on the patient's initial presentation, what are likely diagnostic possibilities?**
- **What additional history would you want to obtain?**
- **How might the past medical history guide your diagnostic decision making?**
- **How can you determine what might be causing her symptoms?**
- **Are there any questions that are crucial to ask before the patient leaves your office?**

INTRODUCTION

Clinical depression is a syndrome characterized by the following cardinal symptoms: depressed mood or anhedonia, additional psychological (eg, decreased concentration) or somatic symptoms (eg, insomnia), and impaired functioning. Depressed mood is very common. In settings where primary care patients are screened systematically, 10% to 30% report depressed mood. The US Preventive Services Task Force recommends a brief 2-item depression screen,[1] the Patient Health Questionnaire 2 (PHQ2), for use in settings where staff-assisted depression care supports are available.[2] Although depressed mood is a cardinal feature of depression, most patients actually present with physical complaints. If systematic screening is not being employed, clinicians should consider clinical depression in patients who present with a "red flag" such as insomnia, fatigue, chronic pain, recent life changes or stressors, fair or poor self-rated health, and unexplained physical symptoms.[3]

KEY TERMS[4]

Anhedonia	Markedly diminished interest or pleasure in almost all activities most of the day, nearly every day.
Appetite or weight change	Substantial change in appetite nearly every day or unintentional weight loss or gain (eg, ≥ 5% of body weight in 1 month).
Decreased concentration	Diminished ability to think or concentrate, or indecisiveness nearly every day.
Decreased energy	Fatigue or loss of energy nearly every day.
Depressed mood	Depressed mood most of the day, nearly every day.
Guilt or feelings of worthlessness	Feelings of worthlessness or excessive guilt nearly every day.
Increased or decreased psychomotor activity	Psychomotor agitation or retardation nearly every day.
Sleep disturbance	Insomnia or hypersomnia nearly every day.
Suicidal ideation	Recurrent thoughts of death or suicide.

ETIOLOGY[5,6]

Female gender, prior depression, chronic medical illness, and depression in a first-degree relative are risk factors for clinical depression. Among patients with depressed mood or a positive depression screen (eg, PHQ2), the prevalence of clinically significant depressive disorders varies depending on the clinical setting and patient characteristics. In primary care settings, approximately 25% to 50% of such patients will have transient dysphoria (eg, feeling down because their sports team lost the big game) or more persistent but mild symptoms that do not impair function and hence do not meet formal criteria for a psychiatric diagnosis. Among the remaining patients, approximately 25% will have major depression, 25% will have dysthymic disorder or depression not otherwise specified (NOS), and a small proportion will have bipolar disorder or general medical causes for the depressive symptoms.

Major depressive disorder is characterized by ≥ 5 of the 9 depressive symptoms, including depressed mood or anhedonia, which impair function and last ≥ 2 weeks. Dysthymic disorder is a chronic but milder depressive disorder characterized by depressed mood that is present more days than not for 2 or more years, in addition to other depressive symptoms. Depressive disorder NOS is a milder depressive disorder that does not meet criteria for major depression or dysthymic disorder. It is characterized by 2 to 4 depressive symptoms, including depressed mood or anhedonia, that impair function and last ≥ 2 weeks. Depressive disorders commonly co-occur with other psychiatric disorders.

Differential Diagnosis[7-11]

	Prevalence[a] in Patients With Depressed Mood	Prevalence in Unselected Primary Care Patients
Bipolar disorder	2%–10%	0.5%–3%
Major depressive disorder	20%–30%	4%–9%
Dysthymic disorder	5%–15%	1%–4%
Depression NOS	10%–15%	4%–6%
Adjustment disorder		2%–10%
Bereavement		1%–2%
Mood disorder due to a general medical condition	Uncertain but < 5%	Uncertain but very low
Premenstrual dysphoric disorder		2%–9% of women of reproductive age
Other psychiatric illness, such as alcohol or anxiety disorders	10%–50% (may co-occur with depressive disorder)	Alcohol use disorder 3%–9% Anxiety disorder 7%–19%
Transient dysphoria or mild symptoms not meeting criteria for a psychiatric diagnosis	25%–50%	5%–30%

[a]Among persons with depressed mood or a positive depression screen; prevalence is unknown when not indicated.

GETTING STARTED WITH THE HISTORY

- It may be useful to begin with a general question, such as "How are things at home or work?" or "How are you doing emotionally?"
- Because clinically significant depression requires 1 of 2 cardinal symptoms, an efficient strategy is to ask specifically about depressed mood and anhedonia. Because patients from different backgrounds use differing terms for depression, it is best to use several synonyms. The screen is considered positive if patients endorse depressed mood or anhedonia; the likelihood ratio for a positive screen (LR+) is 4.0 to 8.3, and likelihood ratio for a negative screen (LR–) is 0.16 to 0.67.[12]

Questions	Remember
Over the past month, have you been feeling down, depressed, or hopeless?	Depressed patients may make the interviewer feel sad. Use your emotional response as a diagnostic clue.
Over the past month, have you been bothered by little interest or pleasure in doing things?	This symptom is often more prominent than depressed mood in older adults.

INTERVIEW FRAMEWORK

- If depressed mood or anhedonia is present, inquire about additional depressive symptoms by clinical interview, or administer a depression questionnaire such as the Patient Health Questionnaire (PHQ).[13] The PHQ is a 9-item, self-report questionnaire that assesses the 9 signs and symptoms specified in the *Diagnostic and Statistical Manual of Mental Disorders* (DSM) to diagnose major depressive disorder. For each question, the patient checks a box corresponding to the level of symptoms experienced in the past 2 weeks (ranging from "not at all" to "nearly every day"); total scores range from 0 to 27. Scores ≥ 10 indicate a probable depressive disorder.
- Ask about impact on daily functioning, because impaired function at home, work, or in interpersonal relationships is required to diagnose clinical depression.
- Assess for alarm symptoms of suicidality.
- Consider secondary causes such as medications, hypothyroidism, malignancy, or autoimmune or central nervous system disorders.
- Consider symptom pattern, duration, and associated symptoms to make a specific diagnosis.

Medications Associated With Clinical Depression

Definite Causal Relationship	Possible Causal Relationship
• High-dose reserpine	• Oral contraceptives
• High-dose glucocorticoids	• Carbamazepine
• Anabolic steroids	• Phenobarbital
• Cocaine or amphetamine withdrawal	• Isotretinoin
• Alcohol	
• Interferon	

IDENTIFYING ALARM SYMPTOMS

Because patients rarely volunteer thoughts of suicide, it is important to ask directly about suicidality. The topic may be introduced by asking, "Have you been feeling that life is not worth living or that you would be better off dead?" Another approach is to ask, "Sometimes when a person feels down or depressed, they might think about dying. Have you been having any thoughts like that?" If patients have suicidal ideation, ask more detailed questions to distinguish passive from active suicidal ideation and to assess risk for suicide. Physical symptoms that are inconsistent with the overall severity of depression, such as marked weight loss with otherwise mild depression, suggest alternative diagnoses such as underlying malignancy.

Alarm Symptoms	Comment
Suicide[14]	
Have you had any thoughts of hurting yourself in some way?	A response of "not at all" puts the patient at low risk.
Have you made any plans or considered a method that you might use to harm yourself?	If yes, ask for details.

—Continued next page

Continued—	
Have you ever attempted to harm yourself?	Past attempts are a risk factor for future attempts.
There's a big difference between having a thought and acting on a thought. Do you think you might actually make an attempt to hurt yourself in the near future?	A positive response puts the patient at very high risk for suicide.
Serious general medical conditions	Think about
Have you lost weight despite having a normal or near-normal appetite?	Malignancy
Have you felt cold when everyone else felt comfortable? Have you noticed dry skin or constipation?	Hypothyroidism
Have you noticed a rash, dry eyes or mouth, difficulty swallowing food, or pain/swelling in the hands or feet?	Autoimmune disorders (eg, Sjögren syndrome)
Have you noticed a tremor or a change in gait? Have you had episodes of weakness on one side of the body?	Central nervous system disorders (Parkinson's disease or recurrent strokes)

FOCUSED QUESTIONS

Assessing DSM Symptoms[4,15,16]

To assess the effects of depressive symptoms on function, ask "How difficult has the *fill in the pertinent symptoms* made it for you to do your work, take care of things at home, or get along with other people?"

QUESTIONS	THINK ABOUT...
How has your mood been lately? Have you been feeling down, depressed, or hopeless? How often does that happen? How long does it last?	Depressed mood
Have you lost interest in your usual activities? Do you get less pleasure from things you used to enjoy?	Anhedonia
How have you been sleeping? How does that compare to your normal sleep?	Sleep disturbance
Has there been any change in your appetite or weight?	Appetite or weight change
Have you noticed a decrease in your energy level?	Decreased energy
Have you been feeling fidgety or had problems sitting still? Have you felt slowed down, like you were moving in slow motion or stuck in mud?	Increased or decreased psychomotor activity
Have you been having trouble concentrating? Is it harder to make decisions than before?	Decreased concentration
Are you feeling guilty or blaming yourself for things? How would you describe yourself to someone who had never met you before?	Guilt or feelings of worthlessness
Have you felt that life is not worth living or that you would be better off dead? *Sometimes when a person feels down or depressed, they might think about dying. Have you been having any thoughts like that?*	Suicidal ideation

Quality	
At least 5 DSM symptoms including depressed mood or anhedonia	Major depressive disorder
Milder severity including depressed mood or anhedonia	Dysthymic disorder
	Depressive disorder NOS
	Adjustment disorder
Mild symptoms that do not impair function	Transient dysphoria
Time course	
Did these symptoms begin after the death of a loved one?	Bereavement
Did these symptoms begin during a time of stress?	Adjustment disorder with depressed mood
Have you ever seen or experienced a traumatic event in which you or someone else's life was in danger? *How about threat of serious injury?*	Posttraumatic stress disorder
Have these symptoms been present on most days for at least 2 years?	Dysthymic disorder or chronic major depressive disorder
Do these episodes occur at a particular time of the year?	Seasonal affective disorder
Do your symptoms begin during the week prior to menses and remit within a few days of menses?	Premenstrual dysphoric disorder
Associated symptoms	
Have you ever had periods where your mood was very good, or too good, for no reason?	Bipolar disorder
Were these periods accompanied by racing thoughts, reduced need for sleep, or increased energy?	Bipolar disorder
Did it get you into trouble, for instance by spending too much money, impulsively traveling, or taking on too many projects?	Bipolar disorder
Have you ever had visions or seen things that other people could not see? Have you heard things that other people could not hear, such as noises or the voices of people whispering or talking?	Depressive disorder with psychotic features
	Psychotic disorders such as schizophrenia or schizoaffective disorder
Have you ever had a panic attack, where out of the blue you experienced intense anxiety, fear, or discomfort for no apparent reason?	Panic disorder
Have you felt nervous, anxious, or on edge on more than half the days in the last month?	Generalized anxiety disorder (see Chapter 63)

—Continued next page

Continued—

Do you drink alcohol? Tell me about your drinking habits.	
• *Was there ever a time when you drank too much?*	Alcohol disorder Substance-induced mood disorder
• *Has drinking alcohol ever caused problems such as missing work, legal problems, or driving while intoxicated?*	Alcohol disorder Substance-induced mood disorder
Modifying symptoms	
Some people find their mood changes frequently—as if they spend every day on an emotional roller coaster. Does this sound like you?	Personality disorder is suggested by frequent mood swings or need to be the center of attention (particularly if bothered by others being in the spotlight).
Some people prefer to be the center of attention, while others are content to remain on the edge of things. How would you describe yourself?	

DIAGNOSTIC APPROACH (INCLUDING ALGORITHM)

Once clinical depression is diagnosed, additional history should be elicited about factors that may affect treatment. First, explore the patient's understanding and acceptance of the diagnosis. Stigmatizing beliefs about depression or outright rejection of the diagnosis may interfere with treatment adherence. Second, ask about prior episodes and response to treatment. The risk of relapse and, hence, the need for longer-term treatment increase with the number of prior episodes. Treatments that have been effective for past episodes are likely to be effective for the current episode. See Figure 64–1 for the diagnostic approach algorithm for depressed mood.

CAVEATS

- Men and adolescents may describe excessive irritability rather than depressed mood.
- Because the psychological and physical symptoms of depression may overlap with other physical illness, diagnosing depression in patients with severe or multiple chronic medical illnesses can be challenging. The DSM criteria suggest counting symptoms toward a clinical depression diagnosis unless the symptom is "clearly and fully accounted for by a general medical condition."
- Distinguishing early dementia from depression may be difficult; in many instances, the conditions co-occur. If the depressive symptoms are at least as prominent as those suggesting dementia, diagnose and treat for depression. If the patient does not respond to depression treatment, further evaluation for dementia is warranted.
- Although depressive disorders are common globally, symptom descriptions (eg, "nervios") and illness attributions (eg, susto, Hwa-byung) vary across cultures.[17]

PROGNOSIS

Major depression is a relapsing illness for many patients; the probability of recurrence is 50% after a single episode, increasing to 90% after 3 episodes. For patients willing to complete stepwise treatment with either antidepressant medication or a depression-specific psychotherapy, the remission rate is about 70%.[18] Chronic major depression (lasting ≥ 2 years) is more treatment resistant, and combined antidepressant therapy and psychotherapy is more effective. For patients with depressive symptoms only, major depression will develop in approximately 25% within 2 years.

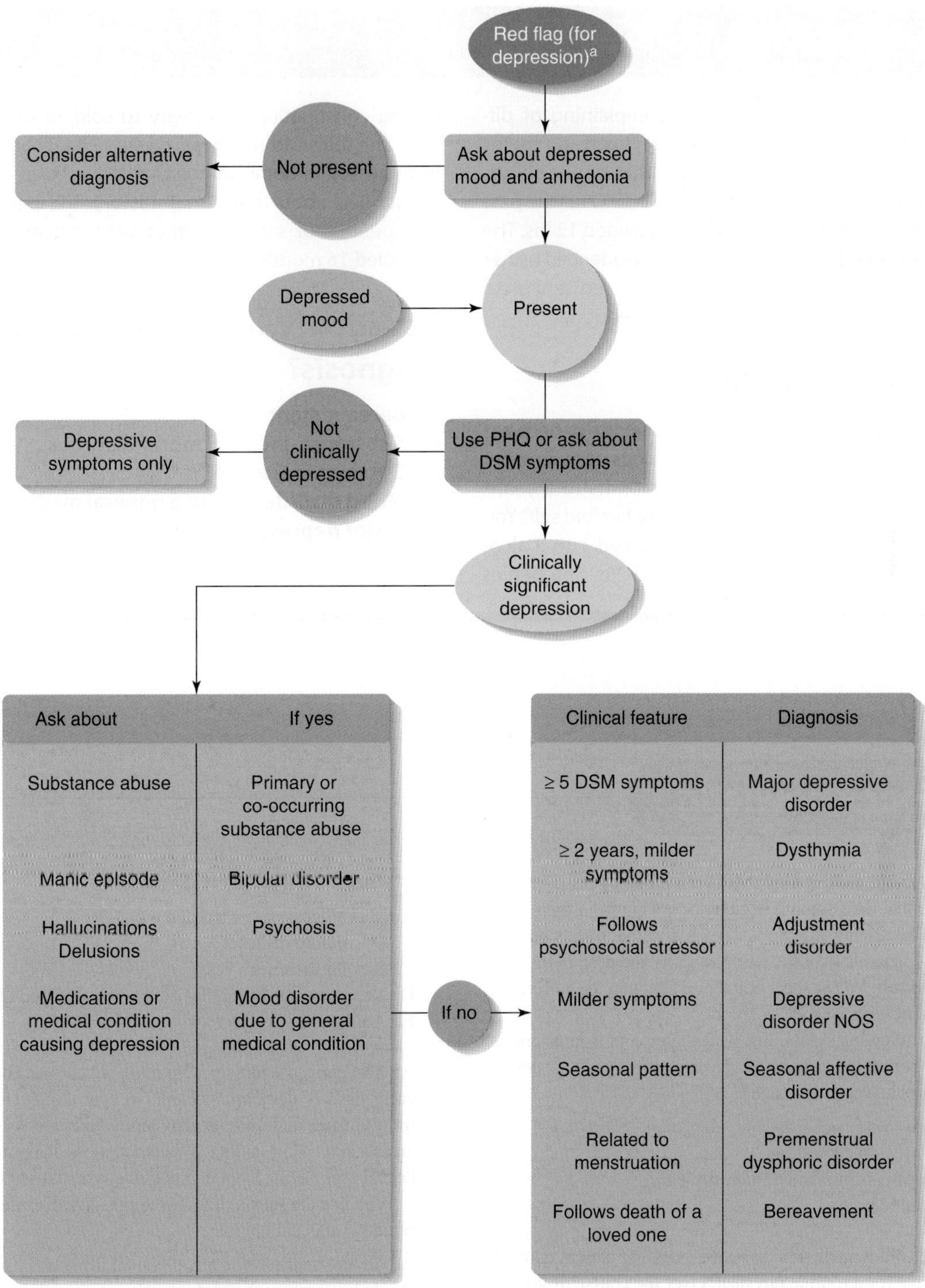

FIGURE 64–1 Diagnostic approach: Depressed mood.

[a]Red flags for clinical depression include insomnia, fatigue, chronic pain, recent life changes or stressors, fair or poor self-rated health, and unexplained physical symptoms. DSM, *Diagnostic and Statistical Manual of Mental Disorders;* NOS, not otherwise specified; PHQ, Patient Health Questionnaire.

CASE SCENARIO | Resolution

A 58-year-old woman comes to you complaining of difficulty sleeping. She reports that her sleep problems began about 2 months ago, and since that time, she has felt "drained, weak, and not like my usual self." Over the past 2 months, she also acknowledges having gained 12 lbs. The patient appears visibly lethargic to you, as evidenced by her slumped posture, sluggish movement, delayed replies to your questions, and difficulty sustaining attention.

ADDITIONAL HISTORY

Upon further questioning, you discover that the patient has developed similar symptoms during previous periods in her life. These periods have lasted from 2 months to 2 years, with the patient eventually getting back to her "old self." You also find out that she has typically consumed 1 to 2 alcoholic beverages each night since her mid-20s. She denies having constipation, sensitivity to cold, or dry skin. However, she feels sad nearly all the time lately and no longer is interested in doing things that she used to enjoy. When questioned about her family history, the patient reports that periods of sadness sometimes affected her mother, who died 16 months ago.

Question: What is the most likely diagnosis?

A. Bereavement
B. Substance-induced mood disorder
C. Dysthymic disorder
D. Mood disorder due to a general medical condition
E. Major depressive disorder

Test Your Knowledge

1. An 18-year-old male is brought to your clinic by his parents, who state that their son has been withdrawing from them and from his friends at school. They report that he has been especially irritable over the past 5 months and prefers to isolate himself. You suspect that the patient may be suffering from a depressive episode.

   Of the following symptoms, which symptom is most crucial to assess before the patient (or any patient that you suspect has depression) leaves your office?

   A. Fatigue
   B. Difficulty concentrating
   C. Anhedonia (diminished interest/pleasure)
   D. Suicidal ideation

2. A 46-year-old woman who is a long-standing patient comes to the office for a routine physical. Over the course of your relationship with this patient, you have noticed that she seems persistently down. She denies most symptoms of depression but acknowledges regularly having low mood, low energy, and low self-esteem, stating "I've pretty much always been this way."

   What is the most likely diagnosis?

   A. Major depressive disorder
   B. Dysthymic disorder
   C. Bipolar disorder
   D. Depressive disorder, not otherwise specified (NOS)
   E. Adjustment disorder

3. An 83-year-old widower with multiple chronic illnesses and early signs of dementia presents to your clinic. He does not have immediate family nearby and is likely to soon move into an assisted living facility. When questioned about his mood, he endorses having 8 out of 9 possible symptoms of depression.

   Why is a diagnosis of major depressive disorder unwarranted in this patient?

   A. He has multiple chronic physical illnesses.
   B. He has early signs of dementia.
   C. He has miserable life circumstances.
   D. All of the above.
   E. None of the above. A diagnosis of depression may be appropriate.

References

1. US Preventive Services Task Force. Screening for depression: recommendations and rationale. *Ann Intern Med.* 2002;136:760–764.
2. US Preventive Services Task Force. Screening for depression in adults: U.S. Preventive Services Task Force recommendation statement. *Ann Intern Med.* 2009;151:784–792.
3. Jackson JL, O'Malley PG, Kroenke K. Clinical predictors of mental disorders among medical outpatients. Validation of the "S4" model. *Psychosomatics.* 1998;39:431–436.
4. American Psychiatric Association. *Diagnostic and Statistical Manual of Mental Disorders: DSM-IV*. Washington, DC: American Psychiatric Association, 1994.
5. US Department of Health and Human Services. Adults and mental health. mood disorders. In. *Mental Health: A Report of the Surgeon General*. Rockville, MD: US Department of Health and Human Services, Substance Abuse and Mental Health Services Administration, Center for Mental Health Services, National Institutes of Health, National Institute of Mental Health, 1999.
6. Williams JW Jr, Pignone M, Ramirez G, Stellato CP. Identifying depression in primary care: a literature synthesis of case-finding instruments. *Gen Hosp Psychiatry.* 2002;24:225–237.
7. Coyne JC, Fechner-Gates S, Schwenk TL. Prevalence, nature, and comorbidity of depressive disorders in primary care. *Gen Hosp Psychiatry.* 1994;16:267–276.
8. Piver A, Yatham LN, Lam RW. Bipolar spectrum disorders: new perspectives. *Can Fam Physician.* 2002;48:896–904.
9. Narrow WE, Rae DS, Robbins LN, Regier DA. Revised prevalence estimates of mental disorders in the United States. *Arch Gen Psychiatry.* 2002;59:115–123.
10. Sherbourne CD, Jackson CA, Meredith LS, Camp P, Wells KB. Prevalence of comorbid anxiety disorders in primary care outpatients. *Arch Fam Med.* 1996;5:27–34.
11. Kessler RC, Chiu WT, Demler O, Merikangas KR, Walters EE. Prevalence, severity, and comorbidity of 12-month DSM-IV disorders in the National Comorbidity Survey Replication. *Arch Gen Psychiatry.* 2005;62:617–627.
12. Gilbody S, Richards D, Brealey S, Hewitt C. Screening for depression in medical settings with the Patient Health Questionnaire (PHQ): a diagnostic meta-analysis. *J Gen Intern Med.* 2007;22:1596–1602.
13. Macarthur Initiative on Depression in Primary Care. Patient Health Questionnaire. Available at: http://www.depression-primarycare.org/clinicians/toolkits/materials/forms/phq9/. Accessed March 8, 2010.
14. Jacobs D, Brewer M. APA practice guideline provides recommendations for assessing and treating patients with suicidal behaviors. *Psychiatr Ann.* 2004;34:373–380.
15. Williams JW Jr, Noel PH, Cordes JA, Ramirez G, Pignone M. Is this patient clinically depressed? *JAMA.* 2002;287:1160–1170.
16. Zimmerman M. *Diagnosing DSM-IV psychiatric disorders in primary care settings. An interview guide for the nonpsychiatrist physician.* East Greenwich, RI: Psych Products Press, 1994.
17. Kirmayer LJ. Cultural variations in the clinical presentation of depression and anxiety: implications for diagnosis and treatment. *J Clin Psychiatry.* 2001;62:22–28.
18. Rush AJ, Trivedi MH, Wisniewski SR, et al. Acute and longer-term outcomes in depressed outpatients requiring one or several treatment steps: a STAR*D report. *Am J Psychiatry.* 2006;163:1905–1917.

Suggested Reading

Depression Management Tool Kit, Macarthur Initiative on depression in primary care at Dartmouth and Duke. Resources for clinicians and organizations. Available at: http://www.depression-primarycare.org/.

Gould MS, Marrocco FA, Kleinman M, et al. Evaluating iatrogenic risk of youth suicide screening programs. *JAMA.* 2005;293:1635–1643. Kaiser Permanente Care Management Institute. *Depression clinical practice guidelines.* Oakland, CA: Kaiser Permanente Care Management Institute, Mar 2006. Available at: http://www.guideline.gov/summary/summary.aspx?doc_id=9632&nbr=5152&ss=6&xl=999.

Mann JJ. The medical management of depression. *N Engl J Med.* 2005;353:1819–1834.

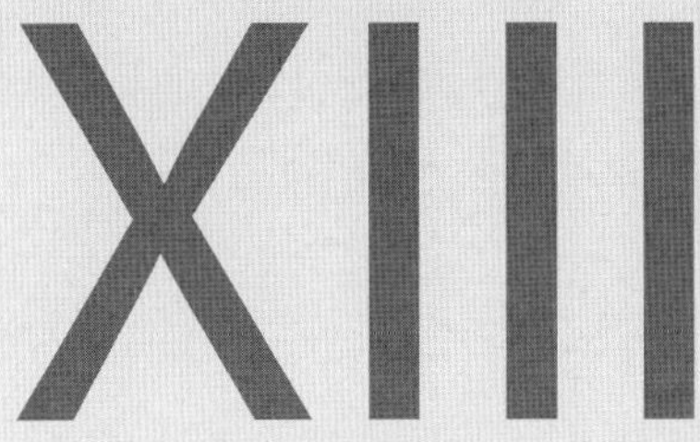

SECTION XIII

COMMUNICATING THE HISTORY

Chapter 65

The Case Presentation

Lawrence M. Tierney, Jr., MD

The spoken case presentation is a concise summary of the history and physical examination. Unlike the written version in a patient's chart, the oral presentation is dynamic and ranges from a brief summary given by phone to a consultant to a more formal presentation to a large medical audience at an academic session. Succinctness and organization are especially important, as the presenter has neither the luxury of omitting important details nor time for repetition. Brevity is of paramount importance; simply reading from a chart defeats the purpose of the exercise. Highlighted in this chapter are the essential components of the presentation: the chief complaint, the history of present illness (HPI), the past medical history, the family and social history, the review of systems, and finally, the physical examination findings.

The chief complaint should be as directed and short as possible, articulating the principal subject under consideration. Invariably, there is one overriding problem in the majority of patients, and a listener is helped enormously by its identification immediately, allowing focus. Indeed, from the first words of a presentation, a listener is formulating possible diagnoses. A lengthy chief complaint including details of past history serves only to confuse and lengthens the presentation—a cardinal sin. The patient's own words need be mentioned only if they illuminate the problem under consideration. The source is always assumed to be the patient, and its content accurate; if considered otherwise by the presenter, this qualification must be made clear. The patient is best identified as a man or woman, which are more respectful designations than male or female. Mentioning the patient's occupation is often helpful medically and certainly socially, because a listener is likely to examine the patient shortly after the presentation.

The HPI is the most important part of the exercise. If the problem is not understood at the conclusion of a properly presented HPI, it is unlikely to be understood after extensive further evaluation. Instead of calendar dates, the duration of time prior to the episode of care should be specified. Calendar dates require a listener to remember the current date and subtract backwards to determine the duration of a problem, an unnecessary distraction.

The initial step in organizing the HPI is to identify the logical parts of the present illness. For example, *beginning* the HPI with a chronic history of hypercholesterolemia is sensible in a middle-aged man with chest pain. Thereafter, events should be given chronologically, up to the present moment. Many presentations are confusing because they include recent information first, followed by previous but relevant data. Instead, the HPI should be related like a story, with a beginning and an end. Again, the value to a listener is significant.

What about the inclusion of pertinent negative historical information in the HPI? Presenting negative data is unnecessary when positives tell the whole story. However, negative data become extremely important in narrowing the differential diagnosis when the positive information leaves the listener uncertain. For example, a 27-year-old woman with crushing substernal chest pain that radiates to both arms and is associated with a sense of impending doom sparks the interest of the listener; the differential diagnosis includes psychiatric, cardiovascular, gastrointestinal, and drug-induced causes. In this case, presenting the absence of symptoms referable to those symptoms helps the listener focus his or her differential diagnosis.

The past medical history, although a crucial component of the patient's written record, adds little to the presentation. If a historical fact is deemed relevant, it likely belongs in the HPI, and some past history may be eliminated entirely in the interest of time. The same is true for the family history; a lengthy pedigree often serves no function, and if important, family history is best consigned to the HPI.

Presenting the social history is always important and is a humanizing endeavor as well. Statements such as "the social history was noncontributory" diminish the practice of medicine by rendering patients pathophysiologic specimens rather than human beings. In addition, such knowledge may facilitate the doctor–patient interaction. Although medications and habits are often included at this point, such items may be more relevant in the HPI.

The review of systems should be as brief as possible, containing only those symptoms felt to be significant enough to merit further investigation. Including numerous positive responses by well-meaning patients only dilutes the significance of truly important symptoms.

It is of utmost importance that in the spoken presentation information not be repeated. The presenter decides where a fact best belongs, and its repetition will only consume time.

Although the physical examination is beyond the scope of this book, a few suggestions are in order. It is best delivered in simple declarative sentences. Qualifiers such as remarkable and unremarkable, although widespread in medical parlance, are clichés that do not assist the listener. A complete examination can be presented in less than 1 minute, and a brief mention of each system tells the listener that they all have been examined. For instance, "the chest was clear" is an entirely appropriate elucidation of the pulmonary examination in a patient whose symptoms do not suggest lung disease. All positive findings, expected or not, are given; whereas negative data focus on signs logically expected by a listener. "There were no spider angiomata" in the patient with liver disease tells the listener that the examiner sought them. Announcing the *system* being presented (for example, "*chest*—he had no wheezes, rales, or rhonchi") is unnecessary because the listener should know what part of the body is being described.

Although laboratory or other diagnostic tests, problem lists, and the assessment are also not the focus of this book, a few points are pertinent. Specific laboratory data presented depend on the setting, such as a hospital or clinic, and the nature of the patient's symptoms or clinical problem. Some listeners prefer that the presentation be concluded with a brief case synthesis, but a lengthy assessment and plan are better placed in the written record. Once again, the issue is time, and it is well known that the captive audience attention span rarely exceeds 7 minutes.

In summary, the best oral presentation resembles a narrative, given chronologically and delivered in language similar to routine conversation. The ability to articulate a crisp, clear presentation requires practice and skill. It is a dying art, but not one that cannot be rekindled.

Answers to Case Study Questions and Test Your Knowledge Questions

CHAPTER 2

TEST YOUR KNOWLEDGE

QUESTION #1

Correct answer: E

Although it can be a tedious task, it is crucial to verify the medication a patient is taking. The chart may be inaccurate, an outside provider may be providing an additional prescription, the patient may be taking an incorrect dose of the prescribed medication, or the patient may have discontinued the medication altogether.

QUESTION #2

Correct answer: C

Often when a patient gives an incomplete answer to a sensitive question, it is useful to gently ask the question in a different way. Pausing briefly might work with some patients, but a truncated answer usually needs further encouragement from the interviewer. Skipping over the question would miss important clinical information, and demanding an answer would alienate the patient and prevent further discussion.

CHAPTER 3

CASE SCENARIO

Correct answer: B

The most efficient way to build rapport and to make patients feel understood and cared for is to use the relationship-building skills outlined in answer B. Agenda setting offers the opportunity to get all of the patient's complaints on the table. Nonfocusing open-ended skills can elicit rich patient-centered data but may not make the patient feel understood and supported unless combined with relationship-building skills.

TEST YOUR KNOWLEDGE

QUESTION #1

Correct answer: D

Patient-centered description of a physical symptom originates from the patient rather than the interviewer. The interviewer facilitates this process with focusing open-ended questioning skills like the echoing and direct request demonstrated in answer D. Option A focuses the patient on emotions, rather than on a *description* of the physical symptom. Answers B and C are closed-ended and clinician-centered questions that are not likely to lead to patient-centered descriptions.

QUESTION #2

Correct answer: A

The phrase "personal story" refers to the part of the patient's story that is neither physical (such as answers B and C) nor emotional (such as answer D).

QUESTION #3

Correct answer: B

Patients feel supported when the interviewer uses emotion-seeking skills followed by NURS. Option B is a "respect" statement (R in NURS). Answers A and C are used to gather data, and answer D is an inappropriate attempt to reassure the patient with insufficient data.

CHAPTER 4

CASE SCENARIO

Correct answer: B

While the clinician-centered part of the interview may seem like a long list of questions, you must remain attuned to the patient and respond to any emotion that arises. The best way to respond to emotion is with one or more statements from the NURS quartet (see Chapter 3). Answer B is an example of a respect statement. Answer A expresses premature reassurance and is never experienced as empathic by the patient. Answer C fails to acknowledge that the patient is having an emotional reaction and is an inappropriately probing question under the circumstances. Answer D is a misguided understanding statement that takes the focus from the patient to the clinician. A better understanding statement would be, "I can understand how this might be upsetting to talk about," which can be followed by answer B and then a support statement such as, "I want to help in any way I can." The patient would feel heard, understood, and cared for.

TEST YOUR KNOWLEDGE

QUESTION #1

Correct answer: D

Each section of the clinician-centered part of the interview should begin with at least one open-ended question. Answers A, B, and C would be appropriate closed-ended follow-up questions. Answer A should be asked as separate or individual questions rather than being stacked together.

QUESTION #2

Correct answer: A

Not all 7 cardinal features pertain to nonpain symptoms. For example, loss of smell, blurry vision, and tinnitus (ringing in the ears) would not be expected to radiate beyond the affected organ.

QUESTION #3

Correct answer: C

A direct inquiry, stated in a caring manner, is most likely to result in a truthful answer. Answer A is incorrect because patients rarely divulge that they are experiencing domestic violence unless directly asked. While patient-centered interviewing skills help to establish a caring and safe clinician–patient relationship, use clinician-centered skills to inquire about sensitive topics. Answer B is negatively worded, so the patient is likely to say "no" even if the answer is "yes," because it seems that "no" is the answer expected by the clinician. It often feels awkward to ask such probing and intimate questions; thus although answer D may be tempting, it fails the patient and puts her at continued risk for violence.

CHAPTER 5

TEST YOUR KNOWLEDGE

QUESTION #1

Correct answer: B

Sensitivity refers to how frequently a clinical finding or test result is present in patients known to have the disease of interest. In this case, nausea is the clinical finding or feature. If 81% of patients with migraine have the clinical finding (nausea), 19% of patients with migraine do not (false-negative rate). In order to know how common nausea occurs among patients *without* migraine, one needs to know the specificity (not stated in this question). For a clinical feature (nausea) to reliably establish a diagnosis (migraine), the specificity would need to be very high.

QUESTION #2

Correct answer: D

The likelihood ratio (LR) is the ratio of the likelihood of a given clinical finding in patients with disease to the likelihood of the *same* finding in patients without disease. In this example, the clinical feature (ferritin = 30) increases the likelihood of iron deficiency, as opposed to other causes of anemia, by 3-fold. LRs are independent of prevalence, so it is impossible to state the frequency or prevalence of iron deficiency in the population without additional information.

QUESTION #3

Correct answer: A

Likelihood ratios (LRs) help clinicians interpret the meaning of a test result because they increase or decrease the probability of disease compared to the prior probability (ie, prior to performing the test). Few tests can reliably rule in or rule out a disease because posttest probability depends strongly on the pretest probability or prevalence of disease, not just the test result. Because LRs are derived from sensitivity and specificity, they are likewise independent of prevalence and apply across clinical settings (where prevalence can vary widely). For example, the prevalence of inflammatory bowel disease is higher in patients referred to a gastroenterology clinic than in a primary care practice. LRs reflect the ability of a test to discriminate between patients with and without a disease and thus can be used to compare the utility of different tests.

CHAPTER 6

CASE SCENARIO

Correct answer: B

These symptoms are typical of benign paroxysmal positional vertigo (BPPV). It is more common in people over the age of 60 years. In addition, similar episodes have occurred in the past with spontaneous resolution. The episodes last less than 1 minute and are most severe when the patient moves her head. If the episodes only occurred upon standing, then it would be more consistent with postural hypotension. She has no alarm symptoms, such as neurologic deficits, which would signal a serious diagnosis. Demonstration of normal gait and absence of any chronic medical diseases, such as Parkinson's disease, would make dysequilibrium less likely.

TEST YOUR KNOWLEDGE

QUESTION #1

Correct answer: B

This patient has presyncope due to volume depletion and concomitant use of antihypertensive medications. The clinical history is consistent with brief periods of diminished cerebral perfusion from orthostatic hypotension.

QUESTION #2

Correct answer: D

This patient has dysequilibrium from the syndrome of multisensory deficits. Peripheral neuropathy from long-standing diabetes mellitus and prior alcohol abuse would decrease his touch and proprioceptive abilities. Additionally, his vision is impaired and he has hearing loss. He does not report any vertiginous symptoms, such as spinning or tilting. The patient does not describe any orthostatic symptoms.

QUESTION #3

Correct answer: B

This patient is having an acute vertebrobasilar infarct and has numerous red flags. He has multiple stroke risk factors, including diabetes mellitus, hypertension, and tobacco use. The sudden onset of dizziness, severe ataxia, and double vision are all alarm symptoms. He requires an urgent evaluation for a serious neurologic cause.

CHAPTER 7

CASE SCENARIO

Correct answer: B

The patient is suffering from depression. Her loss of interest in her usual activities (eg, workout routine), difficulty concentrating, and feelings of sadness and decreased self-worth following her son's departure strongly suggest a diagnosis of depression, which may commonly present with fatigue (see Chapter 64, Depressed Mood).

She reports no physical symptoms, which makes you less concerned about a medical cause for her fatigue. She reports no alarm symptoms. Her normal sleep habits and lack of daytime sleepiness point us away from a diagnosis of obstructive sleep apnea. A diagnosis of chronic fatigue syndrome requires duration of fatigue greater than 6 months and several other symptoms.

TEST YOUR KNOWLEDGE

QUESTION #1

Correct answer: B

This patient meets criteria for chronic fatigue syndrome (CFS), a diagnosis suggested by persistent fatigue of 6 months or greater in duration and presence of at least 4 of the following 8 symptoms at some point during that time period: impaired short-term memory or concentration, sore throat, tender cervical or axillary lymph nodes, myalgias, arthralgias, new or worsening headaches, unrefreshing sleep, and postexertional malaise. She reports the following symptoms:

1. Fatigue impairing her ability to function at home (eg, take care of her children)
2. Onset of fatigue following a viral illness (eg, sore throat)
3. Arthralgias (discomfort in several joints but no evidence of warmth or erythema to suggest arthritis)
4. Fatigue that is worse after exercise or exertion

QUESTION #2

Correct answer: D

This history raises concern for occult gastrointestinal (GI) malignancy. She reports at least one "alarm" symptom (black stools) that should prompt an evaluation for a medical cause of her fatigue. The physical examination also raises concern about GI bleeding, given pale conjunctivae and heme-positive stool on rectal examination. Additional targeted work-up, focusing on the GI tract, should be obtained.

QUESTION #3

Correct answer: C

The patient is likely suffering from hypothyroidism. Fatigue is common in these patients, as is weight gain despite exercise. Patients may also report feeling cold despite warm temperatures, dry skin, coarse hair, and brittle nails. A measurement of serum thyroid-stimulating hormone (TSH) would be warranted at this juncture.

CHAPTER 8

CASE SCENARIO

Correct answer: B

This patient is suffering from an acute febrile illness for 3 days without a discernible pattern to peaks in temperature. Her recent sick contacts and the acute nature of the illness both suggest an infectious etiology rather than an inflammatory condition such as rheumatoid arthritis. Pulmonary symptoms predominate and suggest a respiratory infection. Gastroenteritis is typically viral in etiology and usually presents with significant nausea, vomiting, and/or diarrhea as the main constellation of symptoms. Pulmonary embolism needs to be a consideration in any patient with pleuritic chest pain. She has few risk factors for this condition; she is not on oral contraceptives, has had no recent hospitalization or immobilization, and has no family history of clotting disorders.

This patient has pneumonia; the constellation of fever, cough, and pleuritic pain are characteristic. When considering an infectious etiology for fever, look for symptoms that herald potential complications or signify a critical condition. This patient has no alarm symptoms to suggest meningitis (headache or neck pain), a CNS infection (altered mentation), or sepsis (dizziness, altered mentation.) Causative pathogens for pneumonia include bacteria and viruses and, less frequently, fungi or parasites. Treatment is often guideline driven and utilizes antibiotics, fluid, and oxygenation when needed.

TEST YOUR KNOWLEDGE

QUESTION #1

Correct answer: B

This patient's long duration of fever and arthritic symptoms suggest an inflammatory disorder. Her lack of sick contacts, recent travel, and drug use argue against but do not rule out an infectious process such as bacterial endocarditis. Symptoms that suggest vasculitis include arthritis and jaw claudication, which is the most specific clinical feature of this disease. Up to 42% of patients with giant cell arteritis (GCA) present with fever, and although not typically high, up to 15% of patients develop fever over 39°C. Loss of vision is likely due to a cranial arteritis and is a feared complication of this disease. Prompt recognition and diagnosis of GCA is critical in order to prevent visual loss.

QUESTION #2

Correct answer: A

Acute fever after hospitalization raises concern for nosocomial infection, pulmonary embolism from immobilization, or drug fever due to a new medication. The dysuria and abdominal pain raise the concern of urinary tract infection, and this is most commonly associated with recent catheter placement. Asking a patient whether a catheter was placed can help narrow the search for cause of fever even in patients without dysuria.

Always consider pulmonary embolism after a hospitalization. However, this patient received venous thromboembolism prophylaxis, which makes this less likely. He also denies chest pain or shortness of breath. Recent anesthesia raises the possibility of malignant hyperthermia; however, the time course of fever would be immediate, not delayed, and the peak of temperature is usually higher. Medications such as antibiotics can cause fever even within this short time frame. Drug fever should remain on the differential should the work-up for infection return negative. Evaluation should focus on urinary and blood cultures given that nosocomial urinary infections can quickly progress to sepsis.

QUESTION #3

Correct answer: C

This patient has fever of unknown origin—a fever that lasts 3 weeks or longer with temperatures exceeding 100.9°F with no clear diagnosis despite 1 week of clinical investigation. This fever pattern is consistent with Pel-Ebstein fevers. Sixteen percent of patients with Hodgkin's disease present with this cyclic but unpredictable pattern. She also has several other symptoms that suggest malignancy or chronic inflammation including weight loss and sweats. Interestingly, pruritus is a common feature of Hodgkin's lymphoma at some point in the course of the disease; diagnostic work-up should include an examination for lymphadenopathy and a chest x-ray.

The loose bowel movements in the setting of travel and eating uncooked food raise the possibility of traveler's diarrhea. However, the time course is long even for parasite infections, and gastrointestinal symptoms are not her primary symptom. Weight loss itself is a nonspecific sign of inflammation or infection and thus does not help narrow the differential diagnosis.

CHAPTER 9

CASE SCENARIO

Correct answer: B

The patient has old headaches (ie, they are the same in character as her usual headaches, albeit more severe). Therefore, the diagnosis for her headaches remains the same. Cervicogenic headache is generally a disease of middle-aged or older patients and is uncommon in young women. Occasionally, it can occur in younger patients after whiplash-type neck injuries. It is most commonly a burning or dull pain in the occiput and forehead. Brain tumor is a new headache. The character and description of her pain have not changed, as one would expect if a new source, such as brain tumor, were the cause of the headache.

The unilateral, throbbing nature of the headaches is typical of migraine. The occasional visual aura and associated nausea confidently establish the diagnosis of migraine with great certainty. These 2 features most accurately distinguish migraine from tension-type headache. She has no alarm symptoms. The challenge is to determine why the headaches are more severe and frequent now. Her headaches are likely worse due to a change in her lifestyle including triggers of irregular sleep and excessive caffeine.

TEST YOUR KNOWLEDGE

QUESTION #1

Correct answer: B

Migraine headaches usually begin for the first time in adolescence. Migraine-like headaches that begin for the first time at age 40 raise concern about an arteriovenous malformation (AVM). Although migraines are commonly unilateral, they should vary from one side to the other over a patient's lifetime. Pain always on the same side also suggests the possibility of AVM, although in some patients, this will prove to be an atypical manifestation of ordinary migraine. Pain that worsens over 2 to 3 months is worrisome for a brain tumor. Finally, visual aura should not last for more than 1 hour, so a prolonged aura raises concern for AVM as well. Throbbing pain is a cardinal feature of migraine and by itself is not an alarm symptom.

QUESTION #2

Correct answer: C

While there is some variation of pain location among patients with migraine, most patients will report unilateral pain that is most intense in the temporal area. Occipital and vertex pain raise the possibility of a cervicogenic headache. Periorbital pain can occur with cluster headache and with trigeminal neuralgia. Frontal pain is nonspecific.

QUESTION #3

Correct answer: A

Scalp tenderness and jaw claudication are the most specific features of giant cell arteritis. The pain can be anywhere in the head but is most commonly temporal, not vertex. Photophobia is characteristic of migraine; it may also occur in meningitis, although that would be an acute, rather than recurring, headache. Unilateral pain is nonspecific. It can occur with giant cell arteritis, but also with migraine and cluster headache. Lacrimation is a feature of cluster headache, not giant cell arteritis.

CHAPTER 10

CASE SCENARIO

Correct answer: B

She has multiple causes for her insomnia, most notably probable depression and stimulant use (caffeine). Most cases of insomnia are multifactorial. This is comorbid insomnia related to mental health and caffeine use, not primary insomnia where no obvious cause for the insomnia can be found. She does not have any symptoms of primary sleep disorders, such as obstructive sleep apnea, restless legs syndrome, or PLMD. Her sleep hygiene is good and likely not contributing.

TEST YOUR KNOWLEDGE

QUESTION #1

Correct answer: C

This patient is complaining of nonrestorative sleep with resulting significant daytime symptoms. His sleep patterns seem normal and he has no identifiable comorbid conditions. Given his obesity and significant daytime sleepiness, he has features that are consistent with obstructive sleep apnea. Thus, a bed partner history on snoring and apnea spells would be the next best step. A sleep log is unlikely to help, as he tells you his sleep pattern itself is normal. Formal polysomnography might be undertaken to confirm a sleep-related breathing disorder, but would not be warranted before taking a thorough history.

QUESTION #2

Correct answer: C

Mental health disorders are the most common cause of comorbid insomnias and are present in 30% to 40% of patients. The other conditions listed are also common.

QUESTION #3

Correct answer: B

Insomnia is a significant risk factor for the future development of depression. Heart failure is unlikely to develop in just 6 months if the patient complies with therapy for sleep apnea. Benzodiazepines would be a poor choice of therapy in patients with sleep-disordered breathing or sleep apnea. Advanced sleep phase disorder is an uncommon circadian rhythm disorder and would have no relation to this patient's sleep apnea or insomnia.

CHAPTER 11

CASE SCENARIO

Correct answer: B

The patient has painful cervical lymphadenopathy in addition to systemic features. Infectious mononucleosis (IM) caused by Epstein-Barr virus (EBV) commonly occurs in young adults. About 95% of affected patients have lymphadenopathy affecting the posterior cervical nodes; in a few cases, lymphadenopathy may be generalized. The affected lymph nodes are frequently mobile, tender, and symmetrically enlarged. Constitutional symptoms such as fever, malaise, fatigue, and myalgias are also common. Symptomatic splenomegaly presenting as left upper quadrant abdominal discomfort and fullness may also be seen.

Lymphoma usually presents with painless lymphadenopathy and occurs in older patients, although Hodgkin's lymphoma may also present in young adulthood. In patients with HIV infection, lymphadenopathy is often generalized, and additional history may reveal high-risk behaviors like multiple sexual partners and use of intravenous drugs. In streptococcal pharyngitis, the pharynx commonly shows an exudate, which this patient did not see. Patients with leukemia often complain of swollen lymph nodes in more than one lymph node group and have prominent constitutional symptoms along with a higher likelihood of abnormal bruising or bleeding.

TEST YOUR KNOWLEDGE

QUESTION #1

Correct answer: C

Lymph nodes that demonstrate progressive growth over time are concerning for the possibility of significant underlying disease such as infection or malignancy. His age is not yet greater than 40, when cancer becomes increasingly more prominent in differential diagnosis. Although enlarged lymph nodes in the supraclavicular area or axilla in the absence of trauma are of greater concern, palpable inguinal lymph nodes greater than 1.0 cm in size are relatively common in adults without underlying disease. The absence of tenderness is a nonspecific finding. Finally, associated symptoms such as hoarseness, chronic cough, abdominal pain, hematochezia, melena, or hematuria suggest more serious underlying disease.

QUESTION #2

Correct answer: D

The most likely diagnosis is HIV infection. He has generalized lymphadenopathy in addition to high-risk behaviors (multiple sexual partners and intravenous drug use) that predispose him to HIV infection. Lymphoma, CMV infection, and medications such as phenytoin may also cause lymphadenopathy, but the history of high-risk behaviors makes HIV the most likely diagnosis.

QUESTION #3

Correct answer: A

The presence of alarm features like hoarseness or chronic cough in a patient with supraclavicular lymphadenopathy should increase suspicion for head and neck or thoracic cancers. With a history of exposure to pets, diagnoses like cat-scratch disease should be considered. High-risk behaviors should increase suspicion for HIV. When lymph nodes decrease in size over time without treatment, a benign cause is more likely than a cancer.

CHAPTER 12

CASE SCENARIO

Correct answer: C

Idiopathic hyperhidrosis is usually a long-standing problem that begins in childhood or adolescence; sweating is often focal, occurring in the axillae and on the palms and soles, and a family history is common. Always consider hyperthyroidism in patients with night sweats, but this is most often associated with systemic signs such as increased hunger, weight loss, tachycardia, and anxiety. Obstructive sleep apnea is reported as a cause of night sweats, but the association is unclear, and this should be considered a diagnosis of exclusion.

The patient's report of episodes of intense heat beginning in her face and then spreading to the rest of her body is stereotypical of hot flashes, a symptom that is reported in up to 50% of perimenopausal women. In an otherwise healthy woman with hot flashes and irregular menses, menopause is the most likely diagnosis.

TEST YOUR KNOWLEDGE

QUESTION #1

Correct answer: C

Many people who volunteer for the Peace Corp work in developing countries where they are often exposed to diseases such as malaria and tuberculosis. These infections may lay dormant for years and recrudesce with systemic symptoms such as night sweats. Hypertension is common and is usually essential (idiopathic). However, when hypertension develops in young patients without obvious risk factors (eg, obesity, family history, black race), consider secondary causes, including hormonal and vascular disease. Unintentional weight loss, although nonspecific, can also be a warning sign of more serious disease. Evaluate for possible malabsorption or endocrinopathies in patients who have weight loss despite increased appetite. Weight loss in a patient with anorexia may be due to an undiagnosed psychiatric illness or an occult malignancy.[18]

Excessive sweating with exercise is common. Because sweating is the primary mechanism by which heat is dissipated, it is an appropriate response to an increased metabolic rate, as seen during exercise, and to increased ambient temperature, as occurs with excessive bedding or on a hot day. The amount an individual sweats during exercise is often genetic and/or related to body weight and fitness level.

QUESTION #2

Correct answer: C

Patients often have complicated histories, and it can be difficult to know which elements are most concerning and should be addressed first.

Although marijuana use is sometimes associated with the use of other illicit drugs, it is not associated with the transmission of infections such as hepatitis or HIV. SSRI antidepressants are a very common cause of night sweats, but the night sweats invariably resolve when the medication is discontinued. Working in a healthcare setting increases the risk of exposure to infectious diseases, especially tuberculosis. This is an important consideration, and she should have tuberculin skin testing, if not recently performed. Her report of an extramarital affair raises the possibility of exposure to a sexually transmitted disease, the most concerning being HIV. Although night sweats are most often reported in the first stages of HIV infection, patient may present years later with night sweats due to opportunistic infections; for this reason, HIV testing is reasonable and appropriate.

Her report of red-tinged urine is the most concerning element of the history, because this may be due to blood in the urine, which can be the sole manifestation of a malignancy in the bladder or kidneys. Any patient who reports night sweats and has specific physical symptoms such as bleeding, pain, shortness of breath, or a change in bowel habits should be assumed to have a serious cause of night sweats until proven otherwise.

CHAPTER13

CASE SCENARIO

Correct answer: B

The hallmark of multiple sclerosis is multiple focal central nervous system lesions separated by space and time. Her history of ocular involvement followed several months later by relapsing lower extremity weakness and vertigo fits that description. Multiple sclerosis is thought to be an inflammatory autoimmune disorder caused by axonal demyelination and degeneration. It affects women more than men in an approximately 2:1 ratio. The sharp pain experienced with neck flexion is called Lhermitte phenomenon and occurs commonly in multiple sclerosis; although, similar symptoms may also result from cord disruption caused by disk herniation or trauma. As with this patient, symptoms generally worsen in warm temperatures.

Symptoms of stroke present much more acutely, and the pattern of disability would not involve lesions separated by space and time. Myasthenia gravis initially affects the muscles used most frequently including the extraocular muscles, bulbar muscles, and respiratory muscles. Vertigo may occur as a result of ocular muscle impairment, but should not occur in the absence of diplopia. Although depression is a common illness in young women, the patient does not meet the diagnostic criteria for depression (see Chapter 64). Furthermore, depression is a diagnosis of exclusion in a patient complaining of neurologic symptoms and motor weakness.

TEST YOUR KNOWLEDGE

QUESTION #1

Correct answer: A

The focal nature of the patient's weakness and presence of both sensory and motor findings suggest neuromuscular weakness. The rapid onset of symptoms, lateralization of weakness with an arm and face distribution, and history of atrial fibrillation are highly suggestive of an embolic stroke. If the patient presents within 3 hours of symptom onset, the use of thrombolytic agents should be considered. A seizure with Todd's paralysis is possible, but less likely given the patient's risk factors for stroke and absence of a seizure history. A herniated disk will not present with weakness in the face and arm. Subdural hematomas should be considered in older patients with subacute hemiparesis even without identifiable precedent trauma, but this diagnosis cannot be ruled out on history alone. Imaging studies are imperative to exclude intracranial bleeding before beginning thrombolytic therapy for a suspected stroke. Multiple sclerosis is an unlikely new diagnosis in a patient over 50 years old.

QUESTION #2

Correct answer: D

The patient's age, constitutional symptoms of weight loss and fatigue, and significant smoking history are worrisome for cancer. The proximal pattern of weakness and diagnosis of small-cell lung cancer are typical of Lambert-Eaton myasthenic syndrome (LEMS). Strength improvement after exercise is common in LEMS. Because LEMS affects the neuromuscular junction, ocular findings of ptosis or diplopia may occur, but optic neuritis does not. Muscle fasciculations occur commonly in patients with ALS. Myasthenia gravis classically causes weakness worsening with exercise. Numbness and paresthesias are sensory symptoms that are not associated with neuromuscular junction disorders.

QUESTION #3

Correct answer: C

A careful physical examination should be conducted to confirm that the patient does not have true neuromuscular weakness; however, this patient's history is most consistent with functional weakness resulting from depression. Deconditioning causes easy fatigability, not asthenia. Although patients with hyperthyroidism typically have increased appetite, hyperthyroidism is possible, and so thyroid-stimulating hormone level should be measured. Duchenne muscular dystrophy presents with proximal weakness, so is unlikely.

QUESTION #4

Correct answer: A

The most common cause of acute symmetrical peripheral neuropathy is Guillain-Barré syndrome. It is a diagnosis that must not be missed because the rapidly ascending paralysis may lead to respiratory failure. Furthermore, early treatment with plasmapheresis results in fewer lasting neurologic deficits. Diabetes mellitus may cause a chronic symmetrical peripheral neuropathy, but does not present acutely and tends to have prominent sensory symptoms. Polyarteritis nodosa is a vasculitis that leads to multiple mononeuropathies and thus is less likely to have a symmetrical distribution. Charcot-Marie-Tooth disease is a slowly progressive genetic demyelinating disease causing peripheral neuropathy that may be symmetric. However, patients are usually symptomatic before adulthood and have prominent muscle atrophy. The patient does not have systemic signs of infection or lateralized weakness, which would be expected with a brain abscess.

CHAPTER 14

CASE SCENARIO

Correct answer: A

The pace and time course of weight gain provide valuable insight into contributing factors. In this case, the patient gained weight with each pregnancy and had progressive difficulty returning to her prepregnancy weight. The stepwise pace and long time course do not suggest weight gain due to fluid retention or a secondary endocrine cause. Rather, this history suggests a physiologic predisposition to weight gain from pregnancy consistent with primary weight gain.

TEST YOUR KNOWLEDGE

QUESTION #1

Correct answer: C

Her weight gain is primarily due to a physiologic predisposition related to prior pregnancies. However, secondary causes frequently coexist with primary obesity. She had difficulty losing weight while on medroxyprogesterone acetate. Medication side effects are probably the most common secondary cause of weight gain; hormonal contraceptives are a common offender. Medication side effect likely contributed to her weight gain but was not the primary cause.

QUESTION #2

Correct answer: C

Obesity increases the risk for serious comorbid disease including impaired glucose tolerance or diabetes, hypertension, hyperlipidemia, coronary artery disease, sleep apnea, and osteoarthritis. The medical history should include a directed review of systems to screen for these conditions. This patient's history is even more concerning given the strong family history of type 2 diabetes and coronary artery disease. Her review of systems is positive for polydipsia, polyuria, and visual blurring, which indicate that she has developed impaired glucose tolerance or diabetes.

QUESTION #3

Correct answer: C

This case presents a very different pace and time course than the prior one. Here, there is both an abrupt change in the pattern of weight gain as well as a rapid rise in weight. The acuity of the rise should raise alarm for a decompensation resulting in the accumulation of excess body fluid. The major causes are congestive heart failure, renal failure, and chronic liver disease. When concerned about excess body fluid accumulation, direct the medical history toward alarm symptoms that help elucidate the underlying cause of the accumulation. In this case, the patient's symptoms suggest excess body fluid accumulation due to an exacerbation of congestive heart failure.

CHAPTER 15

CASE SCENARIO

Correct answer: E

Weight loss in older adults, especially the frail elderly, is usually multifactorial including age-related changes, organic pathology, psychosocial issues, and medication side effects. He has clinically significant weight loss. His prepared food is incongruent with his ethnicity, which may contribute to his weight loss. Angiotensin-converting enzyme inhibitors are commonly prescribed medications known to cause dysgeusia. Acetylcholinesterase inhibitors often cause gastrointestinal side effects including anorexia and weight loss in up to 17% of patients. Finally his poorly fitting dentures pose a physical limitation to eating. All these factors are likely contributing to his weight loss.

TEST YOUR KNOWLEDGE

QUESTION #1

Correct answer: C

This is voluntary weight loss from healthy dieting. Her body mass index is within the normal range. She lacks signs and symptoms of an eating disorder. Hyperthyroidism would cause involuntary weight loss.

QUESTION #2

Correct answer: B

She has anorexia and weight loss due to digoxin toxicity. Digoxin requires close monitoring because the therapeutic index is narrow, dosing is based on lean muscle mass, and the drug is principally cleared by the kidney. Older adults are predisposed to digoxin toxicity despite normal plasma levels due in part to diminished lean body mass. The case illustrates the risk factors for digoxin toxicity (eg, age, concomitant use of a potassium-wasting diuretic) and associated signs (eg, bradycardia, blurred vision, confusion, fatigue). She does not have evidence of advanced cardiac disease. Involuntary weight loss is considered pathologic until proven otherwise. Her weight loss cannot be attributed to a normal physiologic process until further evaluation has been completed. She does not have a history supporting worsening dementia.

QUESTION #3

Correct answer: C

She has signs and symptoms consistent with hyperthyroidism. There are a limited number of conditions that cause weight loss with an increase in nutritional intake. Diabetes mellitus could also cause involuntary weight loss with an increased nutritional intake, but she does not report any symptoms suggesting diabetes such as polyuria or polydipsia. Anorexia nervosa is an eating disorder that would cause a voluntary weight loss. Lung cancer would also cause involuntary weight loss but typically with increasing anorexia due to the underlying inflammatory state.

CHAPTER 16

CASE SCENARIO

Correct answer: A

The patient has viral conjunctivitis as suggested by the watery discharge, recent exposure to an ill family member, and lack of alarm symptoms or signs of systemic illness. Nonpurulent discharge is inconsistent with bacterial conjunctivitis.

TEST YOUR KNOWLEDGE

QUESTION #1

Correct answer: A

A gritty feeling is common in conjunctivitis and is not considered an alarm symptom.

QUESTION #2

Correct answer: B

Haloes around lights, decreased visual acuity, headache, and onset in low-light situations (where mydriasis can result in further blocking of the narrow angle, preventing the outflow of aqueous humor) are classic symptoms of acute angle-closure glaucoma. Although scleritis can diminish visual acuity and cause deep pain, it should not result in nausea and vomiting or the appearance of halos around lights.

QUESTION #3

Correct answer: D

The patient has sinusitis and is now presenting with symptoms consistent with orbital cellulitis: fevers, diffuse erythema, diplopia, and pain with eye movement secondary to inflammation of the tissues/muscles in the orbit. Periorbital cellulitis would also cause fevers and swelling but would not result in diplopia because the inflammation is anterior to the orbital septum.

CHAPTER 17

CASE SCENARIO

Correct answer: B

The patient has acute ear pain that is not severe and follows a recent upper respiratory infection. His impaired hearing and the "crackling" he describes are most consistent with serous otitis (eustachian tube dysfunction). Acute otitis media generally causes severe pain and is accompanied by fever. It may cause hearing loss but generally not "crackling" in the ear. TMJ dysfunction can cause chronic ear pain, frequently bilateral, and often worse with chewing. Patients may report clicking in the jaw. Temporal arteritis can also cause pain with chewing. It is a type of claudication: Pain occurs with prolonged chewing and goes away shortly after stopping chewing. It almost never occurs in patients younger than 50. It does not cause hearing loss.

Serous otitis is a very common cause of ear pain in adults. It can be bilateral but is more frequently unilateral. It frequently develops after an upper respiratory infection or in the setting of seasonal allergies. Oral decongestants may be helpful, and the symptoms may take up to 12 weeks to resolve.

TEST YOUR KNOWLEDGE

QUESTION #1

Correct answer: B

Otitis media is the most common cause of ear pain in young children. Typical symptoms include pulling or rubbing the affected ear and crying or irritability. Fever is usually, but not always, present. A foreign body can cause ear pain in a young child but would not typically cause fever. Otitis externa is usually more modest pain, often associated with a discharge from the ear and with exposure to water ("swimmer's ear"). Malignant otitis media is a rare disease, usually seen in older patients with diabetes or a compromised immune system.

QUESTION #2

Correct answer: C

Otitis externa ("swimmer's ear") typically presents with mild to moderate ear pain, which is aggravated by pushing or pulling on the ear. The patient often reports a discharge from the ear (otorrhea) and a recent history of swimming. A patient with a perforated ear drum from otitis media usually reports severe ear pain that suddenly lessened, often immediately followed by purulent discharge from the ear. The patient with a perforated eardrum may report decreased hearing if the perforation is large. The pain of temporomandibular joint (TMJ) dysfunction is generally more chronic and is worsened by chewing. Patients with TMJ dysfunction may report a clicking sensation in the TMJ area, although many asymptomatic individuals note this as well. A patient with an infected molar tooth will report pain with chewing and may report increased pain with exposure to hot or cold foods or liquids.

QUESTION #3

Correct answer: C

Temporomandibular joint dysfunction is a common cause of referred pain to the ear. It is typically chronic in its time course and aggravated by chewing. It can be unilateral or bilateral and is sometimes associated with stress. Although ear pain from serous otitis can be persistent, pain for several months would be unusual. Temporal arteritis occurs almost exclusively in patients over 50 years of age and is nearly always unilateral. Referred pain from tight neck muscles would generally be worse later in the day and is not likely to be worsened by chewing.

CHAPTER 18

CASE SCENARIO

Correct answer: B

He has gradual-onset, slowly progressive hearing loss that is bilateral. The most likely diagnosis is therefore presbycusis. Ménière's disease is typically accompanied by aural fullness, tinnitus, and vertigo. The hearing loss of acoustic neuroma is unilateral and asymmetric. Multiple sclerosis can occasionally cause sudden hearing loss and vertigo.

TEST YOUR KNOWLEDGE

QUESTION #1

Correct answer: C

Sudden sensorineural hearing loss is the sudden onset of unilateral rapidly progressive hearing loss that is often associated with tinnitus and vertigo. The presence of fever is atypical and would raise concern for otitis media or meningitis.

QUESTION #2

Correct answer: B

Acoustic neuroma causes a gradual onset unilateral or asymmetric hearing loss. Fever is typically associated with otitis media or meningitis. Itchy ears raise the possibility of psoriasis. Fluctuating hearing loss can be seen in a variety of conditions but not typically with acoustic neuroma.

QUESTION #3

Correct answer: B

Patients with noise-induced hearing loss may report difficulty hearing high-pitched sounds, the TV, or radio. There will also be difficulty hearing when there is background noise or in a conversation with a group of people. Difficulty hearing low-pitched sounds is more typical of Ménière's disease or migraine as the etiology of hearing loss.

CHAPTER 19

CASE SCENARIO

Correct answer: B

This 75-year-old man has several reasons to have nonpulsatile tinnitus. He was subjected to chronic noise exposure as an airline mechanic, which typically causes *bilateral* high-frequency hearing loss and tinnitus. Otosclerosis causes bilateral tinnitus and progressive conductive hearing loss. Cerumen impaction is associated with unilateral hearing loss and tinnitus but would be obvious on physical examination (eg, wax obscuring the tympanic membrane). In this case, alarm features include the presence of tinnitus associated with progressive unilateral hearing loss. Additionally, the patient is experiencing disequilibrium and has fallen. Magnetic resonance imaging of the head revealed an eighth nerve mass, which on careful resection was a schwannoma, without invasion. The patient's hearing improved, and his tinnitus diminished to tolerable levels.

TEST YOUR KNOWLEDGE

QUESTION #1

Correct answer: C

A variety of medications may cause nonpulsatile tinnitus, usually by damaging the cochlear apparatus of the inner ear. Among these medications are chemotherapeutic agents (especially platinum-based treatment), quinine, antibiotics (eg, gentamicin), diuretics (especially thiazides and high-dose furosemide), benzodiazepines, and NSAIDs or aspirin. Acetaminophen is unlikely to cause tinnitus. In this case, the most likely offending agents are the high-dose diuretics and gentamicin. The ototoxicity associated with these medications is usually reversible but occasionally can be permanent.

QUESTION #2

Correct answer: C

In patulous eustachian tube, the eustachian tube is either permanently open or opens intermittently. Breathing and other physiologic sounds are transmitted unimpeded to the tympanic membrane, often resulting in a "whooshing" sound. In some cases, the patulous eustachian tube is exacerbated by weight loss, as the fatty tissue that helps keep the eustachian tube open recedes. Similarly, decongestants can make this condition worse by drying up the secretions that may hold a partially patent eustachian tube closed. Key questions to ask would be if the "whooshing" sound occurs in time with his respiration and if sounds are muffled (as might be the case with allergies and sinus congestion). The clinician may also perform evocative maneuvers (eg, deep breathing exercises) in the office. These sounds are often amplified in quiet rooms and with vigorous exercise. Myoclonic stapedius muscle spasm usually presents with a clicking sound, up to 150 to 300 spasms per minute. Auditory hallucinations, migraine aura, and malingering are all diagnoses of exclusion.

QUESTION #4

Correct answer: B

This patient has classic presentation of Ménière's disease, described by French physician Prospere Ménière in the 1860s.

This disorder is characterized by episodic vertigo, nonpulsatile tinnitus, and progressive fluctuating sensorineural hearing loss (often to low frequencies). The hearing loss and tinnitus may be unilateral (more commonly) or bilateral. During episodes, the patient typically has nystagmus. Symptoms can be mild to incapacitating. The cause of Ménière's disease is unknown but may be related to endolymphatic hydrops, an excess of fluid and pressure in the middle ear. There is an association with herpes simplex infection and with migraine headaches. Labyrinthitis may also present with episodic tinnitus, vertigo, and hearing loss but typically follows a viral infection and is self-limited. Otosclerosis causes bilateral progressive conductive hearing loss and tinnitus. Arteriovenous malformation or other vascular causes would be associated with pulsatile tinnitus.

CHAPTER 20

CASE SCENARIO

Correct answer: D

This young adult has symptoms of acute infectious pharyngitis, but he has no alarm symptoms. The next step is to assess the likelihood of GAS pharyngitis using the Centor Clinical Prediction Rule. He has 2 points (fever and tonsillar exudates). This Centor score has a likelihood ratio of 0.75. With a pretest probability for GAS infection in adults of 10% to 15%, the posttest probability is 8% to 12%. *Fusobacterium necrophorum* is another possible cause, which typically causes severe pharyngitis and is present in only 10% to 15% of young adults. Viral pharyngitis causes the majority of cases of acute pharyngitis. The acuity of the sore throat and fever make GERD an unlikely cause.

TEST YOUR KNOWLEDGE

QUESTION #1

Correct answer: C

Given his low risk of GAS based on his Centor score, empiric antibiotics are not recommended. Similarly, treatment for possible *F necrophorum* in patients with mild pharyngitis is not recommended. A throat culture will take 2 days to come back, so empirically treating with antibiotics (while awaiting the results) would likely be excessive and unnecessarily expose the patient to the risk of antibiotic side effects. Thus, the correct answer is to perform a rapid strep test and treat if positive.

QUESTION #2

Correct answer: C

This patient presents with chronic sore throat, which makes infectious etiologies unlikely. Common noninfectious causes include postnasal drip from allergic rhinitis or chronic sinusitis, laryngeal irritation from gastroesophageal reflux disease (GERD), and head and neck malignancies. He does have symptoms of GERD but no symptoms of postnasal drip or alarm symptoms for cancer. Add this to the normal examination, and the most likely diagnosis is reflux disease. The next step is an evaluation by ENT to examine his larynx and look for signs of inflammation or malignancy.

QUESTION #3

Correct answer: D

This patient presents with alarm symptoms including drooling, trismus, and neck swelling, suggesting a severe suppurative complication of acute pharyngitis. The causative agent could be GAS, *F necrophorum*, or another anaerobic or streptococcal infection, all of which can cause these symptoms. Emergent ear, nose, and throat evaluation and neck imaging are likely the next steps in the evaluation.

CHAPTER 21

CASE SCENARIO

Correct answer: A

This patient has tinea corporis, likely contracted at her gym. The diagnosis is suggested by the presence of an annular, scaly, pruritic, papulosquamous eruption and could be confirmed by the identification of fungal hyphae on a potassium hydroxide preparation of skin scrapings. The history including her social history, medical history, and lack of additional symptoms also tends to exclude alternate diagnoses.

Psoriasis may present in a similar manner. The characteristic lesions are annular, scaly plaques. This eruption may be triggered by a streptococcal throat infection, tends to be less pruritic than tinea corporis, and often involves the extensor surfaces, the scalp, the umbilicus, and/or the nails. Pityriasis rosea is often preceded by a viral upper respiratory infection. Pityriasis rosea may or may not be pruritic, usually begins with a single herald patch, and tends to follow Langer lines, leading to a "Christmas tree" distribution pattern. Subacute cutaneous lupus erythematosus (SCLE) occurs most commonly in white females. Patients with SCLE may have systemic symptoms including arthralgias or fatigue. The lesions are commonly annular but occur in a photodistributed pattern and have little scale. Secondary syphilis occurs 2 to 10 weeks after the primary chancre. Its appearance may vary but often appears as symmetric pink to brown papules on the trunk and proximal extremities.

In the case of your patient, a negative potassium hydroxide test would rule out tinea corporis. A skin biopsy would then have been helpful to identify the pathohistologic patterns of the other dermatoses in the differential diagnosis.

TEST YOUR KNOWLEDGE

QUESTION #1

Correct answer: D

Allergic contact dermatitis classically occurs in the distribution described in the question and is most commonly due to poison ivy or a similar plant exposure. A linear distribution of lesions is an important clue. Careful patient history taking often reveals recent outdoor hiking, gardening, or playing. A history of physical exposure to plants usually precedes the eruption by 1 to 2 days. Herpes zoster is usually painful and follows a dermatomal distribution. Herpes simplex classically presents as painful vesicles clustered on an erythematous base. Drug eruption is generally more diffuse, not extremely pruritic, and not linear.

QUESTION #2

Correct answer: A

Seborrheic dermatitis is very common. Many patients will not report it as a concern, but you may notice it during your examination. This eruption can present on the scalp, face, and chest. It is easy to treat but cannot be cured. Tinea facie is usually annular in appearance and can occur anywhere on face. The lesions of psoriasis are well-demarcated plaques that have a silver scale. Psoriasis can occur anywhere on the body; however, it favors the scalp, elbows, knees, and buttocks. Atopic dermatitis is always pruritic. If located on the face, then generally it presents as lichenified plaques/hyperlinearity around the eyes and erythematous cheeks.

QUESTION #3

Correct answer: C

Stevens-Johnson syndrome/toxic epidermal necrolysis is typically a consequence of medication exposure. The most common offenders are antibiotics (particularly trimethoprim-sulfamethoxazole), nonsteroidal anti-inflammatory drugs (NSAIDs), anticonvulsants, and allopurinol. This is a life-threatening condition and must be diagnosed and treated. Patients with extensive skin sloughing often require attention in intensive care or burn units. Bullous pemphigoid is an autoimmune blistering disease. Typical lesions are tense bullae on an erythematous base. The mucosa is rarely involved. The uninvolved skin is usually not tender to touch. In scarlet fever, the skin is diffusely erythematous with a "sandpaper" feel. There are no bullae or vesicles. Other features that may be present are petechiae on the hard/soft palate and white exudate with prominent papillae on the tongue ("strawberry tongue").

CHAPTER 22

CASE SCENARIO

Correct answer: B

This patient has generalized pruritus due to xerosis. She has many risk factors for dry skin: her use of an antibacterial soap, the application of witch hazel, scrubbing her skin, taking hot showers, and the cool climate. Her age may make her at risk for pruritus due to senescence, which may be compounding her problem. She has no symptoms to suggest systemic illness as the cause for pruritus. Unless she fails to respond to treatment for xerosis, further work-up is not warranted.

TEST YOUR KNOWLEDGE

QUESTION #1

Correct answer: D

This patient has pruritus due to venous insufficiency. Patients with congestive heart failure may develop edema that is similar to that of venous insufficiency. Some patients with long-standing venous insufficiency may also have rust-colored macules on the anterior lower legs, although many patients with venous insufficiency suffer from pruritus without any rash at all. When diabetes is the cause of localized pruritus, it is more often on the genital area. Renal failure and drug reactions would cause generalized and not localized pruritus. Postherpetic neuralgia would not occur bilaterally.

QUESTION #2

Correct answer: A

Pruritus due to polycythemia vera is often worsened in warm conditions, particularly after taking a hot shower. Occasionally, those with polycythemia vera may also have red hands (erythromelalgia). The patient has no risk factors for hepatitis C or HIV, making these choices less likely. The patient has no other systemic complaints, making Hodgkin's lymphoma less likely. Xerosis could be considered with the history of hot showers, but pruritus is often otherwise worse in cold conditions.

QUESTION #3

Correct answer: B

Light-headedness may be a symptom of iron deficiency anemia. Those who follow low-protein diets, such as vegan diets, are at risk for iron deficiency anemia. Although her age may make her at risk for perimenopausal pruritus, the other symptoms and clues do not lead one to this diagnosis. She has no features to suggest cholestasis, polycythemia vera, or renal failure.

CHAPTER 23

CASE SCENARIO

Correct answer: B

Patients with alopecia areata usually present with patchy hair loss of less than 1 year in duration, and have no associated pruritus, pustules, or scaling. The hairs come out by the roots rather than break; nail pitting or other nail changes may occur. Individuals may have a personal or family history of autoimmune disease.

Scarring alopecia is unlikely due to the lack of pain, itching, or pustules. Telogen effluvium is usually diffuse hair loss, with a preceding emotional or physical stress. Tinea capitis is associated with an itchy scalp and hair breakage. The pattern of hair thinning in androgenetic alopecia is usually temporal or frontal in men or central in women.

TEST YOUR KNOWLEDGE

QUESTION #1

Correct answer: B

Telogen effluvium is often preceded by an emotionally or physically stressful event in the previous several months. Physically stressful events might include crash diets or major surgeries. The psychological distress associated with the death of a family member could precipitate telogen effluvium.

QUESTION #2

Correct answer: A

Androgenetic alopecia is characterized by chronic hair thinning in the temporal regions in men with frontal recession and central thinning in women, with widening of the midline part. Hair breakage occurs in traction alopecia, tinea capitis, and trichotillomania. Patchy hair loss is characteristic of alopecia areata and tinea capitis. Itchy erythematous lesions are typical of tinea capitis and inflammatory alopecias.

QUESTION #3

Correct answer: D

Tinea capitis is common in children and is associated with patchy hair breakage, pruritus, and flaking (which patients often describe as dandruff). Alopecia areata is generally not pruritic, and telogen effluvium is usually a diffuse hair loss. Scarring alopecia is uncommon in children.

CHAPTER 24

CASE SCENARIO

Correct answer: B

In this case, upper airway cough syndrome (UACS) is the most likely diagnosis. He reported a dripping sensation in the back of his throat, and his symptoms responded to an antihistamine medication. UACS, previously known as "postnasal drip syndrome," includes a wide constellation of rhinosinus disorders. Allergic rhinitis is one of the most common disorders. Although his symptoms may mimic a viral infection, the duration of his cough argues against an infectious cause. Asthma and gastroesophageal reflux disease (GERD) are very common causes of cough, but in this case, the patient denied any of the characteristic features of these conditions.

TEST YOUR KNOWLEDGE

QUESTION #1

Correct answer: C

The alarm features in this case are hemoptysis, weight loss, and fever. Although serious causes of cough are not common, the alarm features require immediate action and often additional testing. The duration of the cough provides a guideline for the differential diagnosis, but it is not an alarm feature. Although smoking and his occupation provide additional information, they are not alarm features.

QUESTION #2

Correct answer: C

The most likely diagnosis is tuberculosis. Patients typically report chronic cough with/without hemoptysis, fevers, night sweats, and weight loss. Patients come from endemic areas or are immunosuppressed. Lung cancer can cause similar symptoms, but typically it affects an older population. Acute bronchitis is of short duration and does not cause chronic cough or weight loss. Although the patient is a current smoker, he does not have the characteristic features of COPD or emphysema.

QUESTION #3

Correct answer: B

His symptoms suggest GERD. Heartburn characterized by a midline retrosternal burning is a characteristic feature of GERD. Hoarseness may be a sign of severe disease. The patient should be treated empirically for this diagnosis. Depending on his response to therapy, additional testing might be required to confirm the diagnosis. Although asthma remains a possibility, he had no wheezing or other features to suggest this diagnosis. Based on his symptoms, the likelihood of an infectious cause of his cough is low.

CHAPTER 25

CASE SCENARIO

Correct answer: B

The most common causes of dyspnea are primary cardiac and pulmonary causes, anemia, deconditioning, and functional dyspnea. The patient describes a productive cough for greater than 3 months and an impressive smoking history; both have high likelihood ratios for chronic obstructive pulmonary disease (COPD). The patient's presentation is highly suggestive of the chronic bronchitis variant of COPD.

However, congestive heart failure and COPD frequently occur together; thus a diagnosis of one does not exclude the other. Further evaluation for cardiac causes should be pursued because the patient has several coronary artery disease risk factors (smoking, male sex, and age over 60) and CHF may be contributing to the patient's dyspnea. The classic symptoms of asthma are dyspnea, wheezing, and cough, which overlap with those of COPD, making diagnostic distinction difficult. In this case, the patient's older age of onset makes asthma less likely. Pneumonia is unlikely based on the chronicity of symptoms and lack of systemic symptoms or signs of infection.

TEST YOUR KNOWLEDGE

QUESTION #1

Correct answer: B

Pulmonary embolism (PE) is the most likely cause of dyspnea in this patient. The significant smoking history and suspicious mass on chest radiograph are very concerning for lung cancer. The patient's acute dyspnea is most likely due to a venous thromboembolism (deep venous thrombosis) originating in the leg. The modified Wells criteria are clinical prediction rules that can be used to classify the patient as likely (score > 4) or unlikely (score ≤ 4) to have a PE (see van Belle et al reference in Suggested Reading section of Chapter 25). This patient has a Wells score of 4.5, placing him in the category of likely to have a PE because he has had recent surgery (1.5 points) and does not have an alternative diagnosis that is more likely than PE to explain his symptoms (3 points). If the patient also has lung cancer, leading to a hypercoagulable state, this would further increase his Wells score (1 point). Smoking has also been associated with an increased risk of PE. Rib fractures are generally highly painful and lead to shallow, hesitant respirations and, if displaced, can cause pneumothorax. In this case, rib fracture is unlikely given the delay between the patient's accident and the onset of dyspnea. Anxiety should not be diagnosed until other causes have been ruled out. Deconditioning will be a concern for this patient during his recovery but is unlikely to present acutely.

QUESTION #2

Correct answer: B

After cardiac and pulmonary causes, anemia is the most common cause of shortness in breath. In young women, menorrhagia is a common cause of anemia and should be considered in this case. The prolonged nature of the patient's symptoms is inconsistent with anaphylaxis. Chronic pulmonary embolism is unlikely in this otherwise healthy teenager. Although exposure to asbestos can cause infiltrative lung disease, pleural disease, or malignancy, it typically does not develop for decades.

QUESTION #3

Correct answer: A

The patient has several coronary artery disease risk factors (male sex, age > 55 years, smoking history, diabetes, and hypertension) and describes paroxysmal nocturnal dyspnea, 3-pillow orthopnea, and lower extremity edema, the classic symptoms of congestive heart failure (CHF). The patient's significant smoking history also raises suspicion for chronic obstructive pulmonary disease. Asthma is less likely given the patient's age of onset. The patient's smoking history puts him at increased risk of lung cancer. Pulmonary embolism can be difficult to diagnose. Although the other diagnoses cannot be definitively excluded, the clinical picture is most consistent with CHF.

CHAPTER 26

CASE SCENARIO

Correct answer: B

The patient's most likely diagnosis is acute bronchitis. His hemoptysis was mild, and it was followed by a short period of subjective fever, increased cough, and sputum production. Bronchitis remains the most common cause of hemoptysis. He does not have risk factors for lung cancer such as weight loss, advanced age, or tobacco exposure. He does not have any features suggestive of tuberculosis including exposure to sick contacts, weight loss, or prolonged fevers. He does not have any history of prolonged immobilization or recent surgery to suggest pulmonary embolism.

TEST YOUR KNOWLEDGE

QUESTION #1

Correct answer: B

The history of weight loss, advanced age, and tobacco exposure in the setting of hemoptysis are considered alarm features concerning for malignancy. The quantity of hemoptysis can be considered an alarm feature if it is greater than 200 mL in 24 hours. She does not have additional risks for hemoptysis. Her medications cannot explain the hemoptysis, and there was no exposure to any anticoagulants.

QUESTION #2

Correct answer: C

Weight loss, tobacco exposure, advanced age, and hemoptysis make lung cancer a likely diagnosis.

QUESTION #3

Correct answer: D

The next step is to obtain the vital signs and perform a physical examination to obtain more information. The patient will need a chest x-ray but after she is examined. Depending on the chest imaging, the patient might require additional testing including bronchoscopy. It would not be appropriate to just monitor her symptoms without an intervention.

QUESTION #4

Correct answer: D

The most likely diagnosis is tuberculosis, because of the immunocompromised state associated with HIV infection. Bronchitis typically has a shorter and more benign course. He does not have any history of recurrent pulmonary infections to suggest bronchiectasis. Although he has weight loss and tobacco exposure, he is younger than most patients with lung cancer.

QUESTION #5

Correct answer: B

The most likely diagnosis is pulmonary embolism, which typically presents with acute chest pain and dyspnea. Prolonged immobility and hypercoagulability are risk factors for pulmonary embolism. The patient was immobile for a prolonged period of time during his recent travel. Furthermore, his testicular mass most likely represents a malignancy, which increases his risk for hypercoagulability. Bronchitis and pneumonia are less likely as he did not complain of fevers or increased sputum production. He does not have risk factors for tuberculosis.

CHAPTER 27

CASE SCENARIO

Correct answer: A

The patient presents with acute coronary syndrome. He describes a prodrome of typical exertional angina that has progressed to rest symptoms over the last month (unstable angina). On presentation, the pain is prolonged and exhibits several features consistent with acute myocardial ischemia including an oppressive nature, radiation to the arms and shoulders, and associated dyspnea. These alarm symptoms are occurring on the backdrop of a high probability for coronary artery disease (CAD)—a 56-year-old man with typical angina and risk factors of smoking and high cholesterol has an estimated CAD prevalence of greater than 90%. An electrocardiogram and cardiac biomarkers should be obtained without delay in this patient.

TEST YOUR KNOWLEDGE

QUESTION #1

Correct answer: D

The squeezing, oppressive quality, precipitation by exertion, and associated dyspnea are all consistent with ischemic chest pain. Sharp or stabbing pain, pleuritic pain, localized pain, positional pain, and chest pain reproduced by palpation all decrease the likelihood that the symptoms are secondary to myocardial ischemia.

QUESTION #2

Correct answer: C

Chest pain and dyspnea with syncope should raise consideration for conditions that disrupt global cardiac output including acute myocardial infarction, other serious cardiovascular causes (eg, arrhythmia, valvular heart disease), and large pulmonary embolism that obstructs right ventricular flow. Here, the patient has had recent lower extremity surgery that increases the likelihood of deep venous thrombosis that can lead to pulmonary embolism. The pleuritic nature of chest pain and associated hemoptysis also suggest pulmonary embolism. Pleuritic chest pain can also be a feature of pericarditis, pneumonia, and pneumothorax, although the presentation usually does not include acute chest pain with syncope. The overall constellation points most strongly to pulmonary embolism.

QUESTION #3

Correct answer: A

Although the patient has had a prior myocardial infarction, the features of his current chest pain (nonexertional, pleuritic, and positional) do not suggest myocardial ischemia. The recent flu-like illness and relief of the pain upon sitting up and leaning forward suggest pericarditis.

CHAPTER 28

CASE SCENARIO

Correct answer: D

The patient experienced syncope in association with his palpitations, raising concern for an arrhythmia significant enough to decrease cardiac output and prevent adequate cerebral perfusion. The patient's family history and the association of his syncope with a high catecholamine state (exercise) also suggest a ventricular tachycardia (VT) due to an inherited conduction disturbance, such as an idiopathic VT from the right ventricular outflow tract or the long QT syndrome. Panic disorder can cause palpitations but would not cause syncope, and this patient's panic disorder has been well controlled. Hyperthyroidism can cause atrial arrhythmias (most commonly atrial fibrillation) and could therefore cause syncope, but this would not necessarily happen only during exercise. Premature atrial contractions do not cause syncope.

The patient's physical examination was normal, as was his electrocardiogram (ECG). He underwent Holter monitoring, which was unrevealing. However, during an exercise (treadmill) ECG test, the patient went into VT and experienced syncope.

TEST YOUR KNOWLEDGE

QUESTION #1

Correct answer: B

This patient has no identified alarm symptoms for arrhythmia. Although male gender *may* suggest a cardiac etiology, a history of panic disorder carries a likelihood ratio of 0.5. The other 3 answers all suggest an arrhythmic cause. Polyuria may indicate arrhythmia because of atrial stretch (causing increased release of atrial natriuretic peptide). A family history of long QT syndrome is an obvious red flag, and use of antihistamine can be associated with QT prolongation.

QUESTION #2

Correct answer: C

Atrial fibrillation is the most common arrhythmia in this age group. The patient has several historical features suggesting an arrhythmia including age, cardiac disease (she has symptoms of congestive heart failure), perception of an irregular rhythm, and risk of electrolyte abnormalities (eg, hypokalemia) due to being on a diuretic. Anxiety disorders, while common, would be much less likely in this patient. AVNRT is more likely in young patients, although it is still possible in this age group.

QUESTION #3

Correct answer: B

Many clinicians might overlook this patient's palpitations because they have been chronic. Although stopping caffeine may help, the key point is that she reports a recent presyncopal episode (an alarm symptom) after starting a new medication (erythromycin). Erythromycin is well known to cause QT prolongation, so obtaining an electrocardiogram to measure the QT interval is the most appropriate answer. Clinicians who are uncertain about a medication's effect on the QT interval should consult a pharmacist or online resource.

CHAPTER 29

CASE SCENARIO

Correct answer: D

Loss of consciousness is the sine qua non of syncope. The rapid onset with spontaneous, complete recovery excludes other forms of loss of consciousness such as coma, drug intoxication, and seizure. This is true syncope. The circumstances of a hot, crowded environment with prolonged standing and a previous history are characteristic of vasovagal syncope, as are the premonitory symptoms. The negative family and medical history and absence of palpitations also support that diagnosis. Orthostatic hypotension typically occurs with standing and has an underlying autonomic disorder or history compatible with volume loss.

TEST YOUR KNOWLEDGE

QUESTION #1

Correct answer: D

The first 3 options are typical of vasovagal syncope. Loss of consciousness in the supine position is an alarm symptom suggesting a cardiac cause such as an arrhythmia.

QUESTION #2

Correct answer: A

Transient ischemic attacks (TIAs) are transient and, like syncope, self-limited. However, carotid artery distribution TIAs typically last longer and are associated with localizing neurologic signs and symptoms. Vertebrobasilar TIAs may cause loss of consciousness but are accompanied by hemianopsia or other focal neurologic features such as vertigo, dysarthria, and diplopia. In general, cerebrovascular disease is an unusual cause of syncope and should not be considered unless there are focal neurologic symptoms or signs. Only subclavian steal causes loss of consciousness compatible with syncope, often triggered by arm exercise. All other options are known causes of syncope. Severe aortic stenosis causes exercise-induced syncope via decreased cerebral perfusion due to obstruction of left ventricular outflow and cardiac output in the face of peripheral vascular dilatation in exercising muscles. Pulmonary embolism raises pulmonary arterial pressures causing functional obstruction to right ventricular outflow, which leads to "underfilling" of the left ventricle and decreased cardiac output. Left atrial myxoma causes transient obstruction of inflow to the left ventricle and thus decreased cardiac output, leading to decreased cerebral perfusion that is often positional.

QUESTION #3

Correct answer: D

This is a typical story for vasovagal syncope or, in this case, situational syncope, which is triggered by a painful stimulus. Brief jerking movements can be seen in all forms of syncope and must be differentiated from the tonic-clonic movements of a seizure. The lack of tongue biting or postictal confusion makes seizure less likely. Removal of 75 mL of blood is insufficient to cause orthostatic hypotension. Finally, there is no antecedent, reproducible history of neck turning or a tight collar to suggest carotid sinus syncope.

QUESTION #4

Correct answer: A

Loss of consciousness defines syncope. Sweating and pallor are common symptoms of vasovagal or neural reflex syncope. This patient has a history of significant structural heart disease, which is an alarm feature. The presence of heart disease is a strong independent risk factor for a cardiac cause of syncope with sensitivity approaching 95% in some studies (which means the absence of heart disease may be helpful in excluding a cardiac cause).

CHAPTER 30

CASE SCENARIO

Correct answer: C

This patient likely has edema due to diabetic nephropathy. The loss of albumin in the urine results in decreased intravascular oncotic pressure, enabling third spacing of fluid in the dependent portions of the body. Nephrotic syndrome is characterized by the loss of essential proteins (albumin, lipoproteins, and proteins essential for natural anticoagulation), resulting in the triad of edema, hypercholesterolemia, and hypercoagulability. Although this patient has not had a thrombotic event, the other 2 symptoms in the setting of long-term, poorly managed diabetes makes this the likely diagnosis.

Edema can result from medications such as calcium channel blockers and angiotensin-converting enzyme inhibitors, but diuretics are unlikely to cause peripheral edema. Congestive heart failure is the most common cause of edema, but the absence of additional symptoms such as exertional dyspnea, chest pain, or palpitations makes the diagnosis less likely. Hypothyroidism can cause edema in advanced cases, but this patient has no other symptoms of hypothyroidism, which makes this diagnosis unlikely.

TEST YOUR KNOWLEDGE

QUESTION #1

Correct answer: A

This patient likely has hereditary angioedema. Her age, lack of additional comorbidities, family history, and intermittent pattern of edema with a predilection for the face suggest this diagnosis. Hereditary angioedema results from C1 esterase deficiency, which leads to increased vascular permeability and subsequent edema. Although direct measurement of C1 levels or C1 esterase itself is the gold standard of diagnosis, neither is routinely available. Instead, a decreased C4 level, an indirect marker of C1 activity, is the diagnostic test of choice.

Although an ANA test is sensitive for lupus nephropathy (causing nephrotic syndrome), this patient does not have any additional criteria for lupus, and the time course of the edema is too rapid. Echocardiography would be useful in evaluating suspected heart failure or valvular disease, but the absence of "heart failure" symptoms (ie, dyspnea, orthopnea) makes this a less likely diagnosis. Unlike other cardiac valvular disorders, mitral valve prolapse is an unlikely case of edema. Hypothyroidism can cause edema, usually with advanced disease, but this patient has no other symptoms of hypothyroidism, making this disorder unlikely. Hyperthyroidism due to Graves disease may cause "pseudoedema" due to antibody-induced inflammation of the pretibial muscles, but the patient has no additional symptoms of hyperthyroidism (ie, tremulousness, agitation, ocular disease), so thyroid function testing is unlikely to be helpful.

QUESTION #2

Correct answer: A

May-Thurner disease results from compression of the left iliac vein as it crosses under the aorta en route to the inferior vena cava. The compression results in unilateral increased hydrostatic pressure in the left leg, causing edema. Although May-Thurner is a rare cause of edema, it should be suspected in patients with left leg edema for whom deep vein thrombosis has been excluded. Stenting of the area of obstruction may provide relief of persistent edema.

QUESTION #3

Correct answer: D

Calcium channel blocking medications such as amlodipine can induce idiopathic edema. The diagnostic clue in this patient is the absence of additional signs or symptoms, which would suggest more serious etiologies. The presence of constipation, also a calcium channel blocker effect, further suggests this diagnosis. A simple approach would be to switch the patient to a non–calcium channel blocker antihypertensive agent and see if the edema resolves. If the edema persists, additional evaluation would be warranted.

The absence of ascites makes a liver evaluation unwarranted as the first step. Similarly, the absence of a cardiac history or heart failure symptoms (ie, dyspnea or changes in his exercise tolerance) makes an echocardiogram unlikely to be useful. Again, hypothyroidism cause edema but usually as a late-stage manifestation; the absence of other symptoms associated with hypothyroidism suggests that thyroid function testing is unlikely to be useful.

CHAPTER 31

CASE SCENARIO

Correct answer: D

The patient presents with abdominal pain for 6 months, which puts it into the chronic abdominal pain category. Furthermore, he is a former smoker and has history of hyperlipidemia and coronary artery disease, which raises the suspicion of generalized atherosclerotic disease. Nearly 50% of patients with chronic intestinal ischemia have either peripheral vascular disease or coronary artery disease. His symptoms of nausea, vomiting, weight loss, and pain starting an hour after eating and resolving after emesis are all characteristic of chronic bowel ischemia. About 80% of patients with intestinal ischemia present with weight loss, often ascribed to food aversion because patients associate their pain with meals. Peptic ulcer disease could be chronic and present with epigastric pain, but a 20-lbs weight loss would be unusual for this condition. Pancreatitis and cholecystitis cause nausea and vomiting, but patients with these disorders typically are more acutely ill and often have fever.

TEST YOUR KNOWLEDGE

QUESTION #1

Correct answer: B

This patient is presenting with classic symptoms of appendicitis, which include anorexia, nausea, vomiting, fever, and right lower quadrant (RLQ) pain. The pain of appendicitis classically starts in the periumbilical region and then becomes localized to RLQ. Testicular torsion predominantly occurs in neonates and postpubertal boys, although up to 40% of patients are older than 21 years; the absence of testicular pain makes this diagnosis unlikely. Ischemic colitis most commonly occurs in older patients with history of smoking or atherosclerotic disease. The pain occurs after meals and lessens after emesis. Pancreatitis causes abrupt onset of epigastric pain radiating to the back; RLQ tenderness would be unusual. Approximately 50% of patients with small bowel obstruction have had prior abdominal surgeries. The typical pain of small bowel obstruction is crampy and periumbilical and occurs in paroxysms every few minutes.

QUESTION #2

Correct answer: C

Peptic ulcer disease (PUD) is very common; symptoms may include epigastric "burning" or pain, epigastric fullness, postprandial belching, or bloating. As in this patient, duodenal ulcer pain classically occurs hours after eating on an empty stomach. Gastric ulcer pain classically occurs soon after eating. Pancreatitis and cholecystitis are important considerations in the differential diagnosis of acute epigastric pain. Patients with these disorders are typically more ill-appearing, with fevers and nausea or vomiting. In addition, pancreatitis pain is often severe and may radiate to the back. Aortic dissection most commonly presents with tearing chest pain that radiates to the back and is seen in patients who have severe hypertension, abuse cocaine, or have a connective tissue disorder such as Marfan syndrome. Celiac sprue usually presents with diarrhea, flatulence, weight loss, and bloating; acute pain is unusual in this condition.

QUESTION #3

Correct answer: E

After gallstones, alcohol is the second most common cause of acute pancreatitis and is the most common cause in men. This patient is presenting with many classic features of pancreatitis including epigastric pain radiating to the back associated with nausea and vomiting. Peptic ulcer disease is usually characterized by chronic epigastric burning that occurs after eating and is relieved with antacids. The pain is usually not severe and is rarely associated with nausea and vomiting. Both cholecystitis and appendicitis pains are also acute and severe and can be associated with nausea and vomiting. However, cholecystitis pain is usually localized to right upper quadrant and may radiate to the right shoulder. Appendicitis pain initially starts in the periumbilical region and then localizes to the right lower quadrant. Nephrolithiasis patients may be asymptomatic or have colicky flank pain that radiates to the groin and is often associated with urinary symptoms including dysuria and urgency.

CHAPTER 32

CASE SCENARIO

Correct answer: B

Constipation-predominant irritable bowel syndrome is most likely because the abdominal pain is a significant feature and is relieved by bowel movements; the symptoms increase with psychological stress; and the stools change in consistency (and/or number of bowel movements) with onset of pain. This is a type of normal transit constipation. The absence of alarm symptoms makes inflammatory bowel disease less likely. Daily bowel movements and the presence of pain make slow transit constipation less likely, but the Bristol Stool Scale could be useful to confirm this—lower type has longer transit time. She neither passes soft stools nor has to use manual maneuvers to evacuate, so a defecatory disorder is less likely.

TEST YOUR KNOWLEDGE

QUESTION #1

Correct answer: A

The patient's history suggests a defecatory disorder, such as pelvic floor dyssynergia, particularly because she reports sometimes having to manually evacuate even soft stool. An obstetric history is important to elicit because multiparity and rectovaginal trauma during delivery can disrupt the normal function of the pelvic floor. Specific questions to support the diagnosis of defecatory disorder include: "Do you feel like your bowels are blocked? Do you have difficulty letting go or relaxing your muscles to have a bowel movement?" The possibility of sexual abuse should also be explored. Depression-related constipation is unlikely to require digital manipulation to assist evacuation. A medication history is routine, but medications that cause constipation usually do so by slowing colonic transit, resulting in hard stools.

QUESTION #2

Correct answer: C

This patient has several alarm symptoms worrisome for colon cancer, including advanced age. Other possibilities include diverticulitis, stricture, hypothyroidism, depression, and less likely, a spinal cord process. Focused history should include past history of abdominal radiation leading to stricture; poor concentration, low mood, and disturbed sleep suggesting depression; leg weakness and back pain possibly indicating a spinal cord process; and fever, which is consistent with both colon cancer and diverticulitis. Further evaluation is absolutely essential.

CHAPTER 33

CASE SCENARIO

Correct answer: B

She has 6 weeks of diarrhea. Because this episode lasts longer than 4 weeks, this meets the definition of chronic diarrhea. Ulcerative colitis frequently presents as chronic diarrhea with bleeding and tenesmus.

Given the duration of symptoms, by definition, this cannot be acute infectious diarrhea. Irritable bowel disease does not cause bleeding; patients generally have chronic abdominal pain that improves with defecation, a change in stool frequency, and/or a change in the appearance of stool. Bleeding and tenesmus are not features of celiac disease; common food triggers are wheat, rye, or barley.

TEST YOUR KNOWLEDGE

QUESTION #1

Correct answer: A

This patient meets the definition for irritable bowel syndrome (IBS). She has greater than 6 months of symptoms, accompanied by a change in stool frequency and form, and improvement with defecation. Ulcerative colitis leads to chronic diarrhea and bleeding. Rotavirus infection and *Escherichia coli* infection are acute diarrheal illnesses.

QUESTION #2

Correct answer: C

The ingestion of preformed toxins causes acute nonbloody diarrhea less than 6 hours after exposure to *Staphylococcus aureus* or *Bacillus cereus*. *S aureus* is classically associated with ingestion of mayonnaise (frequently in potato or egg salad), custards, or poultry. Enterohemorrhagic *E coli* (O157:H7) usually causes bloody diarrhea. Fever and often bloody diarrhea accompany *Salmonella* infection. Neither enterohemorrhagic *E coli* nor *Salmonella* would be expected to cause diarrhea so soon after exposure. Irritable bowel syndrome is a cause of chronic, not acute, diarrhea.

CHAPTER 34

CASE SCENARIO

Correct answer: B

The patient has classic symptoms of functional or nonulcer dyspepsia. Symptoms commonly include epigastric discomfort, early satiety, and postprandial nausea. These symptoms have significant overlap with those associated with other diagnoses; thus, it is important to probe for features that might make an organic etiology likely. Gastric malignancy is generally associated with the presence of alarm symptoms, including age over 45 to 55, weight loss, bleeding and/or iron deficiency, or dysphagia. GERD typically manifests as a burning sensation with radiation into the chest and rarely presents with early satiety. Peptic ulcer disease is frequently associated with tobacco, alcohol, or NSAID use, and the discomfort is typically affected by food intake and often associated with vomiting or other alarm signs listed above.

TEST YOUR KNOWLEDGE

QUESTION #1

Correct answer: C

Gastroesophageal reflux is a common condition that is often precipitated by ingestion of spicy foods or alcohol and classically causes a burning sensation in the epigastrium and radiating into the chest. Symptoms are worse upon lying down, and patients often complain of a bitter taste in their mouth. Chronic cough is a common complaint due to reflux of gastric contents. Nausea may occur, but vomiting is rare. Weight loss and flatulence are not features of GERD.

QUESTION #2

Correct answer: C

The patient has several concerning features in his presentation: male sex, age over 45, weight loss, and blood in his stool. Other alarm features in the diagnosis of dyspepsia include dysphagia, the presence of an iron deficiency anemia, and persistent vomiting. These symptoms warrant immediate investigation with an endoscopy to explore the possibility of malignancy versus peptic ulcer disease. Constipation is not an alarm symptom that would prompt additional work-up.

QUESTION #3

Correct answer: D

Peptic ulcer disease can cause significant morbidity, particularly if it is associated with bleeding or perforation. Patients with gastric ulcers generally find their symptoms worsened with food, whereas those with duodenal ulcers generally exhibit decreased symptomatology after eating. NSAID use and *Helicobacter pylori* infection are 2 of the most important risk factors for peptic ulcer disease. Pain that is worse upon lying down is suggestive of reflux. Colicky pain is more suggestive of biliary disease, and difficulty with swallowing or odynophagia is typically associated with an esophageal stricture, irritation, ring, or mass.

CHAPTER 35

CASE SCENARIO

Correct answer: A

He has esophageal (rather than oropharyngeal) dysphagia. He has no difficulty with liquids, suggesting that his symptoms are most likely due to a mechanical obstruction rather than a motor disorder such as esophageal spasm or achalasia. He has had only occasional episodes of heartburn or regurgitation to suggest acid reflux disease, and therefore, although possible, it less likely that he has a peptic stricture of his distal esophagus. Likewise, esophageal cancer is less likely because his symptoms have been present for approximately 5 years and, despite this, he has not lost a significant amount of weight. Patients with esophageal rings usually have intermittent dysphagia to solids, particularly foods greater than 13 mm in diameter. The episodes of dysphagia are usually associated with chest discomfort and relieved by regurgitating the obstructing food bolus. Acute impaction of the esophagus may require endoscopic intervention to remove the food bolus.

TEST YOUR KNOWLEDGE

QUESTION #1

Correct answer: B

Eosinophilic esophagitis (or allergic esophagitis) is an increasingly common disorder of the esophagus that is characterized by eosinophilic infiltration of the esophagus due to allergic or idiopathic causes. Children and young adults are most commonly affected, although it can occur at any age. Patients most commonly report dysphagia that is frequently complicated by food impaction. A history of atopy (eg, rhinoconjunctivitis, asthma, dermatitis) is commonly present. Strictures frequently occur and can be present throughout the esophagus. Multiple mucosa rings are commonly present at endoscopy, and biopsies typically reveal greater than 20 eosinophils per high-power field.

Schatzki ring could be a cause of this patient's symptoms. However, given his age, gender, recent onset, and history of atopy, the most likely diagnosis is eosinophilic esophagitis. Achalasia and esophageal spasm are unlikely to explain his symptoms. These motility disorders rarely present with food impaction, and patients generally have dysphagia to both solids and liquids.

QUESTION #2

Correct answer: A

Achalasia is a motor (motility) disorder of the esophagus in which there is failure of the lower esophageal sphincter (LES) to relax along with abnormal movement of the esophagus in response to swallowing. The impairment of the LES to relax causes a functional obstruction of the esophagus, which is relieved when the pressure of the contents of the esophagus exceed the pressure of the sphincter or through occasional intermittent spontaneous relaxations of the LES. Achalasia is rare; it affects men and women equally. Dysphagia for both solids and liquids is the most common symptom. Other symptoms include regurgitation of food, chronic cough, chest pain, and weight loss.

Peptic stricture is less likely given the duration of symptoms, lack of typical gastroesophageal reflux disease symptoms, and complaints of dysphagia to both liquids and solids, which typically occurs in patients with an esophageal motility disorder. Esophageal cancer is unlikely due to the duration of symptoms and the presence of dysphagia to both liquids and solids. This patient does not have symptoms suggestive of oropharyngeal dysphagia.

CHAPTER 36

CASE SCENARIO

Correct answer: C

The patient's age and therapy with both aspirin and clopidogrel (without any gastroprotective agent) put him at increased risk for peptic ulcer disease. The patient has not had any nausea or vomiting, so a Mallory-Weiss tear is unlikely. The patient denies any reflux symptoms, so esophagitis is less likely. The patient denies dysphagia or weight loss, so esophageal cancer is also unlikely.

TEST YOUR KNOWLEDGE

QUESTION #1

Correct answer: A

This patient is known to have alcoholic cirrhosis and presents with maroon stool, witnessed hematemesis, and evidence of hemodynamic instability (tachycardia and hypotension). These suggest that his hematochezia is due to a brisk upper GI bleed. Given his history of cirrhosis, variceal bleeding is the most likely etiology. Gastritis often presents as iron deficiency anemia, coffee-ground emesis, or melena. Diverticular bleeding and ischemic colitis cause hematochezia but not hematemesis.

QUESTION #2

Correct answer: D

The patient has a history of diverticulosis, with one prior episode of self-limited GI bleeding. Bleeding occurs in less than 5% of patients with diverticulosis. Most diverticular bleeds stop spontaneously but may recur in 25% of cases. Esophagitis and gastric cancer are unlikely to present with hematochezia. Hemorrhoids present with trivial amounts of bright red blood per rectum, such as blood on the toilet paper after wiping or drops of blood in the toilet bowl after a bowel movement. Occasionally, red blood is noted to cover the stool. Hemorrhoidal bleeding does not cause frankly bloody bowel movements with clot.

QUESTION #3

Correct answer: D

Abdominal discomfort with lower GI bleeding indicates 1 of 3 main diagnoses: infectious colitis, ischemic colitis, or inflammatory bowel disease. Ischemic colitis is more likely to occur in elderly patients with underlying vascular disease. Inflammatory bowel disease must be considered in young patients with bloody diarrhea. However, in this case, the patient has a very acute onset of symptoms, recent travel, and sick companions with similar symptoms, all suggesting an infectious etiology. Diverticulosis or gastric cancer at this young age would be rare. She has no risk factors for radiation colitis.

CHAPTER 37

CASE SCENARIO

Correct answer: B

The patient presents with painless jaundice, which should raise the suspicion for pancreatic cancer. Dark urine implies the jaundice is due to elevations in conjugated bilirubin, which is filtered in the urine. Pale stools further suggest that the conjugated hyperbilirubinemia is due to extrahepatic obstruction. Extrahepatic obstruction may result from choledocholithiasis, strictures of the common bile duct, or compression of the common bile duct by neoplasm. Obstructing gallstones would be expected to produce more pain. Primary sclerosing cholangitis is typically seen in younger adults who often have a history of inflammatory bowel disease. Chronic viral hepatitis could cause cirrhosis and jaundice, but should not cause extrahepatic obstruction, and would be unlikely in the absence of risk factors. In this older smoker with painless obstructive jaundice, pancreatic cancer is the most likely etiology.

TEST YOUR KNOWLEDGE

QUESTION #1

Correct answer: A

This patient is presenting with the constellation of findings known as Reynolds pentad: jaundice, abdominal pain, fever, hypotension, and mental status changes. These features strongly point to ascending cholangitis. Acute viral hepatitis C is very uncommon, and this patient has no risk factors for this infection. The acuity of illness argues against chronic viral hepatitis or nonalcoholic fatty liver disease.

QUESTION #2

Correct answer: C

Although the patient's gender, age, and weight place her at increased risk of cholelithiasis, the absence of pain and abdominal tenderness renders acute cholecystitis unlikely. Acute viral hepatitis typically presents with fevers, abdominal pain, nausea, and vomiting, findings that are not present in this well-appearing woman. At age 55, pregnancy is unlikely, thus excluding the HELLP syndrome. Carotenemia spares the sclerae; a dietary history can effectively rule out this diagnosis.

QUESTION #3

Correct answer: C

In this woman with prior episodes of self-limited jaundice associated with illnesses, Gilbert syndrome is the most likely diagnosis. In this patient, checking serum concentrations of aspartate aminotransferase (AST), alanine aminotransferase (ALT), and alkaline phosphatase and acute viral hepatitis serologies would be reasonable although not mandatory given the lack of alarm features other than low-grade fever, which can be attributed to her upper respiratory illness. Gilbert syndrome is the most common form of hereditary jaundice. It is an autosomal dominant disorder linked to a mutation in the gene encoding UGT1. This mutation leads to reduced UGT activity that results in hyperbilirubinemia when the body is under stress. It is important to make the diagnosis because if these patients are identified, unnecessary extensive testing, such as ultrasonography or computed tomography scan, is avoided. Biliary colic is unlikely in the absence of pain. Porphyrias are a group of disorders of heme metabolism that typically do not present with hyperbilirubinemia. Hemochromatosis, a common genetic cause of liver disease in adults, typically presents in older adults with progressive hepatomegaly and elevated hepatic transaminases, in conjunction with diabetes mellitus, skin hyperpigmentation, and elevated iron stores; episodic jaundice starting in childhood would be unusual.

CHAPTER 38

CASE SCENARIO

Correct answer: B

The 4-week duration of nausea and vomiting symptoms suggests a subacute rather than chronic etiology. She has no postural symptoms or other alarm symptoms. The key historical features are the postprandial nausea, followed later by vomiting, as well as the worsening early satiety. An additional clue is the long-term use of NSAIDs, a major risk factor for peptic ulcer disease. Some might consider providing empiric therapy with a proton pump inhibitor, but this patient's significant weight loss merits endoscopic evaluation to confirm the diagnosis.

Most patients with eating disorders do not seek medical attention for nausea and vomiting on their own. Pregnancy should always be considered in a premenopausal woman with vomiting, and a confirmatory urine or serum human chorionic gonadotropin pregnancy test is appropriate. Her history is inconsistent with uncomplicated gastroesophageal reflux.

TEST YOUR KNOWLEDGE

QUESTION #1

Correct answer: A

The rapid onset of severe vomiting after eating strongly suggests food poisoning. The development of diarrhea is not an alarm symptom unless associated with postural symptoms or significant blood.

Any new neurologic finding in association with nausea and vomiting raises the possibility of an ingested neurotoxin (botulism, paralytic shellfish poisoning, ciguatera poisoning) or increased intracranial pressure due to mass effect or metabolic encephalopathy. Abdominal pain that increases with jolting movements is highly suggestive of peritonitis. Large-volume hematemesis is always an alarm symptom that requires immediate therapy.

QUESTION #2

Correct answer: D

No single clinical finding has sufficient diagnostic power to establish or exclude a diagnosis of acute cholecystitis in a patient with upper abdominal pain without further testing. With this patient's clinical presentation, ultrasonographic findings of cholelithiasis, a thickened gallbladder wall, and a gallbladder that is tender when pressed with the ultrasound transducer (sonographic Murphy sign) confirm a diagnosis of cholecystitis.

The differential diagnosis in this case includes acute cholecystitis, acute pancreatitis, and acute cholangitis. The Murphy sign has an LR+ of 2.8 but is subject to examiner bias.

QUESTION #3

Correct answer: D

This patient's history meets criteria for chronic nausea and vomiting. The normal and extensive prior testing has likely ruled out organic causes, so we must focus on possible psychogenic causes for the symptoms. It is particularly important to ask about an inciting event that may result in posttraumatic stress disorder such as sexual abuse or being in combat.

CHAPTER 39

CASE SCENARIO

Correct answer: B

This patient has a thrombosed external hemorrhoid, the cardinal features of which include severe pain, a bluish lump at the rectum, and bleeding. External hemorrhoids are located distal to the dentate line, which is significant because the anal mucosa in this region is innervated by sensory nerve fibers. When hemorrhoidal vessels become engorged and there is stasis of blood, a thrombus can form, resulting in severe pain. Predisposing factors include activities that increase intra-abdominal pressure, such as straining from chronic constipation, diarrhea, or cough, and changes in habitus, such as obesity, pregnancy, and accumulation of ascites.

When a patient presents with anorectal pain and bleeding, there are a number of other conditions that must be considered. Patients with rectal cancer may develop pain and bleeding. Fevers, weight loss, and fatigue each increase the index of suspicion. If the patient is engaging in anorectal intercourse without barrier protection, sexually transmitted proctitis will be higher on the differential diagnosis. In patients with Crohn's disease, fevers and purulent drainage would cause concern for a perianal abscess or fistula. Rectal prolapse is a swollen mass (ie, the rectal mucosa) protruding through the anus: Bleeding may occur from the edematous, friable tissue. Severe pain does not occur unless the rectum becomes strangulated. Lastly, an anal fissure is a tear in the anal mucosa that can cause severe pain with defecation and bleeding. Unlike a thrombosed external hemorrhoid, however, a tender lump is not palpable. No matter the history, a perianal inspection and digital examination are imperative in making the final diagnosis.

TEST YOUR KNOWLEDGE

QUESTION #1

Correct answer: C

There are approximately 40,000 new cases of rectal cancer each year in the United States. The incidence increases with age, becoming more common after age 50. Certain inherited conditions predispose patients to colorectal cancer, and thus obtaining a thorough family history is important. In addition, a number of environmental factors, such as cigarette smoking and alcohol consumption, may increase a person's risk of developing rectal cancer. Patients with rectal cancer may develop blood in their stool, signs of anemia, tenesmus, constipation, small-diameter stools, and weight loss. Typically, if patients feel pain, it is poorly localized. The red flags for rectal cancer are weight loss, fatigue, fever, and anemia.

QUESTION #2

Correct answer: B

This patient is suffering from an anal fissure. The typical presentation includes severe pain during and shortly after defecation, blood-streaked stool or blood on the toilet paper, and secondary constipation. It is caused by a tear in the anal canal, most commonly located in the posterior midline. However, anal fissures associated with pregnancy are most often in the anterior midline. The split in the dermal lining occurs distal to the dentate line where sensory nerve fibers run and is therefore very painful. A thrombosed external hemorrhoid can also cause severe pain and bright red blood per rectum; however, a distinguishing characteristic would be the presence of a tender, swollen lump.

QUESTION #3

Correct answer: B

Proctalgia fugax is characterized by sudden, severe pain in the anorectal region that typically lasts seconds to minutes and then disappears completely. It does not have a well-understood etiology and is a diagnosis of exclusion. In patients with proctalgia fugax, there are no organic explanations for the pain and no other signs or symptoms. It may correlate with stressful life events and anxiety, and the prevalence may be higher in patients with a perfectionistic personality type. Consider the diagnosis in patients with sudden, severe pain that only lasts a short time and no anorectal pain between episodes. A confident diagnosis first requires exclusion of other causes of the pain.

CHAPTER 40

CASE SCENARIO

Correct answer: C

Your patient reports dysuria and urgency, suggesting a lower UTI. Given the prior UTI history, her pretest probability of an acute UTI is 85% to 90%. The absence of vaginal irritation or discharge makes vulvovaginitis less likely and increases the pretest probability of UTI to over 90%. Her sexual history indicates a relatively low risk for STIs, such as herpes or chlamydia urethritis. She does not endorse alarm symptoms suggesting pyelonephritis or pelvic inflammatory disease. Her high pretest probability of UTI and lack of risk factors for a complicated UTI suggest that urine culture is unnecessary. Thus she may be safely managed with telephone advice and empiric antibiotic treatment.

TEST YOUR KNOWLEDGE

QUESTION #1

Correct answer: C

Gross hematuria in an older man is concerning for bladder cancer. Patients with bladder cancer usually experience gross hematuria that is intermittent and painless. Bladder cancer can also cause other bladder storage symptoms, such as urinary frequency and urgency. Although bladder cancer can rarely cause obstructive voiding symptoms, such as urinary hesitancy and weak stream, these symptoms commonly occur in men with benign prostatic hyperplasia and do not necessarily raise suspicion for cancer. Smoking and exposure to aniline dyes are important environmental risk factors for the development of bladder cancer.

QUESTION #2

Correct answer: D

This patient has several risk factors for recurrent UTI. Chronic incontinence increases the risk of recurrent UTI in postmenopausal women. Her symptoms of incontinence also suggest neurogenic bladder, due to multiple sclerosis. With neurogenic bladder, incomplete bladder emptying and retained urine can lead to recurrent UTIs. Although atrophic vaginitis is also a risk factor for UTI in postmenopausal women, this patient does not have symptoms of vaginal dryness or pain with intercourse, making it a less likely explanation. Although a retained kidney stone could serve as a nidus for recurrent infections, her lack of hematuria, flank pain, or symptoms of nephrolithiasis make this an unlikely explanation for her recurrent UTIs.

QUESTION #3

Correct answer: C

Sexually active young women with dysuria are at relatively high risk for urethritis caused by chlamydia or other sexually transmitted infections. In addition to urinalysis, such women should be queried about their risk for sexually transmitted infections. Sexually active women who are less than 25 years old, have a new male sexual partner, or report a prior sexually transmitted infection (STI) are at high risk and should undergo pelvic examination and chlamydia testing. Because condom use reduces, but does not eliminate, the risk of STIs, women who are at high risk should undergo chlamydia screening regardless of their use of barrier contraceptive methods.

QUESTION #4

Correct answer: D

This patient has new-onset dysuria and urinary frequency suggesting bladder irritation or infection. His worsening voiding symptoms are concerning for acute urinary retention. This constellation of symptoms, along with systemic symptoms suggesting acute infection, makes acute bacterial prostatitis the most likely diagnosis. Benign prostatic hyperplasia and recent bladder catheterization are the 2 most common risk factors for acute prostatitis. Although epididymitis can also cause fever and chills and may be seen in patients with bacterial prostatitis, this patient's lack of scrotal swelling and pain make epididymitis less likely. His symptoms are concerning for acute bladder outlet obstruction, which is likely due to a swollen, inflamed prostate rather than benign prostatic hyperplasia alone.

CHAPTER 41

CASE SCENARIO

Correct answer: B

This patient's age, the negative past medical history, and the association of her red urine with dysuria, urgency, and frequency of urination strongly suggest that she has a urinary tract infection. With the additional history that her symptoms occurred after intercourse, she most likely has "honeymoon cystitis." Her symptoms are so characteristic that many physicians would treat her with empiric antibiotic therapy based on history alone, with the caveat that she should return in 7 to 10 days if her symptoms do not resolve.

IgA nephropathy and Goodpasture's disease can cause gross hematuria (which may cause mild to moderate dysuria). However, neither IgA nephropathy nor Goodpasture's disease is accompanied by intense dysuria, urgency, or frequency. Although IgA nephropathy is the most common cause of glomerular hematuria, approximately 50% to 60% of all adult women report that they have had a urinary tract infection at some point. Ureteral calculi often present with severe lower abdominal pain, which was not present in this patient. Bladder cancer most often occurs in patients over the age of 50 and would be extremely unusual in a 17-year-old woman.

TEST YOUR KNOWLEDGE

QUESTION #1

Correct answer: C

Age greater than 40 to 50 years, male sex, and history of smoking are all alarm features for bladder cancer. Because gross hematuria itself can often cause mild to moderate dysuria, its presence alone is not an alarm symptom. Although deafness is associated with hereditary nephritis, this condition most often presents in pediatric or young adult patients and so would not be an alarm symptom in a 75-year-old man. Extended travel to or immigration from tropical Africa, the Middle East, Turkey, or India suggests the possibility of urinary *Schistosoma haematobium* infection or tuberculosis. These infections are not endemic in the Ukraine. This patient's hematuria was not accompanied by intense abdominal or groin pain, which is characteristic of patients with ureteral calculi.

QUESTION #2

Correct answer: C

This patient's symptoms are most characteristic of IgA nephropathy, the most common cause of primary glomerular nephropathy. Characterized pathologically by deposition of IgA in the mesangium of the kidney, it is present in 3% to 9% of biopsies (although not all of these patients are symptomatic). Bladder cancer is extremely rare in female patients under the age of 40, even those with a smoking history. Symptoms associated with urinary tract infections would not be expected to spontaneously resolve without treatment, and renal infarct and ureteral calculus are both accompanied by extreme abdominal or flank pain, which are not present in this patient.

QUESTION #3

Correct answer: A

This patient's family history is positive for kidney disease in his grandfather, father, and paternal aunt, which suggests a familial form of kidney disease. Autosomal dominant polycystic kidney disease (PCKD) is common, occurring in approximately 1 in 500 births. Patients with PCKD can present with recurrent gross hematuria and abdominal pain of one of the multiple cysts found in the grossly enlarged, often football-sized kidneys. Although smoking is an alarm feature for bladder cancer, this disease rarely occurs in patients less than 40 years old. A ureteral calculus would be expected to cause intense flank or abdominal pain, and unlike PCKD, there is not a clear genetic predisposition. Likewise, there is no clear genetic cause for IgA nephropathy. The self-limited nature of the patient's symptoms (without treatment) does not support the diagnosis of urinary tract infection.

CHAPTER 42

CASE SCENARIO

Correct answer: B

This patient is presenting with an infection of the upper urinary tract or pyelonephritis. Pyelonephritis is an infection that most often ascends from the lower urinary tract, which explains her initial complaint of dysuria. In addition to flank pain, pyelonephritis may be associated with high fever, malaise, nausea, and vomiting. The pain of pyelonephritis is often constant as opposed to the colicky pain that is classically associated with nephrolithiasis. Pain from musculoskeletal strain would not be associated with fever, nausea, and vomiting. The patient does not have any risk factors, such as atrial fibrillation, that would increase her risk for renal infarction.

TEST YOUR KNOWLEDGE

QUESTION #1

Correct answer: C

It is unlikely that this patient would tolerate the severe pain of nephrolithiasis for 2 months before seeking medical attention. The pain of pyelonephritis is often described by patients as intense spasm-like pain in the flank. Nephrolithiasis can be associated with gross hematuria. Finally, nephrolithiasis can recur, and a history of nephrolithiasis may prompt suspicion that another kidney stone has formed.

QUESTION #2

Correct answer: B

Sudden onset of severe flank pain in a patient with atrial fibrillation suggests the possibility of a renal embolism or infarction. The patient is also taking warfarin, which increases suspicion for retroperitoneal hemorrhage. Pain radiating to the groin is typical of nephrolithiasis but can also be seen in pyelonephritis. Pain that started after picking up a heavy box suggests musculoskeletal injury. Hematuria can be associated with both pyelonephritis and nephrolithiasis.

QUESTION #3

Correct answer: A

The flank pain associated with herpes zoster, or "shingles," can be severe and, in its earliest stages, may occur before the characteristic dermatomal rash develops. For this reason, it is occasionally mistaken for other causes of flank pain. A patient with herpes zoster may complain of burning pain and may describe a tingling or an electrical sensation. Flank pain that occurs after cardiac catheterization may indicate retroperitoneal hemorrhage and should be evaluated immediately. Pain radiating to the groin and nausea are suggestive of nephrolithiasis or pyelonephritis.

CHAPTER 43

CASE SCENARIO

Correct answer: C

Most patients with erectile dysfunction (ED) have an organic cause, and this patient is no exception. He has no evident psychiatric problems, and his gradual progression of symptoms is consistent with an organic cause. Overt vascular disease, diabetes, and neurologic problems are unlikely given his history, and he has no symptoms of androgen deficiency. Although many physicians would check testosterone levels, significant deficiencies are rare, and treatment of borderline levels is of unproven benefit. His antihypertensive medication is not one that commonly causes ED. His family history and lipid profile do, however, raise concern that his ED may be an indicator of concurrent cardiovascular disease. That risk should be carefully evaluated, with the understanding that the safety of ED treatments will depend on his cardiovascular status.

TEST YOUR KNOWLEDGE

QUESTION #1

Correct answer: B

Clinically evident vascular disease, occurring independent of diabetes, is present in one-third of men with ED. When one also considers diabetes with concomitant vascular disease, it should be clear that vascular disease is a very common accompaniment of ED. Diabetes per se is found in up to a quarter of patients with ED, as is drug effect. Neurologic diseases cause only a small percentage of ED cases.

QUESTION #2

Correct answer: C

This man describes several red flags indicating a possible pituitary tumor. He has headaches, peripheral vision loss suggesting compression of his optic chiasm, and a breast discharge or galactorrhea (likely resulting from elevated serum prolactin). These are classic symptoms of a pituitary tumor, which, if present, could be impairing gonadotropin release with resultant testosterone deficiency and ED. Primary testicular failure should not have these associated symptoms. Drugs that impair hormone function may cause breast discharge but should not cause headache or vision changes. Migraine may cause headache and vision changes (during the aura) but should not cause galactorrhea.

QUESTION #3

Correct answer: A

This patient describes sudden loss of erectile function at the time he began a new relationship. Sudden onset of ED is usually due to psychogenic factors, drugs, or rarely, urologic surgery (eg, prostate surgery). This man is taking no new medications and has had no surgery; so his sudden difficulty is a tip-off that his problem is psychogenic. Difficulty with a new partner is also suggestive of a psychogenic problem. His depressed affect further supports that possibility but by itself is not diagnostic because many men with ED will have secondary emotional difficulty. The persistence of morning erections, long thought an indicator of normal organic physiology, may not be a reliable feature; in one series, 15% of patients with organic disorders still reported satisfactory morning erections. Even in the absence of cardiovascular symptoms, this patient may still have an organic basis for his ED.

CHAPTER 44

CASE SCENARIO

Correct answer: E

The patient has mixed urinary incontinence (UI). She has mild stress UI induced by activity that increases intra-abdominal pressure (ie, exercise). Her principal risk factor for stress UI is 2 vaginal births, but her weight gain could also be contributing. In addition, she has symptoms suggestive of urge incontinence (ie, a sudden, intense need to urinate). By contracting the muscles of her pelvic floor, she has been able to abort the involuntary detrusor contractions before they cause her bladder to empty fully. Hard contraction of the pelvic musculature during a voiding urge (the Kegel maneuver) triggers a reflex relaxation of the detrusor muscle.

TEST YOUR KNOWLEDGE

QUESTION #1

Correct answer: D

This postmenopausal woman has delivered 4 children, increasing her chance of having laxity of the pelvic muscles and stress-type urinary incontinence (UI). The occasional urine loss with standing suggests mild stress UI at baseline. Remaining dry most of the day, together with large leakages, goes against overflow UI. Given her age, it is likely that she has some degree of baseline detrusor overactivity. Since the ankle sprain, she may be becoming incontinent because she can't walk to the bathroom fast enough. In addition, patients who have difficulty with ambulation often choose to ignore the first voiding urge, compounding the risk of an accident. The narcotics may excessively sedate her and prevent her from responding to a full bladder when asleep, accounting for the bed wetting. A urinary tract infection (UTI) can contribute to urinary urgency, and incontinence may be the only manifestation of a UTI in older patients. However, the temporal association of her worsened UI with her sprained ankle and the lack of UTI symptoms make functional incontinence the most likely cause. Cutting back on liquids because of a fear of wetting herself places her at risk of dehydration.

QUESTION #2

Correct answer: E

Mr. S reports symptoms suggesting benign prostatic hyperplasia (BPH). The weak stream, hesitancy, and postvoid dribbling (the cause of the wet mark on his pants after leaving the washroom) are signs of bladder outlet obstruction. Although some degree of urinary retention is possible, he is not experiencing frequent, involuntary, small-volume leakages suggestive of overflow incontinence. Over time, the resistance to urinary outflow produced by BPH results in hypertrophy of the detrusor muscle, leading to an overactive bladder and, in some cases, to urge incontinence. The dribbling does not indicate an incompetent urethral sphincter. His inability to hold urine after an urge to void results from sudden, intense bladder contractions that overwhelm the internal sphincter. A strong external sphincter under voluntary control, coupled with the BPH, may protect him from completely emptying his bladder on these occasions. While the large amount of caffeine he habitually consumes may contribute to his urinary frequency, it is likely not the cause of his UI.

QUESTION #3

Correct answer: B

The patient likely has detrusor hyperactivity with incomplete contraction. The episodes of the patient asking to go to the toilet, but losing her urine if she does not get there right away, suggest urge incontinence. However, in isolated urge incontinence, the bladder empties completely and the diaper should remain dry until the bladder again fills to the threshold volume that triggers involuntary detrusor contractions (which usually takes several hours). The diaper becoming damp within an hour suggests a component of overflow incontinence. A weak detrusor contraction, voluntary or involuntary, leaves most of the urine in the bladder, resulting in progressively increasing urine volumes whose pressures exceed the resistance pressure of the internal sphincter. This leads to leakage of urine until the intravesicular pressure drops below that of the internal sphincter. Clinically, this produces frequent, low-volume leaks that slowly saturate the diaper. A chronically full bladder explains why the patient constantly feels the need to urinate. In Alzheimer's disease, detrusor disinhibition occurs in moderate to severely advanced cases. This patient does have an element of functional incontinence, in that she is wheelchair-bound and cannot get to the toilet by herself, but functional incontinence alone cannot explain her pattern of incontinence.

CHAPTER 45

CASE SCENARIO

Correct answer: A

Gradual-onset, moderate-level, focal pain presenting more than 12 hours after onset in a boy is more likely to be torsion of the testicular appendage or epididymitis. The patient's age and lack of associated features such as dysuria or fever make torsion of a testicular appendage most likely.

TEST YOUR KNOWLEDGE

QUESTION #1

Correct answer: C

Dull, nonacute pain associated with swelling is most likely to be a hydrocele, varicocele, or epididymal cyst. The resolution of swelling with recumbent position is most consistent with varicocele.

QUESTION #2

Correct answer: B

The most likely cause of recurrent episodes of acute scrotal pain in a teenager is a testicular torsion that spontaneously untwists. Torsion of the testicular appendage typically persists until necrosis is complete. Appendicitis typically causes acute right lower quadrant abdominal (not scrotal) pain. Symptoms of epididymitis are more insidious rather than acute.

QUESTION #3

Correct answer: E

Prostatitis or epididymitis is more likely to occur in older patients with recent instrumentation. Each has a more gradual onset and later presentation than testicular torsion and is often accompanied by dysuria and fever. Nephrolithiasis and abdominal aortic aneurysm rupture typically cause pain in the abdomen and perineal area. These entities and inguinal hernia are all less likely to present with fever.

CHAPTER 46

CASE SCENARIO

Correct answer: D

The patient has secondary amenorrhea. Her irregular menstrual cycles interspersed with amenorrhea, obesity, and signs of hyperandrogenism are all consistent with polycystic ovarian syndrome (PCOS). The diagnosis requires 2 of the following criteria: ovulatory dysfunction, hyperandrogenism, and ultrasound evidence of polycystic ovaries. Laboratory abnormalities typically include LH:FSH > 2 and mild elevation in testosterone. Hypothyroidism also causes irregular menstruation, but this patient has no signs or symptoms of hypothyroidism such as cold intolerance, constipation, or coarseness of hair and nails. In addition, hyperandrogenism is not associated with hypothyroidism. Pituitary tumors often can lead to elevated prolactin levels, and alarm symptoms include headaches and vision changes; however, obesity and hyperandrogenism do not commonly occur. A prolactinoma is often caused by medications and can present with galactorrhea. Premature ovarian failure is often associated with estrogen deficiency, and patients usually have related symptoms including hot flashes, vaginal dryness, and decreased libido.

TEST YOUR KNOWLEDGE

QUESTION #1

Correct answer: C

In a woman of reproductive age with amenorrhea, the first step is to rule out pregnancy. A pregnancy test should be obtained before pursuing other potential causes. FSH levels and thyroid function tests are reasonable laboratory tests once pregnancy is ruled out. Emotional stress can cause amenorrhea secondary to hypothalamic dysfunction. Asherman syndrome is also possible given the patient's recent history of instrumentation, so a hysteroscopy should be considered if pregnancy is ruled out.

QUESTION #2

Correct answer: B

The patient has a secondary amenorrhea. An athletic woman with amenorrhea and low body mass index must raise suspicion for exercise-induced hypothalamic dysfunction. Inadequate caloric intake to match energy expenditure can lead to decreased gonadotropin-releasing hormone secretion causing secondary amenorrhea. Consideration of an underlying eating disorder would also be important. She has no signs or symptoms of hyperandrogenism that would suggest polycystic ovarian syndrome. Pregnancy was ruled out as the cause of secondary amenorrhea. Delayed puberty is a type of primary amenorrhea. Finally, it is not "normal" to have secondary amenorrhea.

QUESTION #3

Correct answer: C

She likely has normal development as she has not yet turned 16 and manifests normal secondary sexual characteristics (pubic hair and breast development). Primary amenorrhea is the absence of menarche by age 16 in the presence of otherwise normal secondary sexual characteristics. If she did not have evidence of secondary sexual characteristics, because she is older than 14, this would be considered primary amenorrhea. She does not have secondary amenorrhea because she has never had menses. Premature ovarian failure and polycystic ovarian syndrome are types of secondary amenorrhea.

CHAPTER 47

CASE SCENARIO

Correct answer: C

The most important aspect of her history is the lack of a discrete mass. The majority of breast complaints in the absence of a mass are due to benign causes. In some instances, the patient may feel that her breasts are so lumpy that she cannot tell if there is a discrete mass, and the examination will provide additional information. Moreover, the cyclical nature of her complaint supports the diagnosis of fibrocystic disease. Her breast cancer risk factors are minimal and include nulliparity and a modest family history in a second-degree relative. Her 5-year risk of developing breast cancer, based on the Gail Model, is 0.6% and identical to that of an average 40-year-old woman.

TEST YOUR KNOWLEDGE

QUESTION #1

Correct answer: B

Breast cancer risk factors in this vignette include increasing age; history of a prior breast biopsy, particularly with atypia; exogenous estrogen use (HRT) in postmenopausal woman; and family history, especially in a first-degree relative. A history of fibrocystic disease does not increase a woman's risk of developing breast cancer. However, most women diagnosed with breast cancer do not have these risk factors, with the exception of increasing age. Therefore, a patient who presents with a discrete breast mass needs further work-up regardless of the findings on imaging (see Figure 47–1).

QUESTION #2

Correct answer: C

Bloody nipple discharge is more worrisome for breast cancer than milky, green, black, or brown discharge. The latter is commonly physiologic discharge or due to benign causes. Nipple discharge may continue for months after nursing has ceased. Other alarm symptoms include an underlying breast mass, unilateral breast involvement, discharge from one duct, and spontaneous discharge. The most common cause of bloody nipple discharge is a papilloma; less commonly, the cause may be in situ or invasive breast cancer.

QUESTION #3

Correct answer: A

In a patient with breast skin changes, a history of recent lactation may suggest mastitis. In this case, however, the worrisome features for breast cancer include the partial response to antibiotics and a paternal family history suggestive of hereditary breast and ovarian cancer. The absence of a mass on breast imaging is not reassuring and should not prevent further work-up in patients with persistent skin changes. Frequently, inflammatory breast cancer will cause diffuse skin changes and lack of a discrete mass on imaging.

CHAPTER 48

CASE SCENARIO

Correct answer: C

She has dysmenorrhea complicated by noncyclic chronic pelvic pain. Excessive vaginal bleeding (menorrhagia) is typical of uterine fibroids or adenomyosis. Recent sexual inactivity and the absence of fever make pelvic inflammatory disease unlikely. Endometriosis is a common finding on laparoscopy in patients with noncyclic chronic pelvic pain. However, the absence of infertility and deep dyspareunia make endometriosis less likely to be the cause of this patient's symptoms. A history of childhood abuse and psychosocial stress are common in patients with chronic pelvic pain, and although comorbid functional and psychiatric disorders occur frequently, they do not cause menorrhagia.

TEST YOUR KNOWLEDGE

QUESTION #1

Correct answer: D

This patient has chronic pelvic pain, which virtually rules out causes of acute pelvic pain like ectopic pregnancy, pelvic inflammatory disease, and adnexal torsion. The history of infertility, deep dyspareunia, and irregular menses is characteristic of endometriosis. Absence of fever and vaginal discharge makes pelvic inflammatory disease unlikely, and recent normal period makes pregnancy-related causes like ectopic pregnancy unlikely.

QUESTION #2

Correct answer: C

An intense progressive pain that started as a repetitive transitory pain is a red flag for a surgical emergency like adnexal torsion. Fever and chills are alarm symptoms for serious medical causes like acute pelvic inflammatory disease and urinary tract infection but do not necessarily suggest surgical emergencies. Crampy abdominal pain and deep dyspareunia are typical features of dysmenorrhea and endometriosis, respectively, but they are not red flags for surgical emergencies.

QUESTION #3

Correct answer: B

Abnormal vaginal bleeding in a postmenopausal woman is worrisome for endometrial cancer. Fever and chills in patients with chronic pelvic pain suggest an infectious or inflammatory etiology rather than malignancy. Dyspareunia and sexual promiscuity are not associated with endometrial cancer.

CHAPTER 49

CASE SCENARIO

Correct answer: B

Her vaginal discharge is thin and not clumped. She denies itching. The combination of these findings suggests that she does not have candidal infection; bacterial vaginosis is more common than trichomoniasis, which is a relatively rare infection. Sexual activity is a risk factor for sexually transmitted infection and for bacterial vaginosis, although bacterial vaginosis is not a sexually transmitted disease. Although psoriasis is a common cause of vulvar dermatitis, it does not cause vaginal discharge.

TEST YOUR KNOWLEDGE

QUESTION #1

Correct answer: C

Bacterial vaginosis is not thought to be a sexually transmitted disease but is associated with penile, digital, or sex toy insertion. Trichomoniasis, chlamydia, and gonorrhea are all sexually transmitted and require treatment of the partner as well. These infections imply that one partner has had intercourse with an infected party, although trichomonal infection can remain dormant for many years and does not imply recent other relationships. Consider partner treatment only if a woman has recurrent bacterial vaginosis. *Candida* is not considered sexually transmitted, although males with candidal balanitis can occasionally transmit infection, and *Candida* can be present under an intact foreskin.

QUESTION #2

Correct answer: C

Although candidal vaginitis can occur in completely normal women, recurrent infection should prompt investigation for underlying causes. Diabetes and HIV are particularly common causes. Recent antibiotic use can also cause candidal infection. Hypothyroidism and uterine fibroids are not associated with candidiasis, nor is trichomoniasis infection.

QUESTION #3

Correct answer: D

Atrophic vaginitis is particularly common in postmenopausal women, but other forms of vaginitis, including *Candida* vaginitis, can also occur after menopause. Be sure to obtain a sexual history; do not assume that older women are celibate.

CHAPTER 50

CASE SCENARIO

Correct answer: B

Although the patient's age places her in an age range that might be perimenopausal, she has no symptoms that suggest this, and her cycle is regular. Despite her age, because she is not menopausal, she must be considered to be of reproductive age. Her negative pregnancy test is critical even given the history of her husband's vasectomy. Her bleeding is regular in nature and associated with increased menstrual cramping and pelvic pain, making it ovulatory bleeding. Her history does not include any medications that might lead to menorrhagia, and her history does not suggest that medication use, an endocrine abnormality, or a coagulopathy plays a role.

Although the diagnosis of fibroids would require confirmation with imaging, her history and symptoms point to the category of "uterine lesion or mass," and fibroids is the mostly likely diagnosis among these. Fibroids are common in women in their 40s and commonly cause the increased menstrual cramps she describes.

TEST YOUR KNOWLEDGE

QUESTION #1

Correct answer: C

Although a coagulopathy, especially von Willebrand disease, may be the cause of abnormal bleeding in young women, it would be uncommon for a single episode of light intermenstrual spotting to be the only clinical manifestation. If she had a coagulopathy, one would expect regular heavy bleeding and possibly bleeding from other sites. Any of the other diagnoses are possible in this patient and could cause a single episode of vaginal spotting.

QUESTION #2

Correct answer: B

Cold intolerance suggests hypothyroidism, which, when it causes menstrual irregularities, causes increased bleeding. The other symptoms are all hormonally related to the menstrual cycle and, when present with bleeding, strongly suggest that the bleeding is ovulatory in nature.

QUESTION #3

Correct answer: D

Pregnancy must be excluded in any woman of reproductive age before considering other diagnoses. Although this patient is perimenopausal—by her age and irregular menses—she is not yet menopausal, which requires 12 months of amenorrhea in this age range. Menopause is the second most common time for unplanned pregnancy. Hormonal effect is possible, especially if she was taking hormonal therapy, but would be assessed only after excluding pregnancy. Dysfunctional uterine bleeding is a diagnosis of exclusion that is unlikely to play a role in this patient's presentation of isolated perimenopausal bleeding.

CHAPTER 51

CASE SCENARIO

Correct answer: C

Neck hyperextension (which occurs when viewing a computer screen) or protraction is a common cause of repetitive neck injury, hypertrophy of the facet joints, disk slippage, and nerve root compression. In this case, irritation of the C6 nerve root has caused symptoms radiating to the thumb and first finger. This is the most common nerve root to be irritated by cervical arthritis and is the easiest to remember; C6 irritation radiates to the thumb and forefinger, the "6 shooter" made by children who make an imaginary gun by raising their thumb, extending the forefinger, and drawing the other fingers into a partial grasp. This is the "anchor" dermatome; know this and you can figure out the others. Because the dorsal rami on the cervical nerves innervate the paraspinous muscles, cervical nerve root irritation will cause pain in the upper back along the medial scapula.

TEST YOUR KNOWLEDGE

QUESTION #1

Correct answer: B

Carotid artery dissection is an unusual complication of neck manipulation and can cause a variety of neurologic symptoms in the distribution of the involved carotid artery. In this case, with the absence of any antecedent injury, carotidynia is the most likely diagnosis. This would produce the physical finding of a tender carotid artery. Pain in the thyroid would not radiate to the upper anterior neck. TMJ pain would not radiate below the jaw. Carotidynia is typically on one side only.

QUESTION #2

Correct answer: D

This is a common presentation for shingles or herpes zoster. The pain is in a dermatomal distribution, in this case the C7 nerve root. The pain of shingles can precede the rash by a few days. The case does not suggest cervical spinal cord compression because there is no trauma and no history of chronic neck pain. Although there might be pain with evocative maneuver (she is 85 years old, after all), the presence of the typical rash of shingles makes a concurrent cervical radiculopathy unlikely. For the same reason, there would be no expectation of weakness. Shingles does not affect the motor neurons. A diffuse eczematous rash would not fit with any cause of radicular neck pain.

QUESTION #3

Correct answer: F

The severity of injury, monotonous work, and prior history of neck pain are all associated with a more protracted course. After determining that the spinal cord is not at risk, the next step is to classify the neck pain as axial or radicular. Finally, using your own body as a diagnostic tool can help you to get a better sense of what structures are involved.

CHAPTER 52

CASE SCENARIO

Correct answer: B

Shoulder pain with activity and relieved by rest argues against referred pain, including cervical pain. He has no alarm symptoms. His painting hobby and age increase the likelihood of rotator cuff tendinopathy, and the pain exacerbation with overhead activity (painting) is consistent with this diagnosis. Frozen shoulder typically causes global loss of range of movement, which is not suggested by his history (but will need to be confirmed by examination). Acromioclavicular disease causes anterior pain exacerbated by cross-body adduction. The physical examination would be the next step to confirm the diagnosis.

TEST YOUR KNOWLEDGE

QUESTION #1

Correct answer: C

The absence of pain with movement signifies that this is not "moving parts pain" from the articulations, muscles, or tendons of the shoulder complex. This is likely referred pain. Pain with exertion that is relieved by rest and worsened with cold suggests angina (see Chapter 27).

QUESTION #2

Correct answer: A

Pain exacerbated by cross-body adduction—reaching across the body to grab the opposite shoulder—suggests acromioclavicular (AC) joint disease. Pain when lifting arms above the head would suggest impingement syndrome. A fear of the shoulder popping would suggest intermittent shoulder dislocation, usually in persons with prior shoulder dislocations. Pain radiating from the neck suggests cervical disk disease. Unrelenting pain all day and night suggests an inflammatory arthritis, infection, or malignancy. On his examination, the AC joint was visibly stepped off, and bony enlargement was observed. Stressing the AC joint on examination exacerbated the pain, and radiography confirmed the diagnosis of AC joint osteoarthritis.

QUESTION #3

Correct answer: A

Global loss of range of movement is characteristic of frozen shoulder and other "capsular" diseases—or any inflammatory arthritis involving the entire glenohumeral joint. The absence of swelling (confirmed by physical examination) and morning stiffness goes against rheumatoid arthritis. Polymyalgia rheumatica would be associated with morning stiffness. Pain only with overhead activity suggests rotator cuff disease and not a capsular disorder, which should cause pain in all ranges of motion. Swelling of the hand is not a feature of frozen shoulder. Parenthetically, the association of frozen shoulder with diabetes has recently been challenged.

CHAPTER 53

CASE SCENARIO

Correct answer: C

This patient has a classic presentation of lateral epicondylitis, caused by strain of the wrist extensor attachments. It is called tennis elbow because it can result from poor tennis technique. A similar condition is medial epicondylitis, which is caused by strain of the wrist flexors and associated with poor golf technique. Olecranon bursitis presents as pain and erythema over the olecranon process. This is not de Quervain tenosynovitis, which presents as wrist pain.

TEST YOUR KNOWLEDGE

QUESTION #1

Correct answer: E

This patient has reflex sympathetic dystrophy (RSD), also known as chronic regional pain syndrome (CRPS). Key features include a burning sensation that progresses over time, usually following trauma. Carpal and cubital tunnel syndromes are unlikely because they do not progress to include the entire arm. Intersection syndrome is pain localized to the wrist and is more common in Alpine skiers. Olecranon bursitis presents as pain and erythema over the olecranon process.

QUESTION #2

Correct answer: E

This patient has Raynaud's disorder. Classic features include 3-color changes of the digits exacerbated by cold exposure. Thoracic outlet syndrome presents as pain, weakness, and swelling of the arm and hand. Cubital tunnel syndrome is isolated to the elbow or first 2 or 3 digits, whereas Raynaud's disorder occurs in all fingers. de Quervain tenosynovitis causes soreness on the thumb side of the forearm. Carpal tunnel syndrome is isolated to the first 2 or 3 digits, similar to cubital tunnel syndrome.

QUESTION #3

Correct answer: A

The patient has medial epicondylitis, also known as golfer's elbow. Lateral epicondylitis is not correct because it worsens with repeated wrist extension. There is nothing in this patient's history to suggest that chest pathology is the cause of his elbow pain. Reflex sympathetic dystrophy usually occurs after a trauma and will progress. Olecranon bursitis presents as pain and erythema over the olecranon process.

CHAPTER 54

CASE SCENARIO

Correct answer: C

This patient most likely has nonspecific LBP. Her radiating leg pain is suggestive of radiculopathy and does warrant a comprehensive neurologic examination, but her lack of motor weakness (confirmed by physical examination) and intermittent nature of her leg pain are reassuring; thus, she can be treated for nonspecific LBP. She should be encouraged to resume her normal activities and avoid aggravating activities. If her symptoms persist beyond 4 weeks, physical therapy should be considered. Persistent, bothersome radicular symptoms may warrant magnetic resonance imaging of the lumbar spine. Her high level of function and low fear of activity place her at low risk of developing a chronic disabling condition.

TEST YOUR KNOWLEDGE

QUESTION #1

Correct answer: B

The acute onset, localized distribution, and intermittent nature of the pain strongly suggest a vertebral compression fracture. Patients with chronic obstructive pulmonary disease often require intermittent treatment with corticosteroids, which increases his likelihood of compression fracture. One must also consider abdominal aortic aneurysm in a male patient older than 65 with a smoking history, but the lack of abdominal symptoms and localized mechanical nature make this diagnosis less likely. The next diagnostic step would be plain radiographic imaging with a lumbar posterior-anterior view and lateral x-ray.

QUESTION #2

Correct answer: A

This patient has nonspecific LBP. Her young age and ability to move immediately after the fall, the low impact of the fall, and the fact that stiffness was not apparent until the following day all go against a diagnosis of fracture. The localized distribution of her pain and lack of symptoms suggesting radiculopathy are also reassuring. Of utmost concern for this woman is the lack of activity over the past week and her high avoidance of movement for fear of causing greater symptoms. These are both worrisome predictors for developing a chronic condition. She would benefit from close follow-up, reassurance, and possibly early physical therapy.

CHAPTER 55

CASE SCENARIO

Correct answer: D

This patient has a classic presentation for greater trochanteric bursitis. Trochanteric bursitis presents as pain in the lateral upper thigh that may radiate down the thigh. It may be caused by a leg length discrepancy and improve if the discrepancy is corrected. Patients with trochanteric bursitis often report hip pain. However, true hip pain usually radiates to the groin and does not worsen when lying on the affected side in bed. This patient does not have risk factors for avascular necrosis of the femoral head such as sickle cell anemia or corticosteroid use. Additionally, she denies trauma, making fracture unlikely. Osteoarthritis of the hip is common; however, pain from osteoarthritis usually radiates to the groin and is exacerbated with movement of the joint.

TEST YOUR KNOWLEDGE

QUESTION #1

Correct answer: B

This patient has avascular necrosis of the femoral head. Risk factors for this condition include sickle cell anemia, fracture, corticosteroid therapy, alcohol, gout, diabetes, and Gaucher disease. Avascular necrosis has been associated with prednisone (a corticosteroid) and not ibuprofen, salmeterol, aspirin, or simvastatin.

QUESTION #2

Correct answer: E

The patient has coccydynia, which is present in up to 20% of women after difficult deliveries. Coccydynia usually presents as midline pain at the end of the spinal column. Sciatica and piriformis syndrome are usually unilateral and cause pain in the distribution of the sciatic nerve. Meralgia paresthetica is caused by damage to the lateral femoral cutaneous nerve and usually presents with bilateral lateral thigh pain. Reflex sympathetic dystrophy is characterized by a burning pain that is progressive. It usually has a predisposing event such as injury.

QUESTION #3

Correct answer: D

Meralgia paresthetica is caused by damage or injury to the lateral femoral cutaneous nerves by surgery, diabetic neuropathy, restrictive clothing, or weightlifting belts. Trochanteric bursitis usually causes unilateral pain in the upper lateral thigh. Quadriceps and hamstring strains are usually precipitated by activity. Sciatica usually presents with deep posterior buttock pain with radiation down the posterior thigh and leg.

CHAPTER 56

CASE SCENARIO

Case Scenario 1

Correct answer: E

You never want to miss a septic joint. Although a septic joint cannot be excluded purely on history and physical examination, certain elements of the history increase suspicion for this diagnosis. This patient reports pain, subjective fevers, and recent injection drug use. Therefore, it is imperative to exclude septic joint as a possibility. Gout may also present this way, but septic arthritis must first be excluded. The other diagnoses mentioned do not warrant urgent intervention.

Case Scenario 2

Correct answer: A

Deep venous thrombosis is the most likely diagnosis because of recent immobilization and oral contraceptive use. Muscle strain is less likely because pain is absent with activity. Intermittent claudication is unlikely due to her relatively young age and because the pain is not provoked by walking. Patient did not report fullness behind her knee prior to the pain, making a ruptured Baker cyst less likely.

TEST YOUR KNOWLEDGE

QUESTION #1

Correct answer: B

Ligamentous tear is most likely because the patient had injury by external force and immediate swelling of her knee. Fracture may occur with ligamentous tear, but the immediate swelling strongly suggests ligamentous tear. Meniscal tears usually do not cause immediate swelling (but rather swelling over several hours). Septic joint is unlikely because the symptoms were precipitated by trauma.

QUESTION #2

Correct answer: C

Patellofemoral syndrome is most likely because he has chronic anterior knee pain aggravated by climbing stairs and rising from a chair. There is no swelling or trauma, making fracture and ligamentous tear unlikely. Septic joint is unlikely given the chronic nature of the pain and absence of fever, swelling, or other risk factors.

QUESTION #3

Correct answer: B

The patient has ≥ 3 points per the Wells criteria (1 for recent major surgery, 1 for calf swelling, and 1 for pitting edema) and thus is at high risk for deep venous thrombosis.

CHAPTER 57

CASE SCENARIO

Correct answer: B

An inversion injury with lateral ligament sprain is the most common type of ankle sprain. With an inversion injury of the ankle, a deltoid or medial ligament sprain would not be likely. Plantar fasciitis causes pain on the plantar aspect of the foot at the anterior heel and is not usually associated with trauma. Bunions, although common, do not cause ankle pain; they cause pain at the first metatarsophalangeal (MTP) joint, especially with tight-fitting shoes.

TEST YOUR KNOWLEDGE

QUESTION #1

Correct answer: D

You must not miss a septic arthritis. Although fever is not always present, a painful, red, swollen joint should be considered septic until proven otherwise. A joint with hardware is especially susceptible to septic arthritis. Osteoarthritis and ligamentous strain may cause painful swollen joints, but typically not redness or fever. Plantar fasciitis causes pain without swelling, and the pain is not near the joint.

QUESTION #2

Correct answer: D

The history of pain worse in the morning with the first step is typical of plantar fasciitis. Calcaneal fractures are usually seen after trauma or in long-distance runners. Bunions cause pain at the first MTP joint. Although calluses can occur anywhere on the foot, the pain would not abate with walking in the morning.

QUESTION #3

Correct answer: B

This history is typical for gout, in which the pain is exquisite. The first MTP joint is a common site for gout, known as podagra. Arthritis pain is less severe and tends to be more of an aching pain that comes on slowly over time. Plantar warts can cause pain with weight bearing and walking but are not red or swollen unless infected. Bunions also occur at the first MTP joint and may become red with rubbing from a shoe but do not typically cause acute, severe pain.

CHAPTER 58

CASE SCENARIO

Correct answer: B

The history of trauma in an elderly patient leading to confusion over days to weeks suggests a subdural hematoma. The patient likely also has an underlying dementia, which is both a risk factor for falls and for subdural hematomas. The "acute on chronic" nature of a worsening over days to weeks on a baseline of a gradual decline over months to years is highly suggestive of a delirium in the setting of a decreased cognitive reserve from dementia.

The other causes are less likely; think first of the most likely cause and secondly of treatable causes of confusion. There is no history of fever, so meningitis is less likely. Seizures cause fluctuating symptoms and are of more rapid onset. Stroke is less likely in the absence of weakness but is still a possibility. In particular, a right parietal infarction or lobar small hemorrhage remains possible.

TEST YOUR KNOWLEDGE

QUESTION #1

Correct answer: C

Delirium from any cause leads to disorientation and word finding trouble, but neck pain with neck movement (meningismus) is a warning sign for meningitis. Periodic jerking of the legs might suggest a seizure but is more likely due to toxic myoclonus.

QUESTION #2

Correct answer: B

The presence of even a low-grade fever suggests an inflammatory or infectious process underlying her confusional state. The episodes of "blanking out" are likely complex partial seizures, which are frequent in encephalitis. In particular, herpes simplex encephalitis has an affinity for infecting the temporal lobes, causing both complex partial seizures and confusion in setting of a low-grade fever.

CHAPTER 59

CASE SCENARIO

Correct answer: D

Ischemic and anoxic brain events in the patient's mother and brother imply vascular dementia, which would not be associated with Alzheimer's disease (AD) in the patient. However, the insidious onset of his cognitive decline is consistent with AD or the slowly progressive form of vascular dementia. Depression often accompanies early dementia and could cause both irritability and loss of interest in his hobby. His disinterest could also be due to declining ability to handle the complexity of engine repair (eg, impaired problem solving, forgetting the purpose of parts or how to reassemble them, or apraxia when using tools). The patient's accusations of theft, or paranoid delusions, are common in mild to moderate dementia of any etiology, including AD. These delusions may also represent the patient's rationalization for losing objects in the face of his unacknowledged memory problem, which is common among patients with early dementia. In early dementia, short-term (recent) memory is more likely to be impaired than long-term memory. His lack of in-depth conversations with family members may conceal forgetfulness. Getting lost implies problems with orientation; his limited education is a risk factor for AD. Nonprescription sleeping pills often contain diphenhydramine, an anticholinergic antihistamine that may cause confusion in older persons.

TEST YOUR KNOWLEDGE

QUESTION #1

Correct answer: C

Frontotemporal dementia usually begins by the sixth decade with slow, insidious changes in personality and executive function that precede changes in memory. Early in the disease, patients may score well on standard screening tests for dementia such as the Mini-Mental State Examination. The patient displays hyperorality, manifested by the excessive consumption of snack food. His alcohol use may imply loss of judgment and impulsiveness, as do his buying sprees on the Internet. Disinhibited, inappropriate behavior with a female student, suggestive of frontotemporal dementia, likely resulted in his being fired from his teaching job.

QUESTION #2

Correct answer: D

The patient likely has Lewy body dementia (LBD), in which parkinsonian features and cognitive impairment tend to appear within a year of each other. In Parkinson's disease, dementia is not seen until the late stages of the illness. In early LBD, noticeable fluctuations in the severity of the dementia are seen, and hallucinations are common. Patients with LBD are especially prone to develop extrapyramidal side effects from antipsychotic medication, including the atypical antipsychotics. Judge M's parkinsonism markedly worsened after starting risperidone, further impairing his mobility and balance, leading to his falls. Unfortunately many healthcare providers are quick to attribute cognitive impairment in the elderly to Alzheimer's disease without considering other diagnoses.

QUESTION #3

Correct answer: A

The triad of a wide-based gait, urinary incontinence, and dementia should raise suspicion of idiopathic normal-pressure hydrocephalus (NPH), a rare cause of dementia. A diagnosis of NPH is suggested by a wide-based gait plus either urge-type urinary incontinence or dementia. The presence of all 3 signs in the absence of other explanations increases the probability of NPH. The dementia of NPH classically begins as frontal-subcortical cognitive impairment, with generalized psychomotor slowing and impaired executive function. Depression may also be present. This patient's mental slowing and inability to follow a recipe, a clue to executive dysfunction, are consistent with NPH, as is her gait. Urge-type incontinence could explain her inability to get to the bathroom in time. The differential diagnosis of the gait disturbance in NPH includes diffuse Lewy body disease and vascular parkinsonism, both of which may produce a broad-based, shuffling gait. However, NPH is not associated with increased motor rigidity. A tremor is seen in approximately 40% of cases of NPH, but unlike Parkinson's disease, the tremor is not observed at rest. This patient has significant risk factors for vascular dementia, and well-controlled diabetes, hyperlipidemia, and hypertension do not preclude significant cerebrovascular disease. In older persons, obstructive sleep apnea has been associated with cognitive impairment and may worsen cognitive decline in Alzheimer's disease.

CHAPTER 60

CASE SCENARIO

Correct answer: C

With sudden onset, headache, and pupil involvement, this could be due to compression by an aneurysm at the junction of the internal carotid artery and posterior communicating artery, possibly with a sentinel bleed. One should also look for meningismus or altered consciousness, which could suggest more significant subarachnoid bleeding. Regardless, neuroimaging with some form of angiography is required urgently. This patient did indeed turn out to have such an aneurysm (see Figure), which was treated urgently by neurosurgery. The following image is a lateral view of her cerebral angiogram, showing the aneurysm at the junction of the internal carotid artery and posterior communicating artery (*arrow*). (Image reprinted with permission from www.neuroophthalmology.ca.)

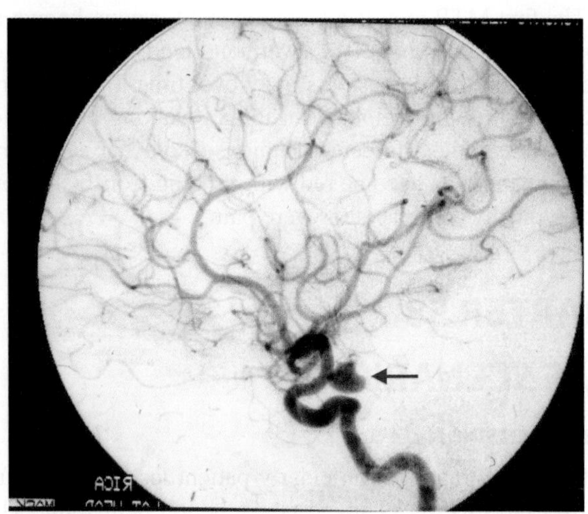

TEST YOUR KNOWLEDGE

QUESTION #1

Correct answers: A, B, C, and D

Double vision at far but not near suggests weakness of one or both of the lateral recti from muscle disease or VI nerve palsies. Ptosis could suggest muscle disease, III nerve palsy, or a Horner syndrome. Therefore, at this point, you would consider the possibility of muscle disease or a combination of VI nerve palsy and Horner syndrome at the top of your list. Hence it would be important to look for a smaller pupil on the side of the ptosis, especially if this is more obvious in the dark than in the light. Combined Horner syndrome and VI nerve palsy can occur from pathology inside the cavernous sinus. If he has a muscle problem instead, weakness of lid closure would confirm this because neuropathic causes of ptosis tend not to cause weakness of the orbicularis oculi too. Fluctuating diplopia related to activity suggests fatigability and should raise suspicion of myasthenia. Increased ptosis after prolonged up gaze would be another sign of excessive fatigability, and dysarthria would indicate that the problem is more extensive than just the ocular muscles and possibly generalized. This man did have ocular myasthenia.

The effect of head tilt on diplopia is really only relevant to vertical or oblique diplopia, not horizontal diplopia, because it is the vertical recti and the oblique muscles that generate the torsional eye movements that are called into play to compensate for head tilt.

QUESTION #2

Correct answers: B and C

Increasing distance between the images is an indication that the ocular motor deficit is worsening. This should not continue to happen over weeks with a microvascular palsy but should raise suspicion of nerve compression by a mass. VI nerve palsies accompanied by other neurologic signs are often due to underlying lesions, particularly compressive masses. Trigeminal symptoms such as facial pain or numbness in this setting strongly suggest a lesion of the skull base, such as nasopharyngeal carcinoma, as in this patient.

Monocular diplopia indicates a refractive problem, not a neurologic one, and usually is more benign in its outlook. Scalp tenderness always raises the possibility of giant cell arteritis, which can cause ocular motor palsies on occasion, but the patient is too young for this condition, and some patients with true migraine do report such tenderness. Diabetes would be a risk factor for a microvascular palsy, but that is not an ominous problem.

QUESTION #3

Correct answer: A

Patients with Graves ophthalmopathy often have lid retraction. If there is ptosis, one should suspect myasthenia gravis, which given the similarities in pathogenetic mechanisms does occur frequently in patients with autoimmune thyroid disease. Red bulging eyes are classic for moderately severe Graves ophthalmopathy but may not be that obvious in all patients. The disorder has a propensity to affect the medial and inferior recti, stiffening them and restricting their movement. Because diplopia is thus often a result of restriction rather than weakness of these muscles, the tendency is to limit the ability of the eyes to abduct (most noticeable in far gaze) or to elevate.

CHAPTER 61

CASE SCENARIO

Correct answer: C

This patient's gait abnormality is likely due to a peroneal nerve palsy secondary to mononeuritis multiplex. The peroneal nerve is responsible for dorsiflexion of the foot, which is necessary to keep the foot from dragging into the ground during ambulation. Damage to this nerve results in a foot drop, necessitating augmented flexion of the hip to raise the foot off of the ground during ambulation. The characteristic "I have to throw my foot forward to walk" suggests the diagnosis. A peroneal nerve palsy can result from any of the causes of peripheral neuropathy but is most commonly seen following trauma or prolonged pressure (as seen in obstetrics patients) to the lateral knee. The addition of sensory abnormalities, as described in this case, distinguishes a peroneal nerve palsy from upper motor neuron disease such as stroke. The presence of 2 nerve palsies not in the same vascular distribution suggests mononeuritis multiplex, a vasculitis of the vasonervosum affecting nerves in different locations of the body. The past history of advanced HIV, which is associated with mononeuritis multiplex, further suggests the diagnosis.

Stroke is less likely given the prolonged time course, but also because of the distribution of the lesions. It would be rare to have only the peroneal nerve as a manifestation of stroke; the presence of sensory abnormalities in the same distribution suggests that this is a peripheral nerve problem, not a central nervous system lesion such as a stroke. The patient has no balance difficulty, and this, in combination with the focal deficit, excludes cerebellar degeneration. Parkinson's disease is the most common disorder of gait, but the patient exhibits none of the characteristic features (eg, hypertonicity, tremor).

TEST YOUR KNOWLEDGE

QUESTION #1

Correct answer: B

This patient has symptoms consistent with spinal cord impingement due to a metastatic cancer. The age of the patient, history of significant tobacco use, and the "red flag" symptoms of incontinence and back pain suggest that this is an upper motor lesion within the spine. Any new gait abnormality in a patient at high risk for malignancy or epidural infection should prompt an immediate evaluation for spinal cord lesions, especially in the context of back pain, fever, or incontinence. MRI is the diagnostic test of choice.

A CT of the head would be useful for evaluating acute stroke or metastatic lesions to the brain. Although both diagnoses would be possible in a patient of this age, especially with the history of smoking, the distribution of the lesions (bilateral) and the associated incontinence make these diagnoses less likely. Nerve conduction studies can be useful in evaluating peripheral neuropathy, but the clinical presentation of bilateral nerve deficits and incontinence suggests spinal cord pathology. Multiple sclerosis can present with spinal cord lesions, but the patient's age and the clinical presentation would be very unusual for a new presentation of multiple sclerosis.

QUESTION #2

Correct answer: C

This patient is suffering from progressive cerebellar (likely vermis) degeneration due to chronic alcohol consumption. Balance abnormalities but no weakness suggest that the gait abnormality is due to inadequate proprioceptive input to adjust the gait. Appropriate proprioceptive input is contingent upon both sensory input from peripheral nerves and interpretation of this input by the cerebellar vermis. Gait abnormalities worse at night are characteristic, because the absence of visual cues results in complete reliance upon the proprioceptive apparatus to maintain gait. Although peripheral neuropathy (from alcohol) can also cause gait abnormality, the presence of "unsteadiness when I walk" and lack of weakness suggest cerebellar (rather than peripheral nerve) origin.

The time course of the abnormality, lack of focal symptoms, and exacerbation while ambulating at night make stroke unlikely. The patient has no symptoms of hypertonicity or tremor, making Parkinson's disease less likely. It would be rare to have new-onset multiple sclerosis after age 50.

QUESTION #3

Correct answer: A

The patient's gait abnormality is highly suggestive of Parkinson's disease. Having "a hard time getting started" and taking "little steps" suggest hypertonicity and spasticity, both characteristic features of Parkinson's disease. The additional historical information of "choking" or "gagging" after eating food suggests a motor dysphasia, also common in this disorder.

Spastic paraplegia is usually associated with upper motor neuron disease such as cerebral palsy. The gait abnormality is typically a "scissors gait," as the knees are brought together to maintain balance because of bilateral spasticity. This description does not match our patient's gait abnormality. Wilson's disease results from excessive copper deposition and usually causes chorea rather than excessive rigidity. Although this patient is the right age for Huntington's disease, the absence of other psychiatric symptoms or motor abnormalities during wakefulness makes this disorder a less likely cause of the gait disturbance.

CHAPTER 62

CASE SCENARIO

Correct answer: C

The tremor is present with use of his hands, so it is an action tremor. He does not have any rest tremor. Patients will often overlook a rest tremor. However, the patient also does not have any other symptoms to suggest Parkinson's disease, such as slowness, stiffness, or gait changes. The tremor is bilateral, which makes early Parkinson's disease less likely. The tremor is present when he does several different tasks, such as pouring milk and building models, so it is unlikely to be a task-specific tremor, which occurs with a specific, usually overlearned, task. There is no suggestion of stress or increased caffeine consumption, which might suggest enhanced physiologic tremor. There are no alarm symptoms, such as acute onset or other associated neurologic symptoms to suggest a stroke or another serious illness.

The characteristics of this tremor that suggest essential tremor include the slow onset, action component, bilaterality, and family history. The additional feature of alcohol responsiveness cannot be determined in this particular patient. He likely is coming to see you now because he has started a hobby that requires very fine motor movements, which can be affected by even a very mild tremor. A tremor may be present for a long time before it affects function sufficiently to seek medical attention. Determine whether the tremor is causing enough dysfunction to require treatment or if the purpose of the visit is instead reassurance that this is not Parkinson's disease or another serious condition.

TEST YOUR KNOWLEDGE

QUESTION #1

Correct answer: C

Rest tremors are most often due to Parkinson's disease or parkinsonism (including secondary causes, like multiple system atrophy, progressive supranuclear palsy, or drug-induced parkinsonism). Patients of older age are at increased risk for both Parkinson's disease and essential tremor, but a younger age does not rule out Parkinson's disease. Both conditions are associated with gradual tremor onset. In early essential tremor, there may be no functional impact of the tremor, even if it is most prominent with action. In addition, with a severe tremor of Parkinson's disease, there may be re-emergence of the tremor with a new posture or with action, which can result in dysfunction. Finally, although stiffness, slowness, and gait difficulties suggest Parkinson's disease, isolated tremor may be the sole presenting symptom.

QUESTION #2

Correct answer: D

The acute onset of this tremor and association with other neurologic symptoms such as slurred speech and "walking like a drunk" are alarm symptoms that suggest an acute cerebellar process, likely a stroke. Tremor is rarely concerning enough to cause patients to go to the emergency room; if they do present in an urgent setting, there is likely a particular reason (acute onset, other new associated symptoms). Tremor with use of the limb is consistent with a cerebellar cause, but action tremors are frequently seen in essential tremor and enhanced physiologic tremor.

QUESTION #3

Correct answer: A

Haloperidol is one of the common typical antipsychotic drugs, all of which are dopamine receptor blockers that can cause parkinsonism and an associated resting tremor. Other dopamine receptor blockers include fluphenazine, chlorpromazine, metoclopramide (a nonantipsychotic drug used for gastric reflux and gastroparesis), and less frequently, the so-called "atypical antipsychotics," such as olanzapine and aripiprazole. Most other medications cause postural tremors, such as lithium, valproic acid, selective serotonin reuptake inhibitors, and tricyclic antidepressants. Benzodiazepines, such as clonazepam, can cause tremors during withdrawal.

CHAPTER 63

CASE SCENARIO

Correct answer: B

The patient's symptoms and time frame are consistent with generalized anxiety disorder (GAD). The patient has had excessive difficulty controlling anxiety along with difficulty concentrating, problems with sleep, and fatigue for at least 6 months. She also has significant impairment in her social life. She does not have any medical conditions or substance abuse history. From the history, it is less likely that she has other anxiety disorders. Patients with panic disorder experience abrupt, recurrent attacks of symptoms, with at least 3 attacks in a 3-week period. The symptoms usually are fear of dying, "air hunger," palpitations, and sweating. Our patient's symptoms are constant and not acute attacks. The patient has significant impairment in social, occupational, and other areas of functioning due to pathologic anxiety. However, she does not have fear of open places and social situations, which makes agoraphobia and generalized social anxiety, respectively, less likely. She has no symptoms or signs suggesting obsession or compulsion and hence no obsessive-compulsive disorder.

TEST YOUR KNOWLEDGE

QUESTION #1

Correct answer: C

The most likely diagnosis is acute stress disorder. The patient's nightmares and avoidance of the associated stimuli (driving or riding in a car) after an identified traumatic life event (motor vehicle accident) are consistent with PTSD, but the time frame of only 3 weeks is insufficient to establish a diagnosis of PTSD, in which symptoms should exist and persist for at least 1 month. Her symptoms are more severe than those of a normal grieving process. The patient has no specific phobia to driving or riding in a car; it is a particular traumatic experience that made her avoid these stimuli. Her symptoms do not suggest panic disorder.

QUESTION #2

Correct answer: B

The most likely diagnosis is social anxiety disorder (social phobia). The patient has an irrational, intense, and consistent fear of being negatively evaluated by others, leading to dysfunctional behaviors. Such patients frequently fear feeling stupid or being embarrassed in social situations (in agoraphobia, fear particularly of open places), which makes them avoid interacting with people or doing things in public settings. This is not generalized anxiety disorder (GAD) because her symptoms occur mainly with social interactions. The patient's nightmares are secondary to his intense fear of embarrassment or looking stupid in social settings but not due to any traumatic life experience, making posttraumatic stress disorder less likely.

QUESTION #3

Correct answer: B

The most likely diagnosis is panic disorder. The abrupt onset of symptoms (palpitations, shortness of breath, sweating, fear of dying) with no clear precipitating factor and the absence of a known history of the medical condition the patient is concerned about (eg, asthma) make panic disorder a likely diagnosis. The patient is also beginning to express a persistent concern about having additional attacks and is making significant changes in behavior (eg, exercise) as a result of the attacks. Recurrent panic attacks of at least 6 months in duration often leave patients hypochondriacal. These patients can also be depressed and agoraphobic following multiple attacks. However, the case description is classical for panic disorder. Her symptoms are not due to a traumatic event, making acute stress disorder less likely. In obsessive-compulsive disorder, patients recognize that their thoughts and repetitive actions are absurd, and they try to resist them. In the given case description, there is no evidence of any obsession or compulsion.

CHAPTER 64

CASE SCENARIO

Correct answer: E

The patient has major depressive disorder. She has symptoms of depressed mood, anhedonia, weight gain, insomnia, psychomotor retardation, fatigue, and diminished ability to concentrate. From the available history, it is unclear whether the patient has feelings of guilt/worthlessness or suicidal ideation. If a major depressive episode is suspected, the clinician should always assess for suicidal ideation and take appropriate steps if the patient has a plan or intent to commit suicide.

Although the patient lost her mother 16 months ago, bereavement should be considered in place of major depressive disorder only if the patient has experienced the loss of a loved one in the past 2 months. Although the patient uses alcohol, her relatively low consumption level and the lack of correlation between alcohol intake and her mood go against a diagnosis of substance-induced mood disorder. Dysthymic disorder does not fit because she has experienced periods of interepisode recovery after prior depressive episodes. Mood disorder due to a general medical condition is not suggested by the data; in particular, the patient denied a number of symptoms suggestive of hypothyroidism.

TEST YOUR KNOWLEDGE

QUESTION #1

Correct answer: D

If a patient appears to be suffering from depression, it is critical to assess for suicidal ideation, plan, and intent. Some clinicians fear that inquiring about suicide may inadvertently introduce the idea and thereby put the patient at higher risk, but evidence does not support this notion (Gould MS, Marrocco FA, Kleinman M, et al. Evaluating iatrogenic risk of youth suicide screening programs. *JAMA*. 2005;293:1635–1643). If a patient endorses having thoughts of death or of hurting himself or herself, a clinician should then inquire as to whether the patient has a plan or method for attempting suicide, whether the patient has a history of previous attempts, and whether the patient intends to carry out the suicide plan. Positive responses to these inquiries put a patient at high risk for suicide, and emergency measures such as inpatient hospitalization should be considered.

QUESTION #2

Correct answer: B

The long-standing symptoms of depressed mood, low energy, and low self-esteem without other more severe depressive symptoms are most suggestive of dysthymic disorder. To increase confidence in this diagnosis, the clinician should ensure that the patient has suffered from these symptoms for at least 2 years, has not had a symptom-free period of more than 2 months, and did not have a major depressive disorder during the first 2 years of the mood disturbance.

QUESTION #3

Correct answer: E

Although diagnosing depression can be more challenging in someone with multiple complex medical conditions, symptoms of depression should only be attributed to other conditions if they can be fully accounted for by such conditions. Clinicians are sometimes reluctant to diagnose depression in the elderly because the circumstances that accompany old age may seem to warrant feelings of depression. However, a diagnosis of depression is often still appropriate for elderly individuals and can be an important aid in signaling the need for interventions to improve quality of life.

Index

Page numbers followed by *f* and *t* indicate figures and tables, respectively.

A

H

M

O

P